Diagnosis and Management of Skin Cancer

Diagnosis and Management of Skin Cancer

Editor: Elizabeth Burns

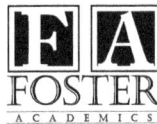

FA
FOSTER
ACADEMICS

www.fosteracademics.com

www.fosteracademics.com

FA
FOSTER
A C A D E M I C S

Cataloging-in-Publication Data

Diagnosis and management of skin cancer / edited by Elizabeth Burns.
   p. cm.
Includes bibliographical references and index.
ISBN 978-1-63242-747-2
1. Skin--Cancer. 2. Skin--Cancer--Diagnosis. 3. Skin--Cancer--Treatment. I. Burns, Elizabeth.
RC280.S5 D53 2019
616.994 77--dc23

© Foster Academics, 2019

Foster Academics,
118-35 Queens Blvd., Suite 400,
Forest Hills, NY 11375, USA

ISBN 978-1-63242-747-2 (Hardback)

Contents

Preface

Skin cancers are the cancers arising from the skin, caused due to an abnormal development of cells, which invade and spread to other parts of the body. These are of three main types, squamous-cell skin cancer, basal-cell skin cancer and melanoma. Melanomas are aggressive cancers. Symptoms vary as per the underlying cancer and may include a painless raised area of skin, a color or shape change in a mole, etc. More than 90% of all cases of skin cancer are caused due to an exposure to ultraviolet radiation from the sun. Its diagnosis is done based on a histopathological examination and through a biopsy. The treatment of skin cancer is designed based on the location of the cancer, the type of cancer and the age of the person. Whether the cancer is primary or a recurrence also determines the treatment modality. Radiation therapy, topical chemotherapy, cryotherapy, surgery and immunotherapy may be used for the management of skin cancer. This book brings forth some of the most innovative concepts and elucidates the unexplored aspects of skin cancer. Some of the diverse topics covered in this book address the varied diagnostic and management strategies of skin cancer. It aims to equip students and experts with the advanced topics and upcoming concepts in this area.

This book is a comprehensive compilation of works of different researchers from varied parts of the world. It includes valuable experiences of the researchers with the sole objective of providing the readers (learners) with a proper knowledge of the concerned field. This book will be beneficial in evoking inspiration and enhancing the knowledge of the interested readers.

In the end, I would like to extend my heartiest thanks to the authors who worked with great determination on their chapters. I also appreciate the publisher's support in the course of the book. I would also like to deeply acknowledge my family who stood by me as a source of inspiration during the project.

Editor

Sun-Tanning Perceptions of a New Zealand Urban Population (1994–2005/6)

A. I. Reeder,[1] G. F. H. McLeod,[2] A. R. Gray,[3] and R. McGee[3]

[1] *Cancer Society of New Zealand Social & Behavioural Research Unit, Department of Preventive & Social Medicine, Dunedin School of Medicine, University of Otago, P.O. Box 913, Dunedin 9054, New Zealand*

[2] *Department of Psychological Medicine, School of Medical and Health Sciences, University of Otago, Christchurch 8140, New Zealand*

[3] *Department of Preventive & Social Medicine, Dunedin School of Medicine, University of Otago, P.O. Box 913, Dunedin 9054, New Zealand*

Correspondence should be addressed to A. I. Reeder; tony.reeder@otago.ac.nz

Academic Editor: Giuseppe Argenziano

Background. Sun-tanning perceptions are monitored to identify changes and help refine targeting of skin cancer prevention messages. *Aim.* To investigate associations between perceptions of sun-tanning and demographic factors among a New Zealand urban population, 1994–2006. *Methods.* A telephone survey series was conducted during summer in 1994, 1997, 1999/2000, 2002/2003, and 2005/2006. Demographic and personal information (sex, age group, skin sun-sensitivity, and self-defined ethnicity) obtained from 6,195 respondents, 50.2% female, 15–69 years, was investigated in relation to six sun-tanning related statements. A total "positive perceptions of tanning" (ProTan) score was also calculated. Regression analyses modelled each component and the ProTan score against survey year and respondent characteristics. *Results.* Statistically significantly higher ProTan scores were found for age group (strong reverse dose-response effect), male sex, residence (highest in Auckland), ethnicity (highest among Europeans), and sun sensitivity (an *n*-shaped association). There was no statistically significant change in total ProTan scores from baseline. *Conclusions.* The development, pretesting, and evaluation of messages for those groups most likely to endorse ProTan statements should be considered for the New Zealand skin cancer prevention program. To achieve and embed significant change, mass media campaigns may require greater intensity and reinforcement with sustained contextual support for settings-based behavioural change.

1. Introduction

In environments where high levels of ambient solar ultraviolet radiation (UVR) are recorded, up to 95% of cutaneous malignant melanoma (melanoma) and 99% of other skin cancers are attributed to excess sun exposure [1]. New Zealand (NZ) has rates among the highest age-standardized incidence and mortality rates for cutaneous malignant melanoma [2], and recent registration rates show an upward trend, 1999–2010 [3]. In 2010, melanoma was the fourth most commonly registered cancer and resulted in 324 deaths among a total population of around 4 million. The most recent official estimate of public melanoma treatment costs is NZ$24.4 M/year [4]. Although the registration of nonmelanoma skin cancers (NMSC) is not required in NZ, there are an estimated 67,000

new cases per year, for which annual health system treatment costs are conservatively estimated to exceed NZ$48 M/year [5]. In addition, there is the cost of treating other solar UVR related diseases, such as cortical cataracts [6]. Although some UVR exposure is required to protect against bone diseases, such as rickets, osteomalacia, and osteoporosis, it has been argued that "there should be no need to accept an increased risk of diseases of excessive exposure, in order to achieve minimal risk of diseases of underexposure" [7].

Perceptions that a suntan is attractive and healthy may reinforce sunbathing and contribute to excessive sun exposure [8]. Perceptions regarding the attractiveness of a tan are strongly correlated with sunbathing [9, 10]. Given the potentially modifiable nature of such perceptions, their conversion into sun protective attitudes among populations at-risk of skin cancer may play an important role in behavioural changes that would help reduce skin cancer risk [11].

Public health campaigns aimed at reducing excessive UVR exposure and increasing the frequency of sun protective behaviours were first developed in Australia. The original campaign slogan, "Slip (on a shirt), Slop (on sunscreen), Slap (on a hat)" was launched in 1981 [12]. Although protanning attitudes continued to be commonly held, especially among males and younger respondents [13], subsequent Victorian survey research concluded that the campaign appeared to be effective, with positive perceptions of tanning decreasing significantly from 1988 to 1990 [14]. By 1998, the percentage of respondents that liked to get a suntan had reduced from 61% in 1988 to 35% [15]. Campaigns using mass media which were initiated in other countries produced inconclusive results regarding attitude change, although there were some encouraging findings [16].

In NZ, national and regional health promotion programs aimed at increasing awareness of skin cancer and reducing excessive solar UVR exposure were implemented in 1988 [17]. Since it was important to evaluate these efforts, the Cancer Society of New Zealand Inc. (CSNZ) and the Health Sponsorship Council (now the Health Promotion Agency, HPA), initiated the Triennial Sun Protection Survey (Sun Survey) series, modelled on Victorian precedent [13], with data collected about the sun protection knowledge, perceptions, and practices of the NZ urban population. Selected findings published from the first two surveys, 1994 and 1997, indicated that appropriate use of sun protection was poor, resulting in high levels of sunburn [18], in particular, among younger age groups [19, 20]. Thereafter, the overall frequency of self-reported, summer weekend sunburn continued to exceed 20% [21].

The five waves of data in this unique Sun Survey database also provide opportunities to investigate perceptions regarding tanning. The aims of the present study were to investigate among the NZ urban population, 1994–2006, (1) six specific dimensions of sun-tanning perceptions, (2) a summed ProTan score, and (3) associations between these measures and respondent characteristics (city of residence, sex, age group, skin sun-sensitivity, and self-reported ethnicity) and survey year. It was hypothesized that population perceptions might change over time and differ by these demographic characteristics, with some groups having more positive perceptions than others and thereby increasing their potential future risk of skin cancer. Insights obtained from the study could potentially inform and help guide the existing SunSmart program and the content and targeting of future skin cancer prevention efforts.

2. Methods

2.1. Sample Selection. Respondents, aged 15–69 years inclusive, were resident in households randomly selected (using random digit dialling in predetermined areas, 1994 and 1997, or telematched from electoral rolls, 1999–2006) in five metropolitan areas: Auckland, Wellington, Hamilton, Christchurch, and Dunedin, which represented approximately 55% of the total NZ resident population in the 2006

Census. The random selection procedure was limited to respondents from around 92% of NZ households with land-line telephone access around this time [22]. Given a primary prevention focus, interview protocols prioritised younger household members, but a quota system ensured that the sample comprised approximately equal numbers of each sex, and that each city contributed 20%, both of adolescents (15–17 years) and adults (18–69 years).

2.2. Procedures. Meteorological data were used to select appropriate survey weekends during southern hemisphere summers, with the main criterion being that the weather had been sufficiently "fine" for potentially harmful sun exposure to have occurred [18]. The telephone questionnaire was administered by market research contractors using computer assisted telephone interviewing (CATI) systems. Interviews were usually conducted on either a Monday or Tuesday evening, following the selected survey weekends.

2.3. Measures. Respondents were administered a questionnaire concerning weekend sun exposure and sun protective behaviours which also included demographic information and measures of sun-tanning perceptions. For the latter, respondents were asked to rate, on a five-point Likert-type scale, their level of agreement or disagreement (1 = Strongly disagree; 2 = Disagree; 3 = Neither agree or disagree; 4 = Agree; 5 = Strongly agree) with six statements: (1) "I feel more healthy with a suntan" (hereafter abbreviated to *More Healthy*); (2) "a suntan makes me feel better about myself" (*Feel Better*); (3) "a suntan makes me feel more attractive to others" (*More Attractive*); (4) "this summer I intend to sunbathe regularly to get a suntan" (*Intention*); (5) "most of my close family think that a suntan is a good thing" (*Family*); and (6) "most of my friends think a suntan is a good thing" (*Friends*). The content of these statements was guided by Australian research [13]. An investigation of the psychometric properties of the summative ProTan scale, constructed from these six items, supported its applicability to the NZ urban population [23]. A higher ProTan score indicates more positive perceptions of tanning.

Self-defined ethnicity was coded according to Level 1 (the highest) of the NZ Ministry of Health ethnicity and data protocols as either Māori, Pacific, Asian, or New Zealand European/European/Other (NZE/O) [24]. Self-reported skin type was based on a modified Fitzpatrick classification of skin sun-reaction: Type I (always burn, never tan), Type II (usually burn, tan with difficulty), Type III (sometimes burn, tan moderately), and Type IV (rarely burn, tan easily) [25].

2.4. Statistical Analyses. Responses to the six statements (*More Healthy, Feel Better, More Attractive, Intention, Friends,* and *Family*) were dichotomised into two categories, one of which included the Strongly disagree and Disagree responses, and the other which included the Strongly agree, Agree, and Neither Agree nor Disagree responses. Noncommittal respondents were included in the latter group because they did not express the preferred response, which was explicit disagreement with each ProTan statement. Responses to the six statements were modelled using logistic regression against survey year and respondent characteristics (city of residence, age, sex, self-defined ethnicity, and skin sun sensitivity). In addition, a total ProTan score was calculated by summing all six statement responses, creating a score between 6 and 30, and modelled using linear regression. All statistical analyses were performed using Stata 12.1 software and a two-sided $P < 0.05$ was considered statistically significant in all cases [26].

2.5. Ethical Approval. Participation in the survey was taken as informed consent. Participants had previously been notified of the survey by mail from the commissioned market research agency. The proposed project analyses, in part reported here, were reviewed and ethical approval granted at the Departmental level, following University of Otago Human Ethics Committee procedures.

3. Results

Data usable for analysis were obtained from 6,195 respondents (Table 1).

There were approximately equal numbers of participants by year, city of residence, and sex but relatively greater numbers of younger than older adults as a result of the primary prevention focus of study protocols. Overall, 80% of participants defined themselves as being either skin type I or II, the two groups most vulnerable to UVR skin damage. Respondents of non-European ethnicity were somewhat underrepresented in relation to the 2006 Census population.

The reference groups, odds ratios, and 95% confidence intervals for the responses to the six statements about sun-tanning perceptions by survey year and respondent characteristics are presented in Tables 2 and 3, both unadjusted and adjusted for all other tabulated variables. We now highlight key results, following the order of tabular presentation of the variables.

3.1. Survey Year and City of Residence. In the unadjusted model, survey year was positively associated with *Friends*, but this association was no longer significant after adjustment and survey year became statistically significantly associated only with the *More Attractive* variable, demonstrating a steadily strengthening positive relationship from 1999-2000 to 2005/6. Statistically significant differences between cities were found for *More Healthy*, *Feel Better* and *Friends*, with higher odds of endorsement of *More Healthy* and *Feel Better* by Auckland residents than those of other cities, with the *Feel Better* association weakening somewhat after adjustment. Christchurch residents were the least likely to endorse these statements. For *Friends*, all cities except Christchurch had higher odds of endorsement than Auckland.

3.2. Personal Characteristics. Compared with males, females had consistently significantly reduced odds of endorsing the *Healthy*, *More Attractive*, *Family*, and *Friends* statements, both before and after adjustment. With respect to age group, the odds of endorsing the *More Healthy*, *Feel Better*, *More*

TABLE 1: Sample demographic and personal characteristics ($n = 6,195$).

Variable	n	%
Survey year		
1994	1,243	20.1
1997	1,188	19.2
1999/2000	1,250	20.2
2002/2003	1,250	20.2
2005/2006	1,264	20.4
City of residence		
North Island		
Auckland	1,254	20.2
Hamilton	1,237	20.0
Wellington	1,230	19.9
South Island		
Christchurch	1,242	20.1
Dunedin	1,232	19.9
Sex		
Male	3,084	49.8
Female	3,111	50.2
Age group (year range)		
15–19	756	12.2
20–29	1,270	20.5
30–39	1,416	22.9
40–49	1,109	17.9
50–59	999	16.1
60–69	645	10.4
Skin type*		
Most sun sensitive		
I	1,494	24.4
II	3,432	56.1
III	1,109	18.1
Least sun sensitive		
IV	84	1.4
Missing data	76	
Self-defined ethnicity		
NZ European	5,326	86.7
Māori	405	6.6
Pacific	123	2.0
Asian	231	3.8
All other	55	0.9
Missing data	55	

*Modified Fitzpatrick sun-sensitivity scale.
Percentages may not total 100% due to rounding.

Attractive, *Friends*, and *Intend* statements demonstrated an almost entirely consistent reverse dose-response effect by decreasing significantly with increasing age, with only a few relatively minor exceptions in point estimate increments. For example, for *More Healthy*, the 20–29 year age group demonstrated slightly higher odds of endorsement than the youngest age group. Reporting the most sun-sensitive skin type was associated with the lowest odds of endorsing each statement, with the exception that the numerically small,

TABLE 2: Unadjusted and adjusted* odds ratios and 95% confidence intervals for personal perceptions by sample characteristics.

| | More healthy | | | | Feel better | | | | More attractive | | | |
	Unadjusted		Adjusted $n = 5,959$		Unadjusted		Adjusted $n = 5,985$		Unadjusted		Adjusted $n = 5,913$	
		$P = 0.637$		$P = 0.524$		$P = 0.524$		$P = 0.633$		$P = 0.797$		$P = 0.023$
Year (summer)												
1994	1.00		1.00		1.00		1.00		1.00		1.00	
1997	1.00	0.85, 1.17	1.03	0.87, 1.21	0.92	0.79, 1.08	0.95	0.80, 1.12	0.93	0.79, 1.10	0.98	0.83, 1.16
1999/2000	1.09	0.93, 1.28	1.23	1.04, 1.45	0.94	0.81, 1.11	1.07	0.91, 1.26	0.92	0.78, 1.08	1.11	0.93, 1.31
2002/2003	0.98	0.84, 1.15	1.08	0.91, 1.27	0.96	0.82, 1.13	1.06	0.90, 1.26	0.95	0.81, 1.11	1.13	0.95, 1.33
2005/2006	0.97	0.83, 1.14	1.11	0.94, 1.31	0.87	0.74, 1.02	1.02	0.87, 1.21	0.99	0.85, 1.16	1.28	1.08, 1.51
		$P < 0.001$		$P < 0.001$		$P = 0.045$		$P = 0.016$		$P = 0.154$		$P = 0.066$
City (N to S)												
Auckland	1.00		1.00		1.00		1.00		1.00		1.00	
Hamilton	0.73	0.62, 0.86	0.71	0.60, 0.84	0.88	0.75, 1.03	0.84	0.71, 0.99	0.92	0.79, 1.08	0.90	0.77, 1.07
Wellington	0.82	0.70, 0.96	0.79	0.67, 0.93	0.91	0.78, 1.07	0.88	0.74, 1.03	0.97	0.83, 1.14	0.95	0.80, 1.12
Christchurch	0.71	0.60, 0.83	0.68	0.58, 0.81	0.78	0.67, 0.92	0.75	0.64, 0.88	0.83	0.70, 0.97	0.79	0.67, 0.93
Dunedin	0.81	0.69, 0.94	0.78	0.66, 0.92	0.91	0.77, 1.06	0.87	0.74, 1.03	0.90	0.77, 1.05	0.87	0.74, 1.03
		$P < 0.001$		$P = 0.009$		$P = 0.066$		$P = 0.149$		$P = 0.001$		$P = 0.009$
Sex												
Male	1.00		1.00		1.00		1.00		1.00		1.00	
Female	0.84	0.76, 0.93	0.87	0.78, 0.97	0.91	0.82, 1.01	0.93	0.83, 1.03	0.85	0.77, 0.94	0.87	0.78, 0.97
		$P < 0.001$		$P < 0.001$		$P < 0.001$		$P < 0.001$		$P < 0.001$		$P < 0.001$
Age group												
15–19	1.00		1.00		1.00		1.00		1.00		1.00	
20–29	1.01	0.84, 1.21	1.04	0.86, 1.25	0.83	0.69, 1.00	0.83	0.69, 1.01	0.91	0.76, 1.09	0.91	0.76, 1.10
30–39	0.84	0.70, 1.01	0.86	0.72, 1.03	0.71	0.59, 0.85	0.68	0.56, 0.82	0.68	0.57, 0.81	0.63	0.53, 0.76
40–49	0.85	0.71, 1.03	0.87	0.72, 1.06	0.63	0.52, 0.76	0.59	0.49, 0.72	0.60	0.50, 0.73	0.54	0.45, 0.66
50–59	0.72	0.59, 0.87	0.72	0.59, 0.88	0.61	0.50, 0.74	0.59	0.48, 0.72	0.52	0.43, 0.63	0.47	0.38, 0.57
60–69	0.62	0.50, 0.76	0.63	0.50, 0.79	0.48	0.38, 0.59	0.44	0.35, 0.55	0.39	0.31, 0.49	0.35	0.27, 0.44
		$P < 0.001$		$P < 0.001$		$P < 0.001$		$P < 0.001$		$P < 0.001$		$P < 0.001$
Skin type												
I	1.00		1.00		1.00		1.00		1.00		1.00	
II	1.78	1.57, 2.02	1.75	1.54, 1.99	1.72	1.52, 1.95	1.71	1.51, 1.94	1.67	1.47, 1.89	1.64	1.44, 1.86
III	2.00	1.70, 2.34	2.03	1.72, 2.40	1.55	1.32, 1.81	1.66	1.41, 1.96	1.45	1.24, 1.70	1.53	1.29, 1.80
IV	1.00	0.62, 1.61	1.13	0.69, 1.84	0.96	0.61, 1.51	1.17	0.73, 1.87	0.74	0.45, 1.21	0.91	0.54, 1.51
		$P = 0.825$		$P = 0.012$		$P < 0.001$		$P < 0.001$		$P < 0.001$		$P < 0.001$
Ethnicity												
NZ European	1.00		1.00		1.00		1.00		1.00		1.00	
Māori	0.98	0.80, 1.21	0.80	0.65, 0.99	0.82	0.67, 1.00	0.66	0.54, 0.82	0.82	0.67, 1.01	0.64	0.52, 0.79
Pacific	1.01	0.70, 1.47	0.72	0.49, 1.05	0.69	0.48, 0.98	0.48	0.33, 0.70	0.79	0.55, 1.14	0.53	0.36, 0.77
Asian	0.86	0.65, 1.13	0.67	0.50, 0.90	0.57	0.43, 0.75	0.45	0.34, 0.61	0.51	0.39, 0.69	0.37	0.27, 0.51
Other	0.85	0.49, 1.46	0.77	0.44, 1.34	0.66	0.38, 1.12	0.60	0.35, 1.04	0.50	0.28, 0.88	0.45	0.25, 0.80

* Adjusted for all six ProTan scale components, that is, all those listed in Tables 2 and 3, inclusive.

least sensitive group had some lower odds, including lower adjusted odds for the adjusted *Friends* and *More Attractive* statements. Respondents of NZ European ethnicity had significantly higher odds of endorsing the *Feel Better* and *More Attractive* statements, for which those of Asian ethnicity had the lowest odds. The association between ethnicity and *Feel Healthy* only became statistically significant after adjustment, with Asians again having the lowest odds. The pattern for

Family was less clear, but those of Māori ethnicity had somewhat higher odds of endorsement than Europeans, in both the unadjusted and adjusted models. Along with those of Pacific ethnicity, Māori had significantly higher odds, both unadjusted and adjusted, of endorsing the statement *Friends*, but the significantly increased unadjusted odds for *Intentions* were not found after adjustment. The odds of endorsing *Friends* were also somewhat higher among Asians

TABLE 3: Unadjusted and adjusted* odds ratios and 95% confidence intervals for perceptions of others and intentions statements.

	Family				Friends				Intentions			
	Unadjusted		Adjusted $n = 5{,}816$		Unadjusted		Adjusted $n = 5{,}738$		Unadjusted		Adjusted $n = 6{,}021$	
	$P = 0.685$		$P = 0.212$		$P < 0.001$		$P = 0.397$		$P = 0.084$		$P = 0.314$	
Year (summer)												
1994	1.00		1.00		1.00		1.00		1.00		1.00	
1997	1.04	0.88, 1.23	1.06	0.89, 1.26	1.10	0.93, 1.30	1.13	0.95, 1.35	1.01	0.81, 1.25	1.04	0.83, 1.30
1999/2000	1.11	0.94, 1.31	1.19	1.00, 1.42	0.81	0.69, 0.96	0.99	0.83, 1.18	1.00	0.81, 1.24	1.26	1.01, 1.58
2002/2003	1.10	0.93, 1.29	1.20	1.00, 1.43	0.84	0.71, 0.99	1.12	0.94, 1.34	0.83	0.67, 1.04	1.07	0.85, 1.35
2005/2006	1.02	0.86, 1.20	1.13	0.95, 1.35	0.77	0.66, 0.91	1.07	0.89, 1.27	0.80	0.64, 1.00	1.10	0.87, 1.39
	$P = 0.512$		$P = 0.815$		$P = 0.002$		$P = 0.004$		$P = 0.468$		$P = 0.588$	
City (N to S)												
Auckland	1.00		1.00		1.00		1.00		1.00			
Hamilton	0.95	0.81, 1.13	0.94	0.80, 1.12	1.12	0.95, 1.32	1.12	0.95, 1.34	0.82	0.66, 1.02	0.88	0.71, 1.11
Wellington	1.04	0.88, 1.22	1.00	0.85, 1.19	1.07	0.91, 1.26	1.07	0.90, 1.27	0.91	0.74, 1.13	0.94	0.75, 1.18
Christchurch	0.90	0.76, 1.06	0.92	0.77, 1.09	0.84	0.71, 0.99	0.89	0.75, 1.06	0.88	0.71, 1.09	0.84	0.67, 1.06
Dunedin	0.97	0.82, 1.14	0.97	0.81, 1.15	1.11	0.95, 1.31	1.23	1.04, 1.47	0.95	0.77, 1.17	0.98	0.78, 1.22
	$P < 0.001$		$P < 0.001$		$P < 0.001$		$P < 0.001$		$P = 0.822$		$P = 0.165$	
Sex												
Male	1.00		1.00		1.00		1.00		1.00		1.00	
Female	0.70	0.63, 0.77	0.71	0.64, 0.80	0.77	0.70, 0.86	0.82	0.73, 0.92	1.02	0.88, 1.17	1.11	0.96, 1.28
	$P < 0.001$		$P < 0.001$		$P < 0.001$		$P < 0.001$		$P < 0.001$		$P < 0.001$	
Age group (yrs)												
15–19	1.00		1.00		1.00		1.00		1.00		1.00	
20–29	0.56	0.47, 0.68	0.57	0.47, 0.69	0.45	0.36, 0.57	0.46	0.37, 0.58	0.53	0.43, 0.65	0.54	0.44, 0.67
30–39	0.41	0.34, 0.50	0.42	0.35, 0.50	0.24	0.20, 0.30	0.25	0.20, 0.32	0.31	0.25, 0.39	0.31	0.25, 0.39
40–49	0.47	0.39, 0.57	0.48	0.39, 0.58	0.21	0.16, 0.26	0.22	0.17, 0.27	0.25	0.19, 0.31	0.25	0.19, 0.32
50–59	0.46	0.38, 0.56	0.47	0.38, 0.57	0.16	0.12, 0.20	0.17	0.13, 0.21	0.25	0.19, 0.32	0.25	0.20, 0.33
60–69	0.43	0.35, 0.54	0.43	0.34, 0.54	0.13	0.10, 0.16	0.13	0.10, 0.17	0.14	0.10, 0.20	0.14	0.10, 0.20
	$P < 0.001$		$P < 0.001$		$P = 0.001$		$P = 0.499$		$P < 0.001$		$P < 0.001$	
Skin type												
I	1.00		1.00		1.00		1.00		1.00		1.00	
II	1.34	1.18, 1.53	1.30	1.14, 1.48	1.13	0.99, 1.28	1.03	0.90, 1.17	1.95	1.60, 2.37	1.88	1.54, 2.30
III	1.50	1.27, 1.76	1.41	1.18, 1.67	1.39	1.18, 1.64	1.12	0.94, 1.34	2.44	1.94, 3.06	2.23	1.75, 2.84
IV	1.16	0.71, 1.88	1.14	0.69, 1.88	0.99	0.62, 1.57	0.86	0.52, 1.42	1.65	0.88, 3.13	1.64	0.85, 3.19
	$P = 0.021$		$P = 0.029$		$P < 0.001$		$P = 0.001$		$P = 0.016$		$P = 0.092$	
Ethnicity												
NZ European	1.00		1.00		1.00		1.00		1.00		1.00	
Māori	1.29	1.05, 1.59	1.08	0.87, 1.34	2.08	1.66, 2.61	1.54	1.22, 1.96	1.26	0.96, 1.64	0.83	0.63, 1.10
Pacific	1.17	0.81, 1.70	0.87	0.59, 1.29	2.10	1.41, 3.13	1.31	0.86, 2.00	1.32	0.84, 2.10	0.73	0.45, 1.19
Asian	0.75	0.56, 1.00	0.62	0.45, 0.84	1.36	1.02, 1.80	1.04	0.76, 1.42	1.46	1.05, 2.04	0.93	0.64, 1.33
Other	1.31	0.76, 2.27	1.15	0.65, 2.02	0.76	0.43, 2.61	0.57	0.32, 1.04	0.33	0.10, 1.08	0.25	0.08, 0.82

*Adjusted or all six ProTan scale components, that is, all those in Tables 2 and 3, inclusive.

than Europeans, also for *Intentions*, but in the latter case not after adjustment.

The associations between each of the six sample characteristics and the total mean ProTan score (range from 6 to 30) are presented in Table 4.

Before adjustment, all six sample characteristics were statistically significantly associated with ProTan score, but this association failed to reach significance for survey year after adjustment for the other five characteristics. In the adjusted model, mean ProTan scores peaked in 1999/2000

TABLE 4: Unadjusted and adjusted* effects with 95% confidence intervals for total Protan scores.

	Unadjusted		Adjusted (n = 5,392)	
	P = 0.004		P = 0.142	
Year (summer)				
1994	0.00		0.00	
1997	−0.04	−0.54, 0.45	0.08	−0.40, 0.56
1999/2000	−0.13	−0.63, 0.37	0.59	0.10, 1.07
2002/2003	−0.49	−0.99, 0.00	0.28	−0.21, 0.76
2005/2006	−0.80	−1.29, −0.31	0.19	−0.29, 0.68
	P = 0.005		P = 0.006	
City (N to S)				
Auckland	0.00		0.00	
Hamilton	−0.30	−0.79, 0.19	−0.36	−0.84, 0.11
Wellington	−0.40	−0.89, 0.09	−0.47	−0.94, 0.01
Christchurch	−0.94	−1.43, −0.45	−0.89	−1.36, −0.42
Dunedin	−0.37	−0.87, 0.12	−0.29	−0.77, 0.19
	P < 0.001		P < 0.001	
Sex				
Male	0.00		0.00	
Female	−0.77	−1.08, −0.46	−0.56	−0.86, −0.26
	P < 0.001		P < 0.001	
Age group (years)				
15–19	0.00		0.00	
20–29	−1.70	−2.23, −1.17	−1.64	−2.16, −1.11
30–39	−3.38	−3.90, −2.86	−3.34	−3.86, −2.82
40–49	−3.72	−4.27, −3.17	−3.69	−4.24, −3.13
50–59	−4.30	−4.86, −3.73	−4.22	−4.80, −3.65
60–69	−5.52	−6.17, −4.87	−5.49	−6.16, −4.83
	P < 0.001		P < 0.001	
Skin type				
(most sun sensitive) I	0.00		0.00	
II	1.83	1.46, 2.20	1.63	1.27, 1.99
III	2.12	1.64, 2.60	1.88	1.40, 2.36
(least sun sensitive) IV	−0.73	−2.21, 0.75	−0.48	−1.93, 0.97
	P = 0.016		P < 0.001	
Ethnicity				
NZ European	0.00		0.00	
Māori	0.67	0.04, 1.30	−0.48	−1.09, 0.14
Pacific	0.62	−0.48, 1.73	−1.19	−2.26, −0.11
Asian	−0.97	−1.82, −0.12	−2.17	−3.02, −1.32
Other	−0.92	−2.60, 0.79	−1.74	−3.35, −0.13

*Adjusted for all other variables in the table.

then declined, but there was no evidence of significantly less endorsement of tanning in 2005/6 than in 1994. Auckland residents had the highest and Christchurch residents the lowest mean ProTan score. Females had a significantly lower mean ProTan score than males, particularly after adjustment, and a strong reverse dose response effect was observed for age. As skin sun sensitivity reduced, ProTan scores increased, except among the relatively numerically small, least sun sensitive group. European ethnicity was the most strongly positively associated with ProTan score, whereas Asian ethnicity was the most strongly negatively associated.

4. Discussion

This is the first published study to report perceptions of sun tanning among the NZ urban population and investigate demographic and personal factors associated with them, based on all five surveys in the Sun Survey series, 1994–2006. Unlike what has been reported for Victoria, Australia [27], there was no evidence of statistically significant overall improvement in perceptions of tanning among the NZ population since baseline.

In multivariable analyses, city of residence, age group, sex, skin type, and ethnicity were each statistically significantly associated with mean ProTan score. Auckland residents were significantly more ProTan than other groups. Since Auckland is NZ's most populous city, is the most northern city surveyed, and has a tendency towards higher UVR levels than the other cities, there would seem to be a specific need for efforts to moderate ProTan perceptions there.

The strong, reverse dose response association between ProTan scores and age group is consistent with Victorian survey findings [27]. In Victoria, the response to this observed pattern was to initiate more "hard-hitting messages with shock value," a mass media approach to targeting young adults which was backed up by local qualitative research. In New Zealand, at least during the survey series period, 1994–2006, the core mass media approach was to target caregivers and young children using animal exemplars and animated cartoons about sun protection. This content was likely to have had little appeal to the young adults most at risk and who, by design, were overrepresented in the survey series. Although some hard-hitting messages were used, these were the exception and mostly disseminated either prior to or early in the survey period.

NZ males expressed significantly more ProTan perceptions than females, both overall, and for four of the six measures, except *Intend* (intention to tan) and *Feel Better*. Respondents of NZ European ethnicity had a significantly higher mean overall ProTan score than all other ethnic groups, with those of Asian ethnicity having the lowest mean scores, consistent with negative social associations with skin darkening in, for example, Chinese culture [28]. Reports from Australia, the region with climatic and social conditions most readily comparable to NZ, have not reported analyses by ethnicity. In NZ, those of European ethnicity, especially males, are a key target group for changing positive perceptions of tanning, in particular, since they are likely to have the skin types most vulnerable to UVR damage.

Higher odds of endorsing positive statements about tanning would not necessarily be problematic, provided that the intention to sunbathe remained low. However, no significant change in intentions was observed since 1994. Sun bathing intentions are factors that will be important to continue to monitor in the Sun Exposure Survey (SES) which superseded the series reported here. In a descriptive report of the 2010 SES survey, around the same percentage of respondents endorsed the sunbathing intentions statement as in 1994 [29], although revised survey procedures limit the appropriateness of direct comparison.

Some limitations of this research need to be considered. First, it may only be appropriate to generalise our findings to the NZ urban population. Nevertheless, the five cities surveyed contributed more than 55% of the total population and, according to the 2006 Census, 73% of the resident population lived in the greater urban areas of NZ. Second, the present study and the Australian studies cited sometimes used slightly differently worded perception and demographic variables which may limit comparability. Third, although the NZ skin cancer awareness programme began in 1988, no baseline measures of perceptions were obtained until 1994, which leaves open the possibility that positive change may have occurred during the first six years of the programme,

after which time it may have become more difficult to change the remaining, perhaps more entrenched, attitudes. This illustrates the need for adequate funding to support essential programme evaluation, including the taking of timely baseline measurements. Finally, it is possible that some questions may have been misinterpreted by some groups, perhaps due to language and cultural differences.

Further analyses are planned, in particular, regression models to identify which factors (in addition to personal characteristics and perceptions) may be most strongly associated with poor sun protection and sunburn experience [21], so that these factors may be targeted in prevention campaigns. These analyses will include climatic variables and contextual data, such as engagement in different types of activity.

5. Conclusions

Overall, NZ population ProTan perceptions in 2006 were not significantly different from those in 1994. Without sustained, significant, targeted public health investment in sun safety interventions, attitudinal and behavioural change is unlikely to occur. However, the guiding Australian SunSmart programme model has demonstrated a positive cost benefit ratio, such that "sustained modest investment in skin cancer control is likely to be an excellent value for money" [30].

Systematic reviews of skin cancer primary prevention interventions indicate that there is convincing evidence for the effectiveness of multicomponent, community-wide programmes with supportive media messages [31], but not mass media campaigns, alone [32]. Media campaigns focused on changing personal perceptions need reinforcement by building contextual support for attitudinal and behavioural change through changes in public policies and practices [33] and settings-based interventions, for example, in primary schools [34] and workplaces—contexts for which there is convincing evidence of effectiveness in improving sun protection behaviours [35, 36].

Finally, since perceptions differed significantly by respondent characteristics, NZ skin cancer prevention programs should consider development and evaluation of efforts specifically targeted towards those groups most likely to endorse and indicate intentions to partake in risky sun exposure behaviours or subscribe to perceived positive social norms for tanning.

Acknowledgments

The data analysed in this research were collected by contractors to the owners of the data, the Health Sponsorship Council (HSC) (now the Health Promotion Agency), SunSmart programme, and the Cancer Society of New Zealand Inc. (CSNZ). Data were collected by Roy Morgan Research Centre Pty Ltd. (1994), MRL Research Group (1997), and

TNS New Zealand Ltd., made up of CM Research and NFO NZ (1999/00–2005/06). The data were analysed by the authors. Geraldine McLeod received support from the Health Sponsorship Council SunSmart Ph.D. Scholarship. Associate Professor Reeder and the Cancer Society Social and Behavioural Research Unit receive support from the CSNZ Inc. and the University of Otago. Professor McGee and Mr. Gray receive support from the University of Otago. The authors would like to thank Nathalie Huston for providing research support services, Helen Glasgow for initial work developing the survey, and Dr Simon Horsburgh for earlier data management assistance. The Cancer Society Social and Behavioural Research Unit's role was primarily limited to the provision of advice about the more recent survey waves, data analysis, and reporting.

References

[1] B. Armstrong, "How sun exposure causes skin cancer: an epidemiological perspective," in *Prevention of Skin Cancer*, D. Hill, J. M. Elwood, and D. R. English, Eds., Kluwer Academic, Dordrecht, The Netherlands, 2004.

[2] International Agency for Research on Cancer, *GLOBOCAN 2012: Estimated Cancer Incidence, Mortality and Prevalence Worldwide in 2012*, IARC, Lyon, France, 2013, http://globocan.iarc.fr/old/bar_sex_site.asp?selection=16120&title=Melanoma+of+skin&statistic=2&populations=5&window=1&grid=1&info=1&color1=5&color1e=&color2=4&color2e=&submit=%C2%A0Execute%C2%A0.

[3] Ministry of Health, *Cancer: New Registrations and Deaths 2010*, Ministry of Health, Wellington, New Zealand, 2013, http://www.health.govt.nz/system/files/documents/publications/cancer-new-registrations-deaths-2010-aug13.pdf.

[4] Ministry of Health, *The Price of Cancer: The Public Price of Registered Cancer in New Zealand*, Ministry of Health, Wellington, New Zealand, 2011.

[5] D. O'Dea, *The Costs of Skin Cancer to New Zealand*, Wellington School of Medicine, University of Otago, Wellington, New Zealand, 2009.

[6] C. Delcourt, I. Carrière, A. Ponton-Sanchez, A. Lacroux, M. Covacho, and L. Papoz, "Light exposure and the risk of cortical, nuclear, and posterior subcapsular cataracts: the pathologies oculaires liees a l'age (POLA) study," *Archives of Ophthalmology*, vol. 118, no. 3, pp. 385–392, 2000.

[7] R. Lucas, A. McMichael, W. Smith, and B. Armstrong, "Solar ultraviolet radiation," in *Global Burden of Disease from Solar Ultraviolet Radiation*, A. Prüss-Üstün, H. Zeeb, C. Mathers, and M. Repacholi, Eds., vol. 13 of *Environmental Burden of Disease Series*, WHO, Geneva, Switzerland, 2006.

[8] K. M. Jackson and L. S. Aiken, "A psychosocial model of sun protection and sunbathing in young women: the impact of health beliefs, attitudes, norms, and self-efficacy for sun protection," *Health Psychology*, vol. 19, no. 5, pp. 469–478, 2000.

[9] L. Wichstrøm, "Predictors of Norwegian adolescents' sunbathing and use of sunscreen," *Health Psychology*, vol. 13, no. 5, pp. 412–420, 1994.

[10] M. R. Leary and J. L. Jones, "The social psychology of tanning and sunscreen use: self-presentational motives as a predictor of health risk," *Journal of Applied Social Psychology*, vol. 23, no. 17, pp. 1390–1406, 1993.

[11] S. Arthey and V. A. Clarke, "Suntanning and sun protection: a review of the psychological literature," *Social Science and Medicine*, vol. 40, no. 2, pp. 265–274, 1995.

[12] J. Rassaby, I. Larcombe, D. Hill, and F. R. Wake, "Slip Slop Slap: health education about skin cancer," *Cancer Forum*, vol. 7, pp. 63–69, 1983.

[13] D. Hill, T. Theobald, R. Borland, V. White, and R. Marks, *Summer Activities, Sunburn, Sun-Related Attitudes and Precautions against Skin Cancer: A Survey of Melbourne Residents in the Summer of 1987/1988*, Anti-Cancer Council of Victoria, Melbourne, Australia, 1990.

[14] P. D. Baade, K. P. Balanda, and J. B. Lowe, "Changes in skin protection behaviors, attitudes, and sunburn: in a population with the highest incidence of skin cancer in the world," *Cancer Detection and Prevention*, vol. 20, no. 6, pp. 566–575, 1996.

[15] M. Montague, R. Borland, and C. Sinclair, "Slip! slop! slap! and sunsmart, 1980–2000: skin cancer control and 20 years of population-based campaigning," *Health Education and Behavior*, vol. 28, no. 3, pp. 290–305, 2001.

[16] R. Bellamy, "A systematic review of educational interventions for promoting sun protection knowledge, attitudes and behaviour following the QUESTS approach," *Medical Teacher*, vol. 27, no. 3, pp. 269–275, 2005.

[17] C. Watts, A. I. Reeder, and H. Glasgow, "A cover-up story: the cancer society melanoma prevention programme," in *UV Radiation and Its Effects—An Update*, Miscellaneous Series 60, Royal Society of New Zealand, Wellington, New Zealand, 2002.

[18] R. McGee, S. Williams, B. Cox, M. Elwood, and J.-L. Bulliard, "A community survey of sun exposure, sunburn and sun protection," *New Zealand Medical Journal*, vol. 108, no. 1013, pp. 508–510, 1995.

[19] R. Richards, R. McGee, and R. G. Knight, "Sun protection practices, knowledge and attitudes to tans among New Zealand adolescents, 1991–1997," *New Zealand Medical Journal*, vol. 114, no. 1132, pp. 229–231, 2001.

[20] R. Richards, R. McGee, and R. G. Knight, "Sunburn and sun protection among New Zealand adolescents over a summer weekend," *Australian and New Zealand Journal of Public Health*, vol. 25, no. 4, pp. 352–354, 2001.

[21] G. F. H. McLeod, A. I. Reeder, A. Gray, and R. McGee, "Summer weekend sun exposure and sunburn among a New Zealand urban population, 1994–2006," *New Zealand Medical Journal*, vol. 126, no. 1381, pp. 12–26, 2013.

[22] Statistics New Zealand, *Housing Indicator—Indicator 18: Access to Telecommunications*, Statistics New Zealand, Wellington, New Zealand, 2013, http://www.stats.govt.nz/Census/2006CensusHomePage/Tables/AboutAPlace/SnapShot.aspx?type=region&tab=Phones,netfax&id=9999999.

[23] G. F. Horsburgh-McLeod, A. R. Gray, A. I. Reeder, and R. McGee, "Applying item response theory (IRT) to a suntan attitudes scale," *Australasian Epidemiologist*, vol. 17, no. 1, pp. 40–46, 2010.

[24] Ministry of Health, *Ethnicity Data Protocols for the Health and Disability Sector*, Ministry of Health, Wellington, New Zealand, 2004.

[25] T. B. Fitzpatrick, "The validity and practicality of sun-reactive skin types I through VI," *Archives of Dermatology*, vol. 124, no. 6, pp. 869–871, 1988.

[26] StataCorp LP, *Stata Statistical Software: Release 12*, StataCorp LP, College Station, Tex, USA, 2011.

[27] M. Montague, R. Borland, and C. Sinclair, *Sunsmart Twenty Years On: What Can We Learn from This Successful Health Promotion Campaign?* Anti-Cancer Council of Victoria, Carlton, Australia, 2001.

[28] H. Qiu, F. Flament, X. Long et al., "Seasonal skin darkening in Chinese women: the Shanghaiese experience of daily sun protection," *Clinical, Cosmetic and Investigational Dermatoloy*, vol. 6, pp. 151–158, 2013.

[29] R. Gray, *Sun Exposure Survey 2010: Topline Time Series Report*, Health Sponsorship Council, Wellington, New Zealand, 2010.

[30] S. T. F. Shih, R. Carter, C. Sinclair, C. Mihalopoulos, and T. Vos, "Economic evaluation of skin cancer prevention in Australia," *Preventive Medicine*, vol. 49, no. 5, pp. 449–453, 2009.

[31] U.S. Centers for Disease Control and Prevention, Guide to Community Preventive Services, *Preventing Skin Cancer: Multicomponent Community-Wide Interventions*, 2012, http://www.thecommunityguide.org/cancer/skin/community-wide/multicomponent.html.

[32] U.S. Centers for Disease Control and Prevention, Guide to Community Preventive Services, *Preventing Skin Cancer: Mass Media*, 2012, http://www.thecommunityguide.org/cancer/skin/community-wide/massmedia.html.

[33] G. F. H. McLeod, A. Insch, and J. Henry, "Reducing barriers to sun protection—application of a holistic model for social marketing," *Australasian Marketing Journal*, vol. 19, no. 3, pp. 212–222, 2011.

[34] A. I. Reeder, A. R. Gray, and J. A. Jopson, "Primary school sun protection policies and practices 4 years after baseline—a follow-up study," *Health Education Research*, vol. 27, no. 5, pp. 844–856, 2012.

[35] U.S. Centers for Disease Control and Prevention, Guide to Community Preventive Services, *Preventing Skin Cancer: Primary and Middle School Interventions*, 2012, http://www.thecommunityguide.org/cancer/skin/education-policy/primaryandmiddleschools.html.

[36] U.S. Centers for Disease Control and Prevention, Guide to Community Preventive Services, *Preventing Skin Cancer: Interventions in Outdoor Occupational Settings*, 2013, http://www.thecommunityguide.org/cancer/skin/education-policy/outdooroccupations.html.

2

Validity and Stability of the Decisional Balance for Sun Protection Inventory

Hui-Qing Yin, Joseph S. Rossi, Colleen A. Redding,
Andrea L. Paiva, Steven F. Babbin, and Wayne F. Velicer

Cancer Prevention Research Center, University of Rhode Island, 130 Flagg Road, Kingston, RI 02881, USA

Correspondence should be addressed to Joseph S. Rossi; jsrossi@uri.edu

Academic Editor: Silvia Moretti

The 8-item Decisional Balance for sun protection inventory (SunDB) assesses the relative importance of the perceived advantages (Pros) and disadvantages (Cons) of sun protective behaviors. This study examined the psychometric properties of the SunDB measure, including invariance of the measurement model, in a population-based sample of $N = 1336$ adults. Confirmatory factor analyses supported the theoretically based 2-factor (Pros, Cons) model, with high internal consistencies for each subscale ($\alpha \geq .70$). Multiple-sample CFA established that this factor pattern was invariant across multiple population subgroups, including gender, racial identity, age, education level, and stage of change subgroups. Multivariate analysis by stage of change replicated expected patterns for SunDB (Pros $\eta^2 = .15$, Cons $\eta^2 = .02$). These results demonstrate the internal and external validity and measurement stability of the SunDB instrument in adults, supporting its use in research and intervention.

1. Introduction

Skin cancer is a major public health concern. Melanoma is the most serious form of skin cancer and accounts for the majority of skin cancer deaths. The American Cancer Society estimates there will be more than 76,000 new cases of melanoma diagnosed in 2014 in the United States. Non-melanoma skin cancers are typically nonfatal but much more prevalent; in 2006, approximately 3.5 million people in the United States were diagnosed with these malignancies, and more than 2 million were treated [1]. The incidence rates for both types of skin cancers have been increasing [1, 2]. Skin cancers lead to substantial direct medical care costs and significant indirect costs associated with premature mortality and morbidity [3, 4]. Preventing all skin cancers is both important and possible by adopting habitual sun protective behaviors such as reducing sun exposure and using sunscreen [5].

Interventions for increasing sun protection behaviors using tailored health communications based on the transtheoretical model of behavior change have been developed and implemented and have demonstrated significant impacts in numerous applications [6–9]. The transtheoretical model (TTM) [10–13] is an integrative model of intentional behavior change underlying numerous effective interventions. Empirically based tailoring is especially relevant in population-based interventions when not everyone is prepared to immediately change their risk behavior(s). Decisional Balance is one of the core constructs integrated within the TTM framework. Based initially on the work of Janis and Mann [14], Decisional Balance reflects the cognitive and motivational shifts in decision making as an individual weighs the relative importance of the Pros and Cons of changing the behavior in question [15]. The theoretical relationship between Decisional Balance and transitions across the stages of change (i.e., readiness to change the problem behavior) has been well documented across a variety of health behaviors [16, 17], and therefore incorporated into intervention programs. Appropriately operationalizing theoretical constructs into psychometrically sound measures is critical for testing and implementing a theoretical model. The Decisional Balance for sun protection inventory has been used in a number of applications [7–9]; however, no published study has evaluated the psychometric properties of this measure.

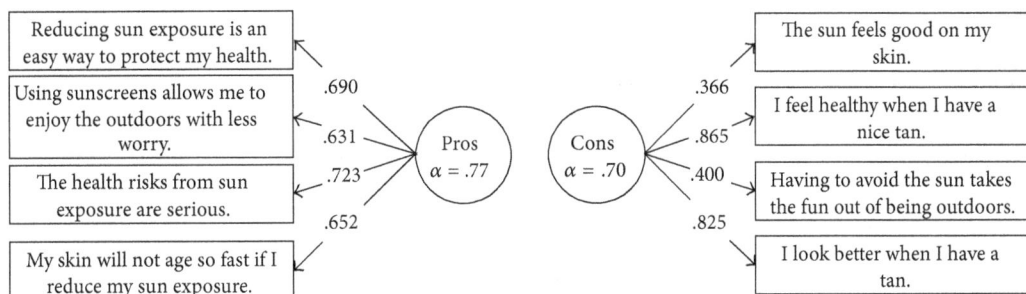

FIGURE 1: Measurement model for uncorrelated Pros and Cons of sun protection with standardized parameter estimates for full sample ($N = 1336$).

The aim of this study was to assess the psychometric properties of the Decisional Balance for sun protection instrument, including confirming the factorial invariance of the measure across population subgroups. Factorial invariance is central to establishing the validity of a measure, as it indicates whether a set of items measures the same theoretical constructs across subgroups, allowing legitimate comparisons between groups on the measure of interest [18]. Three levels of factorial invariance were assessed in sequential order, with increasing levels of restrictiveness or equality constraints on parameters in the model. Configural invariance is an unconstrained model, in which the number of factors and the specific items associated with each factor are assumed to be the same across comparison groups. Pattern identity invariance is the next level of invariance and requires factor loadings for the same items to be equal across groups. Strong factorial invariance is the most restrictive of these three levels and requires factor loadings and error variances to be the same across groups [18, 19]. Meaningful group comparisons can be assumed when a measure has demonstrated strong factorial invariance.

The present study involved secondary analysis of baseline data for a large population-based sample of adults enrolled in a randomized TTM-tailored intervention study targeting sun protection and exercise behaviors. The theoretical structural model of the Decisional Balance for sun protection measure was assessed. The factorial invariance of the measurement model was then tested across population subgroups defined by gender, racial identity, age, education, untanned skin color (a proxy for sun reactivity), and stage of change for sun protection. Mean differences for Decisional Balance by stages of change were also examined to see if expected patterns based on TTM predictions would replicate. Confirming measurement structure and stability, and the functional relationship between the Decisional Balance constructs and stages of change, provides a necessary empirical foundation for TTM-tailored interventions.

2. Method

2.1. Sample.
Participants were population-based adults (age range 18–75 years, 88% white, and 63% female) from across the United States enrolled in a recent intervention study for exercise and sun protection based on the TTM [20]. Participants in the sample were all "at risk" for both behaviors

at baseline based on public health criteria. Participants were identified to be "at risk" for sun exposure if they reported not *consistently* (i) using sunscreens with a sun protection factor (SPF) of 15 or more, (ii) wearing protective clothing, and (iii) avoiding or limiting exposure to the sun during the midday hours. All procedures were approved by the Institutional Review Board at the University of Rhode Island, and participants understood and consented to their voluntary involvement in the study. Data for these analyses were drawn from the baseline assessment collected from April 2009 through September 2011.

2.2. Sun Protection Decisional Balance Instrument.
The 8-item Decisional Balance instrument assessed the perceived advantages (Pros) and disadvantages (Cons) of sun protection. This measure consists of two subscales: a four-item Pros scale and a four-item Cons scale and was developed and successfully employed in a number of previous randomized intervention trials [7–9, 21]. The instrument asked respondents to rate how important each item was in deciding whether or not to protect themselves from too much sun exposure on a 5-point Likert scale from 1 (not important) to 5 (extremely important). The theoretical measurement model for Decisional Balance with two latent Pros and Cons factors (see Figure 1) was assessed for the invariance analyses with this sample.

2.3. Data Analyses.
Three sets of analyses were conducted sequentially on the Decisional Balance for sun protection inventory. The first step tested and confirmed the best-fitting structural model for the Decisional Balance measure. Next, the factorial invariance (stability) of the measurement model was evaluated across multiple population subgroups. All structural equation modeling (SEM) procedures for the first two steps were based on maximum likelihood estimation and performed using EQS 6.1 [22]. The final step determined if the hypothesized functional relationships between each Decisional Balance construct and stages of change would replicate, supporting the known groups and external validity of the measure in this sample [23].

2.3.1. Measurement Structure.
Confirmatory factor analysis (CFA) was conducted to establish the best-fitting structural model for the Decisional Balance measure. Two measurement models were compared, including the correlated and uncorrelated two factor models. Model fit was assessed based

TABLE 1: Sample size by category for each subgroup.

Subgroup	Category	N
Gender	Female	842
	Male	492
Racial identity[a]	White	1143
	Black/African American	84
Ethnicity[b]	Hispanic	56
	Non-Hispanic	1279
Age	18–29 years old	186
	30–39 years old	198
	40–49 years old	346
	50–59 years old	358
	60–75 years old	246
Education level	High school or less (≤12 years)	307
	Some tertiary education (13–15 years)	459
	College graduate or beyond (≥16 years)	569
Untanned skin color	Fair white	291
	Medium white	590
	Dark white/light brown	395
Stage of change for sun protection	Precontemplation	818
	Contemplation	151
	Preparation	367

[a]Not including participants who selected more than one race.
[b]Invariance model could not be assessed across ethnic identity groups due to the low number of participants identified as Hispanic.

on several macrofit indices, including the Comparative Fit Index (CFI), Tucker-Lewis Index (TLI), and Root Mean Square Error of Approximation (RMSEA). For the incremental fit indices, CFI and TLI, values of at least .90 indicate an adequate fit, and values above .95 indicate an excellent fit [24–26]. For RMSEA, smaller values indicate a better fit of the model to the data, with values less than .08 considered acceptable and values below .05 indicating a very good fit [25, 26].

2.3.2. Factorial Invariance. Stability of the Decisional Balance measurement structure was assessed across six subgroups defined by gender, racial identity, age, education level, untanned skin color (a proxy for sun reactivity), and stage of change for sun protection [11, 21]. Three levels of invariance were tested, proceeding from the least to the most restrictive: (1) configural invariance with unconstrained factor loadings; (2) pattern identity invariance with factor loadings for like items constrained to be equal across groups; and (3) strong factorial invariance with equal factor loadings and measurement error variances across groups [19, 27–29]. None of the equality constraints were released to achieve a better fit in any of the invariance models assessed. In addition to the model fit indices (CFI, TLI, and RMSEA) described, the difference in CFI (ΔCFI) values between the model and the previous (less restrictive) invariance model was calculated to test the null hypothesis of noninvariance, with a $|\Delta$CFI$|$ value within .01 indicating model invariance [30]. The χ^2-difference test was also included to assess change in model

fit for the nested invariance model comparisons, although this test tends to be overly sensitive to even small differences in fit between models when sample sizes are large [25–27]. Cronbach's coefficient alphas [31] were calculated and used to assess the internal consistency reliability of both Pros and Cons subscales.

2.3.3. Known Groups Validation. A MANOVA, with follow-up ANOVA and Tukey tests, was conducted to examine functional relationships between Decisional Balance (Pros and Cons subscale means in standardized T-scores) and the three stage of change groups.

3. Results

3.1. Analytic Sample. Participants had complete data on the Decisional Balance for Sun Protection measure. Twenty-eight participants (2%) with extreme response patterns on the Decisional Balance measure were deleted, resulting in the final analytic sample of 1336 participants. Sample sizes by category for each of the six population subgroups assessed by invariance testing are presented in Table 1.

3.2. Measurement Structure. CFA was conducted on the Decisional Balance measure using the full sample. The measurement model with two uncorrelated factors, consisting of four items each for Pros and Cons (Figure 1), provided a good fit for the data, $\chi^2(20) = 138.37$, $P < .001$; CFI = .956; TLI = .939; RMSEA = .057 [90% confidence interval = .053, .061].

TABLE 2: Goodness-of-fit statistics for three nested invariance models.

Model	χ^2	df	CFI	ΔCFI	TLI	RMSEA	[90% CI]
Gender							
Configural invariance	164.489	40	.952	—	.933	.068	[.058, .079]
Pattern identity invariance	179.778	48	.949	−.003	.941	.064	[.054, .074]
Strong factorial invariance	195.002	56	.946	−.003	.939	.061	[.052, .070]
Racial identity							
Configural invariance	148.451	40	.956	—	.939	.067	[.055, .078]
Pattern identity invariance	164.205	48	.953	−.003	.945	.063	[.052, .073]
Strong factorial invariance	192.406	56	.945	−.008	.937	.063	[.053, .073]
Age							
Configural invariance	240.234	100	.948	—	.927	.073	[.061, .084]
Pattern identity invariance	287.769	132	.942	−.006	.939	.067	[.056, .077]
Strong factorial invariance	339.652	164	.935	−.007	.932	.063	[.054, .073]
Education							
Configural invariance	194.881	60	.951	—	.931	.071	[.060, .082]
Pattern identity invariance	232.137	76	.943	−.008	.937	.068	[.058, .078]
Strong factorial invariance	255.272	92	.940	−.003	.935	.063	[.054, .072]
Untanned skin color							
Configural invariance	190.479	60	.948	—	.928	.072	[.060, .083]
Pattern identity invariance	212.751	76	.946	−.002	.940	.065	[.055, .075]
Strong factorial invariance	242.077	92	.941	−.005	.936	.062	[.052, .071]
Stage of change for sun protection							
Configural invariance	205.704	60	.941	—	.917	.074	[.063, .085]
Pattern identity invariance	238.505	76	.934	−.007	.927	.069	[.059, .079]
Strong factorial invariance	309.411	92	.913	−.021	.906	.073	[.064, .082]

An alternative model with correlated latent Pros and Cons factors was also assessed and provided a good fit for the data, $\chi^2(19) = 138.14$, $P < .001$; CFI = .956; TLI = .935; RMSEA = .057 [.052, .061]. The correlation of .016 estimated between the latent Pros and Cons factors was low and not significant, and a χ^2-difference test comparing the nested correlated and uncorrelated models was also not significant ($\chi^2[1] = .23$; $P = .63$), indicating that estimating the extra parameter in the correlated model did not improve model fit. The uncorrelated model was therefore retained for parsimony and used for subsequent invariance testing. Baseline models were assessed in each subsample before the model was tested across subsamples. All baseline models fit well (median CFI = .930; median RMSEA = .068).

3.3. Factorial Invariance. Multiple-sample CFA was used to examine hierarchical factorial invariance for the two Pros and Cons subscales. The fit indices for the invariance models are summarized in Table 2.

3.3.1. Gender. Sample sizes were adequate to test the models across women ($n = 842$) and men ($n = 492$). Strong factorial invariance provided a good fit for the model for gender (CFI = .946; TLI = .939; RMSEA = .061).

3.3.2. Racial Identity. Sample sizes were adequate for comparing subsamples of participants identified as white ($n = 1143$) or black/African American ($n = 84$). Strong factorial invariance provided a good fit across the two racial identity subsamples (CFI = .945; TLI = .937; RMSEA = .063).

3.3.3. Age. Sample sizes were adequate for five age group subsamples, 18 to 29 years old ($n = 186$), 30 to 39 years old ($n = 198$), 40 to 49 years old ($n = 346$), 50 to 59 years old ($n = 358$), and 60 to 74 years old ($n = 246$). Strong factorial invariance provided a good fit for age (CFI = .935; TLI = .932; RMSEA = .063).

3.3.4. Education. Sample sizes were adequate for three subsamples based on the highest level of education attained, 12 years or less ($n = 307$), 13 to 15 years ($n = 459$), and 16 years or more ($n = 569$). Strong factorial invariance provided a good model fit across education levels (CFI = .940; TLI = .935; RMSEA = .063).

3.3.5. Untanned Skin Color. Untanned skin color was used as a proxy indicator of sun reactivity. Sample sizes were adequate to test the models across subgroups of participants who described their untanned skin color as fair white ($n = 291$), medium white ($n = 590$), and dark white/light brown ($n = 395$). Strong factorial invariance provided a good model fit across skin color (CFI = .941; TLI = .936; RMSEA = .062).

3.3.6. Stage of Change for Sun Protection. Sample sizes were adequate to test the models across participants in precontemplation ($n = 818$), contemplation ($n = 151$), and preparation

TABLE 3: Summary statistics for Pros and Cons subscales of Decisional Balance ($N = 1336$).

Subscale	Number of items	Mean[a]	Standard deviation	Coefficient alpha	Skewness	Kurtosis
Pros	4	3.35	0.96	.77	−0.29	−0.52
Cons	4	2.92	0.98	.70	0.11	−0.74

[a]Subscale totals divided by number of items before calculating mean and standard deviations.

TABLE 4: Standardized T-scores (SD) for Decisional Balance by stage of change ($N = 1336$).

Factor	Stage	N	Mean	(SD)	$F(2, 1333)$	η^2	Post hoc Tukey HSD[a]
Pros					114.59*	.147	PC < C, PR
	Precontemplation	818	46.99	(9.60)			
	Contemplation	151	53.27	(8.53)			
	Preparation	367	55.36	(8.71)			
Cons					13.91*	.020	PC, C > PR
	Precontemplation	818	50.87	(10.11)			
	Contemplation	151	50.92	(9.62)			
	Preparation	367	47.68	(9.55)			

*$P < .001$.
[a]PC indicates precontemplation; C: contemplation; PR: preparation.

($n = 367$). This was the only sequence of nested invariance model comparisons that did not support strong invariance, with a $|\Delta$CFI$| > .01$ for the comparison between strong invariance and pattern identity invariance. Pattern identity invariance provided an adequate fit across stage (CFI = .934; TLI = .927; RMSEA = .069).

3.4. Scale Reliabilities. Strong factorial invariance demonstrated good fit for the cross-sample comparisons across gender, racial identity, age, education level, and skin color. Cronbach's coefficient alphas were therefore calculated for each subscale based on the total sample (see Table 3). The coefficient alphas of .77 for the Pros subscale and .70 for the Cons subscale are consistent with the alphas reported previously [32] and indicate good internal consistency reliability of these two subscales. The factor structure for the eight-item Decisional Balance for sun protection measure is reported with standardized parameter estimates for the entire sample in Figure 1.

3.5. Known Groups Validation. A MANOVA was conducted to determine if the Pros and Cons of sun protection differed across the three baseline stage-of-change groups. As predicted [16, 17], there was a significant main effect for stage of change (Wilks' Λ = .83; $F[4, 2664]$ = 67.26; $P < .001$; multivariate η^2 = .17). Follow-up ANOVAs and Tukey tests revealed that both the Pros ($F[2, 1333]$ = 114.59; $P < .001$; η^2 = .147) and Cons ($F[2, 1333]$ = 13.91; $P < .001$; η^2 = .020) differed significantly by stage. Individuals in precontemplation reported significantly lower Pros of sun protection than those in contemplation and preparation. In addition, participants in precontemplation and contemplation reported significantly higher Cons of sun protection than those in preparation. Scale means for the Pros and Cons are shown are Table 4.

4. Discussion

This study replicated an uncorrelated two-factor (Pros and Cons) measurement structure for the Decisional Balance for sun protection instrument in a large national sample of adults at risk for sun exposure, confirming the theoretical model from previous studies [12, 17, 21, 32]. Both Pros and Cons subscales showed good internal consistency as seen by alphas of .70 and .77, and the factor loadings for individual items were adequate to excellent (.366 to .865). These results suggest that participants in this sample discriminated between the positive and negative aspects of adopting sun protective behaviors.

The eight-item Decisional Balance for sun protection inventory with two uncorrelated Pros and Cons subscales demonstrated strong factorial invariance in a large population-based sample of adults who did not meet public health criteria for sun protection behavior. This invariance model required that factor loadings and error terms for individual items were constrained to be equal across comparison groups in the model. Strong factorial invariance provided a good fit across gender, racial identity, age, education level, and untanned skin color, based on CFI values around .95 and RMSEA values below .08. The $|\Delta$CFI$|$ values were consistently within the suggested .01 range as each invariance level was assessed hierarchically, demonstrating a high degree of fit for the strong invariance model across the five subgroups. Results of these analyses indicate a consistent relationship between the Pros and Cons factors and the eight items that serve as measured indicators for these two factors.

The pattern identity invariance model demonstrated a reasonably good fit across the stages of change for sun protection, based on fit indices above .90 (CFI > .93; TLI > .92) and RMSEA below .07. This indicates a consistent relationship between the Pros and Cons factors and equivalent loadings for the eight items on these factors across the stages. However, when the item error terms were restricted to be equal in the strong invariance model, $|\Delta CFI|$ was considerably over the recommended .01 although the CFI, TLI, and RMSEA values still indicated adequate fit for the model (CFI > .91; TLI > .90). This suggests some slight differences in the measurement model across stage, specifically excess variability in responses on individual items that were not consistent across stage groups. This is perhaps not surprising because it was shown previously that stage of change contributes significantly to variation in the Pros and Cons [16, 17].

Decisional Balance varied across baseline stage-of-change groups, and the overall η^2 of .17 could be interpreted as a medium multivariate effect size [33, 34]. As expected, participants in the preparation and contemplation stages endorsed the Pros of sun protection more highly compared to those in precontemplation, with η^2 of .15 representing a large effect of stage of change [34]. Similarly, the Cons of sun protection were rated as less important by participants in preparation compared to those in precontemplation and contemplation. Although the magnitude of the Cons stage effect was small (η^2 = .02), it should be noted that this baseline sample included only participants who were in the three earliest (out of five possible) stages, because they were recruited to be at risk for sun exposure for the intervention study. It is likely that the reduced variability in the sample attenuated the Cons stage effect compared to including the full range of five stages. Meta-analyses of Decisional Balance suggest that most of the change in Cons occurs between the preparation and maintenance stages [16, 17]. The overall patterns for Pros and Cons across the first three stages of change were consistent with the expected functional relationships based on previous studies [16, 17].

This study has several limitations. First, because there was limited demographic variability in this sample, especially for racial and ethnic identity categories, invariance of the Decisional Balance measurement model could not be assessed across ethnic identity groups. When attempted, the invariance model failed to converge due to too few participants identified as Hispanic (n = 56 with complete data). A future sample that is more diverse, with adequate numbers representing additional racial and ethnic groups, would allow more comprehensive assessment of the invariance of this measure beyond white and black racial groups. The sample sizes used in analyses were also unbalanced across racial identity groups, although the invariance models were still indicative of good fit. Second, only the first three (out of five possible) stages of change for sun protection were represented in the baseline sample, which was recruited for an intervention study targeting only at-risk individuals. As described above, this likely restricted the magnitudes of the observed stage effects, especially for the Cons, although the expected cross-sectional differences across the three stages for Decisional Balance were replicated in this sample. Future research is also needed to examine the stability of this measure over time. Third, since this study used a nonclinical, population-based sample, this instrument should undergo additional validation to be utilized with individuals with skin cancer. Finally, the generalizability of the measurement properties of this Decisional Balance instrument is limited to the adult population from which the validation sample was drawn.

5. Conclusion

The results of the present study demonstrate that the measurement model for the two uncorrelated factors representing Decisional Balance (Pros and Cons) for sun protection has a consistent relationship across multiple population subgroups, while providing empirical support for the internal and external validity and internal consistency reliability of the measure. The two subscales have demonstrated invariance in factor loadings and measurement error variances across the subgroups assessed and can be used in multiple subgroups, allowing meaningful comparisons to be made across different samples in the target population for these constructs. The cross-sectional relationship between Decisional Balance and the stages of change demonstrated in previous samples was replicated. These findings add to the evidence supporting the use of the Decisional Balance for sun protection inventory in research and intervention.

Acknowledgments

This study was supported in part by the National Institutes of Health Grants R01CA119195 from the National Cancer Institute, R01DA023191 from the National Institute of Drug Abuse, and G20RR030883 from the National Center for Research Resources. NIH had no role in the study design, collection, analysis or interpretation of the data, writing the paper, or the decision to submit the paper for publication.

References

[1] H. W. Rogers, M. A. Weinstock, A. R. Harris et al., "Incidence estimate of nonmelanoma skin cancer in the United States, 2006," *Archives of Dermatology*, vol. 146, no. 3, pp. 283–287, 2010.

[2] A. Jemal, M. Saraiya, P. Patel et al., "Recent trends in cutaneous melanoma incidence and death rates in the United States, 1992–2006," *Journal of the American Academy of Dermatology*, vol. 65, no. 5, pp. S17.e1–S17.e11, 2011.

[3] G. P. Guy Jr. and D. U. Ekwueme, "Years of potential life lost and indirect costs of melanoma and non-melanoma skin cancer," *PharmacoEconomics*, vol. 29, no. 10, pp. 863–874, 2011.

[4] G. P. Guy Jr., D. U. Ekwueme, F. K. Tangka, and L. C. Richardson, "Melanoma treatment costs: a systematic review of the literature, 1990–2011," *The American Journal of Preventive Medicine*, vol. 43, no. 5, pp. 537–545, 2012.

[5] American Cancer Society, *Cancer Prevention & Early Detection Facts & Figures 2014*, American Cancer Society, Atlanta, Ga, USA, 2014.

[6] G. J. Norman, M. A. Adams, K. J. Calfas et al., "A randomized trial of a multicomponent intervention for adolescent sun protection

behaviors," *Archives of Pediatrics and Adolescent Medicine*, vol. 161, no. 2, pp. 146–152, 2007.

[7] J. O. Prochaska, W. F. Velicer, J. S. Rossi et al., "Multiple risk expert systems interventions: impact of simultaneous stage-matched expert system interventions for smoking, high-fat diet, and sun exposure in a population of parents," *Health Psychology*, vol. 23, no. 5, pp. 503–516, 2004.

[8] J. O. Prochaska, W. F. Velicer, C. Redding et al., "Stage-based expert systems to guide a population of primary care patients to quit smoking, eat healthier, prevent skin cancer, and receive regular mammograms," *Preventive Medicine*, vol. 41, no. 2, pp. 406–416, 2005.

[9] M. A. Weinstock, J. S. Rossi, C. A. Redding, and J. E. Maddock, "Randomized controlled community trial of the efficacy of a multicomponent stage-matched intervention to increase sun protection among beachgoers," *Preventive Medicine*, vol. 35, no. 6, pp. 584–592, 2002.

[10] J. O. Prochaska and W. F. Velicer, "The transtheoretical model of health behavior change," *American Journal of Health Promotion*, vol. 12, no. 1, pp. 38–48, 1997.

[11] J. S. Rossi, L. M. Blais, and M. A. Weinstock, "The Rhode Island Sun Smart Project: skin cancer prevention reaches the beaches," *The American Journal of Public Health*, vol. 84, no. 4, pp. 672–674, 1994.

[12] J. S. Rossi, L. M. Blais, C. A. Redding, and M. A. Weinstock, "Preventing skin cancer through behavior change: implications for interventions," *Dermatologic Clinics*, vol. 13, no. 3, pp. 613–622, 1995.

[13] W. F. Velicer, J. O. Prochaska, J. L. Fava et al., "Using the trans-theoretical model for population-based approaches to health promotion and disease prevention," *Homeostasis in Health and Disease*, vol. 40, no. 5, pp. 174–195, 2000.

[14] I. L. Janis and L. Mann, *Decision Making: A Psychological Analysis of Conflict, Choice, and Commitment*, Macmillan, London, UK, 1977.

[15] W. F. Velicer, C. C. DiClemente, J. O. Prochaska, and N. Brandenburg, "Decisional balance measure for assessing and predicting smoking status," *Journal of Personality and Social Psychology*, vol. 48, no. 5, pp. 1279–1289, 1985.

[16] K. L. Hall and J. S. Rossi, "Meta-analytic examination of the strong and weak principles across 48 health behaviors," *Preventive Medicine*, vol. 46, no. 3, pp. 266–274, 2008.

[17] J. O. Prochaska, W. F. Velicer, J. S. Rossi et al., "Stages of change and decisional balance for 12 problem behaviors," *Health Psychology*, vol. 13, no. 1, pp. 39–46, 1994.

[18] W. Meredith and J. A. Teresi, "An essay on measurement and factorial invariance," *Medical Care*, vol. 44, no. 11, pp. S69–S77, 2006.

[19] W. Meredith, "Measurement invariance, factor analysis and factorial invariance," *Psychometrika*, vol. 58, no. 4, pp. 525–543, 1993.

[20] W. F. Velicer, C. A. Redding, B. Blissmer et al., "Using relational agents to increase engagement in computer-based interventions: preliminary outcomes," *International Journal of Behavioral Medicine*, vol. 21, supplement 1, p. S206, 2014.

[21] M. A. Weinstock, J. S. Rossi, C. A. Redding, J. E. Maddock, and S. D. Cottrill, "Sun protection behaviors and stages of change for the primary prevention of skin cancers among beachgoers in Southeastern New England," *Annals of Behavioral Medicine*, vol. 22, no. 4, pp. 286–293, 2000.

[22] P. M. Bentler, *EQS 6 Structural Equations Program Manual*, Multivariate Software, Encino, Calif, USA, 2006.

[23] C. A. Redding, J. E. Maddock, and J. S. Rossi, "The sequential approach to measurement of health behavior constructs: issues in selecting and developing measures," *California Journal of Health Promotion*, vol. 4, no. 1, pp. 83–101, 2006.

[24] P. M. Bentler, "Comparative fit indexes in structural models," *Psychological Bulletin*, vol. 107, no. 2, pp. 238–246, 1990.

[25] R. B. Kline, *Principles and Practice of Structural Equation Modeling*, The Guilford Press, New York, NY, USA, 3rd edition, 2011.

[26] L.-T. Hu and P. M. Bentler, "Cutoff criteria for fit indexes in covariance structure analysis: conventional criteria versus new alternatives," *Structural Equation Modeling*, vol. 6, no. 1, pp. 1–55, 1999.

[27] S. F. Babbin, M. Harrington, C. Burditt et al., "Prevention of alcohol use in middle school students: psychometric assessment of the decisional balance inventory," *Addictive Behaviors*, vol. 36, no. 5, pp. 543–546, 2011.

[28] M. Harrington, S. Babbin, C. Redding et al., "Psychometric assessment of the temptations to try alcohol scale," *Addictive Behaviors*, vol. 36, no. 4, pp. 431–433, 2011.

[29] H. A. McGee, S. F. Babbin, C. Redding et al., "Prevention of smoking in middle school students: psychometric assessment of the temptations to try smoking scale," *Addictive Behaviors*, vol. 37, no. 4, pp. 521–523, 2012.

[30] G. W. Cheung and R. B. Rensvold, "Evaluating goodness-of-fit indexes for testing measurement invariance," *Structural Equation Modeling*, vol. 9, no. 2, pp. 233–255, 2002.

[31] L. J. Cronbach, "Coefficient alpha and the internal structure of tests," *Psychometrika*, vol. 16, no. 3, pp. 297–334, 1951.

[32] J. E. Maddock, C. A. Redding, J. S. Rossi, and M. A. Weinstock, "Development and validation of an appearance motivation attitudes scale for sun protection," *Psychology & Health*, vol. 20, no. 6, pp. 775–788, 2005.

[33] J. Cohen, "A power primer," *Psychological Bulletin*, vol. 112, no. 1, pp. 155–159, 1992.

[34] J. S. Rossi, "Statistical power analysis," in *Handbook of Psychology*, J. A. Schinka, W. F. Velicer, and I. B. Weiner, Eds., vol. 2 of *Research Methods in Psychology*, pp. 71–108, John Wiley & Sons, 2nd edition, 2013.

3

Kaposi's Sarcoma-Associated Herpesvirus Subversion of the Anti-Inflammatory Response in Human Skin Cells Reveals Correlates of Latency and Disease Pathogenesis

Judith M. Fontana,[1] Justin G. Mygatt,[1] Katelyn L. Conant,[1]
Chris H. Parsons,[2] and Johnan A. R. Kaleeba[1]

[1] Department of Microbiology and Immunology, Uniformed Services University of the Health Sciences, 4301 Jones Bridge Road, Bethesda, MD 20814, USA
[2] Department of Medicine and Microbiology, Stanley S. Scott Cancer Center, Louisiana State University Health Science Center, New Orleans, LA 70112, USA

Correspondence should be addressed to Johnan A. R. Kaleeba; kaleebajar@gmail.com

Academic Editor: Iris Zalaudek

KSHV is the etiologic agent for Kaposi's sarcoma (KS), a neoplasm that manifests most aggressively as multifocal lesions on parts of human skin with a propensity for inflammatory reactivity. However, mechanisms that control evolution of KS from a benign hyperplasia to the histologically complex cutaneous lesion remain unknown. In this study, we found that KSHV induces proteomic and morphological changes in melanocytes and melanoma-derived cell lines, accompanied by deregulation of the endogenous anti-inflammatory responses anchored by the MC1-R/α-MSH signaling axis. We also identified two skin-derived cell lines that displayed differences in ability to support long-term KSHV infection and mapped this dichotomy to differences in (a) NF-κB activation status, (b) processing and expression of KSHV latency-associated nuclear antigen isoforms putatively associated with the viral lytic cycle, and (c) susceptibility to virus-induced changes in expression of key anti-inflammatory response genes that antagonize NF-κB, including MC1-R, POMC, TRP-1, and xCT. Viral subversion of molecules that control the balance between latency and lytic replication represents a novel correlate of KSHV pathogenesis and tropism in skin and underscores the potential benefit of harnessing the endogenous anti-inflammatory processes as a therapeutic option for attenuating cutaneous KS and other proinflammatory outcomes of KSHV infection in high-risk individuals.

1. Introduction

Kaposi's sarcoma (KS) is a highly angioproliferative neoplasm etiologically linked to infection with Kaposi's sarcoma-associated herpesvirus (KSHV), also formally known as human herpesvirus 8 (HHV-8) [1, 2]. Four epidemiological forms of KS have been described and distinguished based on age, sex, geographical location, socioeconomic status, previous exposure to parasitic infections, coinfection with HIV, and the extent of iatrogenic organ transplant-associated immune suppression [3–5]. Although the precise trigger(s) for KS are currently not known, all forms of the lesion display histopathological characteristics consistent with a shared requirement for chronic inflammation, leading to the notion that a preexisting or virus-induced state of inflammation is essential for creating the physiologic conditions necessary for KS development and progression. Indeed, at the early patch stage, the lesion produces and/or paracrinally responds to pro-inflammatory cytokines and growth factors including interferon-γ (IFN-γ), tumor necrosis factor-α (TNF-α), interleukin-1β (IL-1β), IL-2, and IL-6 [6–9] that support expression of adhesion molecules and chemokines that mediate recruitment of circulating monocytes to the lesion. The early stage is also associated with secretion of protumorigenic mediators such as vascular endothelial growth factor (VEGF) that drives the angiogenic increase in hyperproliferating spindle cells, which in turn form the basic slit-like frame-work for erythrocyte extravasation, neovascularization, and plasma cell infiltration; together, these biologic processes are believed to contribute to the complex cellularity found in KS lesions [6, 7, 10–14].

Generally, expression of pro-inflammatory proteins within and around the KS lesion is primarily controlled by the nuclear factor-κ-B (NF-κB) transcription factor, an important mediator of inducible gene expression during cellular growth, immune reactivity, and pathological inflammation [15]. Although the list of molecules that comprise the definitive NF-κB signaling axis is rapidly expanding [16], the classical transactivating form of NF-κB is comprisesd of RelA (p65)/p50 heterodimers which, in unstimulated cells, are sequestered in an inactive form in the cytoplasm via physical association with one of several inhibitors, designated IκB [15]. Upon extracellular stimulation, signal transduction events rapidly lead to activation of the IκB kinase (IKK) complex composed of two catalytic subunits (IKKα and β) and a regulatory "NF-κB essential modulator subunit" (NEMO). Activated IKK (mainly IKKβ) phosphorylates IκBα, triggering its polyubiquitination and proteasomal degradation; this liberates the active NF-κB homo- or heterodimers, which subsequently translocate to the nucleus where they drive transcription of NF-κB-responsive genes [15].

The role of NF-κB in KSHV pathogenesis was brought into focus by the observation that sustained, virus-induced activation of NF-κB following infection is required not only for establishment and maintenance of latency [17, 18] but also for oncogenic transformation [19, 20]. Accordingly, KSHV commits a large portion of its coding potential towards NF-κB activation, primarily via the functions of the viral FADD-like interleukin-1-β-converting enzyme [FLICE/caspase-8]-inhibitory protein (vFLIP) [21], the viral G-protein-coupled receptor (vGPCR) [22, 23], K1 [24], K13 [25], K15 [26], the viral tegument protein encoded by open reading frame-75 [25], as well as a cluster of microRNAs, many of which are linked to regulation of immune reactivity, cell survival, and the tumorigenic potential of KSHV [27–29]. Ironically, NF-κB activation is associated with viral latency, whereas its inhibition results in viral entry into the lytic cycle [17, 18]. It was recently reported, for example, that NF-κB not only activates expression of KSHV latent genes including LANA, v-FLIP, and v-Cyclin, but also negatively regulates the transactivating potential of the KSHV major lytic switch regulator, RTA [17, 30, 31]. NF-κB inhibits RTA recruitment to viral promoters either through direct competition with RBP-Jκ (which cooperatively enhances RTA transactivation by binding DNA adjacent to low-affinity RTA-binding sites within RTA-responsive genes [32–34]) or by sequestering RTA from RBP-Jκ, both of which were shown to depend on the relative amount and activation status of NF-κB [35].

Clearly, the pro-inflammatory function of NF-κB controls the balance between viral latency and lytic replication by regulating accessibility of the KSHV genome to transactivating factors, and is therefore a fundamental determinant of KS development in skin and other target sites. Given this regulatory control, it is intriguing that the host anti-inflammatory mechanisms that are normally activated to

attenuate inflammation in skin somehow fail to control disease induction in this target organ. To explore the molecular basis for this paradoxical outcome, we tested the hypothesis that KSHV infects and subverts the local anti-inflammatory processes of skin cells so that they are unable to overcome the virus-induced pro-inflammatory reactions that support KS histogenesis. We now present the first evidence that melanocytes can be infected by KSHV and in turn may be co-opted as an important cellular determinant of KSHV pathogenesis in skin. Importantly, we have identified two cell lines that displayed dichotomous properties with respect to their ability to support the KSHV latency program and mapped these cytologic attributes to (a) differences in the state of virus-induced NF-κB activation immediately following primary infection and upon establishment of latency, (b) expression of unique LANA isoforms associated with lytic replication, and (c) susceptibility of persistently infected cells to viral impairment of key components of the endogenous anti-inflammatory response pathways. Together, our findings represent the first delineation of the important role that skin cells may play in KSHV pathogenesis and reveal both the cellular correlates for maintenance of viral latency and the nature of interactions between KSHV and the host anti-inflammatory axis that could serve as predictive markers for cutaneous KS.

2. Materials and Methods

2.1. Cell Culture. Vero cells (ATCC; Manassas, VA) and rKSHV.219-infected Vero cells (a kind gift from Jeffrey Vieira, University of Washington, Seattle, WA) were cultured in DMEM (Quality Biological, Inc., Gaithersburg, MD) supplemented with 10% fetal bovine serum (FBS; HyClone Laboratories, Logan, UT) and puromycin (10 μg/mL; Calbiochem, EMD Chemicals, Inc., Gibbstown, NJ). As described previously [36], rKSHV.219 expresses enhanced green fluorescent protein (GFP) under the control of the strong cellular elongation factor 1-α promoter and the Ds-red fluorescent protein (RFP) from the KSHV lytic polyadenylated nuclear (PAN) RNA promoter, in addition to the gene for puromycin resistance as a selectable marker for maintenance of the viral episome in rKSHV.219-infected cells [36]. Normal human adult epidermal primary melanocytes (NHEM-Ad; Lonza Walkersville, Inc., Walkersville, MD) were cultured in 254CF media supplemented with 0.1 mM CaCl$_2$ and human melanocyte growth supplement with PMA (Cascade Biologics, Invitrogen, Carlsbad, CA). MeWo, a highly-pigmented cell line derived from a nodular lymph node metastasis in a patient with malignant melanoma [37], was obtained from ATCC and cultured in EMEM (Quality Biological, Inc.) supplemented with 10% FBS. Mel1700, a benign human melanoma-derived cell line, was provided by Maurice Zauderer (Vaccinex, Inc., Rochester, NY) and cultured in RPMI-1640 (Quality Biological, Inc.) supplemented with 20% FBS. rKSHV.219-infected MeWo and Mel1700 cells were derived in our laboratory and maintained under selection with puromycin at concentrations of 0.5 μg/mL and 1 μg/mL, respectively. The immortalized human keratinocyte cell line,

HaCat [38], was cultured in DMEM supplemented with 10% FBS. rKSHV.219-infected HaCat cells were also maintained in DMEM supplemented with 10% FBS and puromycin (0.5 μg/mL). The body cavity-based lymphoma cell line, BCBL-1, that is persistently infected with KSHV, was obtained from Michael McGrath and Don Ganem via the NIH AIDS Research and Reference Reagent Program, Division of AIDS (NIAID, NIH, Bethesda, MD), and was cultured in RPMI-1640 supplemented with 10% FBS.

2.2. Virus Infections. For infection studies, cultures of rKSHV.219-infected Vero cells were induced with 6 mM sodium *n*-butyrate (NaB; Sigma, St. Louis, MO) and monitored for expression of RFP. Four days after induction, cells were scraped, resuspended in spent media, and collected by centrifugation at 4°C, as previously described [36]. The supernatant containing concentrated KSHV particles was maintained on ice while the cell pellet was resuspended in 2 mLs of DMEM and frozen and thawed two times to release cell-associated viral particles. The resulting lysate was centrifuged at 2500 rpm for 10 minutes at 4°C to remove debris and the clarified supernatant was combined with the original culture supernatant, sterile-filtered through a 0.45 μm membrane filter, and stored at −80°C. Uninfected Vero cells were treated with 6 mM NaB and harvested in parallel to be used for mock infection.

To generate chronically rKSHV.219-infected cells, uninfected cells were plated in T-25 flasks in their respective growth media supplemented with 10% FBS. At 70% confluency, media were removed from each flask and 2 mLs of the Vero-derived rKSHV.219 supernatant was added. After one hour of incubation at 37°C, 3 mLs of media (with 5% FBS) was added and further incubated at 37°C and monitored for the expression of GFP. Subsequently, a progressively increasing concentration (0.1–10 μg) of puromycin/mL was added to the culture in order to enrich for rKSHV.219-infected cells over time. Mock infections were performed in parallel using uninfected Vero cell supernatant and cells were harvested for further analysis at the time of puromycin addition for rKSHV.219-infected cells. For infection of HaCat cells, a T-75 flask of rKSHV.219-infected Mel1700 cells was induced with 6 mM NaB for two days to achieve optimal amounts of RFP positive cells (reactivation conditions were determined empirically). Cell supernatants containing reactivated KSHV were collected, spun at 2500 rpm for 10 minutes at 4°C to remove floating cells and other debris, sterile-filtered through a 0.45 μm membrane filter, and added to uninfected HaCat cells. HaCat cells infected with Mel1700-derived rKSHV.219 were monitored for the appearance of GFP and selected with puromycin (0.5 μg/mL starting at day 3 postinfection).

2.3. Antibodies and Reagents. The following antibodies were purchased from Santa Cruz Biotechnology, Inc. (Santa Cruz, CA): polyclonal anti-GAPDH (L-20), monoclonal anti-TRP-1 (H-90), anti-Melan A (FL-118), anti-MC1R (H-60), and HRP-labeled goat anti-rat secondary antibody. Rat anti-LANA monoclonal antibody LN35 was purchased from Abcam (Cambridge, MA). AlexaFluor-647-labeled chicken anti-rat

IgG secondary antibody (Cat no. A21472) and AlexaFluor-568-labeled goat anti-rat IgG secondary antibody (Cat no. A11077) were purchased from Molecular Probes (Invitrogen, Carlsbad, CA). Unless otherwise indicated, all rabbit monoclonal antibodies against key components of the NF-κB pathway, as well as a polyclonal rabbit antibody to phosphorylated NF-κB p65, were purchased from Cell Signaling Technology (Danvers, MA). Additional antibodies to total NF-κB p65 were purchased from Biosource International (Camarillo, CA) and used in western blot assays with HRP-labeled sheep anti-mouse (Amersham Biosciences, GE Healthcare Life Sciences, Piscataway, NJ) or HRP-labeled donkey anti-rabbit (Chemicon, Millipore, Billerica, MA) secondary antibodies, respectively. Western blot analysis or human xCT was carried out using a previously described polyclonal rabbit antibody to the N-terminal peptide of human SLC7A11 (xCT) [39], or with polyclonal anti-xCT antibody NB300-318 from Novus Biologicals, (Littleton, CO). Recombinant alpha-MSH was purchased from EMD-Calbiochem (La Jolla, California).

2.4. Microscopy. Images were captured using an AxioCam MRm digital camera (Carl Zeiss, Inc.) attached to a Zeiss Axio Observer.A1 inverted fluorescent microscope (Carl Zeiss, Inc.). Pseudocoloring and other image analyses were performed using AxioVision Release 4.6 software.

2.5. Flow Cytometry. Cells were washed, trypsinized, resuspended in FACS Buffer (sterile filtered 1% FBS in PBS without Ca^{2+} or Mg^{2+}), and counted. 1×10^6 cells were fixed with 2% paraformaldehyde (Electron Microscopy Sciences, Fort Washington, PA) and transferred into 12×75 FACS tubes (Falcon, #352063) for analysis by flow cytometry. Cell measurements were acquired using the BD Biosciences LSRII Cell Analyzer and FACSDiva software. Data was analyzed using FlowJo software (version 8.7.3).

2.6. PCR Amplification. Total DNA was extracted from 5×10^5 rKSHV.219-infected or uninfected cells using the DNeasy Blood and Tissue Kit (Qiagen, Valencia, CA), and PCR amplification was performed with Platinum PCR SuperMix High Fidelity (Invitrogen), as recommended by the manufacturer. For detection of viral DNA by PCR, the KS330 primer pair derived from KSHV ORF26 (Table S1) was used to amplify a 232 bp (nt 987–1218) fragment using the following conditions: 94°C for two minutes, then 35 cycles of 94°C for one minute, 58°C for one minute, and 72°C for one minute, followed by 72°C for five minutes, as previously described [1]. Samples were analyzed by gel electrophoresis on 2% agarose gels stained with ethidium bromide.

2.7. RT-PCR. Total RNA was extracted from cell pellets using Trizol Reagent (Invitrogen), digested with the RNase-free DNase set (Qiagen) and quantified using a ND-1000 NanoDrop spectrophotometer supported by the associated software, version 3.1.2. RT-PCR was performed on 0.5 μg DNase-digested RNA using the SuperScript One-Step RT-PCR with Platinum Taq kit (Invitrogen) with primer sets specific for viral or cellular genes (Table S1). Amplification products were analyzed by gel electrophoresis on 1% agarose gels stained with ethidium bromide.

2.8. Immunofluorescence.

Cells were seeded in eight-well chamber slides (Lab-Tek Chamber Slide System, Nalge Nunc) at a concentration of 1×10^5 cells per well and allowed to adhere overnight at 37°C. For direct immunofluorescence, the cells were fixed the next day in 2% paraformaldehyde (Electron Microscopy Sciences, Fort Washington, PA) in PBS for 30 minutes and then permeabilized in 2% paraformaldehyde and 0.1% Triton X-100 (Calbiochem, La Jolla, CA) in PBS for an additional 30 minutes. After fixation, the cells were washed once with PBS and incubated in blocking buffer (2% FBS in PBS) for one hour at 37°C. Blocking buffer was then removed and the cells were further incubated with anti-LANA primary antibodies in fresh blocking buffer for one hour at 37°C. Cells were washed five times with PBS and then incubated with fluorescently-labeled secondary antibodies for one hour at 37°C. After five washes with PBS to remove unbound antibody, coverslips were mounted onto the slides using Vectashield Mounting Medium for Fluorescence with DAPI (Vector Laboratories, Burlingame, CA) and cells were visualized using fluorescence microscopy.

2.9. Western Blot.

Cell pellets (1×10^6 cells per pellet) were lysed in RIPA buffer (0.1% SDS, 1% NP-40, 150 mM NaCl, 1 mM EDTA, 50 mM Tris-HCl pH 7.5, 0.5% deoxycholate, 50 μg/mL BSA) and electrophoresed under reducing conditions on a NuPAGE 4–12% Bis-Tris gel with MES SDS Running Buffer (Invitrogen). Resolved proteins were transferred from the gel to a PVDF membrane (Invitrogen) and blocked overnight in PBS containing 5% nonfat powdered milk and 0.1% Tween-20. Primary and secondary antibodies were each diluted in blocking buffer and incubated with the blots for one hour, rocking at room temperature. Blots were washed three times (0.05% NP-40 in PBS) for 15 minutes after incubation with each antibody and developed using SuperSignal West Femto substrate (Thermo Scientific, Rockford, IL).

3. Results

3.1. Human Melanocytes Can Be Infected by KSHV.

We determined the susceptibility of skin cells to KSHV by innoculating primary adult melanocytes (NHEM-Ad) and two melanoma-derived cell lines (MeWo and Mel1700) with rKSHV.219 and then analyzed: (i) postentry expression of virus-encoded GFP, (ii) viral genome content by PCR, (iii) viral gene expression by RT-PCR, and (iv) productive release of infectious virus upon lytic reactivation. Compared to controls, infected melanocytes (NHEM-Ad) and MeWo cells lost their elongated morphology and acquired a stubby, dedifferentiated phenotype (Figures 1(b) and 1(c)). Persistently infected MeWo cells also formed large, multinucleated syncytia (Figures 1(c) and S1A; yellow asterisks), possibly induced by viral glycoprotein-mediated cell fusion [40]. On the other hand, persistently infected Mel1700 cells did not become stubby but instead expressed outgrowths of elongated dendritic spines (Figures 1(d) and S1C; arrows). These

morphologic changes are reminiscent of the neuroendocrine-like features characteristically associated with subskin lesions [41–43] and may be the first indication of hitherto unexplored aspects of virus-host interactions that contribute to pathology in skin. After a series of a selective passage of infected cells in the presence of puromycin, we were able to generate long-term cultures (almost 100% infection rate) of persistently infected KSHV-infected cells (see Figure S1 in Supplementary Material available online at http://dx.doi.org/10.1155/2014/246076), allowing us to further characterize the virologic outcomes of KSHV infection in these cells.

3.2. Differential Induction of the KSHV Lytic Cycle in Skin Cells Suggests Cell Line-Specific Correlates of Viral Tropism.

Long-term infection of skin cells was confirmed by PCR amplification of viral DNA isolated from cells treated with increasing amounts of n-butyrate (NaB), a histone deacetylase inhibitor known to induce viral reactivation [44]. As shown in Figure 2, the template from uninduced Mel1700-KSHV cells produced a more intense viral DNA product compared to the target template from uninduced MeWo-KSHV cells (Figures 2(a) and 2(b); compare lane 2 in each case), implying that Mel1700-KSHV cells may harbor more viral genome copies than MeWo-KSHV cells, which we confirmed by dilutional analysis against preset standards of viral DNA from KSHV$^+$ BCBL-1 cells previously determined to contain approximately 100 genome copies per cell [45]. To determine whether the putative difference in viral genome content reflected a difference in the replicative potential of the virus in these cells, we used epifluorescence to analyze spontaneous or NaB-induced virus reactivation based on expression of RFP, which is transcribed under the control of a strictly lytic viral PAN promoter [36]. As shown in Figure 2(c), RFP was virtually undetectable in untreated MeWo-KSHV cells, but increased slightly after treatment with 2 mM NaB. In contrast, the already high level of spontaneous RFP expression in Mel1700-KSHV cells was further increased by NaB (Figure 2(d)), further suggesting that Mel1700 cells may have a higher propensity for supporting viral lytic reactivation. However, we were mindful of the fact that differences in cell density could also influence the timing and/or robustness of viral reactivation in confluent cultures of infected cells, so we used flow cytometry to more accurately quantitate the time-dependent increase in RFP+ cells following NaB treatment. As shown in Figure S2A, approximately 0.9% of untreated MeWo-KSHV cells were RFP+, compared to 7.9% of untreated Mel1700-KSHV. At each time point after NaB treatment, the number of RFP+ cells in MeWo and Mel1700 cells increased to approximately 30% versus 36% after 1 day, 41% versus 45% after 2 days, and to 46% versus 57% after 2 days, respectively. This temporal change in RFP expression is also illustrated in various formats (Figures S2B–S2D), all of which reveal that Mel1700 cells support a higher level of spontaneous and/or drug-induced KSHV reactivation than MeWo cells. Furthermore, virions from the highly inducible Mel1700-KSHV cells were infectious for human HaCat keratinocytes, which subsequently maintained

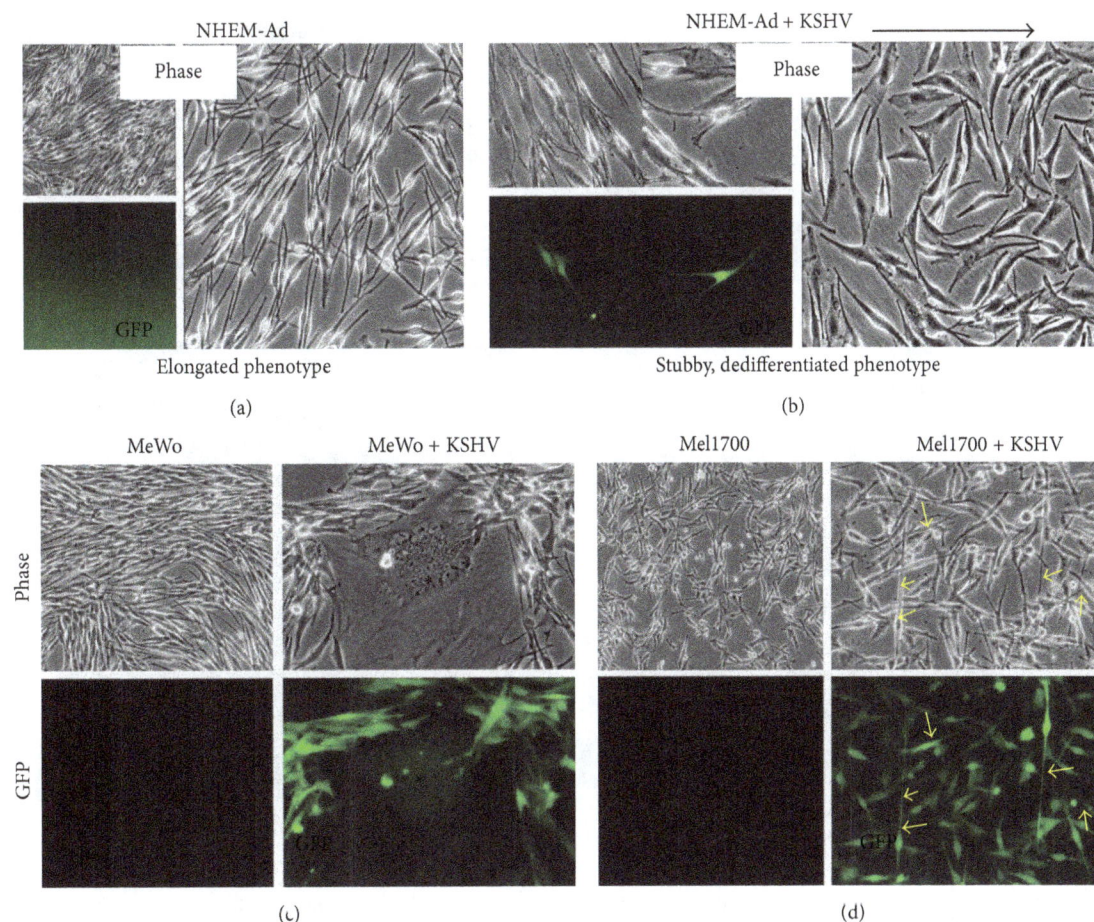

FIGURE 1: KSHV infection of primary melanocytes and melanoma-derived cells is associated with virus-induced morphological changes. (a) (b): Representative phase and GFP images of uninfected (a) or rKSHV.219-infected (b) primary NHEM-Ad melanocytes at day two after infection. Rightmost panels are enlarged (20x) phase contrast views of uninfected and infected cultures, respectively. (c) (d): Representative images of uninfected or rKSHV.219-infected MeWo cells (c) and Mel1700 cells (d). Multinucleated cells in infected MeWo cells are denoted with asterisks, whereas yellow arrows in infected Mel1700 cells point to elongated dendritic spines putatively induced by the virus.

GFP expression (Figure S3A) and viral DNA after more than 48 days of continuous culture in presence of puromycin (Figure S3B). Moreover, infected HaCat-KSHV cells could also support viral lytic replication, as evidenced by foci of RFP-expressing cells upon treatment with a low dose of NaB (Figure S3C).

3.3. KSHV-Infected Skin Cells Support the Full Spectrum of Viral Gene Expression. To determine whether differences in viral lytic replication in MeWo and Mel1700 cells (Figure 2) also reflected patterns of viral gene expression in these cells, we analyzed the transcriptional profile of selected viral genes belonging to each of the three previously described classes of viral transcription in KSHV-infected cells [46–48]. Thus, class I genes include LANA, v-FLIP, and v-Cyclin that are constitutively expressed, while class II genes include the immediate early master switch regulator of the KSHV viral lytic cycle, RTA, as well as Orf74 (v-GPCR), and K2 (v-IL-6), which are constitutively expressed but highly inducible regulators of viral gene expression and the host

microenvironment. On the other hand, class III genes include strictly lytic genes such as gB, gH, and K8.1 that encode viral structural proteins. Viral gene transcription was assessed by semiquantitative RT-PCR; all RNA samples were treated with DNase I prior to the RT-PCR reaction, and as a consequence no amplification product was detected in a pre-RT-PCR control experiment in which *Reverse-Transcriptase* (RT) was omitted from the reactions (Figure S4A). In addition, no viral DNA was detected in DNase I-treated RNA samples (Figure S4B), confirming that we had successfully removed contaminating viral DNA. As shown in Figure 3, all genes tested were expressed in both cell lines, especially following NaB treatment. However, an important distinction was evident in the expression of key markers of stage-specific replication, most notably the immediate early RTA, the early/late vGPCR, and the strictly late K8.1. While these transcripts were expressed only in NaB-treated (but not in uninduced) MeWo-KSHV cells, they were abundantly expressed in untreated Mel1700-KSHV cells (Figure 3, compare lanes 2 and 5). Given that RTA transactivates the promoters of several lytic KSHV genes including its own [46–48], the difference in RTA expression

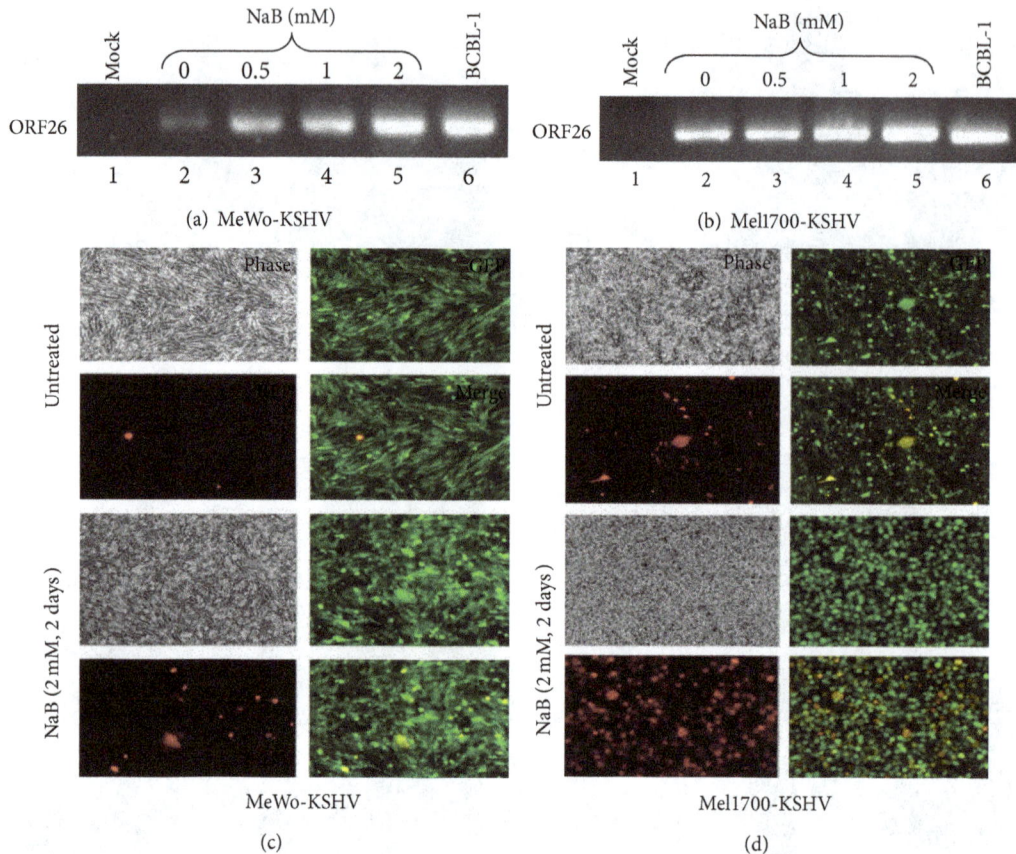

FIGURE 2: Differential induction of viral lytic cycle in skin cells reveals cell line-specific correlates of latency. (a) and (b): Total DNA was extracted from 5×10^5 rKSHV.219-infected MeWo-KSHV cells (a) or Mel1700-KSHV cells (b) either mock-treated or treated with increasing concentrations of NaB, as indicated. An equal amount of normalized viral DNA was then used for PCR amplification of the virus genome using ORF26-specific primers (Table S1). Approximately 10 ng of DNA from KSHV-infected BCBL-1 cells was used as a positive control. (c) and (d): Representative phase, GFP, RFP, and color-merged images of infected MeWo-KSHV (c) or Mel1700-KSHV cells (d) either untreated or treated with 2 mM NaB for two days.

in the absence of drug induction could explain the higher level of spontaneous viral reactivation and virion output in infected Mel1700-KSHV cells compared to their MeWo-KSHV counterparts.

3.4. Differential Expression of LANA in KSHV-Infected Cells Highlights Diffuse Nuclear LANA Expression as a Marker of Viral Lytic Replication. KSHV LANA maintains viral latency in part by tethering episomal DNA to the host chromosome and by suppressing RTA-controlled lytic genes [49]. Consistent with this function, LANA is often detected as punctate nuclear speckles depicting discrete foci of LANA-mediated tethering of viral episomes to host DNA [49]. In light of our finding that RTA is robustly expressed in Mel1700-KSHV cells even in the absence of drug induction, we speculated that deregulated expression of LANA might relieve RTA repression, resulting in the relatively higher level of virus reactivation in Mel1700, but not in MeWo cells. Consistent with this prediction, all infected MeWo-KSHV cells exhibited punctate nuclear LANA staining that is also typically seen in latently-infected endothelial cells and PEL-derived cell lines

[49], whereas LANA staining was predominantly "diffuse" in Mel1700-KSHV cells (Figure 4 and supplementary Figure S5). The "punctate" versus "diffuse" distinction was not due to antibody cross-reactivity or artifacts associated with the IFA, because similar results were obtained in a parallel experiment in which we used a goat anti-rat secondary IgG conjugated to a different fluorophore (Figure S6). Moreover, no background fluorescence was seen in control experiments in which only primary or secondary antibody was used (Figure S7), and, in this case the RFP signal is a result of NaB treatment, which induces a higher level of RFP expression in Mel1700-KSHV cells compared to MeWo-KSHV cells (as illustrated in Figure 2).

To confirm whether diffuse LANA staining directly correlates with lytic replication, we treated both MeWo-KSHV and Mel1700-KSHV cells with NaB and then attempted to simultaneously capture both punctate (unreactivated) and diffuse (reactivated) LANA images in the same cell population. Figure S8 is a representative set of RFP, GFP, DAPI, and LANA images from two separate visual fields I and II (panel A, for MeWo-KSHV) and III and IV (panel B, for Mel1700-KSHV). In MeWo-KSHV cells, diffuse LANA staining was

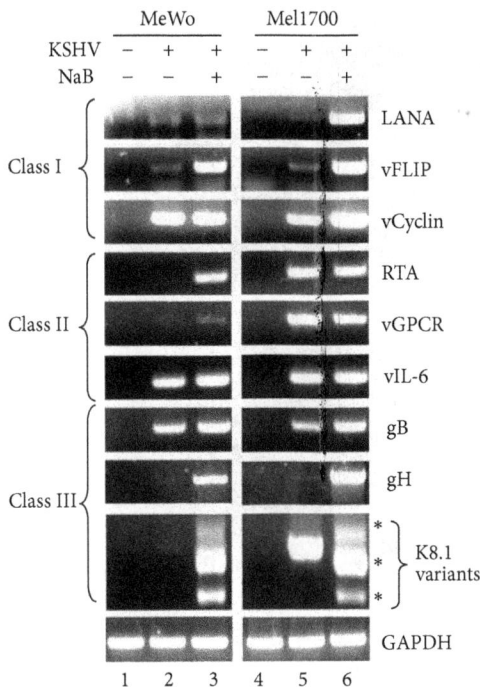

FIGURE 3: rKSHV.219-infected melanoma cells support the full spectrum of latent and lytic viral gene expression. Total RNA from mock (−) or rKSHV.219-infected (+) MeWo and Mel1700 cells either left untreated (−) or induced (+) with 2 mM NaB for two days was used as template for RT-PCR amplification of viral transcripts using primer sets specific for genes belonging to the latent class I (LANA, vFLIP, vCyclin), latent/inducible class II (RTA, vGPCR, vIL6), or the strictly lytic class III (gB, gH, K8.1) (Table S1). GAPDH was used as a template loading control.

detected only in reactivated (RFP+) cells nos.10, 11, and 12 that are surrounded by apparently nonreactivated (RFP−) cells nos.1–9 in which LANA is indeed punctate (Figure S8A). On the other hand, cells nos.1–6 in the Mel1700-KSHV fields appear to be reactivated, and accordingly exhibit diffuse LANA staining (Figure S8B), confirming that diffuse nuclear LANA staining may be a marker for lytic replication, while punctate LANA expression may reflect viral genomes in a predominantly latent state. Surprisingly, we also detected cytoplasmic LANA staining in a small number of reactivated cells (e.g., MeWo-KSHV cells #10–12) and Mel1700-KSHV cells (#1 and 3). Although the molecular basis for extranuclear LANA staining in reactivated cells is not known, it reveals important new perspectives on hitherto unrecognized regulatory functions for novel LANA isoforms that may control the timing, robustness, and molecular threshold for the mechanisms that control viral reactivation.

3.5. Differential Processing and Expression of KSHV LANA Reveal Novel Mechanisms for Regulation of the Viral Lytic Cycle in Skin-Derived Cells. Since the LANA genome-tethering function depends on its ability to bind host DNA, and since entry into the viral lytic cycle may disrupt these interactions in a manner that could, in theory, result in delocalized

(diffuse) LANA staining, we tested the hypothesis that diffuse LANA staining during lytic replication reflects a disproportionate accumulation of C-terminally truncated LANA isoforms that lack the capacity to bind DNA and are, therefore, diffusely expressed throughout the nucleus and possibly the cytoplasm as well. Interestingly, KSHV LANA (1,162 aa) has a predicted molecular weight of 135 kDa, yet various studies have often detected the protein as a doublet of approximately 220–230 kDa in addition to two NaB-inducible 150–180 kDa and 130 kDa bands [49], underscoring the potential for multiple posttranscriptional regulation. In the current study, we also detected the 220 kDa band in uninduced MeWo-KSHV lysates (Figure 5(a), lane 1), in addition to a 130 kDa band that was induced by NaB (Figure 5(a), lane 2) but became clearly visible in uninduced MeWo-KSHV samples only after a 30 min exposure (Figure 5(b), lane 1). Mel1700-KSHV cells also contained the ~220 and 130 kDa bands in addition to three more bands at ~180, 160, and 90 kDa (Figure 5(a), lane 3), all of which were expressed in absence of NaB induction. Although the β-actin control band suggests that less total protein may have been loaded for the MeWo samples, additional repeats and longer exposures confirmed that the MeWo samples expressed the ~180, 160, or 90 kDa bands only after NaB treatment (Figure 5(b), compare lanes 1 and 2), in contrast to Mel1700-KSHV cells in which they were clearly present even in absence of NaB induction, giving us reason to believe that the ~180, 160, and 90 kDa LANA bands may be uniquely associated with lytic replication. We note that the reduction in LANA-specific bands in NaB-treated Mel1700-KSHV cells (Figure 5(a), lane 4) may be either due to NaB cytotoxicity or cell lysis potentially associated with infectious virus release. Another insightful finding was that the pattern of LANA expression in infected MeWo cells was analogous to BCBL-1 cells in which LANA is often detected as punctate speckles [49], a fact that is even more demonstrable in the side-by-side western blots (Figure S9A) and LANA IFA images (Figure S9B). Together, these results imply that punctate LANA staining marks strong latency, whereas the switch to diffuse staining may represent entry into the viral lytic phase.

3.6. NF-κB Activation and the Overall Inflammatory Status of Infected Cells Regulate KSHV Latency in Skin Cells. A number of studies have shown that a preexisting state of inflammation or direct KSHV-mediated activation of the NF-κB pathway early following infection may be necessary for successful establishment of viral latency [50, 51]. To examine this concept in skin cells, we analyzed the activation status of key components of the classical NF-κB pathway in relation to intrinsic cellular attributes that support specific virologic outcomes during both de novo (or acute) and persistent (or chronic) infection. Similar to previous reports, KSHV rapidly induced phosphorylation of NF-κB p65 and IkBα within 20 minutes of infection (Figures 6(a) and 6(b)), an effect that correlated with changes in expression of the NF-κB-controlled intracellular adhesion molecule 1 (ICAM-1) [52]. Interestingly, while phosphorylated p65 remained relatively unchanged for several hours postinfection of MeWos, it

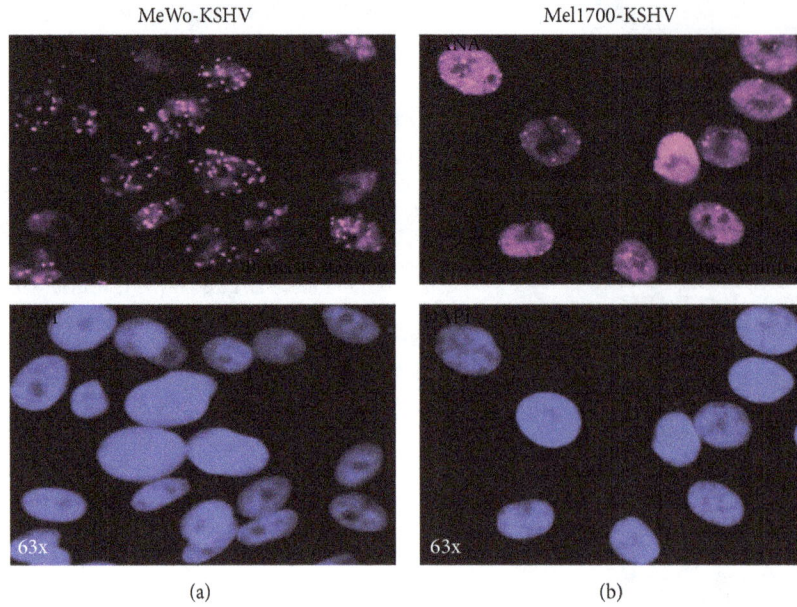

FIGURE 4: Differential expression of LANA in KSHV-infected MeWo and Mel1700 cells reveals diffuse nuclear staining as a marker of spontaneous or drug-induced lytic replication. Infected MeWo-KSHV (a) and Mel1700-KSHV cells (b) were plated in chamber slides and allowed to adhere overnight, then fixed, permeabilized, and stained with the LANA-specific LN35 primary antibody, followed by chicken anti-rat secondary antibody conjugated to Alexa-Fluor-647 (Cy5). Shown are 63x magnification (oil immersion) images of infected MeWo-KSHV (a) and Mel1700-KSHV cells (b) showing LANA (top image) along with the corresponding DAPI nuclear counter-stain (bottom image), respectively. Note the predominantly discrete "punctate" LANA staining in MeWo-KSHV cells (a) in contrast to the more diffuse LANA staining in almost all Mel1700-KSHV cells (b).

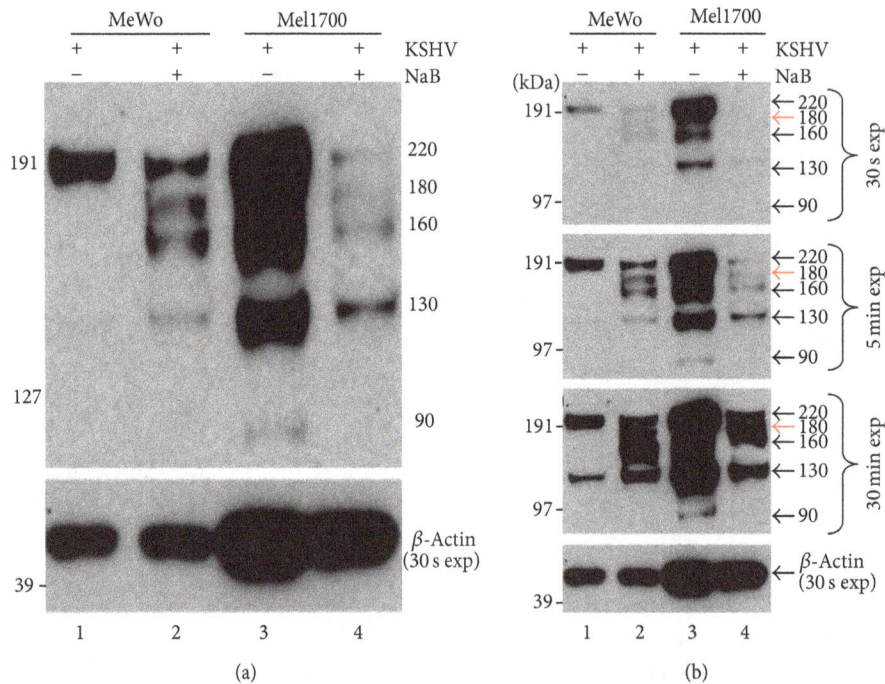

FIGURE 5: Differential expression of specific LANA isoforms in KSHV-infected MeWo and Mel1700 cells is associated with differences in viral lytic replication. (a) RIPA buffer lysates of rKSHV.219-infected MeWo and Mel1700 cells either untreated (−) or treated with NaB (+) for four days were resolved in SDS-PAGE and probed with anti-LANA antibody LN35. Blots were visualized with anti-rat-horse radish peroxidase (HRP)-conjugated secondary antibody. (b) 30 sec, 5 min., and 30 min. exposure times for the blot in (a), revealing "fine" differences between the samples with respect to expression of specific LANA bands. β-Actin (30 sec. exposure) was used as loading control, and the estimated LANA band sizes are on the right side of the blot(s).

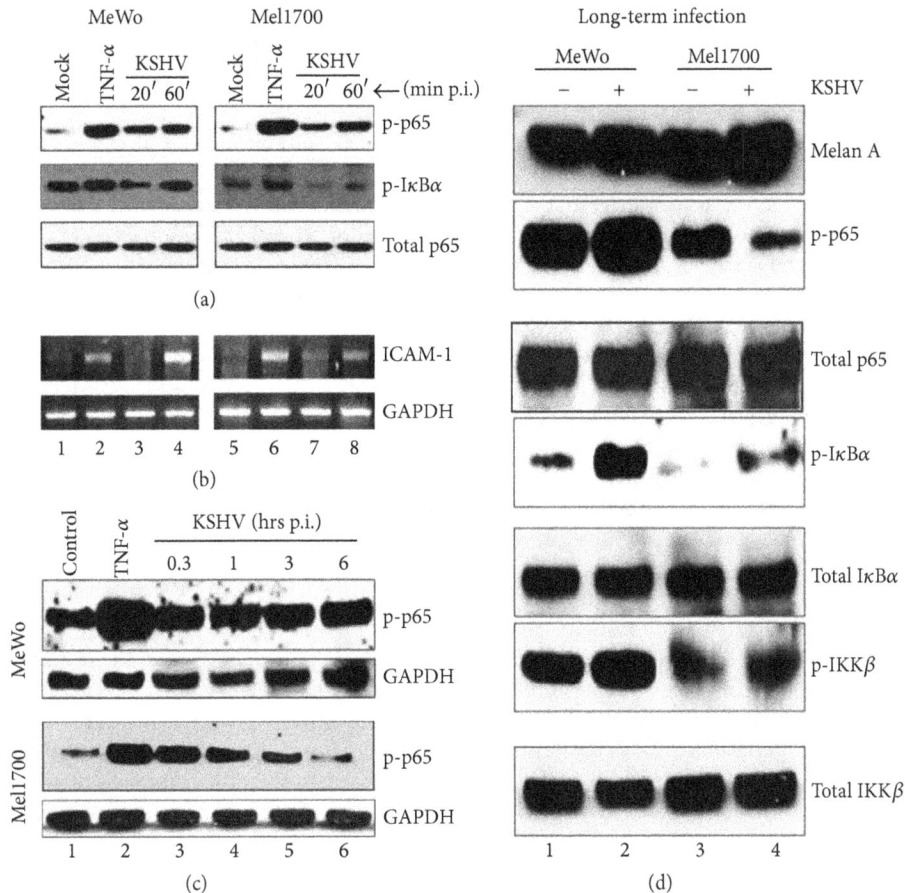

FIGURE 6: Early activation of NF-κB signaling during acute infection with rKSHV.219 is sustained in MeWo cells, but subsequently limited in Mel1700 cells following long-term infection. (a) MeWo and Mel1700 cells either mock-infected, treated for 20 min. with TNF-α, or infected with rKSHV.219 for 20 and 60 min. were used in western blot analysis for phosphorylated NF-κB p65. Mock-infected cell lysates were used to determine baseline levels of phosphorylated NF-κB p65, whereas lysates from cells treated with TNF-α served as positive controls for activation of NF-κB p65. Total NF-κB protein was used as an internal loading control. (b) Total RNA from half of the same cells used in (a) was used for RT-PCR amplification of the NF-κB-controlled ICAM-1 gene. (c) MeWo cells (top) and Mel1700 cells (bottom) either mock-infected (control), TNF-α-treated, or infected with rKSHV.219 for 0.3 h, 1 h, 3 h, or 6 h were used in western blot analysis for phosphorylated NF-κB p65. (d) Western blot analysis of the phosphorylation levels of key components of the NF-κB-signaling pathway in long-term cultures of uninfected (−) and infected (+) MeWo and Mel1700 cells.

was short-lived and in fact began to decline within one hour postinfection of Mel1700 cells (Figure 6(c)). Since NF-κB activation represses RTA while its inhibition relieves RTA repression [17, 18], the fact that NF-κB activation is curtailed in KSHV-infected Mel1700 cells implies that Mel1700 cells likely express endogenous mechanisms that function in an adaptive manner to attenuate NF-κB activity, a process that could explain the relatively higher propensity for virus reactivation in these cells. Consistent with this view, we found that after several days of selective passage in presence of puromycin (designed to maintain stable replicative viral genomes in persistently infected cells), key components of the NF-κB signaling axis were differentially impacted by the virus, even though both MeWo and Mel1700 cells retained their melanoma phenotype, as indicated by sustained expression of Melan-A (Figure 6(d)). For example, while phosphorylated p65, IkBα, and IKKβ were elevated in persistently infected MeWos, the level of phosphorylated

p65 was dramatically reduced, and the relative increase in phosphorylated IkBα and IKKβ was also much more modest in long-term cultures of infected Mel1700 cells (Figure 6(d), compare lanes 2 and 4, resp.). Therefore, we have found that, in comparison to MeWo cells, Mel1700 cells (a) support a more robust viral lytic replication program (Figure 2), (b) express higher levels of RTA (Figure 3), (c) display diffuse nuclear LANA staining (Figure 4(b)) that correlates with stage-specific expression of specific LANA isoforms including the 180 kDa band that is associated with lytic replication (Figure 5), and (e) have reduced NF-κB activation (Figure 6). These dichotomous properties are consistent with a model whereby sustained activation of NF-κB (as in MeWo cells) correlates with maintenance of latency whereas a reduction in activated NF-κB p65 (as in Mel1700) correlates with a higher propensity for viral reactivation, a paradigm supported by findings in other cell types as well [17, 18, 50, 51].

3.7. KSHV Blocks Expression of Anti-Inflammatory Response Proteins to Maintain a Latent State in MeWo Cells, but Fails to Do so in Mel1700 Cells That Support Robust Lytic Replication. The control of inflammation within the epidermal unit of skin is orchestrated by anti-inflammatory responses primarily initiated by alpha-melanocortin stimulating hormone (α-MSH), a potent peptide derived from pro-opiomelanocortin (POMC) by posttranslational proteolytic processing [53]. The effects of α-MSH are transduced through the melanocortin 1 receptor (MC1-R) [54], which is expressed by skin-resident melanocytes, keratinocytes, microvascular endothelial cells, and other monocytic infiltrates [54]. Upon binding to MC1-R, α-MSH triggers a signaling cascade that effectively blunts inflammatory reactivity by preventing activation of NF-κB and the associated expression of pro-inflammatory cytokines and adhesion molecules that mediate infiltration of pro-inflammatory cells into the vascular endothelial environment [53, 55–57]. α-MSH also regulates pigment production and deposition through activation of tyrosinase, the enzyme that catalyzes synthesis of dopaquinone, the first step in melanogenesis [58]; in turn, dopaquinone reacts with intracellular cystine (supplied by the cystine/glutamate transporter, xCT) to produce cysteinyl-dopa, a rate-limiting step in the synthesis of pheomelanin during inflammation [59]. Since establishment of a persistent state is determined by the overall inflammatory status of infected cells, we asked whether establishment of strong KSHV latency (in MeWo and not in Mel1700) is controlled by differential deregulation of endogenous anti-inflammatory mediators that would otherwise be expressed to prevent establishment of latency in these cells. We measured the temporal changes in NF-κB activation in relation to key components of the anti-inflammatory α-MSH/MC1-R signaling axis, and found that within the first 1 hr of infection KSHV induced a rapid increase in phosphorylated NF-κB p65 in MeWo cells (Figure 7(a)). This was in contrast to Mel1700 cells in which the increase in NF-κB activation did not occur until at least 3 hrs postinfection (see Figure 7(b) and the ImageJ quantitation of phosphorylated p65 band intensities in Figure 7(c)). During the rapid increase in NF-κB activation in MeWos cells, MC1-R was not expressed while there was a progressive abrogation of endogenous tyrosinase-related protein-1 (TRP-1), which is involved in pigment synthesis and deposition during inflammation (Figure 7(a)). By contrast, MC1-R protein was induced almost immediately after infection of Mel1700 cells, but there was no appreciable impact on the already high baseline level of TRP-1 (Figure 7(b)); instead, there was a virus-induced increase in mRNA for MC1-R, POMC (the precursor of α-MSH), and xCT (gene name SLC7A11) (Figure 7(d)). This effect correlated with the amount of virus used, as marked by the correspondingly dose-dependent expression of viral GPCR, LANA, and vFLIP (Figure 7(e)).

When infection was monitored over a longer period of time, it was evident that phosphorylated p65 remained high in MeWos, whereas in Mel1700 cells it was consistently detected much later (Figure S10A). Moreover, the kinetics of phosphorylated p65 in both cell lines overlapped with expression of xCT (Figure S10B), which not only forms a

receptor complex that mediates KSHV entry [39], but also supplies cystine for the manufacture of glutathione (GSH), a potent anti-inflammatory mediator [60]. Interestingly, we recently discovered that KSHV microRNAs target a transcriptional inhibitor of xCT in infected cells, ostensibly to promote virus dissemination while protecting infected cells from inflammatory stress [61]. Therefore, the fact that the kinetics of NF-κB activation overlap with xCT expression in KSHV-infected skin cells is consistent with cellular induction of anti-inflammatory responses as an adaptive response to inflammation during the latent state. In accordance with this link, we detected a significant reduction in the expression levels of xCT, MC1-R, and TRP-1 in persistently infected MeWos, but in Mel1700 cells expression of MC1-R and TRP-1 was sustained in conjuction with an increase in xCT (Figure 7(f)). Together, these findings suggest that the differential influences of KSHV in MeWo and Mel1700 that we observed following *de novo* infection are also maintained after establishment of latency.

3.8. KSHV Latency Correlates with Impairment of the Overall Anti-Inflammatory Response in Infected Skin Cells. To determine the biological significance of the impact of KSHV on mediators of the endogenous melanogenic response, we treated both uninfected and KSHV-infected MeWo or Mel1700 with α-MSH and assessed the cellular redistribution of TRP-1, a known downstream marker for the effector function of MC1-R activity. TRP-1 is expressed exclusively in melanosomes where it plays a role in the maintenance of melanosome structure. As shown in Figure 8, untreated MeWo cells express weak but detectable levels of TRP-1 that is predominantly associated with the ER/Golgi network (Figure 8(a), top-left quadrant). However, treatment with α-MSH resulted in a slight change in the distribution of the TRP-1 from being exclusively associated with the ER/Golgi to other aspects of the cell (Figure 8(a), lower-left images), indicating that these cells are capable of responding to the anti-inflammatory effects of α-MSH. However, in KSHV-infected MeWos, the basal expression of TRP-1 was abrogated (Figure 8(a), top-right image), consistent with western blot data in Figure 7(a). Remarkably, treatment of KSHV-infected MeWo-KSHV cells with α-MSH restored TRP-1 expression to levels analogous to those in uninfected samples (Figure 8(a), white arrows), revealing a direct influence of KSHV on the MC1-R/α-MSH axis in these cells. On the other hand, we found that unlike MeWo and their infected counterparts in which not all cells expressed TRP-1, Mel1700 cells expressed high basal levels of TRP-1 (Figure 8(b), top-left image), and in this case KSHV actually did not abrogate but instead induced a noticeable increase in TRP-1 expression (Figure 8(b), top-right image; also see TRP-1 blot in Figure 7(b)). Moreover, α-MSH treatment of Mel1700-KSHV cells resulted in a dramatic alteration in TRP-1 expression from being primarily associated with the supranuclear ER/Golgi network to what appeared, at higher magnification, to resemble melanogenic vesicles arrayed along dendritic spines (Figures 8(b) and S11B, green arrows, and additional data not shown). At a functional level, it is reasonable to conclude that in MeWos

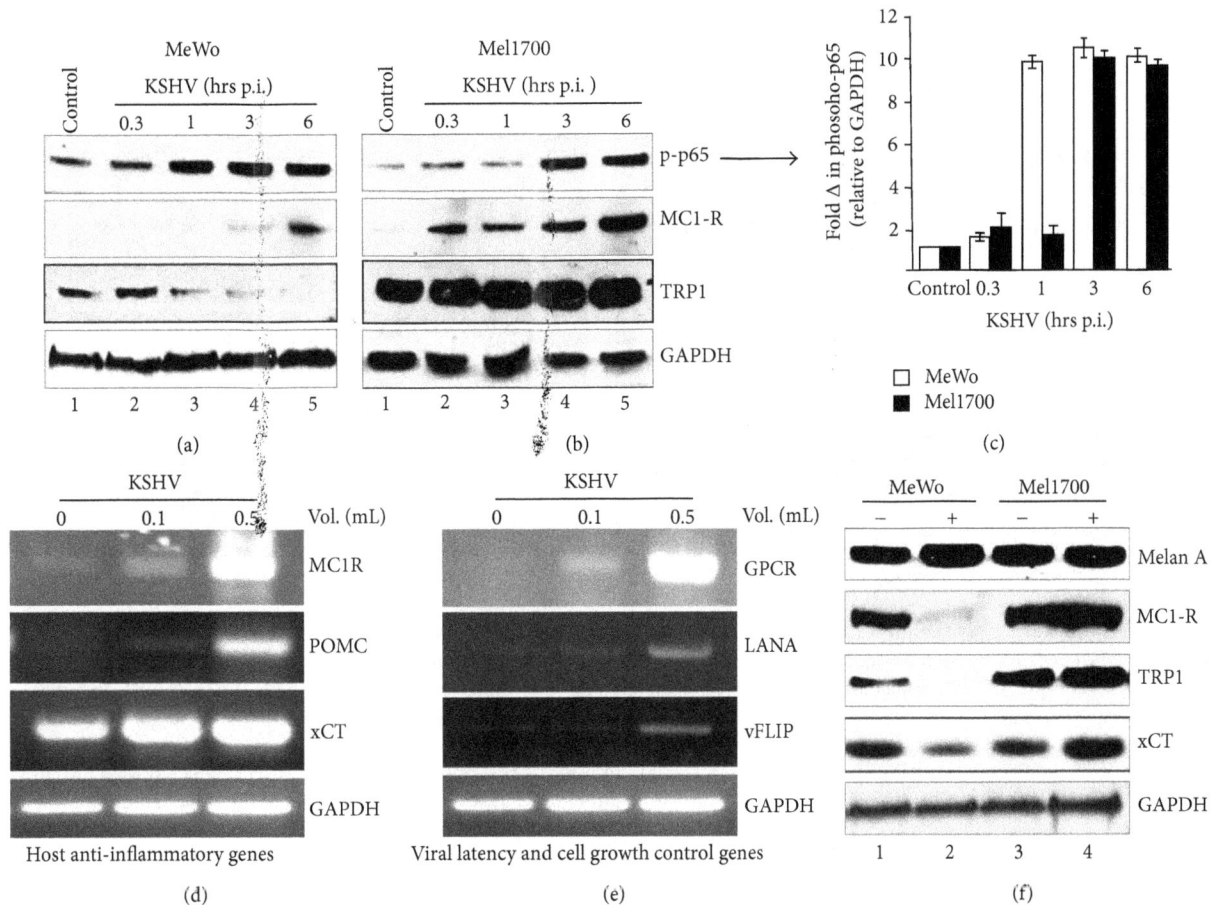

FIGURE 7: A link between KSHV latency and the MC1-R signaling axis in skin-derived cell lines. (a) Western blot analysis of phosphorylated NF-κB p65, MC1-R, and TRP-1 in total cell lysates extracted from MeWo (a) or Mel1700 (b) cells either uninfected (control) or acutely infected with KSHV for 0.3 h, 1 h, 3 h, or 6 h. GAPDH was used as loading control. (c) ImageJ quantitation of the p65 band intensities in (a) and (b) relative to GAPDH controls. (d) Mel1700 cells were infected in 6-well plates with increasing volumes (mL/well) of concentrated supernatant containing infectious KSHV, and total RNA from infected cells was subjected to RT-PCR using primer sets for host anti-inflammatory MC1R, POMC, and SLC7A11. (e) Equal aliquots from the same RNA used in (d) were subjected to RT-PCR analysis for select viral latency and cell growth control genes (i.e., GPCR, LANA, and v-FLIP). (f) Western blot analysis of the melanoma cell marker, Melan A, and anti-inflammatory genes MC1-R, TRP1, and SLC7A11 in total cell lysates of uninfected (−) or chronically infected (+) long-term cultures of MeWo-KSHV and Mel1700-KSHV cells. GAPDH was used as an internal control for both the RT-PCR (e) and western blot assays.

that fail to express the necessary anti-inflammatory mediators in the context of infection, viral latency is the more likely outcome, whereas the rapid increase in expression of MC1-R and other anti-inflammatory molecules in infected Mel1700 cells blocks NF-κB [53, 55–57], which would consequently limit establishment of a latent state and/or result in a greater propensity for Mel1700 cells to support lytic replication.

4. Discussion

In this study, we investigated the infectious process of KSHV in skin-derived cells in order to identify pathogenetic themes that underlie the ability of KSHV to induce cutaneous KS lesions in skin, a highly specialized site whose endogenous anti-inflammatory processes presumably fail to overcome this pathologic outcome. Using primary melanocytes as well as established melanoma-derived cells, we examined key

markers of virus/host interactions that control KSHV tropism and pathogenesis in skin and identified important correlates that link the replicative program of KSHV with the underlying inflammatory status of infected cells. Specifically, we identified two cell lines—MeWo and Mel1700—that consistently displayed differences in (a) susceptibility to productive infection, (b) timing and robustness of virus replication, (c) expression of KSHV latency-associated nuclear antigen, LANA, (d) replication phase-specific expression of viral genes, and (e) susceptibility to virus-induced perturbation of the anti-inflammatory melanogenic response. We found that underlying these differences are cell-type specific markers that operate at the level of KSHV interactions with the host genome, chief among them being differential expression of KSHV LANA.

LANA maintains viral latency in part by tethering episomal viral DNA to host chromosomes and by blocking RTA expression [49]. We found that diffuse nuclear LANA staining

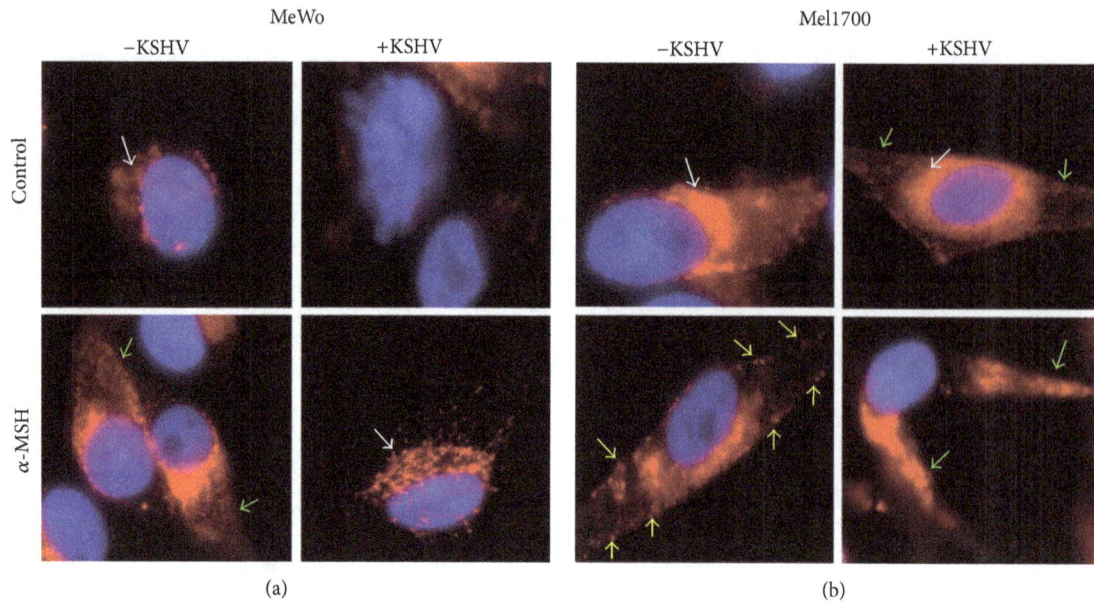

FIGURE 8: KSHV impairment of the melanogenic response is a virologic correlate of latency in skin cells. Uninfected (−) and rKSHV.219-infected (+) MeWo cells (a) or Mel1700-cells (b) were plated on chamber slides without (control) or with α-MSH and allowed to adhere overnight. Cells were then fixed, permeabilized, and stained with anti-TRP-1 antibody and counterstained with DAPI nuclear stain. Shown are representative 63x magnification (oil immersion) images of representative cells from each field of view. White arrows depict ER/Golgi-associated TRP-1 (apparently present in untreated MeWo and in α-MSH-treated MeWo-KSHV cells), whereas green arrows point to outgrowths of promelanogenic dendritic spines induced by α-MSH in MeWos ((a) bottom left) and in KSHV-infected Mel1700, in which they appear to increase even more profoundly upon treatment with α-MSH (b). For wide-view 20x images of the same treatments, please see Figure S11.

was associated with lytic replication, whereas punctate staining marked a state of latency, leading us to hypothesize that diffuse LANA staining reflects the accumulation of "untethered" LANA isoforms that are unable to block RTA. Consistent with this view, NaB induced a switch from punctate to diffuse LANA staining; moreover, RTA expression was higher in spontaneously reactivated Mel1700-KSHV cells in which LANA staining was diffuse, in contrast to MeWo-KSHV cells in which RTA was expressed only after NaB treatment, further supporting our hypothesis.

Although the mechanisms that control nuclear LANA expression at different stages of the virus life cycle are not fully known, it was recently observed that when the N- and C-termini of LANA (that contain nuclear localization signals, NLS) were expressed individually in KSHV-infected cells, the C-terminus (which binds terminal repeats of KSHV DNA) formed discrete nuclear speckles, whereas the N-terminus (which binds host chromosomes) exhibited diffuse nuclear staining [62–64]. However, when full length LANA was expressed by itself in uninfected cells, it exhibited diffuse nuclear staining that became speckled when a bacterial artificial chromosome containing the KSHV terminal-repeat region was introduced [65]. Furthermore, a naturally occurring LANA isoform (with a 76 amino acid truncation at the C-terminal end) was detected in KSHV-infected primary effusion lymphoma (PEL) cell lines, BCP-1 and BC-3, but this isoform was incapable of binding to KSHV episomes and therefore exhibited diffuse nuclear staining [66]. Together,

these findings support the conclusion that diffuse LANA staining reflects the accumulation of LANA isoforms that may still be associated with host chromatin but are not tethered to viral genomes presumably undergoing a state of lytic replication. Surprisingly, we also detected diffuse LANA staining in the cytoplasm of a few reactivated Mel1700-KSHV cells, and although there is currently no published evidence for nucleo-cytoplasmic shuttling of functional LANA in KSHV-infected cells, one study showed that the LANA amino acids 1–323 region, which lacks a NLS, is retained in the cytoplasm [67]. Whether this short form of LANA is generated and shuttled to the cytoplasm in some lytically replicating cells remains to be determined.

Various studies have consistently shown that depending on the cell type and the state of viral reactivation, the LANA-specific LN35 antibody used in this study can detect at least five distinct LANA bands at approximately 220, 180, 160, 130, and 90 kDa, that are potentially generated by alternative initiation [68], truncations [66], or post-translational modifications [69–71]. Because the epitope recognized by LN35 has not yet been mapped, the identity and amino-acid sequence(s) of each of these bands requires systematic proteomic analysis beyond the scope of the current study. Nonetheless, we and others have now shown that appearance of the ~180, 130, and 90 kDa LANA-specific bands correlates with lytic replication [72, 73], which leads us to believe that the ~220 kDa band likely corresponds to full-length LANA, while the ~180 kDa band may be the C-terminally truncated form associated with diffuse LANA staining [66] because it is present only in lytically replicating cells. One prediction from these findings is that the ratio of the 180 kDa band relative to full length LANA regulates the switch from the latent to the lytic phase. Interestingly, Toptan et al. recently described complex LANA isoforms analogous to those that we have detected and proposed that these bands may result from noncanonical translation initiation [68]. While these independent findings reveal an emerging new perspective on the complexity of LANA function(s), they also raise several new questions. (a) What factors trigger non-canonical translation initiation and/or differential processing of LANA into products that may be shuttled to the cytoplasm? (b) Do cells such as Mel1700 that display a higher propensity for supporting lytic replication express host restriction factors that induce the generation of cytoplasmic LANA isoforms that are unable to mediate host chromosomal tethering to the virus genome? (c) What regulatory mechanisms control the accumulation of specific LANA isoforms in relation to full length LANA? Clearly, the pathogenetic implications of these regulatory themes cannot be over-emphasized, but they are not unprecedented among the gammaherpesviruses. For example, during infection with Epstein-Barr virus (EBV), a gammaherpesvirus closely related to KSHV, at least eight different transcripts of the EBV latency-associated nuclear antigen (i.e., EBNA-1, 2, 3A, 3B, 3C, 4, 5, 6), are expressed to control various states of the EBV latency program [74]. Since EBNA is the functional homolog of KSHV LANA, it is conceivable that LANA analogs of the various EBNA isoforms may also be expressed at specific stages of the KSHV life cycle, although further investigation will be required in order to isolate replication phase-specific functions of the protein in a given cellular context.

Our study also revealed a direct link between the NF-κB activation status and virus reactivation, consistent with previous findings that NF-κB activation early following KSHV infection is required for establishment and maintenance of latency [17, 18] and for oncogenic transformation [19, 20]. Interestingly, the KSHV latency program in MeWo cells was accompanied by sustained activation of NF-κB, coincident with reduced expression of key markers of the endogenous anti-inflammatory response. Conversely, in Mel1700 in which the virus readily undergoes spontaneous lytic replication, phosphorylated NF-κB p65 remained low, concomitant with sustained expression of anti-inflammatory proteins, leading us to conclude that KSHV may persist in skin cells both by regulating its replicative program through activation of NF-κB, while also exerting virus-induced subversion of the anti-inflammatory axis. Therefore, it would be reasonable to speculate that in order for KSHV to persist and cause cutaneous disease in skin, it must infect and then either directly or paracrinally overcome the endogenous anti-inflammatory reactions of skin-resident cells in favor of conditions that support development of KS. Indeed, we found that KSHV can indeed infect and induce cytologic reprogramming in melanocytes, the key cellular sensors of inflammatory injury in skin.

Prior to this study, melanocytes were not known to be targets for KSHV infection, which might have led some

to question their relevance during KSHV pathogenesis. However, it can be argued that the anatomical location and function of melanocytes as sentinels of inflammation at the interface of microbial offense and host immunity [58, 75] support the expectation that these cells might regulate KSHV pathogenesis in skin. In response to infections and other pro-inflammatory cues, melanocytes express a wide range of signaling peptides including α-MSH. Upon binding to MC1-R, α-MSH transduces signals that prevent activation of NF-κB and the associated expression of pro-inflammatory cytokines, tumor growth factors, and adhesion molecules that mediate transmigration of inflammatory cells through the vessel wall during angiogenic neovascularization [56, 58]. Given the fundamental role of inflammation in KSHV pathogenesis, and the fact that α-MSH antagonizes NF-κB [56, 58], the ability of KSHV to infect melanocytes may have profound implications for KS development in skin. If impairment of the expression of anti-inflammatory molecules (such as MC1-R, TRP-1, and xCT) represents an important virologic correlate for establishment of KSHV latency in skin cells, it is likely that settings in which sustained inflammation cannot be overcome would support virus-associated disease, whereas approaches that enhance the anti-inflammatory response (e.g., via α-MSH-dependent disruption of NF-κB activation [76]) may disfavor viral persistence in skin and should, therefore, be explored as a potential new option for clinical management of cutaneous KS or other virus-induced dermatologic conditions that may depend on chronic inflammation [77]. Specifically, chronic inflammation in skin may trigger increased vascular permeability, upregulated expression of cell-adhesion molecules on vascular endothelium, and chemokine-mediated recruitment of KSHV-infected cells from the underlying blood vessels to the site of inflammation where seeding of KS might occur (Figure 9), and the fact that monocytes, macrophages, and activated dendritic cells make up a large proportion of the inflammatory infiltrate often present in cutaneous KS lesions [6, 7] supports this model. Additionally, our finding of efficient transmissibility of Mel1700-derived virions to keratinocytes *in vitro* underscores the high probability of a pathophysiologic framework for virus dissemination in and out of skin, which is plausible given the close proximity and dynamic communication networks that naturally exist between melanocytes and keratinocytes in the human epidermal unit [75]. Ironically, such a framework could be exploited by the virus since the anti-inflammatory melanogenic processes of melanocytes that are generally induced as an adaptive response to virus infection could be co-opted for virion transfer. This phenomenon, referred to as "melanosome hijacking", has already been described for varicella-zoster virus, another herpesvirus that displays tropism for human skin [78].

5. Conclusions

Inherently persistent viruses such as KSHV must manipulate infected host cells to support mechanisms that favor either long-term infection within the target organ or inducible

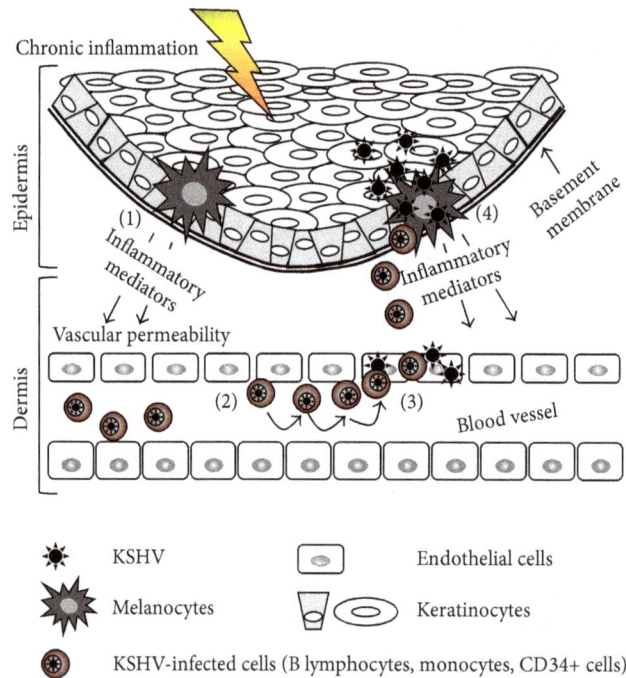

FIGURE 9: Hypothetical model of immunophysiologic mechanisms that control transmission of KSHV from latently infected cellular reservoirs to cells within skin. (1) Chronic activation of NF-κB in the skin induces expression of adhesion molecules on the surfaces of endothelial cells, increased vascular permeability, and secretion of inflammatory cytokines and chemokines by melanocytes and other resident cells of the skin, (2) recruitment of immune cells and other KSHV-infected monocytes to the vascular endothelium, and (3) extravasation of infected cells from the blood vessels into the underlying dermis, where virus may be transmitted to vascular endothelial cells through cell-to-cell contact or other mechanisms. (4) Accumulation of cell-free and KSHV-infected cells at the superficial dermis, where they interact with and infect resident melanocytes and keratinocytes in the basal membrane.

productive lytic replication that promotes viral dissemination to other permissive aspects of the host. Consequently, understanding mechanisms that control the balance between viral latency and lytic replication is an important goal that should guide development of strategies for limiting the pathogenesis of KS and other virus-associated diseases that emerge during the persistent state. Here, we found that the balance between underlying inflammation and lytic replication is a fundamental correlate of KSHV latency and, by extension, KSHV-associated pathology. Although the specific cellular and molecular determinants that control the intrinsic ability of certain cell types to support KSHV latency are not fully defined, our study represents an important first step in our understanding of the nature and biologic impact of KSHV-mediated impairment of the anti-inflammatory function in skin cells, with implications for pathologic outcomes such as cutaneous KS whose progression relies on inflammatory reactivity. Unfortunately, we cannot fully explain why the cell lines used in this study displayed such profound differences in the outcomes of KSHV infection. One clue may be revealed by the fact that unlike Mel1700, MeWo is a highly-pigmented cell line with a high level of underlying inflammation [37], which is consistent with their ability to support a strong latency program. Alternatively (or in addition), it is possible that mechanisms for virus reactivation such as virus-induced apoptosis [79, 80] may be expressed in Mel1700 cells and

not MeWo cells, an interesting concept that should be the focus of follow-on studies beyond the scope of the current study. In addition, isolation and characterization of correlates that control the timing and aggressiveness of KS at a population level may provide predictive power with respect to stratification of individuals at high risk for development of the lesion based on differential exposure to pro-inflammatory cofactors that foment inflammation, including toxins, UV radiation, allergens, trauma, or persistent infections [81]. We note, for example, that in KSHV/HIV coinfected individuals who are generally at a greater risk of developing the most aggressive form of KS, HIV serves as a cofactor for KS not only through establishment of an immunosuppressed environment but also through upregulation of the KSHV receptor, xCT [82], to facilitate KSHV dissemination. Interestingly, HIV replication also requires NF-κB activity [83], while the anti-inflammatory activity of xCT is directly linked to the balance between the NF-κB and α-MSH/MC1-R signaling pathways, which this study has revealed to be important for the KSHV life cycle [84]. Therefore, the ability of KSHV to overcome α-MSH-mediated inhibition of NF-κB activity in MeWos (in which the virus establishes strong latency), would not only promote HIV replication [85] but could also establish conditions that support cutaneous KS development. Future evaluation of these indicators in high-risk individuals with KS compared to those who are KSHV seropositive but never develop KS may provide insight into which cellular dynamics predispose an individual to cutaneous KS and which host responses to infection could be harnessed to help prevent lesional histogenesis.

Acknowledgments

The authors express special thanks to Dr. Jeff Vieira for providing recombinant virus rKSHV.219 and to current and past members of the Kaleeba laboratory for helpful discussions, technical assistance, and critical reading of the paper. Financial support was obtained from the intramural award program of the Uniformed Services University of the Health Sciences. The content of this paper is the sole responsibility of the authors and does not necessarily represent the official views of the University or the Department of Defense.

References

[1] Y. Chang, E. Cesarman, M. S. Pessin et al., "Identification of herpesvirus-like DNA sequences in AIDS-associated Kaposi's sarcoma," *Science*, vol. 266, no. 5192, pp. 1865–1869, 1994.

[2] P. S. Moore, S.-J. Gao, G. Dominguez et al., "Primary characterization of a herpesvirus agent associated with Kaposi's Sarcoma," *Journal of Virology*, vol. 70, no. 1, pp. 549–558, 1996.

[3] D. Bubman and E. Cesarman, "Pathogenesis of Kaposi's sarcoma," *Hematology/Oncology Clinics of North America*, vol. 17, no. 3, pp. 717–745, 2003.

[4] L. A. Dourmishev, A. L. Dourmishev, D. Palmeri, R. A. Schwartz, and D. M. Lukac, "Molecular genetics of Kaposi's sarcoma-associated herpesvirus (human herpesvirus 8) epidemiology and pathogenesis," *Microbiology and Molecular Biology Reviews*, vol. 67, no. 2, pp. 175–212, 2003.

[5] H. W. Haverkos, "Multifactorial etiology of Kaposi's sarcoma: a hypothesis," *Journal of Biosciences*, vol. 33, no. 5, pp. 643–651, 2008.

[6] B. Ensoli, C. Sgadari, G. Barillari, M. C. Sirianni, M. Stürzl, and P. Monini, "Biology of Kaposi's sarcoma," *European Journal of Cancer*, vol. 37, no. 10, pp. 1251–1269, 2001.

[7] B. Ensoli and M. Stürzl, "Kaposi's sarcoma: a result of the interplay among inflammatory cytokines, angiogenic factors and viral agents," *Cytokine and Growth Factor Reviews*, vol. 9, no. 1, pp. 63–83, 1998.

[8] V. Fiorelli, R. Gendelman, M. C. Sirianni et al., "γ-Interferon produced by CD8+ T cells infiltrating Kaposi's sarcoma induces spindle cells with angiogenic phenotype and synergy with human immunodeficiency virus-1 Tat protein: an immune response to human herpesvirus-8 infection?" *Blood*, vol. 91, no. 3, pp. 956–967, 1998.

[9] M. C. Sirianni, L. Vincenzi, V. Fiorelli et al., "γ-Interferon production in peripheral blood mononuclear cells and tumor infiltrating lymphocytes from Kaposi's sarcoma patients: correlation with the presence of human herpesvirus-8 in peripheral blood mononuclear cells and lesional macrophages," *Blood*, vol. 91, no. 3, pp. 968–976, 1998.

[10] G. Barillari, C. Sgadari, V. Fiorelli et al., "The Tat protein of human immunodeficiency virus type-1 promotes vascular cell growth and locomotion by engaging the $\alpha5\beta1$ and $\alpha v\beta3$ integrins and by mobilizing sequestered basic fibroblast growth factor," *Blood*, vol. 94, no. 2, pp. 663–672, 1999.

[11] G. Barillari, C. Sgadari, C. Palladino et al., "Inflammatory cytokines synergize with the HIV-1 Tat protein to promote angiogenesis and Kaposi's sarcoma via induction of basic fibroblast growth factor and the $\alpha(v)\beta3$ integrin," *Journal of Immunology*, vol. 163, no. 4, pp. 1929–1935, 1999.

[12] V. Fiorelli, G. Barillari, E. Toschi et al., "IFN-γ induces endothelial cells to proliferate and to invade the extracellular matrix in response to the HIV-1 Tat protein: implications for AIDS-Kaposi's sarcoma pathogenesis," *Journal of Immunology*, vol. 162, no. 2, pp. 1165–1170, 1999.

[13] V. Fiorelli, R. Gendelman, F. Samaniego, P. D. Markham, and B. Ensoli, "Cytokines from activated T cells induce normal endothelial cells to acquire the phenotypic and functional features of AIDS-Kaposi's sarcoma spindle cells," *Journal of Clinical Investigation*, vol. 95, no. 4, pp. 1723–1734, 1995.

[14] F. Samaniego, P. D. Markham, R. Gendelman et al., "Vascular endothelial growth factor and basic fibroblast growth factor present in Kaposi's sarcoma (KS) are induced by inflammatory cytokines and synergize to promote vascular permeability and KS lesion development," *American Journal of Pathology*, vol. 152, no. 6, pp. 1433–1443, 1998.

[15] M. S. Hayden and S. Ghosh, "Shared Principles in NF-κB Signaling," *Cell*, vol. 132, no. 3, pp. 344–362, 2008.

[16] S. Ghosh and M. S. Hayden, "New regulators of NF-κB in inflammation," *Nature Reviews Immunology*, vol. 8, no. 11, pp. 837–848, 2008.

[17] H. J. Brown, M. J. Song, H. Deng, T.-T. Wu, G. Cheng, and R. Sun, "NF-κB inhibits gammaherpesvirus lytic replication," *Journal of Virology*, vol. 77, no. 15, pp. 8532–8540, 2003.

[18] C. Grossmann and D. Ganem, "Effects of NFκB activation on KSHV latency and lytic reactivation are complex and context-dependent," *Virology*, vol. 375, no. 1, pp. 94–102, 2008.

[19] D. Dadke, B. H. Fryer, E. A. Golemis, and J. Field, "Activation of p21-activated kinase 1-nuclear factor κB signaling by Kaposi's sarcoma-associated herpes virus G protein-coupled receptor during cellular transformation," *Cancer Research*, vol. 63, no. 24, pp. 8837–8847, 2003.

[20] Q. Sun, S. Zachariah, and P. M. Chaudhary, "The human herpes virus 8-encoded viral FLICE-inhibitory protein induces cellular transformation via NF-κB activation," *The Journal of Biological Chemistry*, vol. 278, no. 52, pp. 52437–52445, 2003.

[21] P. M. Chaudhary, A. Jasmin, M. T. Eby, and L. Hood, "Modulation of the NF-κB pathway by virally encoded death effector domains-containing proteins," *Oncogene*, vol. 18, no. 42, pp. 5738–5746, 1999.

[22] S. Pati, M. Cavrois, H.-G. Guo et al., "Activation of NF-κB by the human herpesvirus 8 chemokine receptor ORF74: evidence for a paracrine model of Kaposi's sarcoma pathogenesis," *Journal of Virology*, vol. 75, no. 18, pp. 8660–8673, 2001.

[23] M. Schwarz and P. M. Murphy, "Kaposi's sarcoma-associated herpesvirus G protein-coupled receptor constitutively activates NF-κB and induces proinflammatory cytokine and chemokine production via a C-terminal signaling determinant," *Journal of Immunology*, vol. 167, no. 1, pp. 505–513, 2001.

[24] F. Samaniego, S. Pati, J. E. Karp, O. Prakash, and D. Bose, "Human herpesvirus 8 K1-associated nuclear factor-kappa B-dependent promoter activity: role in Kaposi's sarcoma inflammation?" *Journal of the National Cancer Institute Monographs*, no. 28, pp. 15–23, 2001.

[25] A. Konrad, E. Wies, M. Thurau et al., "A systems biology approach to identify the combination effects of human herpesvirus 8 genes on NF-κB activation," *Journal of Virology*, vol. 83, no. 6, pp. 2563–2574, 2009.

[26] M. M. Brinkmann, M. Glenn, L. Rainbow, A. Kieser, C. Henke-Gendo, and T. F. Schulz, "Activation of mitogen-activated protein kinase and NF-κB pathways by a Kaposi's sarcoma-associated herpesvirus K15 membrane protein," *Journal of Virology*, vol. 77, no. 17, pp. 9346–9358, 2003.

[27] E. Gottwein, "Kaposi's sarcoma-associated herpesvirus microRNAs," *Frontiers in Microbiology*, vol. 3, article 165, 2012.

[28] J. M. Ziegelbauer, "Functions of Kaposi's sarcoma-associated herpesvirus microRNAs," *Biochimica et Biophysica Acta*, vol. 1809, no. 11-12, pp. 623–630, 2011.

[29] Z. Qin, P. Kearney, K. Plaisance, and C. H. Parsons, "Pivotal Advance: Kaposi's sarcoma-associated herpesvirus (KSHV)-encoded microRNA specifically induce IL-6 and IL-10 secretion by macrophages and monocytes," *Journal of Leukocyte Biology*, vol. 87, no. 1, pp. 25–34, 2010.

[30] D. M. Lukac, J. R. Kirshner, and D. Ganem, "Transcriptional activation by the product of open reading frame 50 of Kaposi's sarcoma-associated herpesvirus is required for lytic viral reactivation in B cells," *Journal of Virology*, vol. 73, no. 11, pp. 9348–9361, 1999.

[31] R. Sun, S.-F. Lin, L. Gradoville, Y. Yuan, F. Zhu, and G. Miller, "A viral gene that activates lytic cycle expression of Kaposi's sarcoma-associated herpesvirus," *Proceedings of the National Academy of Sciences of the United States of America*, vol. 95, no. 18, pp. 10866–10871, 1998.

[32] Y. Liang and D. Ganem, "RBP-J (CSL) is essential for activation of the K14/vGPCR promoter of Kaposi's sarcoma-associated herpesvirus by the lytic switch protein RTA," *Journal of Virology*, vol. 78, no. 13, pp. 6818–6826, 2004.

[33] Y. Liang and D. Ganem, "Lytic but not latent infection by Kaposi's sarcoma-associated herpesvirus requires host CSL protein, the mediator of Notch signaling," *Proceedings of the National Academy of Sciences of the United States of America*, vol. 100, no. 14, pp. 8490–8495, 2003.

[34] Y. Liang, J. Chang, S. J. Lynch, D. M. Lukac, and D. Ganem, "The lytic switch protein of KSHV activates gene expression via functional interaction with RBP-Jκ (CSL), the target of the Notch signaling pathway," *Genes and Development*, vol. 16, no. 15, pp. 1977–1989, 2002.

[35] Y. Izumiya, C. Izumiya, D. Hsia, T. J. Ellison, P. A. Luciw, and H.-J. Kung, "NF-κB serves as a cellular sensor of Kaposi's sarcoma-associated herpesvirus latency and negatively regulates K-Rta by antagonizing the RBP-Jκ coactivator," *Journal of Virology*, vol. 83, no. 9, pp. 4435–4446, 2009.

[36] J. Vieira and P. M. O'Hearn, "Use of the red fluorescent protein as a marker of Kaposi's sarcoma-associated herpesvirus lytic gene expression," *Virology*, vol. 325, no. 2, pp. 225–240, 2004.

[37] J. Fogh, J. M. Fogh, and T. Orfeo, "One hundred and twenty seven cultured human tumor cell lines producing tumors in nude mice," *Journal of the National Cancer Institute*, vol. 59, no. 1, pp. 221–226, 1977.

[38] P. Boukamp, R. T. Petrussevska, D. Breitkreutz, J. Hornung, A. Markham, and N. E. Fusenig, "Normal keratinization in a spontaneously immortalized aneuploid human keratinocyte cell line," *Journal of Cell Biology*, vol. 106, no. 3, pp. 761–771, 1988.

[39] J. A. R. Kaleeba and E. A. Berger, "Kaposi's sarcoma-associated herpesvirus fusion-entry receptor: cystine transporter xCT," *Science*, vol. 311, no. 5769, pp. 1921–1924, 2006.

[40] J. A. R. Kaleeba and E. A. Berger, "Broad target cell selectivity of Kaposi's sarcoma-associated herpesvirus glycoprotein-mediated cell fusion and virion entry," *Virology*, vol. 354, no. 1, pp. 7–14, 2006.

[41] K. Takeda, N.-H. Takahashi, and S. Shibahara, "Neuroendocrine functions of melanocytes: beyond the skin-deep melanin maker," *Tohoku Journal of Experimental Medicine*, vol. 211, no. 3, pp. 201–221, 2007.

[42] A. Slominski, J. Wortsman, L. Kohn et al., "Expression of hypothalamic-pituitary-thyroid axis related genes in the human skin," *Journal of Investigative Dermatology*, vol. 119, no. 6, pp. 1449–1455, 2002.

[43] M. Alegre, L. Puig, R. Carreño et al., "Primary neuroendocrine carcinoma of the skin expresses tyrosinase mRNA: detection by a specific nested PCR technique," *Dermatology*, vol. 194, no. 4, pp. 334–337, 1997.

[44] J. R. Davie, "Inhibition of histone deacetylase activity by butyrate," *Journal of Nutrition*, vol. 133, no. 7, pp. 2485S–2493S, 2003.

[45] V. Lacoste, J. G. Judde, G. Bestetti et al., "Virological and molecular characterisation of a new B lymphoid cell line, established from an AIDS patient with primary effusion lymphoma, harbouring both KSHV/HHV8 and EBV viruses," *Leukemia and Lymphoma*, vol. 38, no. 3-4, pp. 401–409, 2000.

[46] R. G. Nador, L. L. Milligan, O. Flore et al., "Expression of Kaposi's sarcoma-associated herpesvirus G protein-coupled receptor monocistronic and bicistronic transcripts in primary effusion lymphomas," *Virology*, vol. 287, no. 1, pp. 62–70, 2001.

[47] R. Sarid, O. Flore, R. A. Bohenzky, Y. Chang, and P. S. Moore, "Transcription mapping of the Kaposi's sarcoma-associated herpesvirus (human herpesvirus 8) genome in a body cavity-based lymphoma cell line (BC- 1)," *Journal of Virology*, vol. 72, no. 2, pp. 1005–1012, 1998.

[48] F. X. Zhu, T. Cusano, and Y. Yuan, "Identification of the immediate-early transcripts of Kaposi's sarcoma- associated herpesvirus," *Journal of Virology*, vol. 73, no. 7, pp. 5556–5567, 1999.

[49] S. C. Verma, K. Lan, and E. Robertson, "Structure and function of latency-associated nuclear antigen," *Current Topics in Microbiology and Immunology*, vol. 312, pp. 101–136, 2007.

[50] S. A. Keller, E. J. Schattner, and E. Cesarman, "Inhibition of NF-κB induces apoptosis of KSHV-infected primary effusion lymphoma cells," *Blood*, vol. 96, no. 7, pp. 2537–2542, 2000.

[51] S. Sadagopan, N. Sharma-Walia, M. V. Veettil et al., "Kaposi's sarcoma-associated herpesvirus induces sustained NF-κB activation during de novo infection of primary human dermal microvascular endothelial cells that is essential for viral gene expression," *Journal of Virology*, vol. 81, no. 8, pp. 3949–3968, 2007.

[52] K. A. Collins and W. L. White, "Intercellular adhesion molecule 1 (ICAM-1) and bcl-2 are differentially expressed in early evolving malignant melanoma," *American Journal of Dermatopathology*, vol. 17, no. 5, pp. 429–438, 1995.

[53] A. Catania and J. M. Lipton, "α-Melanocyte stimulating hormone in the modulation of host reactions," *Endocrine Reviews*, vol. 14, no. 5, pp. 564–576, 1993.

[54] T. A. Luger, T. Brzoska, T. E. Scholzen et al., "The role of α-MSH as a modulator of cutaneous inflammation," *Annals of the New York Academy of Sciences*, vol. 917, pp. 232–238, 2000.

[55] J. M. Lipton and A. Catania, "Anti-inflammatory actions of the neuroimmunomodulator α-MSH," *Immunology Today*, vol. 18, no. 3, pp. 140–145, 1997.

[56] J. W. Haycock, M. Wagner, R. Morandini, G. Ghanem, I. G. Rennie, and S. Mac Neil, "α-Melanocyte-stimulating hormone inhibits NF-κB activation in human melanocytes and melanoma cells," *Journal of Investigative Dermatology*, vol. 113, no. 4, pp. 560–566, 1999.

[57] J. W. Haycock, M. Wagner, R. Morandini, G. Ghanem, I. G. Rennie, and S. Macneil, "α-MSH immunomodulation acts via Rel/NF-κB in cutaneous and ocular melanocytes and in melanoma cells," *Annals of the New York Academy of Sciences*, vol. 885, pp. 396–399, 1999.

[58] G.-E. Costin and V. J. Hearing, "Human skin pigmentation: melanocytes modulate skin color in response to stress," *The FASEB Journal*, vol. 21, no. 4, pp. 976–994, 2007.

[59] G. Hunt, C. Todd, J. E. Cresswell, and A. J. Thody, "α-Melanocyte stimulating hormone and its analogue Nle4DPhe7α-MSH affect morphology, tyrosinase activity and melanogenesis in cultured human melanocytes," *Journal of Cell Science*, vol. 107, part 1, pp. 205–211, 1994.

[60] M. Conrad and H. Sato, "The oxidative stress-inducible cystine/glutamate antiporter, system x (c) (-) : cystine supplier and beyond," *Amino acids*, vol. 42, no. 1, pp. 231–246, 2012.

[61] Z. Qin, E. Freitas, R. Sullivan et al., "Upregulation of xCT by KSHV-encoded microRNAs facilitates KSHV dissemination and persistence in an environment of oxidative stress," *PLoS Pathogens*, vol. 6, no. 1, Article ID e1000742, 2010.

[62] J. Friborg Jr., W.-P. Kong, M. O. Hottiger, and G. J. Nabel, "p53 Inhibition by the LANA protein of KSHV protects against cell death," *Nature*, vol. 402, no. 6764, pp. 889–894, 1999.

[63] M. Glenn, L. Rainbow, F. Auradé, A. Davison, and T. F. Schulz, "Identification of a spliced gene from Kaposi's sarcoma-associated herpesvirus encoding a protein with similarities to latent membrane proteins 1 and 2A of Epstein-Barr virus," *Journal of Virology*, vol. 73, no. 8, pp. 6953–6963, 1999.

[64] M. Schalling, M. Ekman, E. E. Kaaya, A. Linde, and P. Biberfeld, "A role for a new herpes virus (KSHV) in different forms of Kaposi's sarcoma," *Nature Medicine*, vol. 1, no. 7, pp. 707–708, 1995.

[65] S. Sakakibara, K. Ueda, K. Nishimura et al., "Accumulation of heterochromatin components on the terminal repeat sequence of Kaposi's sarcoma-associated herpesvirus mediated by the latency-associated nuclear antigen," *Journal of Virology*, vol. 78, no. 14, pp. 7299–7310, 2004.

[66] M. Canham and S. J. Talbot, "A naturally occurring C-terminal truncated isoform of the latent nuclear antigen of Kaposi's sarcoma-associated herpesvirus does not associate with viral episomal DNA," *Journal of General Virology*, vol. 85, no. 6, pp. 1363–1369, 2004.

[67] C. Lim, H. Sohn, Y. Gwack, and J. Choe, "Latency-associated nuclear antigen of Kaposi's sarcoma-associated herpesvirus (human herpesvirus-8) binds ATF4/CREB2 and inhibits its transcriptional activation activity," *Journal of General Virology*, vol. 81, no. 11, pp. 2645–2652, 2000.

[68] T. Toptan, L. Fonseca, H. J. Kwun, Y. Chang, and P. S. Moore, "Complex alternative cytoplasmic protein isoforms of the Kaposi's sarcoma-associated herpesvirus latency-associated

nuclear antigen 1 generated through noncanonical translation initiation," *Journal of Virology*, vol. 87, pp. 2744–2755, 2013.

[69] B. G. Bajaj, S. C. Verma, K. Lan, M. A. Cotter, Z. L. Woodman, and E. S. Robertson, "KSHV encoded LANA upregulates Pim-1 and is a substrate for its kinase activity," *Virology*, vol. 351, no. 1, pp. 18–28, 2006.

[70] F. Lu, L. Day, S.-J. Gao, and P. M. Lieberman, "Acetylation of the latency-associated nuclear antigen regulates repression of Kaposi's sarcoma-associated herpesvirus lytic transcription," *Journal of Virology*, vol. 80, no. 11, pp. 5273–5282, 2006.

[71] G. M. Platt, G. R. Simpson, S. Mittnacht, and T. F. Schulz, "Latent nuclear antigen of Kaposi's sarcoma-associated herpesvirus interacts with RING3, a homolog of the Drosophila female sterile homeotic (fsh) gene," *Journal of Virology*, vol. 73, no. 12, pp. 9789–9795, 1999.

[72] S.-J. Gao, L. Kingsley, D. R. Hoover et al., "Seroconversion to antibodies against Kaposi's sarcoma-associated herpesvirus-related latent nuclear antigens before the development of Kaposi's sarcoma," *The New England Journal of Medicine*, vol. 335, no. 4, pp. 233–241, 1996.

[73] J. K. Hyun, S. R. Da Silva, I. M. Shah, N. Blake, P. S. Moore, and Y. Chang, "Kaposi's sarcoma-associated herpesvirus latency-associated nuclear antigen 1 mimics Epstein-Barr virus EBNA1 immune evasion through central repeat domain effects on protein processing," *Journal of Virology*, vol. 81, no. 15, pp. 8225–8235, 2007.

[74] G. Klein, E. Klein, and E. Kashuba, "Interaction of Epstein-Barr virus (EBV) with human B-lymphocytes," *Biochemical and Biophysical Research Communications*, vol. 396, no. 1, pp. 67–73, 2010.

[75] J. J. Nordlund, "The melanocyte and the epidermal melanin unit: an expanded concept," *Dermatologic Clinics*, vol. 25, no. 3, pp. 271–281, 2007.

[76] A. Catania, S. Gatti, G. Colombo, and J. M. Lipton, "Targeting melanocortin receptors as a novel strategy to control inflammation," *Pharmacological Reviews*, vol. 56, no. 1, pp. 1–29, 2004.

[77] A. J. Friedman, J. Phan, D. O. Schairer et al., "Antimicrobial and anti-inflammatory activity of chitosan-alginate nanoparticles: a targeted therapy for cutaneous pathogens," *Journal of Investigative Dermatology*, vol. 133, pp. 1231–1239, 2013.

[78] R. Harson and C. Grose, "Egress of varicella-zoster virus from the melanoma cell: a tropism for the melanocyte," *Journal of Virology*, vol. 69, no. 8, pp. 4994–5010, 1995.

[79] A. Prasad, J. Remick, and S. L. Zeichner, "Activation of human herpesvirus replication by apoptosis," *Journal of Virology*, vol. 87, no. 19, pp. 10641–10650, 2013.

[80] A. Prasad, M. Lu, D. M. Lukac, and S. L. Zeichner, "An alternative Kaposi's sarcoma-associated herpesvirus replication program triggered by host cell apoptosis," *Journal of Virology*, vol. 86, pp. 4404–4419, 2012.

[81] L. S. Marks, A. W. Partin, J. I. Epstein et al., "Effects of a saw palmetto herbal blend in men with symptomatic benign prostatic hyperplasia," *Journal of Urology*, vol. 163, no. 5, pp. 1451–1456, 2000.

[82] C. C. Bridges, H. Hu, S. Miyauchi et al., "Induction of cystine-glutamate transporter Xc- by human immunodeficiency virus type 1 transactivator protein Tat in retinal pigment epithelium," *Investigative Ophthalmology and Visual Science*, vol. 45, no. 9, pp. 2906–2914, 2004.

[83] W. Barcellini, G. Colombo, L. La Maestra et al., "α-Melanocyte-stimulating hormone peptides inhibit HIV-1 expression in

chronically infected promonocytic U1 cells and in acutely infected monocytes," *Journal of Leukocyte Biology*, vol. 68, no. 5, pp. 693–699, 2000.

[84] S. Chintala, W. Li, M. L. Lamoreux et al., "Slc7a11 gene controls production of pheomelanin pigment and proliferation of cultured cells," *Proceedings of the National Academy of Sciences of the United States of America*, vol. 102, no. 31, pp. 10964–10969, 2005.

[85] A. Catania, L. Airaghi, L. Garofalo, M. Cutuli, and J. M. Lipton, "The neuropeptide α-MSH in HIV infection and other disorders in humans," *Annals of the New York Academy of Sciences*, vol. 840, pp. 848–856, 1998.

4

Extended UVB Exposures Alter Tumorigenesis and Treatment Efficacy in a Murine Model of Cutaneous Squamous Cell Carcinoma

Erin M. Burns,[1] Kathleen L. Tober,[1] Judith A. Riggenbach,[1] Donna F. Kusewitt,[2] Gregory S. Young,[3] and Tatiana M. Oberyszyn[1]

[1] Department of Pathology, The Ohio State University, 1645 Neil Avenue, 129 Hamilton Hall, Columbus, OH 43210, USA
[2] Department of Molecular Carcinogenesis, Science Park, UT MD Anderson Cancer Center, 1808 Park Road 1C, Smithville, TX 78957, USA
[3] Center for Biostatistics, The Ohio State University, 2012 Kenny Road, Columbus, OH 43221, USA

Correspondence should be addressed to Tatiana M. Oberyszyn; oberyszyn.1@osu.edu

Academic Editor: Mark Lebwohl

Epidemiological studies support a link between cumulative sun exposure and cutaneous squamous cell carcinoma (SCC) development. However, the presumed effects of extended ultraviolet light B (UVB) exposure on tumorigenesis in the sexes have not been formally investigated. We examined differences in ultimate tumorigenesis at 25 weeks in mice exposed to UVB for either 10 or 25 weeks. Additionally, we investigated the effect of continued UVB exposure on the efficacy of topical treatment with anti-inflammatory (diclofenac) or antioxidant (C E Ferulic or vitamin E) compounds on modulating tumorigenesis. Vehicle-treated mice in the 25-week UVB exposure model exhibited an increased tumor burden and a higher percentage of malignant tumors compared to mice in the 10-week exposure model, which correlated with increases in total and mutant p53-positive epidermal cells. Only topical diclofenac decreased tumor number and burden in both sexes regardless of UVB exposure length. These data support the commonly assumed but not previously demonstrated fact that increased cumulative UVB exposure increases the risk of UVB-induced SCC development and can also affect therapeutic efficacies. Our study suggests that cessation of UVB exposure by at-risk patients may decrease tumor development and that topical NSAIDs such as diclofenac may be chemopreventive.

1. Introduction

Epidemiological studies where patients self-report the amount of sun they have been exposed to over their lifetime have been the main source of the described link between cumulative, lifetime sunlight exposure and the development of cutaneous squamous cell carcinoma. While informative, with patients historically developing these lesions in their seventies, these self-reports may not accurately reflect the actual lifetime exposure history. Interestingly, we could not find any controlled studies reporting the effects of the length of lifetime UVB exposure on the extent of tumor development.

Skin carcinogenesis experiments utilizing animal models, especially hairless mice, have contributed greatly to understanding how skin tumorigenesis depends on the wavelength of UV radiation, dose, and time [1]. The Skh-1 hairless mouse model has proven to be an appropriate and accepted model for experimental skin carcinogenesis [2]. Because the Skh-1 mice are hairless, tumors can be easily observed and their progression was tracked over time with relatively no discomfort for the mice. Importantly, after chronic UV exposure, shaved, haired mice can develop fibrosarcomas originating from the dermis [3], whereas the induction of tumors in hairless mice via chronic exposure of non-burn-inducing low UVB levels leads almost exclusively to epidermal squamous cell carcinoma and precursor development [4], which correlates to what is observed in UV-induced skin cancer in humans.

Skin tumors induced by chronic exposure to UV radiation progress from focal epithelial hyperplasia to papillomas and finally squamous cell and spindle cell carcinomas [4]. Previous studies in our laboratory using female mice have demonstrated that papilloma growth begins following 10–12 weeks of three times weekly UVB exposures. Approximately 90% of both male and female mice develop at least one tumor with a diameter greater than 1 mm after 16 weeks of three times weekly UVB exposures, with males having approximately 50% more tumors than females [5]. Squamous cell carcinoma development has been observed following 25–30 weeks of three times weekly UVB exposures [6], with males having more malignant tumors compared to females [5]. However, the effect of increased cumulative UVB exposure on tumorigenesis, while it presumed to increase in both sexes, has not been formally investigated.

Previous murine studies have demonstrated that decreasing the daily UVB exposure dose results in the delay of tumor onset, indicating that patients at risk for developing cutaneous SCC may benefit from decreasing further UV exposure in order to inhibit or delay the development of tumors [7, 8]. Further, patients self-reporting high lifetime UV exposure had increased tumor multiplicity and severity compared to those self-reporting low lifetime UV exposure [9]. While these studies suggest that cumulative lifetime UV exposure may be correlated with the extent of cutaneous tumor development, no study to date has clearly demonstrated this relationship. Thus, we were interested in using the Skh-1 hairless mouse to model men and women who were exposed to UVB during childhood and early adolescence but made efforts to stay out of the sun in adulthood (10-week UVB exposure model) compared to individuals who continue sun worshiping habits throughout adult life (25-week UVB exposure model). Our goal was to determine if limiting the length of chronic UVB exposure (10 weeks versus 25 weeks) would affect the number of tumors that ultimately developed at 25 weeks.

Previously, we demonstrated that the topical anti-inflammatory drug, diclofenac, applied preventatively to chronically UVB-damaged skin of male and female mice, prior to the appearance of lesions, with no further UVB exposure, significantly decreased tumor number and burden compared to vehicle-treated, UVB-exposed mice [10]. We also previously demonstrated in female mice that while the combination antioxidant, C E Ferulic, exerted potential benefits in terms of decreased tumor number and burden, topical vitamin E treatment increased overall DNA damage, cutaneous proliferation and angiogenesis, and tumor growth rate, number, and burden [11]. In the current study, we compared the efficacy of anti-inflammatory (diclofenac) and antioxidant (C E Ferulic (CE) or vitamin E) treatments in male and female mice between the 10-week and 25-week UVB exposure models.

Our results demonstrate that both male and female mice in the 25-week UVB exposure model developed more tumors, larger tumors, and a higher percentage of malignant tumors compared to mice in the 10-week UVB exposure model. Further, in the 25-week UVB exposure model only topical diclofenac treatments effectively decreased both the tumor number and total tumor area in male and female mice. These data demonstrate the commonly assumed fact that longer periods of UVB exposure increase the risk of UVB-induced SCC development in both sexes and suggest that eliminating sun exposure later in life, even after significant prior exposure, may ultimately decrease tumor development in patients. Furthermore, while treatment with topical diclofenac during continued UVB exposure was an effective chemopreventive agent, continued UVB exposure can negatively affect other therapeutic intervention strategies.

2. Materials and Methods

2.1. Animal Treatments and Experimental Design. Outbred, male and female Skh-1 mice (6–8 weeks old, Charles River Laboratories, Wilmington, MA) were housed in the vivarium at The Ohio State University according to the requirements established by the American Association for Accreditation of Laboratory Animal Care. All procedures were approved by the Institutional Animal Care and Use Committee before the initiation of any studies. Mice were dorsally exposed to 2240 J/m^2 UVB, previously determined to be 1 MED, 3× weekly on nonconsecutive days for 10 (10-week UVB exposure model) or 25 (25-week UVB exposure model) weeks. UVB dose was calculated using a UVX radiometer and UVB sensor (UVP, Upland, CA) and delivered using Philips TL 40W/12 RS SLV UVB broadband bulbs emitting 290–315 nm UVB light (American Ultraviolet Company, Lebanon, IN). Following 10 weeks of UVB exposure, mice in the 10-week UVB exposure model were treated topically with vehicle (Surgilube inert surgical lubricant; Savage Laboratories, Melville, NY, $n = 20$ of each sex), 500 μg diclofenac (Solaraze, $n = 10$ of each sex) in vehicle, 5 mg vitamin E (d-alpha tocopherol; Sigma-Aldrich, St. Louis, MO, $n = 10$ of each sex) in vehicle, or 0.1 mL C E Ferulic (SkinCeuticals, $n = 10$ of each sex) for 15 weeks with no additional UVB exposure. After 10 weeks of UVB exposure, mice in the 25-week UVB exposure model were treated topically with the aforementioned agents immediately following each UVB exposure for the remaining 15 weeks of the study. Tumors larger than 2 mm in diameter were counted and measured in two directions with calipers each week. Average tumor number per mouse, per treatment group was calculated for tumors larger than 2 mm in diameter. Tumor burden was calculated based on the average total tumor area per mouse, per treatment group. Mice in both the 10- and 25-week exposure models were sacrificed 25 weeks following the initial UV exposure. After sacrifice, 0.5 cm^2 section of dorsal skin and all tumors were fixed in 10% neutral buffered formalin for 2 (skin) or 4 hours (tumors) while remaining dorsal skin was snap frozen in liquid nitrogen.

2.2. Tumor Grading. Hematoxylin and eosin-stained tissue sections of tumors isolated from mice were graded in a blinded manner by a board-certified veterinary pathologist (DFK) as previously described [5]. Briefly, papillomas were exophytic tumors (tumors that grow outward from the originating epithelium) that showed no invasion of the stroma. Microinvasive squamous cell carcinomas were distinguished by the depth of penetration into the dermis. Fully invasive squamous cell carcinomas were tumors that invaded the panniculus carnosus. Papillomas were considered benign while microinvasive and fully invasive squamous cell carcinomas were considered malignant. Average malignant tumor

TABLE 1: Average percentage of malignant tumors per treatment group after 10 and 25 weeks of UVB exposure in male and female mice.

		10-week UVB	25-week UVB	P value (25 weeks Tx versus Veh)	P value (10 weeks versus 25 weeks)
Male	UVB/vehicle	19.3	37.7	—	0.0467*
	UVB/diclofenac	5.9	57.9	0.1016	0.0262*
	UVB/CE	31.2	45.6	0.3391	0.0087*
	UVB/vitamin E	8.2	34.1	0.6251	0.0028*
Female	UVB/vehicle	10.3	31.7	—	0.0319*
	UVB/diclofenac	25.0	61.3	0.0227*	0.1565
	UVB/CE	0.0	31.4	0.7544	0.0196*
	UVB/vitamin E	2.9	40.5	0.2816	0.0087*

*: The comparison of the percentage of malignant tumors in male mice treated with vehicle in the 25 weeks compared to the 10 weeks of UVB exposure model. For clarity, all of the P values in the final column of Table 1 refer to 25 versus 10 weeks of tumor malignancy within a treatment group and gender.

percentages were calculated using the total number of graded tumors per treatment group.

2.3. Immunohistochemistry

p53. Skin sections were examined for epidermal p53 via immunohistochemistry as previously described [10, 11].

Mutant p53. After rehydration, slides were incubated in 3% H_2O_2 in water for 10 minutes at room temperature to block endogenous peroxidase activity. Slides were subjected to antigen retrieval in a microwave, after which they were blocked with avidin D and biotin (Vector Laboratories), each for 15 minutes, 1× Casein for 30 minutes, and incubated with primary mutant p53 antibody (Novus Biologicals) at a 1:3000 dilution in 1× Casein at 4°C overnight. Slides were then incubated with biotinylated F (ab)' (Accurate Chem) at a 1:250 dilution in 1× Casein, followed by ABC Elite. Slides were incubated in DAB solution (Vector Laboratories) for 10 minutes at RT. Positively stained area in the epidermis was examined at 10x and 20x magnification using ImageJ software (NIH).

2.4. Statistical Analysis.

The results presented in this paper were part of two separate experiments, starting approximately 1 year apart, each involving four treatment groups and a single control group. Considering the results for the 25-week UVB exposure model only, Dunnett's adjustment [12, 13] for multiplicity was used for comparing the primary outcome of tumor burden at 24 weeks between the groups in order to control the probability of a type I error at 5%. The number of control mice was inflated compared to the treatment groups to increase the power of the comparison [12]. Residual plots verified the model assumptions of normality and homoscedasticity and a logarithmic transformation was utilized if necessary. Continuous outcome data were analyzed using an ANOVA approach with linear contrasts for testing the comparisons of interest. For count data, the Poisson regression was used. All analyses were conducted in SAS version 9.2 (SAS Institute, Cary, NC). P values ≤ 0.05 were considered statistically significant. No adjustments were made for multiple comparisons between the studies. The major limitations of

comparisons between the two studies are that mice were not randomized to the two exposure protocols and the studies were run at different times. Thus, the exposure effect is aliased with any batch effect of the mice selected for the particular study. However, as Skh-1 mice were used for both studies, we believe any batch effect to be minimal.

3. Results

3.1. Effects of UVB Exposure Regime Length on Tumorigenesis, Malignancy, and p53 Status in Male and Female Mice.

To examine the effects of increased UVB protocol length on tumor development, we exposed Skh-1 hairless mice to 2240 J/m² UVB three times weekly for 10 (10-week UVB exposure model) or 25 (25-week UVB exposure model) weeks to model chronic sun exposure. Nonirradiated mice did not develop tumors with any topical treatments. Male mice treated with vehicle in the 25-week UVB exposure model developed a 2.7-fold increase in tumor number (P < 0.0001, Figure 1(a)) and a 4.2-fold higher tumor burden (P = 0.0006, Figure 1(b)) compared to vehicle-treated mice in the 10-week UVB exposure model. Female mice in the 25-week model treated with vehicle displayed a 6.75-fold increase in tumor number (P < 0.0001, Figure 1(a)) and a 15.3-fold increase in tumor burden (P < 0.0001, Figure 1(b)) compared to vehicle-treated mice in the 10-week UVB exposure model.

Tumors were isolated from mice at the end of 25 weeks from both the 10-week and 25-week UVB exposure models, formalin fixed, paraffin embedded, H&E stained, and scored by a board-certified veterinary pathologist (DFK). Male and female mice treated topically with vehicle in the 25-week model developed more malignant tumors per mouse compared to vehicle-treated mice in the 10-week model, with males developing 1.9-fold more malignant tumors and females developing 3.05-fold more tumors (19.3% versus 37.7%, P = 0.0467 and 10.3% versus 31.7%, P = 0.0319, resp., Table 1).

As a measure of overall DNA damage, tumor-free, dorsal skin sections were examined for epidermal p53-positive cells via immunohistochemical analysis. Male mice in the 25-week UVB exposure model treated with vehicle exhibited a 3.74-fold increase in p53-positive compared to vehicle-treated

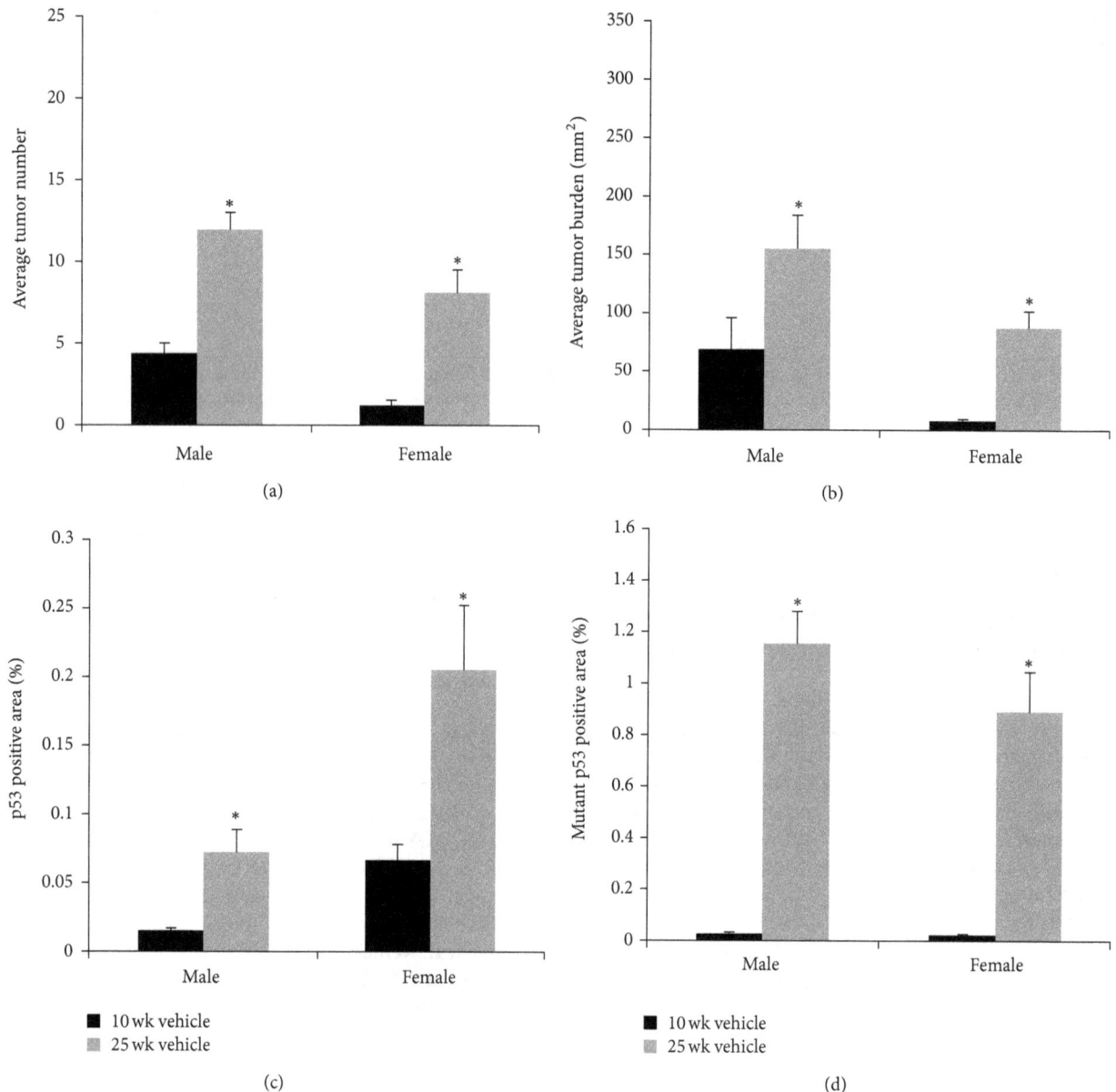

FIGURE 1: *Effect of length of UVB treatments on tumor number, tumor burden, and p53 status in male and female mice.* (a) Vehicle-treated male and female mice developed more tumors in the 25-week exposure model ($^*P < 0.0001$) compared to the 10-week model. (b) Male ($^*P = 0.0006$) and female ($^*P < 0.0001$) vehicle-treated mice in the 25-week exposure model exhibited increased tumor burden compared to the 10-week model. (c) Male ($^*P = 0.0002$) and female ($^*P = 0.011$) mice treated with vehicle in the 25-week model exhibited elevated epidermal p53 staining compared to the 10-week exposure model. (d) Male and female mice treated with vehicle in the 25-week exposure model exhibited elevated epidermal mutant p53 staining ($^*P < 0.0001$) compared to the 10-week UVB model. Error bars = mean+/−SEM.

mice in the 10-week UVB exposure model ($P = 0.0002$, Figure 1(c)), while females in the 25-week UVB exposure model exhibited a 2.52-fold increase compared to female mice in the 10-week UVB exposure model ($P = 0.011$, Figure 1(c)).

To further investigate DNA damage, tumor-free, dorsal skin sections were examined for epidermal mutant p53-positive cells via immunohistochemistry. Both male and female mice in the 25-week UVB exposure model treated with vehicle displayed 45.25- and 33.94-fold increased levels of mutant p53-positive cells, respectively, compared to mice in the 10-week UVB exposure model ($P < 0.0001$, Figure 1(d)).

3.2. Efficacy of Diclofenac on Tumor Number, Burden, and p53 Status in Male and Female Mice. To determine the effect of topical application of the anti-inflammatory drug diclofenac on tumor development in both the 10-week and 25-week UVB exposure models, Skh-1 hairless mice were exposed to 2240 J/m² UVB three times weekly for 10 weeks. Mice in the 10-week UVB exposure model were then treated topically with diclofenac for 15 weeks without further UVB exposure whereas mice in the 25-week UVB exposure model continued to be exposed to UVB three times a week and were treated topically with diclofenac immediately after each UVB

(a)

(b)

(c)

(d)

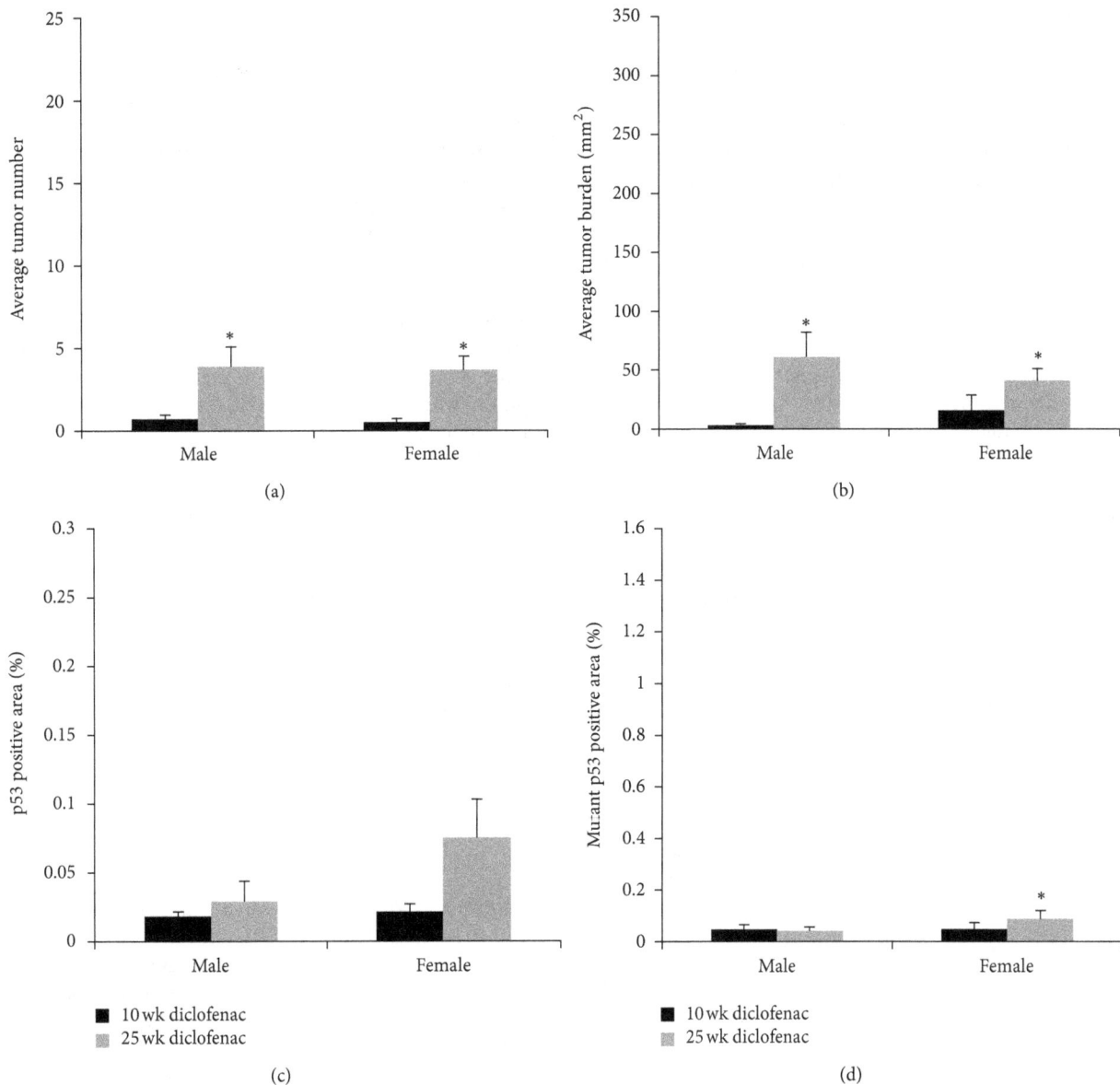

FIGURE 2: *Efficacy of diclofenac on tumor number, burden, and p53 status in male and female mice.* (a) Male and female diclofenac treated mice developed significantly more tumors in the 25- compared to the 10-week model ($^*P < 0.0001$). (b) Male ($^*P < 0.0001$) and female ($^*P = 0.0005$) diclofenac-treated mice in the 25-week UVB model developed significantly larger tumor burden compared to mice in the 10-week model. (c) Male and female mice treated with diclofenac in the 25-week exposure model did not exhibit significantly altered epidermal p53-positive area compared to the 10-week exposure model. (d) Female mice treated with diclofenac exhibited increased epidermal mutant p53-positive area ($^*P = 0.0060$) in the 25- compared to the 10-week model. Error bars = mean+/−SEM.

exposure for the remaining 15 weeks. Compared to male mice in the 10-week UVB exposure model, 25-week male mice displayed a 5.57-fold increase in tumor number ($P < 0.0001$ Figure 2(a)) and a 9.52-fold increase in tumor burden ($P < 0.0001$; Figure 2(b)). Female mice in the 25-week UVB exposure model displayed a 7.33-fold increase in tumor number ($P < 0.0001$; Figure 2(a)) and a 7.06-fold increase in tumor burden ($P = 0.0005$; Figure 2(b)).

Importantly, in the 25-week model, compared to vehicle-treated mice, male mice treated topically with diclofenac developed 77% fewer tumors ($P < 0.0001$, Figures 1(a) and 2(a)) and exhibited an 80% reduction in tumor burden ($P = 0.0002$, Figures 1(b) and 2(b)) while female mice treated topically with diclofenac developed 55% fewer tumors ($P < 0.0001$, Figures 1(a) and 2(a)) and exhibited a 68% reduction in tumor burden ($P = 0.0186$, Figures 1(b) and 2(b)) compared to vehicle-treated mice. These results demonstrate that, even with continued UVB exposure, topical treatment with this anti-inflammatory drug continued to be effective in reducing tumor development.

However, male mice topically treated with diclofenac in the 25-week exposure model developed 9.79-fold more malignant tumors (5.9% versus 57.9%, $P = 0.0262$) compared to male mice treated with diclofenac in the 10-week model. Female mice treated topically with diclofenac developed 2.43-fold more malignant tumors (25% versus 61.3%) in the 25-week model compared to the 10-week model (Table 1), but due to both the smaller amount of tumors developed and the inherent variable nature of this outbred strain, this difference was not statistically significant ($P = 0.1565$). When compared to vehicle-treated mice, male mice in the 25-week UVB model treated topically with diclofenac exhibited a 53.6% increase in malignancy rate, which, due to the variability observed in this outbred mouse strain, was not statistically significant ($P = 0.1016$). Furthermore, in the 25-week UVB model, female mice treated topically with diclofenac displayed an 89% higher malignancy rate compared to vehicle-treated mice ($P = 0.0227$, Table 1). These data suggest that while topical treatment with the anti-inflammatory compound decreased tumor development, it did not decrease malignancy rates observed with continued UVB exposure.

Male mice treated topically with diclofenac exhibited no significant alterations in epidermal p53-positive area between the two models and although female mice treated topically with diclofenac exhibited a 2-fold increase in p53-positive area, this difference was not statistically significant ($P = 0.1683$, Figure 2(c)).

Male mice in the 25-week UVB exposure model did not exhibit significantly altered epidermal mutant p53 staining with topical diclofenac treatment compared to male mice in the 10-week exposure model. In contrast, female mice treated with diclofenac in the 25-week exposure model exhibited a 4.58-fold increase in mutant p53-positive cells compared to female mice in the 10-week UVB exposure model ($P = 0.0060$, Figure 2(d)).

3.3. Efficacy of C E Ferulic on Tumor Number, Burden, and p53 Status in Male and Female Mice.

The effect of topical treatment with the stable antioxidant compound C E Ferulic on tumor development was determined in both the 10- and 25-week UVB exposure models by exposing Skh-1 hairless mice to 2240 J/m² UVB three times weekly for 10 weeks. Mice in the 10-week UVB exposure model were then treated topically with C E Ferulic for 15 weeks without further UVB exposure whereas mice in the 25-week UVB exposure model were treated immediately after each UVB exposure for 15 weeks. Male mice in the 25-week UVB exposure model treated topically with C E Ferulic displayed a 5.68-fold increase in tumor number ($P < 0.0001$, Figure 3(a)) and a 30.05-fold increase in average tumor burden ($P < 0.0001$, Figure 3(b)) compared to mice in the 10-week model. Female mice in the 25-week model treated topically with C E Ferulic displayed a 28.2-fold increase in average tumor number ($P < 0.0001$, Figure 3(a)) as well as a 30.69-fold increase in average tumor burden ($P < 0.0001$, Figure 3(b)) compared to mice in the 10-week model.

Compared to vehicle-treated mice, male mice in the 25-week UVB exposure model treated topically with C E Ferulic did not exhibit a significant alteration in tumor number (Figures 1(a) and 3(a)) but displayed a 60% increase in tumor burden compared to vehicle-treated mice, which possibly due

to the variability in this outbred mouse strain did not reach statistical significance ($P = 0.5590$, Figures 1(b) and 3(b)). Female mice in the 25-week UVB model treated topically with C E Ferulic did not exhibit a significant alteration in tumor number (Figures 1(a) and 3(a)) or average tumor burden (Figures 1(b) and 3(b)) compared to vehicle-treated mice.

Isolated tumors were analyzed as described above. Male mice in the 25-week UVB model treated with C E Ferulic developed 3.46-fold more malignant tumors (31.2% versus 45.6%, $P = 0.0087$, Table 1) while female mice treated developed 10.71-fold more malignant tumors (0 versus 31.4%, $P = 0.0196$, Table 1) compared to mice treated with C E Ferulic in the 10-week model. Compared to vehicle-treated mice, neither male nor female mice in the 25-week model treated topically with C E Ferulic exhibited significant alterations in tumor malignancy ($P = 0.3391$ and $P = 0.7544$, respectively, Table 1). These data suggest that topical C E Ferulic treatment is not effective with continued UVB exposure.

Interestingly, male mice treated with topical C E Ferulic exhibited a 3.71-fold increase in epidermal p53-positive cells ($P = 0.0062$, Figure 3(c)) while female mice exhibited no statistically significant alterations in p53-positive area in the 25-week UVB exposure model compared to the mice in the 10-week model (Figure 3(c)).

Male mice did not exhibit significantly altered epidermal mutant p53 staining with topical C E Ferulic treatment. In contrast, female mice treated with C E Ferulic in the 25-week exposure model exhibited a 8.07-fold increase in mutant p53-positive cells ($P = 0.0001$, Figure 3(d)) compared to female mice treated with C E Ferulic in the 10-week model.

3.4. Efficacy of Vitamin E on Tumor Number, Burden, and p53 Status in Male and Female Mice.

The effect of topical treatment with the classical antioxidant vitamin E on tumor development was determined in both the 10- and 25-week UVB exposure models by exposing Skh-1 hairless mice to UVB as described above. Mice in the 10-week UVB exposure model were then treated topically with vitamin E for 15 weeks without further UVB exposure whereas mice in the 25-week UVB exposure model were treated immediately after each UVB exposure for 15 weeks. Male mice in the 25-week model treated topically with vitamin E demonstrated a 3.84 fold increase in tumor number ($P < 0.0001$, Figure 4(a)) and a 9.44-fold increased tumor burden ($P < 0.0001$, Figure 4(b)) compared to mice in the 10-week model. Female mice in the 25-week model treated topically with vitamin E had a similar 4.11-fold increase in tumor number ($P < 0.0001$, Figure 4(a)), and demonstrated a 11.4-fold increased tumor burden ($P < 0.0001$, Figure 4(b)) compared to mice in the 10-week model.

Compared to vehicle-treated mice, there were no statistically significant differences in tumor number ($P = 0.0813$; Figures 1(a) and 4(a)) or burden ($P = 0.9100$; Figures 1(b) and 4(b)) in male mice treated with vitamin E in the 25-week UVB model. Likewise, compared to vehicle treated mice, topical vitamin E treatment of female mice in the 25-week UVB model did not statistically significantly alter tumor number ($P = 0.9150$; Figures 1(a) and 4(a)) or burden ($P = 0.7961$; Figures 1(b) and 4(b)).

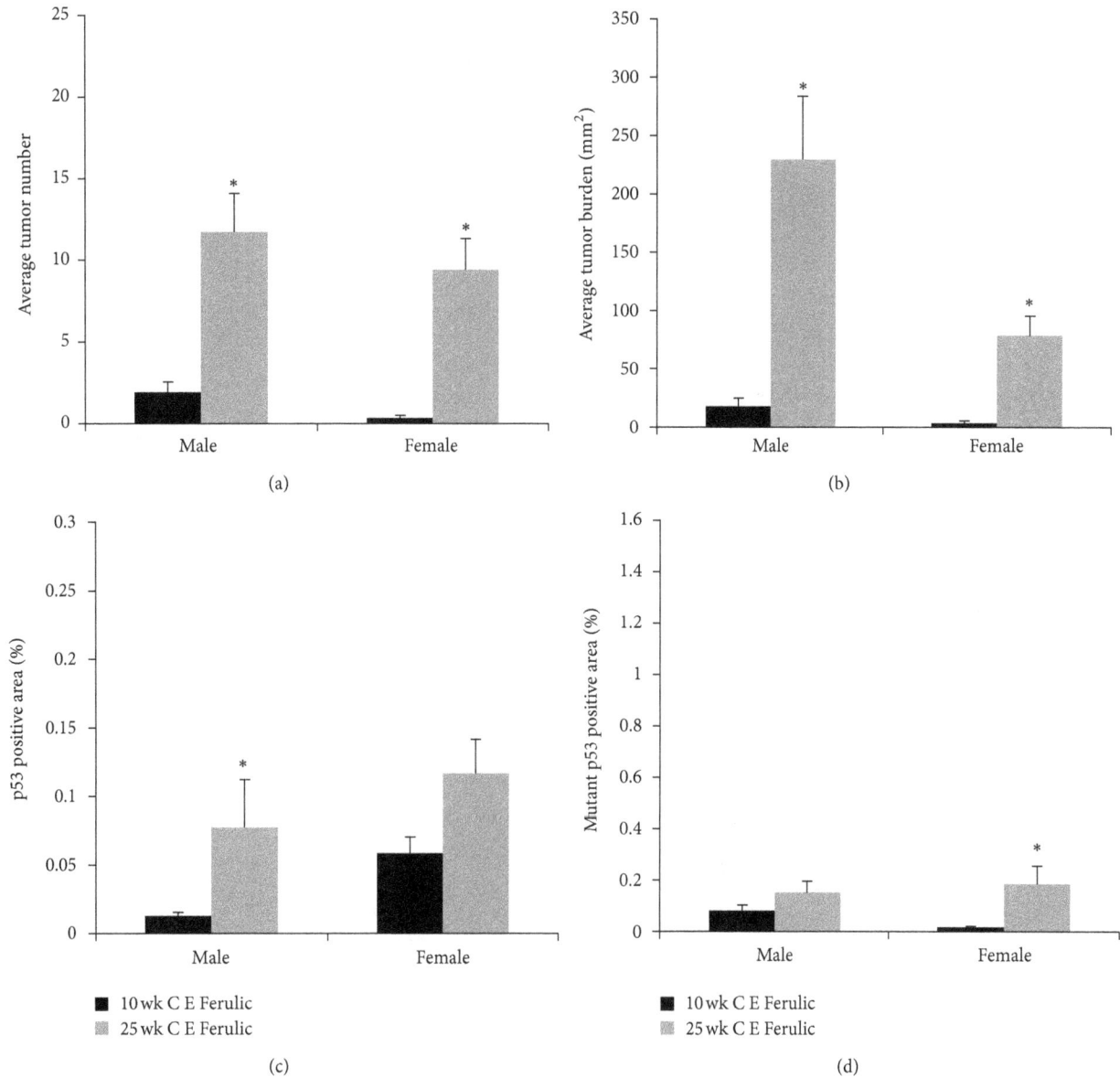

FIGURE 3: *Efficacy of C E Ferulic on tumor number, burden, and p53 status in male and female mice.* (a) Male and female mice topically treated with *C E Ferulic* developed more tumors in the 25- compared to the 10-week model ($^{*}P < 0.0001$). (b) Male and female mice topically treated with *C E Ferulic* developed increased tumor burden in the 25- compared to the 10-week model ($^{*}P < 0.0001$). (c) Male mice treated topically with *C E Ferulic* exhibited increased levels of epidermal p53-positive area in the 25- compared to the 10-week model ($^{*}P = 0.0062$). (d) Female mice treated topically with *C E Ferulic* exhibited increased levels of epidermal mutant p53-positive area in the 25- compared to the 10-week model ($^{*}P = 0.0001$). Error bars = mean+/−SEM.

Isolated tumors were analyzed as described above. Male mice in the 25-week UVB model treated topically with vitamin E developed 4.08-fold more malignant tumors (8.2% versus 34.1%, $P = 0.0028$, Table 1) compared to male mice treated with vitamin E in the 10-week model. Female mice in 25-week UVB model treated topically with vitamin E developed 14.38-fold more malignant tumors (2.9% versus 40.5%, $P = 0.0087$, Table 1) compared to female mice treated topically with vitamin E in the 10-week model. Neither male nor female mice in the 25-week model treated topically with vitamin E exhibited significant alterations in tumor malignancy

compared to vehicle-treated mice ($P = 0.6251$ and $P = 0.2816$, resp.). These data demonstrate that with continued UVB exposure, compared to vehicle-treated mice of either sex, topical treatment with vitamin E was not effective in modulating either tumor development or progression.

Interestingly, male mice in the 25-week UVB exposure model treated with topical vitamin E exhibited a 3.92-fold increase in epidermal p53-positive cells compared to the 10-week model ($P = 0.0023$, Figure 4(c)). However, female mice in the 25-week UVB model exhibited no significant alterations in p53-positive area compared to the 10-week model.

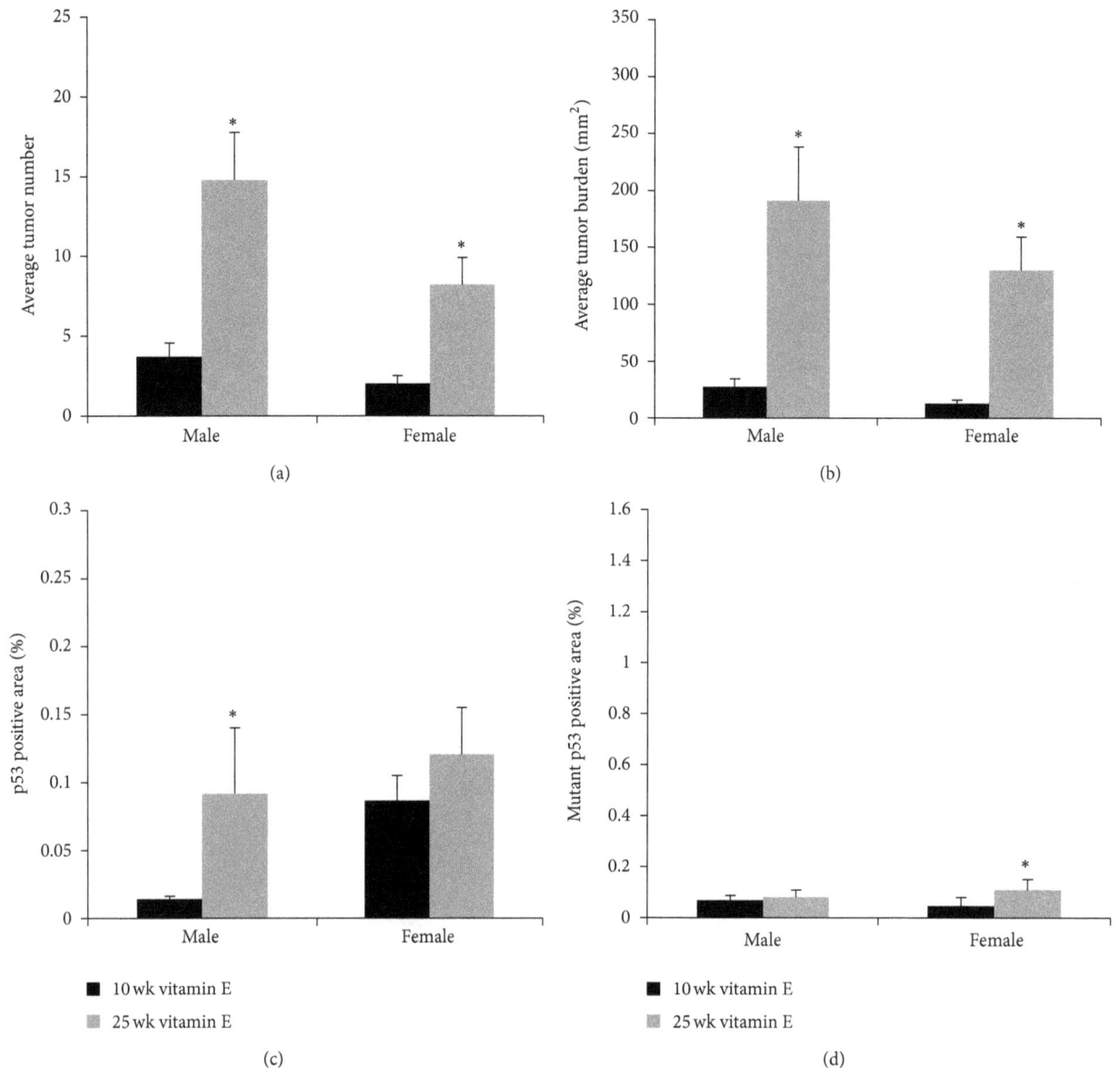

FIGURE 4: *Efficacy of vitamin E on tumor number, burden, and p53 status in male and female mice.* (a) Male and female mice treated with topical vitamin E developed more tumors in the 25-week compared to the 10-week model ($^*P < 0.0001$). (b) Male and female mice treated with topical vitamin E exhibited increased tumor burden in the 25- compared to the 10-week model ($^*P < 0.0001$). (c) Male mice treated with vitamin E exhibited increased epidermal p53-positive area in the 25- compared to the 10-week model ($^*P = 0.0023$). (d) Female mice treated with vitamin E exhibited significantly increased epidermal mutant p53-positive area in the 25- compared to the 10-week model ($^*P = 0.0134$). Error bars = mean+/−SEM.

Male mice in the 25-week UVB exposure model treated topically with vitamin E did not exhibit significantly altered epidermal mutant p53 staining compared to those in the 10-week model. In contrast, female mice treated topically with vitamin E in the 25-week UVB model exhibited a 3.78-fold increase in mutant p53-positive cells ($P = 0.0134$, Figure 4(d)) compared to female mice in the 10-week exposure model.

4. Discussion

Epidemiological studies have suggested a correlation between UV exposure and skin cancer development due to a higher frequency of disease among patients with a self-reported history of significant sun exposure. We were interested in determining the extent to which being compliant versus noncompliant with doctors' orders to stay out of the sun could affect cutaneous tumor development in subjects who have accumulated a significant amount of UVB-mediated skin damage over their lifetime. To that end, male and female Skh-1 mice were used to model compliant versus noncompliant patients, that is, to evaluate the effects of 10 weeks versus 25 weeks of UVB exposure on cutaneous tumor number, burden, grade and p53 status. We were also interested in the effect that continued 25-week UVB exposure had on the efficacy of potential topical therapeutic strategies compared to the effect on skin that was chronically UVB damaged but no longer being actively exposed to UVB. In this study where the extent of UVB exposure was directly monitored and recorded, we demonstrated an increased tumor number, burden, and grade at 25 weeks in in both male and female Skh-1 mice exposed to 2240 J/m^2 UVB three times weekly for 25 weeks compared to 10 weeks. While previous reports have demonstrated that increasing UV doses resulted in a shorter latency period, increased DNA damage and p53 mutations, and increased tumor number, the current study demonstrates that the length of repetitive nonburning amounts of UVB exposure likewise enhances the carcinogenesis process [14, 15]. The increases in tumor burden, tumor grade, and malignancy rate in both male and female mice correlated with increased epidermal p53 and mutant p53 protein in mice exposed to 25 compared to 10 weeks of UVB exposure.

Our previous study demonstrated significantly decreased tumor number and burden in diclofenac-treated mice of both sexes, compared to vehicle-treated 10-week UVB-exposed mice [10]. The current study found that despite the overall increases in tumor number and burden observed in the 25-week model, topical diclofenac treatment continued to effectively decrease tumor number and burden in both male and female mice compared to mice treated with vehicle. In contrast, male and female mice treated with topical antioxidants did not exhibit any beneficial effects in terms of tumor number or burden and in fact demonstrated increases in both parameters. Surprisingly, our previously reported increased malignancy rate in female mice treated topically with diclofenac [10] was exacerbated in the current study, where female mice exposed to UVB for 25 weeks and treated topically with diclofenac exhibited a 90% increase in malignancy rate compared to vehicle-treated mice despite having fewer tumors. Previously we had shown that male mice exposed to UVB and treated with topical diclofenac displayed a decreased malignancy rate compared to vehicle-treated mice [10]. However, with 25 weeks of UVB exposure, male mice treated with diclofenac actually exhibited a 50% increase in malignancy rate compared to vehicle-treated mice. The unexpected observed increases in malignancy rates for both sexes in the 25-week UVB exposure model suggest that the more benign tumors may be more affected by the topical treatment while the malignant tumors are escaping the chemopreventive treatment by an as of yet unexplained mechanism. Many previous studies that examine possible therapeutics or preventative treatments for cancers examine the number and size of tumors that appear but do not report the histologic grade of tumors that did develop, especially if they are small. Our current studies highlight the importance of histologically examining all tumors, including those that develop in groups where treatment may have been effective in decreasing tumor number or burden but may be not effective against eradicating/preventing the more malignant tumors.

We previously demonstrated that the combination of the antioxidants vitamin E, vitamin C, and ferulic acid found in C E Ferulic exerted potential benefits in terms of decreased tumor number and burden in both male and female mice. In contrast, while moderate benefits were observed with vitamin

E topical treatment alone in male mice, female mice treated topically with vitamin E exhibited significantly increased overall DNA damage, cutaneous proliferation, and angiogenesis, as well as increased tumor growth rate, number, and burden [11]. The current study demonstrated that, with continued, prolonged chronic UVB exposure, any observed benefits of topical antioxidant treatment were lost in both sexes. These data highlight not only the detrimental effects of continued UVB exposure on ultimate tumor development and progression but also the importance of limiting UVB exposure to obtain the optimal efficacy of therapeutic interventions.

5. Conclusions

These studies illustrate that, in terms of tumor number and burden, both males and females benefit from topical diclofenac treatment, regardless of overall length of UVB exposure regime. However, especially in females, the elevated malignancy rate of mice treated topically with diclofenac may overshadow the benefits. Further, while we previously demonstrated potential benefits of combination antioxidant topical treatment for decreasing tumor burden and tumor malignancy rates [11], these effects were lost in the 25-week UVB exposure model, indicating that sun exposure must be limited in both males and females in order to benefit from antioxidant treatments. Overall, these data support the commonly assumed, but not demonstrated, fact that cumulative length of UVB exposure is a risk factor for UVB-induced SCC and highlight the fact that changing sun worshiping habits, even after early chronic sun exposure and skin damage, may ultimately decrease tumor development in patients.

Acknowledgments

The authors thank Jonathan Schick, Katie Samijlenko, Keith Lamping, and Paul Cipriani for excellent technical support. This work was funded by NIH grant CA133629.

References

[1] F. R. de Gruijl, "Action spectrum for photocarcinogenesis," *Recent Results in Cancer Research*, vol. 139, pp. 21–30, 1995.

[2] F. R. de Gruijl and P. D. Forbes, "UV-induced skin cancer in a hairless mouse model," *BioEssays*, vol. 17, no. 7, pp. 651–660, 1995.

[3] F. Stenback, "Life history and histopathology of ultraviolet light-induced skin tumors," *National Cancer Institute Monograph*, vol. NO 50, pp. 57–70, 1978.

[4] F. Benavides, T. M. Oberyszyn, A. M. VanBuskirk, V. E. Reeve, and D. F. Kusewitt, "The hairless mouse in skin research," *Journal of Dermatological Science*, vol. 53, no. 1, pp. 10–18, 2009.

[5] J. M. Thomas-Ahner, B. C. Wulff, K. L. Tober, D. F. Kusewitt, J. A. Riggenbach, and T. M. Oberyszyn, "Gender differences in UVB-induced skin carcinogenesis, inflammation, and DNA damage," *Cancer Research*, vol. 67, no. 7, pp. 3468–3474, 2007.

[6] T. A. Wilgus, A. T. Koki, B. S. Zweifel, D. F. Kusewitt, P. A. Rubal, and T. M. Oberyszyn, "Inhibition of cutaneous ultraviolet light B-mediated inflammation and tumor formation with topical celecoxib treatment," *Molecular Carcinogenesis*, vol. 38, no. 2, pp. 49–58, 2003.

[7] F. R. de Gruijl and J. C. van der Leun, "Development of skin tumors in hairless mice after discontinuation of ultraviolet irradiation," *Cancer Research*, vol. 51, no. 3, pp. 979–984, 1991.

[8] K. Togsverd-Bo, C. M. Lerche, T. Poulsen, M. Hoedersdal, and H. C. Wulf, "Reduced ultraviolet irradiation delays subsequent squamous cell carcinomas in hairless mice," *Photodermatology Photoimmunology and Photomedicine*, vol. 25, no. 6, pp. 305–309, 2009.

[9] J. Ramos, J. Villa, A. Ruiz, R. Armstrong, and J. Matta, "UV dose determines key characteristics of nonmelanoma skin cancer," *Cancer Epidemiology Biomarkers and Prevention*, vol. 13, no. 12, pp. 2006–2011, 2004.

[10] E. M. Burns, K. L. Tober, J. A. Riggenbach et al., "Preventative topical diclofenac treatment differentially decreases tumor burden in male and female Skh-1 mice in a model of UVB-induced cutaneous squamous cell carcinoma," *Carcinogenesis*, vol. 34, no. 2, pp. 370–377.

[11] E. M. Burns, K. L. Tober, J. A. Riggenbach, D. F. Kusewitt, G. S. Young, and T. M. Oberyszyn, "Differential effects of topical vitamin e and C e ferulic(R) treatments on ultraviolet light B-induced cutaneous tumor development in skh-1 mice," *PLoS ONE*, vol. 8, no. 5, Article ID e63809, 2013.

[12] C. W. Dunnett and R. Crisafio, "The operating characteristics of some official weight variation tests for tablets," *The Journal of pharmacy and pharmacology*, vol. 7, no. 5, pp. 314–327, 1955.

[13] J. C. Hsu, "The factor analytic approach to simultaneous inference in the general linear model," *Journal of Computational and Graphical Statistics*, vol. 1, no. 2, pp. 151–168, 1992.

[14] H. Rebel, L. O. Mosnier, R. J. W. Berg et al., "Early p53-positive foci as indicators of tumor risk in ultraviolet-exposed hairless mice: kinetics of induction, effects of DNA repair deficieney, and p53 heterozygosity," *Cancer Research*, vol. 61, no. 3, pp. 977–983, 2001.

[15] H. J. van Kranen and F. R. de Gruijl, "Mutations in cancer genes of UV-induced skin tumors of hairless mice," *Journal of Epidemiology*, vol. 9, supplement 6, pp. S58–S65, 1999.

5

Sentinel Lymph Node Biopsy in Nonmelanoma Skin Cancer Patients

Marie-Laure Matthey-Giè,[1] **Ariane Boubaker,**[2] **Igor Letovanec,**[3]
Nicolas Demartines,[1] **and Maurice Matter**[1]

[1] Department of Visceral Surgery, University Hospital CHUV, Lausanne, Switzerland
[2] Department of Nuclear Medicine, University Hospital CHUV, Lausanne, Switzerland
[3] Department of Pathology, University Hospital CHUV, Lausanne, Switzerland

Correspondence should be addressed to Maurice Matter; maurice.matter@chuv.ch

Academic Editor: Günther Hofbauer

The management of lymph nodes in nonmelanoma skin cancer patients is currently still debated. Merkel cell carcinoma (MCC), squamous cell carcinoma (SCC), pigmented epithelioid melanocytoma (PEM), and other rare skin neoplasms have a well-known risk to spread to regional lymph nodes. The use of sentinel lymph node biopsy (SLNB) could be a promising procedure to assess this risk in clinically N0 patients. Metastatic SNs have been observed in 4.5–28% SCC (according to risk factors), in 9–42% MCC, and in 14–57% PEM. We observed overall 30.8% positive SNs in 13 consecutive patients operated for high-risk nonmelanoma skin cancer between 2002 and 2011 in our institution. These high rates support recommendation to implement SLNB for nonmelanoma skin cancer especially for SCC patients. Completion lymph node dissection following positive SNs is also a matter of discussion especially in PEM. It must be remembered that a definitive survival benefit of SLNB in melanoma patients has not been proven yet. However, because of its low morbidity when compared to empiric elective lymph node dissection or radiation therapy of lymphatic basins, SLNB has allowed sparing a lot of morbidity and could therefore be used in nonmelanoma skin cancer patients, even though a significant impact on survival has not been demonstrated.

1. Introduction

20 years ago [1], sentinel lymph node biopsy (SLNB) was introduced for melanoma patients and later for numerous other tumors with lymphatic metastatic propensity. Even though surgical oncology community is divided in believers and nonbelievers regarding its application, data show that SLNB has already changed the treatments modalities in melanoma and breast cancer patients, at least with respect to TNM classification. It has allowed a better understanding of disease progression and response to treatment in patients with comparable staging groups.

Nonmelanoma skin cancer with potential metastatic spreading to regional lymph nodes regroups skin lesions like high-risk squamous cell carcinoma (SCC), Merkel cell carcinoma (MCC), and pigmented epithelioid melanocytoma (PEM). Because of the low incidence of nonmelanoma skin cancer with potential metastatic spread and the lack of large clinical trials, the use of SLNB in these cases is not well established, and no guidelines are currently available. Previous studies conducted about this subject reported a high rate of positive sentinel nodes (SNs) in nonmelanoma skin cancer: 4.5–28% for SCC [2–4], 16–42% for MCC [5–7], and 14–46% for PEM [8, 9]. In this context, the role of SLNB in nonmelanoma skin cancer should be accepted as a standard staging procedure assuming that N status is a strong predictive factor for survival.

2. Material and Methods

Over a 10-year period from January 2002 to December 2011, a total number of thirteen patients underwent a SLNB for nonmelanoma skin cancer at the University Hospital of Lausanne, Switzerland. The patients were identified and registered in parallel of a melanoma patients' registry (550 SLNB during the same time), and a retrospective analysis was performed. Data were retrieved form patient's files and imaging database. The study protocol and data collection were approved by our audit department.

Based on established protocol published earlier [10], a triple technique was used to identify SNs. Briefly, a 99^m Tc nanocoll lymphoscintigraphy was performed preoperatively (day before or same day), followed by intraoperative injection of 2 mL. patent blue V intradermally around the primary tumor or in the scar. SN was localized using hand-held gamma-probe guidance. Histopathology followed standardized analysis for melanoma patients: serial sectioning, H.-E, and corresponding immunohistochemistry (S100 protein and Melan-A or cytokeratins)

Data retrieved included demographics, type of primary tumor, number of SN removed, number of positive SNs, completion lymph node dissection (CLND), nonsentinel lymph nodes (NSNs), and oncological followup including local recurrence, lymphatic extension, metastasis, disease-free, and overall survival.

The aim of our present study was to analyze the rate of positive SNs and reliability regarding false negative rate during followup in nonmelanoma skin cancer patients in our series and compare our data with a review of the current literature.

3. Results

3.1. Patient's Demographics. Thirteen patients with non-melanoma skin cancer underwent SLNB. Of these, eight presented a squamous cell carcinoma (SCC), three a Merkel cell carcinoma (MCC), and two a pigmented epithelioid melanocytoma (PEM). The median age was 68 years (range 25–92 years; mean ± SD: 61.5 ± 21.2). There were 8 males and 5 females. Clinical details are summarized in Table 1.

3.2. Biopsy Results, Outcomes of Surgery, and Followup. The rate of positive SN for the 13 patients was 31% (4/13). The median followup was 23 months (range 2–76 months). Fifty SNs were removed, and 7 were positive in 4 patients.

Patient 1 with MCC of right buttock had one micrometastatic (<2 mm deposit) in 4 examined SNs. Radiation therapy was given to the buttock and inguinal areas. Patient 4 with MCC of the left leg had one metastatic SN (6 mm) out of 2. She refused any further adjuvant therapy. Both MCC N+ patients are free of recurrent disease with a follow-up period of 20 and 54 months, respectively.

Patient 7 with a high-risk SCC of left thumb had 2 metastatic SNs (1.5 cm and 1 cm) out of 3. Two deep suspicious nonsentinel nodes (NSNs) were also removed during the same intervention, and one showed a 3 cm metastasis. The patient was preoperatively investigated only by MRI of the arm, and clinically no axillary node was palpable. ELND was performed, and 2 NSNs out of 10 were positive. He had adjuvant radiation therapy (50 Gy) and chemotherapy (carboplatin) following axilla recurrence. Unfortunately the patient ultimately needed an amputation with disarticulation

15 months after the diagnosis because of further progression of the disease in the axilla. He is still alive 23 months after the diagnosis.

Patient 11 with a deep (11 mm) PEM of the middle of the back had SLNB in both axillas. On the right side, 1 SN showed only one capsular focus of metastatic cells and following a second opinion of an international expertise center we decided not to proceed with ELND. One NSN was negative. On the left side, one SN had a parenchymal focus of PEM and was considered positive. Three other NSNs were negative and ELND showed 12 other negative NSNs. She had no evidence of disease within a followup of 5 years.

Nine patients were found to be SN negative. Seven patients had SCC: patients 6 and 13 were lost during the followup, after 2 and 6 months, respectively. Patient 2 with epidermolysis bullosa developed other SCC lesions on the upper and lower limbs 9 months, respectively 4 years after the excision of the primary tumor of the lower limb. Patient 5 with an initial SCC of the right vulva underwent an excision of the contralateral vulva for a VIN 3 tumor 3 years later. Patient 8 died from an aggressive locoregional progression of the disease six months after the diagnosis. Patients 9 and 10 showed no recurrence after a followup of 9 and 15 months. Patient 12 with PEM was lost during followup after 11 months, and patient 3 with MCC did not recur after a followup of 6 years.

Patient 13 presented a 3.5 cm large poorly differentiated SCC, and lymphoscintigraphy identified four different SN basins (3 interval nodes): humeral lateral, and medial, axilla and cervical (Figure 1). All 7 SNs were negative.

Overall no postoperative complication at the SLNB site was registered. No patient with negative SN had a nodal recurrence.

4. Discussion

Our experience confirms results of other series regarding feasibility and reliability (false negative rate) of SLNB. This cohort of patient with heterogeneous group of rare primary skin carcinomas reflects the experience in the literature. The rate of 30.8% positive SNs observed in the current study is comparable to those of similar studies published on non-melanoma skin cancer patients. For instance, Cecchi et al. [18] and Wagner et al. [19] reported a rate of positive SNB of 20% (2/10) and 31.8% (7/22), respectively. Of note, majority of series describe a pretty limited number of patients. In our own study, patients who were SN positive or negative had no nodal recurrence and disease recurred or progressed regionally independently of SN status (one patient in each group of SN positive or SN negative).

Following potential advantages of SNB must be under-lined.

(1) Detection of regional lymph node basins at risk for N+ status: lymphatic mapping using lymphoscintigraphy is useful in defining lymphatic basins at risk, which is very important in complex lymphatic network in head and neck surgery for example [20].

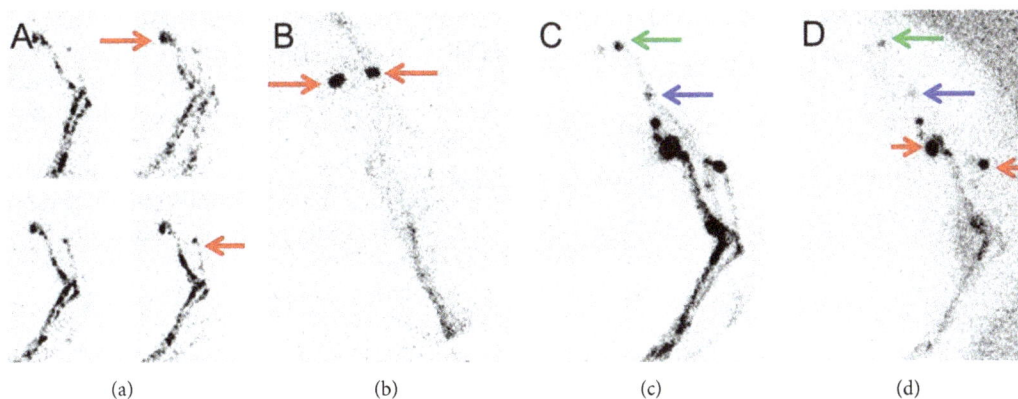

FIGURE 1: Patient 13 had a 3.5 cm large poorly differentiated SCC on the dorsal side of left hand that was reaching subcutaneous level with perineural invasion but with no lymphovascular invasion. Dynamic lymphoscintigraphy of the upper left limb demonstrated multiple drainage pathways on the dynamic views (a), and accessories lymph nodes were immediately visualized in the humeral lateral and medial regions (red arrows). These were confirmed not to be only ectatic lymphatic vessels but 2 different sentinel nodes corresponding to 2 basins (b). Delayed views of the arm and shoulder (c, d) showed 2 more SNs in 2 basins: in the axilla (blue arrow) and basicervical (green arrow). All 7 SNs in 4 basins were negative.

TABLE 1: Patient characteristics, sentinel lymph nodes results, and followup.

Patient	Age	Sex	Type	Primary site	SLN region	Risk factor	SLN total	SLN+	Clearance	Adjuvant therapy	Follow-up (months)	Recurrence
1	78	M	Merkel	Buttock	Inguinal	4 cm large	4	1	No	Yes	20	No
2	39	M	SCC	Leg	Inguinal	EBD	3	0	No	No	75	No
3	72	M	Merkel	Buttock	Inguinal	2.2 cm large	2	0	No	No	76	No
4	84	F	Merkel	Leg	Inguinal	LVI	4	1	No	No	54	No
5	33	M	SCC	Vulva	Inguinal Iliac	2 cm large 7 mm deep	3	0	No	No	52	No
6	92	F	SCC	Leg	Inguinal	5 cm large 7 mm deep	5	0	No	No	2	?
7	72	M	SCC	Thumb	Axillary	Recurrent, 3 cm large Bone infiltration	6	3	Yes	Yes	23	Yes
8	51	F	SCC	Thigh	Iliac	Chronic scar	3	0	No	Yes	6	Yes
9	83	M	SCC	Leg	Inguinal	1.7 cm large 5 mm deep	1	0	No	No	15	No
10	61	F	SCC	Forearm	Axillary	Chronic scar	3	0	No	No	9	No
11	25	F	PEM	Back	Axillary Bilateral	11 mm deep	7	1	Yes	No	61	No
12	46	M	PEM	Back	Axillary Bilateral	Other skin carcinoma	3	0	No	No	41	?
13	68	M	SCC	Hand	Humeral twice axillary, cervical	3.5 cm large Poor differentiation	7	0	No	No	6	?

EBD: epidermolisis bullosa dystrophyca, LVI: lymphovascular invasion.

(2) Staging of real N0 patients, in whom unnecessary CLND or radiation therapy and their significant morbidity can be spared, meaning that false negative assessment (CLND or node recurrence during follow-up) must be as low as possible. It should be assumed that removing early metastatic node improves significantly the prognosis compared with removing advanced nodal disease.

(3) Detection of metastatic and micrometastatic diseases in clinically and radiologically N0 patients. Overstaging is possible (uncertain meaning of isolated tumor cells), but false negative N0 patients (clinically negative and H-E negative) can be detected and their staging is correctly assessed for directing appropriate treatment.

(4) Detection of interval SNs (lymph nodes outside usual basins) that are at the same metastatic risk as other SNs and that can be otherwise misinterpreted as intransit metastases [10, 17, 21–23] (Figure 1).

On the other hand SNLB has a price: a hospital stay and surgery and its own morbidity. Adverse effects of SLNB were observed in 25% compared with 70% with SLNB and CLND

TABLE 2: Criteria for high-risk cutaneous squamous cell carcinoma [12, 22, 24–26].

Histopathologic factors
Size >2 cm
High-risk location (head and neck)
In-transit metastatic lesion
Poor differentiation
Perineural invasion
Tumour thickness >5-6 mm
Desmoplastic growth
Other factors
Radiation field
Patients with immunosuppression (transplantation and others)
Recurrence
Multiple SCCs
Marjolin's ulcer (carcinoma in burn scar or chronic ulcer)

in the Z0011 breast cancer trial (6% lymphedema versus 11% at one year) [24]. In the Sunbelt Melanoma Trial overall morbidity was 4.6% for SLNB alone compared with 23.2% for SLNB and CLND. Lymphedema following SLNB was 0.3% in the axilla and 1.5% in the groin [25]. Incidence of adverse reactions to different blue dyes used for SLNB is 1–3% [26].

5. Squamous Cell Carcinoma (SCC)

SCC represents the second most frequent skin cancer after melanomas [3, 4] and its incidence in the population reaches approximately 1% [4]. Incidence of SCC varies widely according to patients' risk like sun exposure or immunosuppression. Most of these patients will not develop nodal disease, but in some patients it represents the first metastatic step. The reported metastatic rate of high-risk SCC reaches 11–47.3% [27], and the regional lymph nodes are the first involved. Patient with clinical detectable nodal metastasis has a poor prognosis with a reported 5-year survival rates of 26% [27].

Risk factors for metastasis or local recurrence of SCC have been described in the literature and are summarized in Table 2 [19, 28–31]. They should be used to select patients eligible for SLNB. Despite the absence of controlled studies, guidelines about the staging for high-risk SCC in immunosuppressed patients or patients planned for a transplantation recommend to perform a SLNB [32].

Recently the French Dermatology Recommendations Association (aRED) suggested a prognostic classification including 2 groups defined as low-versus-significant metastatic risk [33]. Unlike previously published guidelines reviewed by Veness [29] that proposed no recommendation for the management of lymph nodes in high-risk patients, aRED stated that SLNB may be envisaged for clinical trials and evaluation studies. Their proposal was ultrasound surveillance and no routine ELND or radiation therapy [33].

The low rate of false negative SLNB reported in the literature [2, 34] is an essential quality marker for SLNB

efficacy. False negative rate seems to depend on SCC location: all sites 15.4%, head and neck 0% and truncal/extremity 22.2% [35]. In the absence of consensus in high-risk SCC patients, 46% of surgeons proposed SLNB in Jambsaria-Pahlanjani's survey [36].

They are only a few studies published about high-risk patients presenting SCC arising from a burn scar or a chronic ulcer (Marjolin's ulcer) [22, 37] (patient 8), locally recurrent SCC [38], and patients with recessive-type epidermolysis bullosa (patient 2) [39].

6. Merkel Cell Carcinoma (MCC)

MCCs are rare and aggressive neuroendocrine tumors arising from cutaneous Merkel cells. Their incidence seems to be rising; they affect more elderly and immunosuppressed people with a correlation to sun exposure. They tend to spread locally before developing distant metastasis, and at time of diagnosis up to 68% of patients already present lymph node involvement [40]. The presence of clinically palpable nodes and visible lymphadenopathy on CT scan is an indicator of poor survival rate [13] so that early detection of lymph node involvement is the most important prognostic factor.

MCC is known to be radiosensitive, but the systematic use of radiotherapy to the primary tumour and/or the lymph node basin is still debated. Eich et al. [41] have reported a significant higher disease-free survival rate and Mojica et al. have reported [42] a higher overall survival rate after adjuvant radiotherapy. However, Allen et al. could not demonstrate that an adjuvant radiotherapy was necessary if the primary tumor and the lymph node basin were surgically controlled (ELND, SLNB, and CLND) [5]. Conversely in patient without nodal control (SLNB/ELNB) metastatic lymph node will appear in 45% of cases and radiotherapy is mandatory.

Already in 2002, Goessling et al. listed 49 patients with MCC and concluded that the SLNB could be a useful tool for their staging [43]. Since then, the use of SLNB for MCC has been the subject of several reviews which are summarized in Table 3 [5, 7, 11–17]. The cumulated rate of positive SNs was 31% (101/326). Only half of the SN positive patients underwent a CLND, and the rate of positive NSNs after CLND was 35% (19/54). It seems that despite the absence of guidelines, the number of patients undergoing SLNB followed by CLND is increasing.

Criteria for a high risk of metastatic sentinel node in Merkel cell carcinoma are presented in Box 1. However, patients without these criteria still have a 23–36% risk for positive SN [41, 42, 49].

One of the largest monocentric study was presented by Fields et al. [16]. From 153 patients who underwent SLNB, 45 of them presented positive SN. CLND was consecutively performed in 21 patients, and 6 of them presented metastatic NSNs. During a median followup of 41 months 8/99 SN-negative patients developed nodal recurrence which corresponds to a false negative rate of 15%. The presence of lymphovascular invasion (LVI) was highly predictive for the disease-free and overall survival but not for the SN status. Interestingly 71% of the patients with positive SN and 92% of the patients with negative SN did not receive any adjuvant

TABLE 3: Review of studies with sentinel lymph node biopsy in patients with MCC.

Author	Reference Number	Year	patients with SLNB	H-E ± IHC	+SN	CLND	+ NSN	Nodal recurrence in SN patients	Median followup (months)
Allen et al.	[5]	2005	54	NS	12	8	2	Not detailed*	40
Maza et al.	[11]	2006	23	Both	11	8	4	2	36.1
Gupta et al.	[7]	2006	30/61	Both	7	?	—	Not detailed	—
Ortin-Perez et al.	[12]	2007	8	Both	3	3	0	0	55
Warner et al.	[13]	2008	11/17	Both	3	2	?	5	16
Shnayder et al.	[14]	2008	10/15	Both	4	1	1	1	24
Bajetta et al.	[15]	2009	21/95	NS	8	8	4		65
Fields et al.	[16]	2011	153	Both	45	21	6	8/108	41
Howle and Veness	[17]	2012	16	Both	8	3	2	2/8	19.5
Total			326		101	54	19		

*One out of 21 SN negative patients results published in a previous article (20) with a median followup of 19 months.
NS: not specified.

Greatest horizontal diameter ≥3.75 mm
Histopathologic factors
Infiltrative tumour growth pattern
Mitotic rate >10
Size > 1 cm/>2 cm
Tumour thickness >2 mm

Box 1: Criteria for a high-risk of metastatic sentinel node in Merkel cell carcinoma.

---

therapy. In this study, the author recommends to perform routinely SLNB even by patients who are clinically staged as N0. However, this staging procedure remains a subject of controversies in the recent published studies [15, 44, 45].

The use of immunohistochemistry (pancytokeratin and CK-20 antibodies) can significantly upstage false negative SNs [46, 47] and should be the role for SN examination.

In summary up to 68% of MCC patients present nodal metastases at time of diagnosis. 20–30% of clinically N0 patients can be upstaged if a SLNB is performed. Nodal status is an important prognostic factor. The exact role and benefit of radiation therapy on lymphatic basins are not definitively assessed (clinically negative or after SLND, CLND, and ELND) [5, 13, 14, 42]. New attempts for improving standardized histopathology report [48] and treatment algorithm [49] would be helpful.

MCC has a higher incidence in transplanted patients. These patients are younger and their 5-year overall survival of 46% [50] is slightly lower than the 54% observed in a large MCC data base regarding matched population [51].

7. Nonmelanoma Pigmented Tumors

Some patients with Spitz naevi may present with a difficult differential diagnosis for other melanocytic tumors including melanoma. A review of the literature about spitzoid tumors showed that 37.7% of patients presented metastatic SNs, and 14% of the patients with CLND had metastatic NSNs [52]. Metastatic propensity will define malignancy, but in SN negative patients only the followup can exclude it. These results were published by Magro et al. who reviewed their experience with SLNB in borderline melanocytic tumors (BMTs) [9].

Pigmented epitheloid melanocytoma, also called equine or animal-type melanoma, is a rare melanocytic tumor with frequent metastatic spreading to local lymph nodes and occurs mainly during childhood and in young adults [8].

However, Mandal et al. observed that patients with positive SN had an excellent outcome. They concluded that, while sparing risk for progressive bulky metastatic lymph node, SLNB would not change the prognosis in this low-grade melanocytic neoplasm. As no high-risk PEM has been identified, simple surveillance of the lymphatic basin with ultrasound seems to be a safe solution [53].

8. Other Rare Skin Neoplasms

SLNB has also been evaluated for cutaneous apocrine adenocarcinoma [54] and for aggressive digital papillary adenocarcinoma [55]. As both of them have a high propensity for lymphatic invasion, the systematic use of SLNB should be recommended.

Because of their lymph node metastatic risk, some soft tissue sarcomas may also been concerned by SLNB. Lymph node dissection is recommended in clinically or radiologically N+ patients [56], but the role of SNB has not been clearly established yet.

Lymph node metastatic rate for epithelioid sarcoma and angiosarcoma ranges from 17 to 80% and 11 to 40%, respectively.

Regarding skin lymphomas a large recent series of patients with mycosis fungoides and Sezary syndrome showed that 91% of patients are clinically N0 [57]. As TNM plays a role in prognosis and treatment, SLNB could find its place for detecting patients with early stages (IA-IB) who adversely progress. In cutaneous T-cell lymphoma, SLNB can prove the primary cutaneous origin and avoid a systemic treatment [58].

9. Conclusion

Management of high-risk nonmelanoma skin tumor patients is still a matter of debate in the absence of randomized trials. Randomized studies are difficult to conduct because of the rarity of these tumors; the best option is therefore to pool these patients in multicentric cohort in order to support the guidelines defined by consensus. Definition of high-risk parameters and standardization of examination protocols could allow such studies of these rare but life-threatening malignancies. SLNB has its price and has its own morbidity; it represents, however, the best way for assessing N stage in clinically and radiologically negative patients. It must be remembered that a definitive survival benefit with SLNB in melanoma patients has not been proven (yet) and is currently evaluated by the MSLT 2 trial. However, because of its low morbidity compared with empiric ELND or radiation therapy on lymphatic basins, SLNB has already spared a lot of morbidity in many patients, before this survival advantage can also be demonstrated in nonmelanoma skin cancer patients. Thus, until better data demonstrate the opposite, SLNB should be recommended in nonmelanoma skin tumors.

Abbreviations

SLNB: Sentinel lymph node biopsy
CLND: Completion lymph node dissection
ELND: Elective lymph node dissection
MCC: Merkel cell carcinoma
SCC: Squamous cell carcinoma
PEM: Pigmented epithelioid melanocytoma
SN: Sentinel lymph node
NSN: Nonsentinel lymph node.

References

[1] D. L. Morton, D. R. Wen, J. H. Wong et al., "Technical details of intraoperative lymphatic mapping for early stage melanoma," *Archives of Surgery*, vol. 127, no. 4, pp. 392–399, 1992.

[2] A. S. Ross and C. D. Schmults, "Sentinel lymph node biopsy in cutaneous squamous cell carcinoma: a systematic review of the English literature," *Dermatologic Surgery*, vol. 32, no. 11, pp. 1309–1321, 2006.

[3] Y. Y. Liu, W. M. Rozen, and R. Rahdon, "Sentinel lymph node biopsy for squamous cell carcinoma of the extremities: case report and review of the literature," *Anticancer Research*, vol. 31, no. 4, pp. 1443–1446, 2011.

[4] C. Renzi, A. Caggiati, T. J. Mannooranparampil et al., "Sentinel lymph node biopsy for high risk cutaneous squamous cell carcinoma: case series and review of the literature," *European Journal of Surgical Oncology*, vol. 33, no. 3, pp. 364–369, 2007.

[5] P. J. Allen, W. B. Bowne, D. P. Jaques, M. F. Brennan, K. Busam, and D. G. Coit, "Merkel cell carcinoma: prognosis and treatment of patients from a single institution," *Journal of Clinical Oncology*, vol. 23, no. 10, pp. 2300–2309, 2005.

[6] S. E. Ames, D. N. Krag, and M. S. Brady, "Radiolocalization of the sentinel lymph node in Merkel cell carcinoma: a clinical analysis of seven cases," *Journal of Surgical Oncology*, vol. 67, no. 4, pp. 251–254, 1998.

[7] S. G. Gupta, L. C. Wang, P. F. Peñas, M. Gellenthin, S. J. Lee, and P. Nghiem, "Sentinel lymph node biopsy for evaluation and treatment of patients with Merkel cell carcinoma: the Dana-Farber experience and meta-analysis of the literature," *Archives of Dermatology*, vol. 142, no. 6, pp. 685–690, 2006.

[8] A. Zembowicz, J. A. Carney, and M. C. Mihm, "Pigmented Epithelioid Melanocytoma: a low-grade melanocytic tumor with metastatic potential indistinguishable from animal-type melanoma and epithelioid blue nevus," *American Journal of Surgical Pathology*, vol. 28, no. 1, pp. 31–40, 2004.

[9] C. M. Magro, A. N. Crowson, M. C. Mihm, K. Gupta, M. J. Walker, and G. Solomon, "The dermal-based borderline melanocytic tumor: a categorical approach," *Journal of the American Academy of Dermatology*, vol. 62, no. 3, pp. 469–479, 2010.

[10] M. Matter, M. N. Lalonde, M. Allaoua et al., "The role of interval nodes in sentinel lymph node mapping and dissection for melanoma patients," *Journal of Nuclear Medicine*, vol. 48, no. 10, pp. 1607–1613, 2007.

[11] S. Maza, U. Trefzer, M. Hofmann et al., "Impact of sentinel lymph node biopsy in patients with Merkel cell carcinoma: results of a prospective study and review of the literature," *European Journal of Nuclear Medicine and Molecular Imaging*, vol. 33, no. 4, pp. 433–440, 2006.

[12] J. Ortin-Perez, M. C. van Rijk, R. A. Valdes-Olmos et al., "Lymphatic mapping and sentinel node biopsy in Merkel's cell carcinoma," *European Journal of Surgical Oncology*, vol. 33, no. 1, pp. 119–122, 2007.

[13] R. E. Warner, M. J. Quinn, G. Hruby, R. A. Scolyer, R. F. Uren, and J. F. Thompson, "Management of Merkel cell carcinoma: the roles of lymphoscintigraphy, sentinel lymph node biopsy and adjuvant radiotherapy," *Annals of Surgical Oncology*, vol. 15, no. 9, pp. 2509–2518, 2008.

[14] Y. Shnayder, D. T. Weed, D. J. Arnold et al., "Management of the neck in Merkel cell carcinoma of the head and neck: University of Miami experience," *Head and Neck*, vol. 30, no. 12, pp. 1559–1565, 2008.

[15] E. Bajetta, L. Celio, M. Platania et al., "Single-institution series of early-stage merkel cell carcinoma: long-term outcomes in 95 patients managed with surgery alone," *Annals of Surgical Oncology*, vol. 16, no. 11, pp. 2985–2993, 2009.

[16] R. C. Fields, K. J. Busam, J. F. Chou et al., "Recurrence and survival in patients undergoing sentinel lymph node biopsy for merkel cell carcinoma: analysis of 153 patients from a single institution," *Annals of Surgical Oncology*, vol. 18, no. 9, pp. 2529–2537, 2011.

[17] J. Howle and M. Veness, "Sentinel lymph node biopsy in patients with Merkel cell carcinoma: an emerging role and the Westmead hospital experience," *The Australasian Journal of Dermatology*, vol. 53, no. 1, pp. 26–31, 2012.

[18] R. Cecchi, L. Buralli, and C. De Gaudio, "Sentinel lymphonodectomy in non-melanoma skin cancers," *Chirurgia Italiana*, vol. 58, no. 3, pp. 347–351, 2006.

[19] J. D. Wagner, D. Z. Evdokimow, E. Weisberger et al., "Sentinel node biopsy for high-risk nonmelanoma cutaneous malignancy," *Archives of Dermatology*, vol. 140, no. 1, pp. 75–79, 2004.

[20] F. J. Civantos, F. L. Moffat, and W. J. Goodwin, "Lymphatic mapping and sentinel lymphadenectomy for 106 head and neck lesions: contrasts between oral cavity and cutaneous malignancy," *Laryngoscope*, vol. 116, no. 3, pp. 1–15, 2006.

[21] K. U. Sian, J. D. Wagner, R. Sood, H. M. Park, R. Havlik, and J. J. Coleman, "Lymphoscintigraphy with sentinel lymph node biopsy in cutaneous merkel cell carcinoma," *Annals of Plastic Surgery*, vol. 42, no. 6, pp. 679–682, 1999.

[22] F. C. Cobey, L. H. Engrav, M. B. Klein, C. N. Isom, and D. R. Byrd, "Brief report: sentinel lymph node dissection and burn scar carcinoma. Sentinel node and burn scar carcinoma," *Burns*, vol. 34, no. 2, pp. 271–274, 2008.

[23] N. Hatta, R. Morita, M. Yamada, K. Takehara, K. Ichiyanagi, and K. Yokoyama, "Implications of popliteal lymph node detected by sentinel lymph node biopsy," *Dermatologic Surgery*, vol. 31, no. 3, pp. 327–330, 2005.

[24] A. Lucci, L. M. McCall, P. D. Beitsch et al., "Surgical complications associated with sentinel lymph node dissection (SLND) plus axillary lymph node dissection compared with SLND alone in the American College of Surgeons Oncology Group trial Z0011," *Journal of Clinical Oncology*, vol. 25, no. 24, pp. 3657–3663, 2007.

[25] W. R. Wrightson, S. L. Wong, M. J. Edwards et al., "Complications associated with sentinel lymph node biopsy for melanoma," *Annals of Surgical Oncology*, vol. 10, no. 6, pp. 676–680, 2003.

[26] Y. Masannat, H. Shenoy, V. Speirs, A. Hanby, and K. Horgan, "Properties and characteristics of the dyes injected to assist axillary sentinel node localization in breast surgery," *European Journal of Surgical Oncology*, vol. 32, no. 4, pp. 381–384, 2006.

[27] M. J. Reschly, J. L. Messina, L. L. Zaulyanov, W. Cruse, and N. A. Fenske, "Utility of sentinel lymphadenectomy in the management of patients with high-risk cutaneous squamous cell carcinoma," *Dermatologic Surgery*, vol. 29, no. 2, pp. 135–140, 2003.

[28] K. D. Brantsch, C. Meisner, B. Schönfisch et al., "Analysis of risk factors determining prognosis of cutaneous squamous-cell carcinoma: a prospective study," *The Lancet Oncology*, vol. 9, no. 8, pp. 713–720, 2008.

[29] M. J. Veness, "Defining patients with high-risk cutaneous squamous cell carcinoma," *The Australasian Journal of Dermatology*, vol. 47, no. 1, pp. 28–33, 2006.

[30] J. T. Mullen, L. Feng, Y. Xing et al., "Invasive squamous cell carcinoma of the skin: defining a high-risk group," *Annals of Surgical Oncology*, vol. 13, no. 7, pp. 902–909, 2006.

[31] B. S. Cherpelis, C. Marcusen, and P. G. Lang, "Prognostic factors for metastasis in squamous cell carcinoma of the skin," *Dermatologic Surgery*, vol. 28, no. 3, pp. 268–273, 2002.

[32] F. O. Zwald and M. Brown, "Skin cancer in solid organ transplant recipients: advances in therapy and management: part I. Epidemiology of skin cancer in solid organ transplant recipients," *Journal of the American Academy of Dermatology*, vol. 65, no. 2, pp. 263–279, 2011.

[33] J. J. Bonerandi, C. Beauvillain, L. Caquant et al., "Guidelines for the diagnosis and treatment of cutaneous squamous cell carcinoma and precursor lesions," *Journal of the European Academy of Dermatology and Venereology*, vol. 25, supplement 5, pp. 1s–51s, 2011.

[34] H. Demir, T. Isken, E. Kus et al., "Sentinel lymph node biopsy with a gamma probe in patients with high-risk cutaneous squamous cell carcinoma: follow-up results of sentinel lymph node-negative patients," *Nuclear Medicine Communications*, vol. 32, no. 12, pp. 1216–1222, 2011.

[35] S. Kwon, Z. M. Dong, and P. C. Wu, "Sentinel lymph node biopsy for high-risk cutaneous squamous cell carcinoma: clinical experience and review of literature," *World Journal of Surgical Oncology*, vol. 9, p. 80, 2011.

[36] A. Jambusaria-Pahlajani, S. D. Hess, K. A. Katz, D. Berg, and C. D. Schmults, "Uncertainty in the perioperative management of high-risk cutaneous squamous cell carcinoma among Mohs surgeons," *Archives of Dermatology*, vol. 146, no. 11, pp. 1225–1231, 2010.

[37] A. L. Eastman, W. A. Erdman, G. M. Lindberg, J. L. Hunt, G. F. Purdue, and J. B. Fleming, "Sentinel lymph node biopsy identifies occult nodal metastases in patients with Marjolin's ulcer," *Journal of Burn Care and Rehabilitation*, vol. 25, no. 3, pp. 241–245, 2004.

[38] R. Cecchi, L. Buralli, and C. De Gaudio, "Lymphatic mapping and sentinel lymphonodectomy in recurrent cutaneous squamous cell carcinomas," *European Journal of Dermatology*, vol. 15, no. 6, pp. 478–479, 2005.

[39] M. Yamada, N. Hatta, K. Sogo, K. Komura, Y. Hamaguchi, and K. Takehara, "Management of squamous cell carcinoma in a patient with recessive-type epidermolysis bullosa dystrophica," *Dermatologic Surgery*, vol. 30, no. 11, pp. 1424–1429, 2004.

[40] K. B. Calder and B. R. Smoller, "New insights into merkel cell carcinoma," *Advances in Anatomic Pathology*, vol. 17, no. 3, pp. 155–161, 2010.

[41] H. T. Eich, D. Eich, S. Staar et al., "Role of postoperative radiotherapy in the management of Merkel cell carcinoma," *American Journal of Clinical Oncology*, vol. 25, no. 1, pp. 50–56, 2002.

[42] P. Mojica, D. Smith, and J. D. I. Ellenhorn, "Adjuvant radiation therapy is associated with improved survival in merkel cell carcinoma of the skin," *Journal of Clinical Oncology*, vol. 25, no. 9, pp. 1043–1047, 2007.

[43] W. Goessling, P. H. McKee, and R. J. Mayer, "Merkel cell carcinoma," *Journal of Clinical Oncology*, vol. 20, no. 2, pp. 588–598, 2002.

[44] J. B. Stokes, K. S. Graw, L. T. Dengel et al., "Patients with Merkel cell carcinoma tumors ≤ 1.0 cm in diameter are unlikely to harbor regional lymph node metastasis," *Journal of Clinical Oncology*, vol. 27, no. 23, pp. 3772–3777, 2009.

[45] J. L. Schwartz, K. A. Griffith, L. Lowe et al., "Features predicting sentinel lymph node positivity in merkel cell carcinoma," *Journal of Clinical Oncology*, vol. 29, no. 8, pp. 1036–1041, 2011.

[46] L. D. Su, L. Lowe, C. R. Bradford, A. I. Yahanda, T. M. Johnson, and V. K. Sondak, "Immunostaining for cytokeratin 20 improves detection of micrometastatic Merkel cell carcinoma in sentinel lymph nodes," *Journal of the American Academy of Dermatology*, vol. 46, no. 5, pp. 661–666, 2002.

[47] P. J. Allen, K. Busam, A. D. K. Hill, A. Stojadinovic, and D. G. Coit, "Immunohistochemical analysis of sentinel lymph nodes from patients with Merkel cell carcinoma," *Cancer*, vol. 92, no. 6, pp. 1650–1655, 2001.

[48] T. S. Wang, P. J. Byrne, L. K. Jacobs, and J. M. Taube, "Merkel cell carcinoma: update and review," *Seminars in Cutaneous Medicine and Surgery*, vol. 30, no. 1, pp. 48–56, 2011.

[49] J. H. Ruan and M. Reeves, "A Merkel cell carcinoma treatment algorithm," *Archives of Surgery*, vol. 144, no. 6, pp. 582–585, 2009.

[50] J. F. Buell, J. Trofe, M. J. Hanaway et al., "Immunosuppression and merkel cell cancer," *Transplantation Proceedings*, vol. 34, no. 5, pp. 1780–1781, 2002.

[51] B. D. Lemos, B. E. Storer, J. G. Iyer et al., "Pathologic nodal evaluation improves prognostic accuracy in Merkel cell carcinoma: analysis of 5823 cases as the basis of the first consensus staging system," *Journal of the American Academy of Dermatology*, vol. 63, no. 5, pp. 751–761, 2010.

[52] R. Murali, R. N. Sharma, J. F. Thompson et al., "Sentinel lymph node biopsy in histologically ambiguous melanocytic tumors with spitzoid features (so-called atypical spitzoid tumors)," *Annals of Surgical Oncology*, vol. 15, no. 1, pp. 302–309, 2008.

[53] R. V. Mandal, R. Murali, K. F. Lundquist et al., "Pigmented epithelioid melanocytoma: favorable outcome after 5-year follow-up," *American Journal of Surgical Pathology*, vol. 33, no. 12, pp. 1778–1782, 2009.

[54] K. L. Hollowell, S. C. Agle, E. E. Zervos, and T. L. Fitzgerald, "Cutaneous apocrine adenocarcinoma: defining epidemiology, outcomes, and optimal therapy for a rare neoplasm," *Journal of Surgical Oncology*, vol. 105, no. 4, pp. 415–419, 2012.

[55] H. C. Hsu, C. Y. Ho, C. H. Chen, C. H. Yang, H. S. Hong, and Y. H. Chuang, "Aggressive digital papillary adenocarcinoma: a review," *Clinical and Experimental Dermatology*, vol. 35, no. 2, pp. 113–119, 2010.

[56] M. Beyeler, W. Kempf, J. Hafner, G. Burg, and R. Dummer, "The spectrum of mesenchymal skin neoplasms reflected by the new WHO classification," *Onkologie*, vol. 27, no. 4, pp. 401–406, 2004.

[57] E. S. T. Tan, M. B. Y. Tang, and S. H. Tan, "Retrospective 5-year review of 131 patients with mycosis fungoides and Sézary syndrome seen at the National Skin Centre, Singapore," *The Australasian Journal of Dermatology*, vol. 47, no. 4, pp. 248–252, 2006.

[58] C. H. Wang, H. C. Nien, M. F. Hou, G. S. Chen, and S. T. Cheng, "Sentinel lymphadenectomy for circumscribed cutaneous T-cell lymphoma," *Dermatologic Surgery*, vol. 30, no. 6, pp. 952–956, 2004.

6

Sunscreen Use on the Dorsal Hands at the Beach

Donald B. Warren,[1] Ryan R. Riahi,[2] Jason B. Hobbs,[1] and Richard F. Wagner Jr.[1]

[1] Department of Dermatology, The University of Texas Medical Branch, 301 University Boulevard, Galveston, TX 77555-0783, USA
[2] Department of Dermatology, Louisiana State University, New Orleans, LA 70112-2865, USA

Correspondence should be addressed to Richard F. Wagner Jr.; rfwagner@utmb.edu

Academic Editor: Giuseppe Argenziano

Background. Since skin of the dorsal hands is a known site for the development of cutaneous squamous cell carcinoma, an epidemiologic investigation was needed to determine if beachgoers apply sunscreen to the dorsal aspect of their hands as frequently as they apply it to other skin sites. *Aim.* The aim of the current study was to compare the use of sunscreen on the dorsal hands to other areas of the body during subtropical late spring and summer sunlight exposure at the beach. *Materials and Methods.* A cross-sectional survey from a convenience sample of beachgoers was designed to evaluate respondent understanding and protective measures concerning skin cancer on the dorsal hands in an environment with high natural UVR exposure. *Results.* A total of 214 surveys were completed and analyzed. Less than half of subjects (105, 49%) applied sunscreen to their dorsal hands. Women applied sunscreen to the dorsal hands more than men (55% women versus 40% men, $P = 0.04$). Higher Fitzpatrick Skin Type respondents were less likely to protect their dorsal hands from ultraviolet radiation ($P = 0.001$). *Conclusions.* More public education focused on dorsal hand protection from ultraviolet radiation damage is necessary to reduce the risk for squamous cell carcinomas of the hands.

1. Introduction

Sunlight exposure, particularly ultraviolet radiation (UVR), is recognized as a risk factor for skin cancer. Photoprotection may reduce the risk of developing skin cancer. However, what efforts are made to protect the dorsal aspect of hands from UVR is unknown.

There are over a million cases of skin cancer diagnosed each year in the United States (US), and this number is expected to double in the next 30 years [1–3]. About 2000 deaths occur each year from nonmelanotic skin cancers in the US. The cost of care for nonmelanoma skin cancers is the fifth highest for all cancers in the US Medicare population [4]. Many factors contribute to the risk for developing skin cancer including UV exposure, low Fitzpatrick Skin Types, male gender, and advanced age. However, unprotected UVR exposure is the single most important environmental risk factor for developing most nonmelanocytic skin cancers.

Several studies have evaluated photoprotective behaviors on anatomic regions that are frequently partially or completely unprotected from UVR damage, such as the scalp, lips, and eyelids [5–7]. The dorsal hands, along with the face,

forearms, neck, and legs receive the most sunlight exposure, but unlike the forearms and legs, the hands are often unprotected by clothing. In lower latitudes during the midday hours, the dorsal hands are exposed to more sunlight than any other body part [8]. This additional UVR exposure may put skin of the dorsal hand at increased risk for developing skin cancer. Squamous cell carcinoma (SCC) is more common than basal cell carcinoma on the dorsal hand. It has been estimated that 58–90% of all hand malignancies are due to SCC [9]. Some investigators cite metastasis rates of 2–5% for SCC, while others estimate 10–28% [10, 11]. Local recurrence rates for SCC on the dorsal hands are as high as 22–28% [11, 12]. Men have a much higher incidence of cancer on the dorsal hands than women. One study found that the ratio of male to female SCC is 3 : 1 in this location [13]. Contributing factors to the current male predominance of dorsal hand SCC are the historic male predominance in many outdoor professions and some outdoor recreational activities such as fishing and golf. Men might also be less likely to wear sunscreen on their hands or use lotions with a sun protection factor (SPF) rating.

The primary goal of this survey was to determine if beachgoers protected the dorsal skin of their hands as frequently as other areas of their skin. The secondary goal of this study was to collect additional information about subject demographics and knowledge about skin cancer to determine if these variables were significantly correlated with UVR dorsal hand protection.

2. Materials and Methods

Following approval of the study protocol by The University of Texas Institutional Review Board, three of the authors (DW, RR, and JH) distributed anonymous questionnaires developed by authors (the appendices) to a convenience sample of beachgoers on Galveston Island, TX, public beaches who were at least 18 years of age. Data were gathered from late May to early September during 2011 on days with an average temperature greater than 80 F and with less than 50% cloud coverage. Data were collected about subjects' age, gender, Fitzpatrick Skin Type (FST), UVR skin and hand protection behaviors, duration of time spent at the beach when the survey was performed, and other protective behaviors including hats, umbrellas, shirts, and lip protection, and baseline knowledge questions regarding skin and hand cancer. In order to assess dorsal hand protection among different age ranges, participants were grouped into one of the 4 categories: 18–34 years old, 35–49 years old, 50–64 years old, and 65 years old or older. Associations between two factors were assessed using the Pearson chi-square test. The chi-square test was assessed at the 0.05 level of significance. Data analyses were carried out using PROC FREQ in the SAS system, release 9.2 [14].

3. Results

A total of 214 questionnaires were completed and analyzed. The average age of respondents was 40 years old and ranged from 18 to 86 years. The self-reported FSTs among the study population were 4% Type 1, 19% Type 2, 41% Type 3, 22% Type 4, 9% Type 5, and 5% Type 6. The questionnaires included data from 149 participants (70%) who reported sunscreen use somewhere on their bodies and 65 (30%) who did not apply sunscreen anywhere. Among those who used a sunscreen while being at the beach, 65% applied a lotion-based sunscreen and 35% applied a spray. However, the rate of photoprotection to the dorsal hand was not significantly different when comparing lotions versus sprays ($P = 0.81$). Reapplication of sunscreen to the hand was also not affected by the type of sunscreen used ($P = 0.52$). Fewer than 65% of all responders applied sunscreen to their forearms while 35% did not.

Regarding the dorsal hands, 105 (49%) applied sunscreen while 109 (51%) did not. There was a significant difference ($P = 0.009$) between men and women with rates of sunscreen use in general (60% men versus 77% women) and sunscreen use to the dorsal hands (40% men versus 55% women, Table 1, $P = 0.04$).

Only 21% of the respondents reapplied sunscreen during their stay at the beach, but less (13%) reapplied it to the dorsal hands. Length of stay at the beach affected rates of overall

TABLE 1: Gender differences in dorsal hand UVR protection (women are more likely to apply sunscreen to their dorsal hands than men, $P = 0.04$).

Gender	Sunscreen %	No sunscreen %
Women	55.37	44.63
Men	40.23	59.77
Total	49.04	50.96

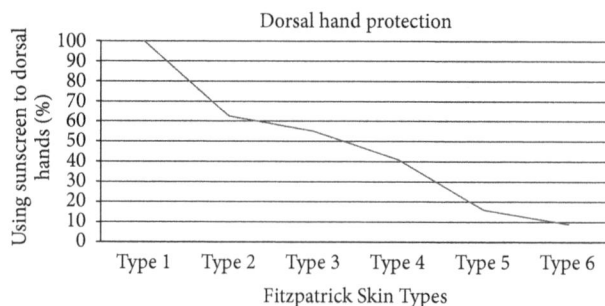

FIGURE 1: UVR dorsal hand protection in relation to Fitzpatrick Skin Types.

sunscreen use: 57% of those who stayed less than 2 hours applied sunscreen compared to 89% of those who stayed longer than 4 hours ($P = 0.0002$) but was not significantly different for dorsal hand protection. Those who stayed less than 2 hours exhibited a 45% dorsal hand protection rate, while 49% of those staying longer than 4 hours protected their hands ($P = 0.46$). When the forearm, an adjacent area, had received photoprotection, 21% of that group did not protect the dorsal hands. The most common reason given for not protecting the back of the hands was "did not think about it," followed by "did not like the feel of it." Higher FST respondents were less likely to protect their dorsal hands from UVR ($P = 0.001$). The rates of dorsal hand protection among each FST were 100% of Type 1 respondents who used photoprotection, 62.5% among Type 2 respondents, 55% among Type 3 respondents, 41% among Type 4 respondents, 16% among Type 5 respondents, and 9% among Type 6 respondents (Figure 1).

Photoprotection rates for the dorsal hands among self-identified ethnicities were the highest in Whites (57%), followed by Hispanics (44%), Asians (43%), other (27%), and the lowest in Blacks (7%, $P = 0.007$). Comparing age groups, the 18–34-year-old group was the least likely to protect the dorsal hands (37%, $P = 0.005$). Rates of other photoprotective measures such as cap/hat (45%), umbrella/shade (44%), lip protection (28%), and eyewear (71%) were also analyzed. Of these additional modes of photoprotective behavior, only umbrella/shade use correlated with dorsal hand protection ($P = 0.001$). Rates for hand protection associated with behaviors such as tobacco use and alcohol use were also surveyed. The data demonstrated that subjects engaging in these behaviors were less likely to protect their dorsal hands from UVR. Only 35% of tobacco users applied sunscreen to the backs of their hands compared to 54% of people who did not use tobacco products ($P = 0.01$). Respondents who drank more than 5 alcoholic beverages a week and applied dorsal hand protection (32%) were less likely to apply sunscreen to the hands than those who drank less (56%, $P = 0.001$). Other factors such as sunburns during the year ($P = 0.21$), outdoor occupations ($P = 0.18$), tanning salon use ($P = 0.89$), and personal or family history of skin cancer ($P = 0.32$) did not significantly influence rates of UVR dorsal hand protection.

Four baseline knowledge questions were also conducted during the survey. Question 1 asked if women were more likely to have skin cancer than men (correct answer is no), and 42% responded yes, 36% chose no, and 22% did not know. Question 2 asked if excessive sun exposure is linked to increased incidence of skin cancer (correct answer is yes) with 91% responding yes, 4% responding no, and 5% not knowing. Question 3 inquired if hand cancer is more common in younger people than older people (correct answer is no), and 51% said no, 16% said yes, and 33% did not know. Question 4 asked if hand cancer is more common in men than women (correct answer is yes), and 16% responded no, 46% said yes, and 38% did not know. Correct knowledge of any of the 4 baseline questions was not associated with significantly higher rates of UVR dorsal hand protection (Q1 $P = 0.52$, Q2 $P = 0.78$, Q3 $P = 0.07$, Q4 $P = 0.62$).

4. Discussion

Hand cancer is an important skin disease, and its potential outcomes on morbidity and mortality can be substantial [15]. Treatment often requires surgery [16]. Skin cancers on the hand are more likely to metastasize when compared to other nonmelanoma skin cancers affecting different skin areas. Cancers in this location may also be more likely to recur following treatment. UVR has been shown to be a risk factor in the development of nonmelanoma skin cancers involving the dorsal hands. This location typically receives higher amounts of UVR than most other body surface areas and depending on the time of day and latitude and may receive the most amount of UVR compared to all other skin areas. As with other skin areas like the scalp and lips, this study demonstrates that the dorsal hands are a neglected body area for photoprotection when compared to other areas where sunscreen is applied more frequently.

Our study population showed a low rate of dorsal hand photoprotection (49%) in an environment of high UVR exposure, the beach. Statistically significant differences were observed based on FST, ethnicity, gender, and age. Participants with low FSTs were more likely to apply sunscreen and on the dorsal hands compared to higher FST participants. With regards to ethnicity, the highest rates of dorsal hand protection were found in Whites and the lowest in Blacks. Women were more likely to use sunscreen in general and on the dorsal hands compared to their male counterparts. This later finding is important because hand cancer historically affects males more than females by a 3 : 1 ratio. Several factors are likely responsible for this skewed incidence, including traditional workforce gender imbalances. Inadequate photoprotective behaviors by men also may play a role in their higher rates of dorsal hand cancer compared to women.

Total skin protection from UVR exposure is the best primary prevention for decreasing the incidence of UVR related skin cancers, but previous research indicates that specific anatomic locations such as the lips, eyelids, and scalp are less protected by beachgoers. More public education focused on dorsal hand protection from UVR damage is necessary to reduce skin cancers in this location. This educational need is also evident based on responses to the baseline knowledge survey regarding hand cancer. Although the majority of people understand that UVR is a risk factor for skin cancer (91%), only 51% were aware that hand cancer is more common in the elderly and that men are more affected than women (46%). Protection of the dorsal hands from sunlight may also delay or prevent the appearance of photoaging in this anatomic location. Helpful strategies to inform the public about hand cancer could come from pamphlets about skin cancer found in healthcare providers' offices and other health promotion activities. Sunscreen manufacturers could also list commonly neglected areas of photoprotection with the directions for product use. Media campaigns should focus on reaching younger demographics as this study found that the 18–34-year-old population was the least likely to protect the dorsal hands (37%). This younger population would potentially benefit the most from such photoprotective intervention due to less lifetime cumulative exposure to this frequently encountered environmental carcinogen. These preventative efforts may improve public awareness and hopefully lower the future incidence of hand cancers.

5. Conclusions

Surveyed Galveston beachgoers were less likely to protect their dorsal hands from UVR injury than other areas of skin. UVR protection of the dorsal hands deserves emphasis in public health messages about skin cancer protection, along with other identified body locations such as the scalp, lips, and eyelids.

Appendices

Age (must be 18 or older for survey)

Gender:

(1) Female
(2) Male

Skin Type:

(1) Pale white; always burns, does not tan
(2) White; burns easily, tans with difficulty
(3) Cream/Light Brown; tans after initial sunburn
(4) Brown; burns minimally, tans easily
(5) Dark Brown; rarely burns, tans easily
(6) Black; never burns, tans easily

Ethnicity

(1) Asian/Pacific Islander
(2) Black
(3) Hispanic
(4) White
(5) Other

A. Sun Protection

Do you currently have sunburn anywhere?

(1) No
(2) Yes

How many hours have you been at the beach today?

(1) 0–2 hours
(2) More than 2 hours but less than 4 hours
(3) More than 4 hours but less than 6 hours
(4) More than 6 hours

Did you apply sunscreen on today? What is SPF?

(1) No
(2) <15 SPF
(3) 15–30 SPF
(4) >30 SPF
(5) Yes, but I don't know what is SPF

If yes, what type of sunscreen did you use?

(1) Lotion
(2) Spray

Did you apply sunscreen to the *back of your hands*?

(1) No
(2) Yes
(3) Not sure

If No, why not?

(1) Did not think about it
(2) Did not like feel of it (oily, greasy, etc.)
(3) Other

Did you apply sunscreen to your *forearms*?

(1) No
(2) Yes
(3) Not sure

If No, why not?

(1) Did not think about it
(2) Did not like feel of it (oily, greasy, etc.)
(3) Other

How many applications of sunscreen did you use on your skin today?

1   2   3   4 or more

How many applications of sunscreen did you use on the *back of your hands* today?

1   2   3   4 or more

How many applications of sunscreen did you use on your *forearms* today?

1   2   3   4 or more

Why did you *reapply* sunscreen to your skin today?

(1) Did not reapply
(2) Time for another application
(3) Sweating/swimming
(4) Skin redness
(5) Other reason? Please tell us

Why did you *reapply* sunscreen to the *back of your hands* today?

(1) Did not reapply
(2) Time for another application
(3) Sweating/swimming
(4) Skin redness
(5) Other reason? Please tell us

Why did you reapply sunscreen to your *forearms* today?

(1) Did not reapply
(2) Time for another application
(3) Sweating/swimming
(4) Skin redness
(5) Other reason? Please tell us

Did you use any of the following forms of skin sun protection today:

Clothing:

(1) only bathing suit
(2) short-sleeved shirt or shorts
(3) long-sleeved shirt or pants

Hat:

(1) none
(2) Cap (no ear protection from sun)
(3) Hat with brim of 3 inches or less
(4) Hat with brim of more than 3 inches

Umbrella/Shade:

(1) No
(2) Yes

Lipstick or Lip Balm with SPF:

(1) No
(2) Yes

Eyewear:

(1) No
(2) Yes

B. Skin Cancer Risk Factors

How many sunburns have you had this summer?

Sunburn = redness > 24 hours and/or peeling, pain, swelling, blistering

Do you use tobacco products?

(1) No
(2) Yes

Do you have more than 5 alcoholic drinks per week?

(1) No
(2) Yes

While at work, do you spend part of your time outdoors?

(1) No
(2) Yes

Did you use indoor tanning salons in the past year?

(1) No
(2) Monthly
(3) Weekly
(4) Daily

Did you or a family member ever have a skin cancer?

(1) No
(2) Self
(3) Immediate Family
(4) Extended Family
(5) I don't know

Did you or a family member ever have a skin cancer on the *back of the hand*?

(1) No
(2) Self
(3) Immediate Family
(4) Extended Family
(5) I don't know

Did you or a family member ever have a skin cancer on the *forearm*?

(1) No
(2) Self
(3) Immediate Family
(4) Extended Family
(5) I don't know

C. Baseline Knowledge

(1) Women are more likely to get skin cancer than men?

(1) No
(2) Yes
(3) I don't know

(2) Excessive sun exposure to the skin can increase the risk of skin cancer?

(1) No
(2) Yes
(3) I don't know

(3) Hand cancer is more common in younger people than older people?

(1) No
(2) Yes
(3) I don't know

(4) Men get more hand cancer than women?

(1) No
(2) Yes
(3) I don't know

References

[1] H. W. Rogers, M. A. Weinstock, A. R. Harris et al., "Incidence estimate of nonmelanoma skin cancer in the United States, 2006," *Archives of Dermatology*, vol. 146, no. 3, pp. 283–287, 2010.

[2] American Cancer Society, *Cancer Facts & Figures 2010*, American Cancer Society, Atlanta, Ga, USA, 2010.

[3] J. S. Rhee, B. A. Matthews, M. Neuburg, B. R. Logan, M. Burzynski, and A. B. Nattinger, "The skin cancer index: clinical responsiveness and predictors of quality of life," *Laryngoscope*, vol. 117, no. 3, pp. 399–405, 2007.

[4] T. S. Housman, S. R. Feldman, P. M. Williford et al., "Skin cancer is among the most costly of all cancers to treat for the Medicare population," *Journal of the American Academy of Dermatology*, vol. 48, no. 3, pp. 425–429, 2003.

[5] D. J.) Heiner, D. B. Warren, T. Uchida, and R. F. Wagner Jr., "Preventing ultraviolet radiation scalp injury in men," *Household and Personal Care Today*, vol. 4, pp. 18–20, 2011.

[6] T. L. Busick, T. Uchida, and R. F. Wagner Jr., "Preventing ultraviolet light lip injury: beachgoer awareness about lip cancer risk factors and lip protection behavior," *Dermatologic Surgery*, vol. 31, no. 2, pp. 173–176, 2005.

[7] P. M. Houghtaling, T. Foster, D. J. Heiner, T. Uchida T, and R. F. Wagner Jr., "Eyelid protection from ultraviolet radiation injury at the beach," *HPC Supplement Focus on Sun Care*, vol. 3, pp. 12–14, 2010.

[8] N. Downs and A. Parisi, "Measurements of the anatomical distribution of erythemal ultraviolet: a study comparing exposure distribution to the site incidence of solar keratoses, basal cell carcinoma and squamous cell carcinoma," *Photochemical and Photobiological Sciences*, vol. 8, no. 8, pp. 1195–1201, 2009.

[9] J. A. Fink and E. Akelman, "Nonmelanotic malignant skin tumors of the hand," *Hand Clinics*, vol. 11, no. 2, pp. 255–264, 1995.

[10] C. R. W. Rayner, "The results of treatment of two hundred and seventy-three carcinomas of the hand," *Hand*, vol. 13, no. 2, pp. 183–186, 1981.

[11] M. Schiavon, F. Mazzoleni, A. Chiarelli, and P. Matano, "Squamous cell carcinoma of the hand: fifty-five case reports," *Journal of Hand Surgery*, vol. 13, no. 3, pp. 401–404, 1988.

[12] F. C. Ames and R. C. Hickey, "Metastasis from squamous cell skin cancer of the extremities," *Southern Medical Journal*, vol. 75, no. 8, pp. 920–932, 1982.

[13] I. Chakrabarti, J. D. Watson, and D. H. Dorrance, "Skin tumors of the hand: a 10-year review," *Journal of Hand Surgery* , vol. 18, no. 4, pp. 484–486, 1993.

[14] SAS Institute Inc., *SAS/STAT 9.2 User's Guide*, SAS Institute Inc., Cary, NC, USA, 2008.

[15] R. F. Wagner Jr. and W. I. Cottel, "Treatment of squamous and basal cell carcinomas of the hand with Mohs micrographic surgery: analysis of 53 consecutive patients," *Skin Cancer*, vol. 4, no. 2, pp. 73–77, 1989.

[16] K. S. Joyner, B. Wilson, R. F. Wagner Jr., and S. F. Viegas, "Marginal excision of squamous cell carcinomas of the hand," *Orthopedics*, vol. 31, no. 1, article 79, 2008.

7

Locally Advanced and Unresectable Cutaneous Squamous Cell Carcinoma: Outcomes of Concurrent Cetuximab and Radiotherapy

Robert M. Samstein,[1] Alan L. Ho,[2] Nancy Y. Lee,[1] and Christopher A. Barker[1]

[1] Department of Radiation Oncology, Memorial Sloan Kettering Cancer Center, 1275 York Avenue, Box 22, New York, NY 10065, USA
[2] Department of Medicine, Memorial Sloan Kettering Cancer Center, New York, NY 10065, USA

Correspondence should be addressed to Christopher A. Barker; barkerc@mskcc.org

Academic Editor: Arash Kimyai-Asadi

Background. Advanced age and immune dysfunction are risk factors for cutaneous squamous cell carcinoma (cSCC) and often render patients with locally-advanced disease medically inoperable or surgically unresectable, but potentially curable with radiotherapy. Concurrent chemotherapy and radiotherapy may not be well tolerated in this population, but another systemic therapy may improve disease control. *Objective.* Determine the tolerance and efficacy of concurrent cetuximab and radiotherapy (CRT) for patients with locally advanced and unresectable cSCC. *Methods.* Retrospective analysis of 12 patients treated with CRT for locally advanced and unresectable cSCC. *Results.* Patients were elderly and 75% had moderate-to-severe comorbidities, while 42% had immune dysfunction. Grades 3-4 adverse events were noted in 83% of patients; 67% required hospital admission for adverse events. Complete and partial response was noted in 36% and 27% (response rate, 64%). Stable and progressive disease was noted in 3 and 1 patients, respectively (disease control rate, 91%). Median progression-free and overall survival were 6.4 and 8.0 months, respectively. *Limitations.* Retrospective small-cohort, single-institution analysis. *Conclusion.* Patients selected for CRT were elderly, with comorbidities and immune dysfunction, but treatment responses were observed. Patients selected for this treatment approach have a poor prognosis with limited capacity for therapy; more effective treatment is needed.

1. Introduction

Cutaneous squamous cell carcinoma (cSCC) is one of the most common cancers in the United States with an increasing incidence over the past few decades. The disease often presents at an early stage and is controlled with surgical, radiation, topical, or photodynamic therapy. Advanced age and immune dysfunction are risk factors for cSCC and render some patients medically unfit for surgery at diagnosis or recurrence. Moreover, some patients present with extensive local invasion or metastasis, rendering the cSCC surgically unresectable. Patients with locally advanced cSCC that are medically inoperable or surgically unresectable have a poor prognosis but can be cured with radiotherapy [1, 2].

Improving the outcome of radiotherapy through the use of concurrent systemic therapy has been demonstrated in several locally advanced cancer-treatment paradigms. Platinum (e.g., cisplatin, carboplatin) and halogenated pyrimidine (e.g., 5-fluorouracil) chemotherapies are frequently used in conjunction with radiotherapy to improve treatment efficacy but may not be well tolerated by patients of advanced age, or those who are immunosuppressed or harbor significant comorbidities [3]. For this particular patient population, a systemic therapy to combine with radiotherapy that is effective and well tolerated is needed.

Cetuximab (Erbitux, Genentech) is a monoclonal chimeric IgG1 antibody that binds and blocks the epidermal growth factor receptor (EGFR). EGFR, a transmembrane tyrosine kinase, has been shown to be upregulated in a variety of squamous cell carcinomas and its downstream antiapoptotic signaling cascade has been well studied [4]. In cSCC, series have reported EGFR overexpression in 43–100% of patients studied [5–8], and overexpression appears to be more common in patients with metastasizing cSCC [9]. Reports from small clinical trials have indicated that cetuximab has activity in metastatic or unresectable cSCC, either alone or in combination with other therapies [10, 11].

Cetuximab has been approved by the Food and Drug Administration for use in combination with radiotherapy for mucosal squamous cell carcinoma of the head and neck based on a large randomized trial demonstrating improved survival compared with radiotherapy alone [12, 13]. Cetuximab is thought to function as a radiosensitizer contributing to a synergistic effect when it is combined with radiotherapy [14]. The combination of cetuximab and radiotherapy (CRT) has also been tested in several other EGFR-expressing squamous cell carcinomas including lung, anal, esophageal, and uterine cervix squamous cell carcinoma [15–18]. There is little data available on the safety and effectiveness of CRT in patients with advanced cSCC. We thus sought to retrospectively study the toxicity and efficacy of combination CRT in patients with advanced cSCC treated at our institution.

2. Methods

2.1. Patients. Review of medical records was conducted with permission of the institutional review board (WA0552-11). Patients with cSCC that were selected for treatment with CRT were identified. Only patients that underwent concurrent treatment with both modalities were included in the study.

Patient demographics, comorbidities, and details of cSCC diagnosis and stage at the time of CRT were recorded. Comorbidities were classified according to the Adult Comorbidity Evaluation-27 (ACE-27). This system identifies 27 common medical ailments among 12 organ systems or disease processes and provides criteria to grade the comorbidity on a scale of 0–3 (0, ailment not present; 1, mild decompensation; 2, moderate decompensation; 3, severe decompensation) [19]. Staging was performed according to the cutaneous squamous cell carcinoma system in the American Joint Committee on Cancer Staging Manual, version 7 [20].

2.2. Treatment and Adverse Events. Details of prior treatment including surgery, radiotherapy, and systemic therapy were reviewed and recorded. Common Terminology Criteria for Adverse Events version 4.0 (CTCAE v4.0) was used to assess, characterize, and grade adverse events observed during both cetuximab and radiotherapy [21].

2.3. Treatment Response. Treatment response within and outside the irradiated volume was assessed at the first posttreatment clinical and radiographic evaluations, 4–12 weeks after the completion of therapy. Formal imaging response assessment was not possible in some patients who were followed clinically (without imaging) after therapy and because of heterogeneous follow-up imaging. Operational

definitions based on the Response Evaluation Criteria in Solid Tumors (RECIST) and PET Response Criteria in Solid Tumors (PERCIST) were used and included complete response (CR, disappearance of lesion), partial response (PR, 30% decrease in longest dimension of lesion), stable disease (SD, no evidence of response or progression), and progressive disease (PD, 20% increase in longest dimension of the lesion). Overall and cSCC-specific survival were recorded.

2.4. Statistical Analysis. Kaplan-Meier curves were generated and used to estimate survival rates (with asymmetric 95% confidence intervals) and median survival times and to compare between groups of patients. Statistical analysis was conducted using Graphpad Prism v6.0c.

3. Results

3.1. Patients. Twelve patients were selected for treatment with concurrent cetuximab and radiotherapy for locally advanced or unresectable cSCC between 2007 and 2013. Three patients were excluded from analysis: one received induction systemic therapy with cetuximab, carboplatin, and paclitaxel, followed by radiotherapy alone; two patients received palliative cetuximab for distant metastases and received a brief course of palliative radiotherapy directed at a site of distant metastasis. As detailed in Table 1, most patients were elderly (median age, 78 years; range, 47–90), all were white, and all but one was male. Median Karnofsky performance score was 80 (range, 50–90). Most patients had moderate (42%) or severe (33%) comorbidities. Almost half (42%) of patients had identifiable immune dysfunction (chronic lymphocytic leukemia in 4, solid organ transplant in 1, and acquired immunodeficiency syndrome in 1).

The stage and presentation of cSCC is presented in Table 2. Most patients (75%) received CRT for recurrent cSCC. All but two patients with known primary tumors (82%) underwent excision; 4 of 9 patients had nodal recurrence after prior lymphadenectomy. No patients received prior chemotherapy for cSCC. All but one patient (who was given adjuvant CRT after surgical resection) had gross disease present at the start of treatment. All patients had locally advanced cSCC (T4 tumors) or regional nodal metastases. Two patients had distant metastases at the start of CRT.

3.2. Treatment and Adverse Events. All patients were treated with static-field intensity modulated radiation therapy using dynamic multileaf collimation. Treatment was delivered by a linear accelerator producing 6 MV photons or 6–9 MeV electrons, depending on the treatment target. One patient (number 3) was initially selected for concurrent cisplatin and radiotherapy but did not tolerate this and was switched to CRT. Conversely, one patient (number 6) was initially selected for CRT but did not tolerate this and was switched to carboplatin and paclitaxel concurrent with radiotherapy. The duration and relationship between cetuximab administration and radiotherapy are plotted in Figure 1. Radiation doses ranged between 12 and 80 Gy with a median dose of 60 Gy in 30 fractions (range, 3–38). Patients received cetuximab

TABLE 1: Patient characteristics.

Patient	Age	Sex	Race	Overall comorbidity severity	Moderate and severe comorbidities	KPS	Immune dysfunction
1	83	M	W	Mild		80	
2	82	F	W	Mild		80	CLL
3	70	M	W	Moderate	Respiratory	80	
4	59	M	W	Moderate	Cardiovascular (congestive heart failure, arrhythmia)	70	Heart transplant
5	78	M	W	Moderate	Obesity	80	
6	85	M	W	Moderate	Cardiovascular (arrhythmia)	80	
7	47	M	W	Severe	Immunologic (AIDS)	70	AIDS
8	78	M	W	Moderate	Malignancy (leukemia)	70	CLL
9	75	M	W	Severe	Endocrine (diabetes), respiratory, malignancy (leukemia)	90	CLL
10	77	M	W	Mild		80	
11	90	M	W	Severe	Malignancy (solid tumor)	50	
12	86	M	W	Severe	Malignancy (solid tumor)	60	

Demographic, comorbidity, and immune system dysfunction for each of the patients ($n = 12$) studied.
KPS: Karnofsky performance status, M: male, F: female, W: white, CLL: chronic lymphocytic leukemia, and AIDS: acquired immunodeficiency syndrome.

TABLE 2: Disease characteristics and treatment response.

Patient	Stage*	Recurrent	Gross disease	Posttreatment response within the irradiated volume	Months until PD (in or out of irradiated volume)
1	T4N2bM0	No	Yes	PR	6.4 (in)
2	T0N2bM0	Yes	Yes	CR	14.7 (in), 16.3 (out)
3	T0N2bM0R0	Yes	No	N/A	(Died with NED)
4	T4N0M0	Yes	Yes	SD	(Died without PD)
5	T0N1M0	Yes	Yes	CR	(Alive with NED)
6	T4N0M0	Yes	Yes	SD	(Alive with NED)
7	T2N2bM0	No	Yes	PD (during treatment)	1.7 (in and out)
8	T0N2bM1	Yes	Yes	CR	2.1 (out), 5.0 (in)
9	T2N2bM0	Yes	Yes	CR	4.4 (out)
10	T4N0M0	Yes	Yes	SD	52.2 (in)
11	T0N3M1	Yes	Yes	PR	1.6 (out)
12	T4N0M0	No	Yes	PR	4.4 (out), 4.7 (in)

Disease status at the start of therapy and investigator assessed response 4–12 weeks after therapy are presented.
*All patients were staged clinically, except patient 3, who was staged pathologically.
PR: partial response, CR: complete response, SD: stable disease, PD: progressive disease, NED: no evidence of disease, IV: irradiated volume, and N/A: not applicable (because patient received adjuvant therapy [no measureable disease for response assessment]).

at $400 \, \text{mg/m}^2$, followed by weekly treatment at $250 \, \text{mg/m}^2$ through the end of radiotherapy, if they tolerated this treatment approach. Median cetuximab dose was $1525 \, \text{mg/m}^2$ (range, 400–2400). Treatment was delayed in 5 patients due to adverse events, and 2 patients had radiotherapy terminated early due to progression of disease. Eight patients were hospitalized during or soon after treatment. The frequency of grades 2–4 adverse events is shown in Table 3; no patient developed a grade 5 adverse event although 83% of patients experienced a grade 3 or higher event. The most common adverse events observed included fatigue, acneiform rash, radiation dermatitis, and infection.

3.3. *Treatment Response.* The best clinical response in the irradiated volume among the 11 patients treated for gross

disease (i.e., not adjuvantly) was CR in 4 patients (36%) and PR in 3 (27%), for an overall response rate of 64% (95% confidence interval, 35–92%). Median time to progression within the irradiated volume for patients achieving CR and PR was 9.9 and 6.4 months, respectively. Within the irradiated volume, SD was noted in 3 patients and PD in another patient, for a disease-control rate (DCR) of 91% (95% confidence interval, 74–100%). Both of the patients with distant metastases at the start of CRT had PD outside of the irradiated volume. Among patients without distant metastases at the start of CRT, PD occurred within the irradiated volume in 5 and outside the irradiated volume in 4. The patient treated with adjuvant CRT died 4.8 months after treatment of noncancer-related causes with no evidence of recurrent cSCC.

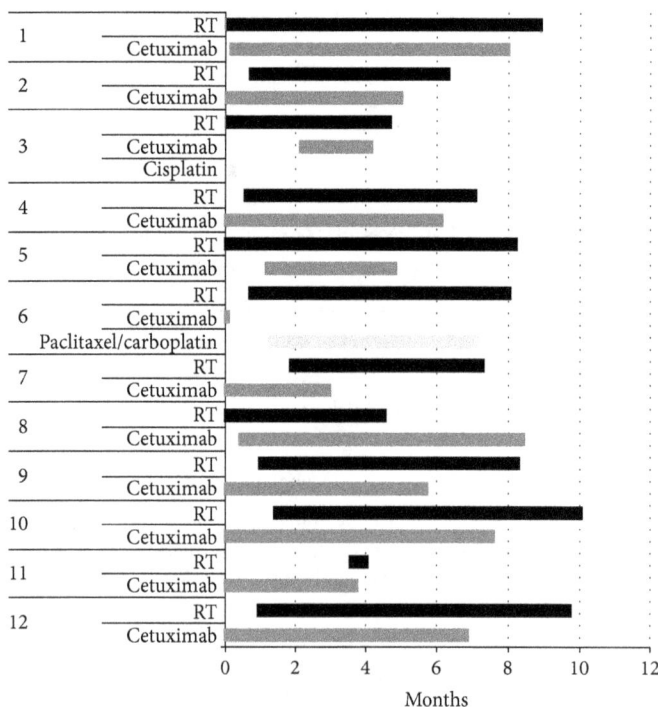

FIGURE 1: Relationship of cetuximab and radiotherapy. The duration of treatment and relationship in time for radiotherapy, cetuximab, and other systemic therapies is presented.

TABLE 3: Grades 2–4 adverse events occurring during cetuximab and radiotherapy classified according to the Common Terminology Criteria for Adverse Events, version 4.0; no grade 5 adverse events were observed.

Adverse event	Grade 2		Grade 3		Grade 4	
	N	(%)	N	(%)	N	(%)
Infusion reaction	1	(8)	0	(0)	0	(0)
Acneiform rash	5	(42)	0	(0)	0	(0)
Radiation dermatitis	5	(42)	3	(25)	0	(0)
Mucositis	3	(25)	2	(17)	0	(0)
Pneumonitis	0	(0)	1	(8)	1	(8)
Anemia	1	(8)	1	(8)	0	(0)
Thrombocytopenia	1	(8)	0	(0)	0	(0)
Neutropenia	0	(0)	1	(8)	0	(0)
Fatigue	7	(58)	1	(8)	0	(0)
Weight loss	2	(17)	0	(0)	0	(0)
Xerostomia	2	(17)	1	(8)	0	(0)
Dysphagia	3	(25)	1	(8)	0	(0)
Infection	2	(17)	3	(25)	0	(0)

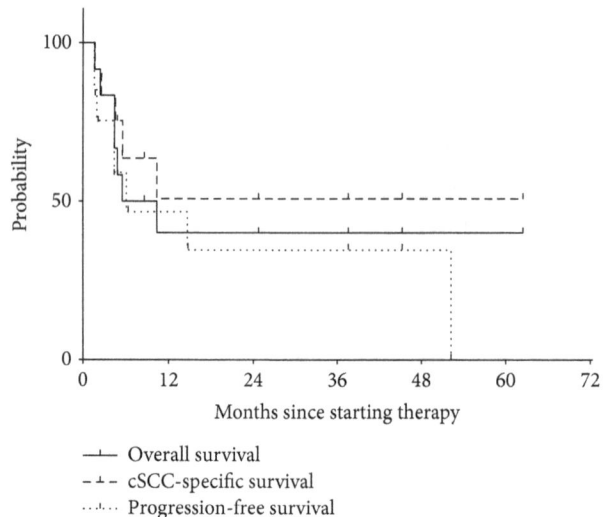

FIGURE 2: Overall, disease-specific, and progression-free survival. Median progression-free and overall survival were 6.4 and 8.0 months, respectively. Median cutaneous squamous cell carcinoma- (cSCC-) specific survival was not reached. cSCC-specific and overall survival were 51% (95% confidence interval, 26–85%) and 40% (95% confidence interval, 14–66%) at 2 years.

As noted in Figure 2, at the time of analysis, 7 of 12 (58%) patients studied had died. Five of 7 (71%) died of cSCC. Median follow-up for the entire cohort was 7.0 months but was 37.6 months for the 5 surviving patients. Median progression-free and overall survival were 6.4 and 7.95 months, respectively. Median cSCC-specific survival was not reached. cSCC-specific and overall survival were 51% (95% confidence interval, 26–85%) and 40% (95% confidence

interval, 14–66%) at 2 years. Median progression-free and overall survival were 2.1 and 3.6 months in patients with distant metastases at the start of CRT compared with 14.7 and 10.4 without distant metastases, respectively. Median overall survival of patients with immune dysfunction was 4.4

TABLE 4: Reported cases of cSCC treated with CRT.

Study design	First author	Publication year	Case number	Age	Sex	Radiotherapy dose (Gy)	Duration of therapy (weeks)	Response	Disease-free survival (months)
Case report	Kanakamedala MR	2010	—	78	M	n/r	8	CR	5
Case report	Goppner D	2010	—	85	F	45	n/r (<12)	CR	14
Case report	Wollina U	2011	—	77	M	60	6	CR	3
Case series	Giacchero D	2011	2	67	M	50	7	CR	3
Case series	Giacchero D	2011	3	72	M	60	7	CR	5
Case series	Giacchero D	2011	4	79	M	70	18	CR	21
Case series	Giacchero D	2011	8	78	M	70	7	PR	n/r
Case series	Alter M	2013	2	61	M	24	5	PR	5
Phase II trial	Preneau S	2014	8	62	M	60–70	n/r	PR	8
Phase II trial	Preneau S	2014	11	63	M	60–70	n/r	PR	8
Phase II trial	Preneau S	2014	16	83	F	60–70	n/r	PR	4
Phase II trial	Preneau S	2014	17	86	F	60–70	n/r	PR	5
Phase II trial	Preneau S	2014	20	77	M	60–70	n/r	SD	5

M: male, F: female, n/r: not reported, PR: partial response, CR: complete response, SD: stable disease, and PD: progressive disease.

months, while it was not reached among patients without immune dysfunction. Likewise, median survival of patients with moderate and severe comorbidities was 5.5 and 3.4 months, respectively, while it was not reached in patients with mild comorbidities.

4. Discussion

This study was designed to assess the efficacy and safety of the combination of cetuximab and radiotherapy in patients with advanced cSCC. We found that this treatment strategy yielded a response in 64% of patients, although disease progression after response was common and survival was limited. We found that patients selected for this treatment strategy were often elderly, with comorbidities and immune dysfunction. Despite the development of moderately severe adverse events, many patients required hospitalization in the period of time surrounding treatment. These results suggest that the patients we have selected for this treatment approach have a poor prognosis and limited capacity for therapy.

A multicenter phase II study of cetuximab monotherapy for unresectable cSCC was published in 2011. Thirty-six patients were accrued from 2005 to 2008, all of whom had performance status ≥2 and no immune dysfunction. Median age of the group was 79 years (range, 32–95). Unresectable cSCC was present at the site of the primary tumor, regional lymph nodes, and distant metastasis in 47, 44, and 8% of the group, respectively. Six weeks after receiving cetuximab (400 mg/m^2, then 250 mg/m^2 weekly), 3% of patients had a CR, 8% of patients had a PR, and 58% had SD, for a DCR of 69% (95% confidence interval, 52–84%). The best overall response rates were CR in 6%, PR in 22% (response rate, 28%; 95% confidence interval, 14–45%), and SD in 42% (DCR, 69%; 95% confidence interval, 52–84%). Median progression-free survival was 4.1 months (95% CI 1.7–5

months). Twenty-three patients (64%) experienced a serious adverse event (grades 3-4). Acneiform rash (but not genetic polymorphisms) was associated with favorable progression-free survival [10].

A single-center phase II study of cetuximab for unresectable cSCC was recently published. Among 20 patients accrued between 2009 and 2011, 5 were selected for treatment with radiotherapy (60–70 Gy) in conjunction with cetuximab (400 mg/m^2, followed by 250 mg/m^2 weekly for 3 weeks). One of the 5 patients receiving CRT was immunosuppressed, and the median age of this subgroup was 77 years. After 2 cycles of therapy (8 weeks) using RECIST criteria the authors observed no patient to have a CR, 4 of 5 (80%) a PR, and 1 of 5 (20%) SD, for a DCR of 100%. Median progression-free survival was 5 months. Four (80%) patients experienced a serious adverse event (grade 3-4). Patients selected to receive radiotherapy appeared to have a higher response rate (80%) than patients selected to receive carboplatin with cetuximab (response rate, 44%) or cetuximab alone (response rate, 33%) [11].

Between 2010 and the present, we have identified 10 patients with cSCC treated with CRT and reported in the medical literature as case reports or small case series. Table 4 provides details of 8 of these patients, in addition to the 5 patients treated with CRT from the phase II trial noted above. The median age of patients is 77 years (range, 61–85). Immune dysfunction was present in at least 1 patient. All had recurrent, unresectable cSCC. Most patients received cetuximab (400 mg/m^2, then 250 mg/m^2 weekly) for a median of 7 weeks and median radiation dose was 60 Gy. Six of eight (75%) patients from case reports or series were reported to have a complete response, while 2 of 8 (25%) were reported to have a partial response [22–26]. One patient treated for unresectable cSCC with CRT was described in another case series, but details were not reported [27]. Yet another case series reported a 62-year-old man treated with adjuvant CRT after resection of a locally advanced cSCC, with no evidence of recurrence 2 years after treatment [28].

The results of CRT described above are generally consistent with those in the present study. The studies have all reported groups of elderly patients, with a median age in the late eighth decade. Immune dysfunction was less common in the previously reported studies (0–20% of patients), compared with the present analysis (46.1%). Importantly, the prior studies of CRT did not report the presence of comorbidities, which were found to be moderate or severe in the majority (76%) of patients studied. Disease stage (and, specifically, the presence of distant metastasis) varied across the studies and is likely to be associated with the outcome of treatment. For these reasons, comparing the present results to prior studies is challenging. Nevertheless, the observed response rate of 64% is similar to the subset of patients in the recently published phase II study (80%).

Our study has several potential limitations. First, the number of patients studied was small ($n = 12$). However, to our knowledge, the present report is the largest single-institution experience of CRT of cSCC and nearly doubles the number of patients reported after treatment for cSCC with CRT in the medical literature. Second, the treatment approach varied among patients studied. This is a function of the extended time period during which this study took place, as well as the nuances of the specific patient and disease characteristics confronted by clinicians at our center. Nevertheless, cetuximab was given in a consistent fashion ($400 \, \text{mg/m}^2$, followed by $250 \, \text{mg/m}^2$ weekly), and radiotherapy was generally given to curative doses in conventional fractionation (60–70 Gy in 30–35 fractions) using standard static-field intensity-modulated techniques. Third, the methods for assessing response were not standardized. However, all patients underwent clinical evaluation and imaging within a relatively limited window of time after the completion of treatment, consistent with the prospective studies on this subject. Finally, the retrospective nature of this study with inherent selection biases and lack of a control group limits the strength of the conclusions that can be made. This study should therefore be used to generate hypotheses for future testing.

5. Conclusion

Our study was designed to assess the safety and efficacy of CRT for patients with locally advanced or metastatic unresectable cSCC. We found that the treatment was delivered to a group of elderly patients with moderate-to-severe comorbidities who often harbored immune dysfunction. Nevertheless, the majority of patients exhibited response to treatment. However, progression of disease typically followed soon thereafter. Progression-free and overall survival were limited, probably as a cumulative result of advanced age, comorbidities, immune dysfunction, and advanced cancer. Additional studies are needed to further improve outcomes by reducing the morbidity and increasing the efficacy of treatment.

Abbreviations

ACE-27:	Adult Comorbidity Evaluation-27
CI:	Confidence interval
CR:	Complete response
CRT:	Concurrent cetuximab and radiotherapy
cSCC:	Cutaneous squamous cell carcinoma
CTCAE:	Common Terminology Criteria for Adverse Events
DCR:	Disease control rate
EGFR:	Epidermal growth factor receptor
PD:	Progressive disease
PERCIST:	PET Response Criteria in Solid Tumors
PR:	Partial response
RECIST:	Response Evaluation Criteria in Solid Tumors
SD:	Stable disease.

Acknowledgment

Part of this study was presented at the 2014 Multidisciplinary Head and Neck Symposium in Scottsdale, Arizona, February 20, 2014.

References

[1] M. Alam and D. Ratner, "Cutaneous squamous-cell carcinoma," *The New England Journal of Medicine*, vol. 344, no. 13, pp. 975–983, 2001.

[2] M. O. F. Al-Othman, W. M. Mendenhall, and R. J. Amdur, "Radiotherapy alone for clinical T4 skin carcinoma of the head and neck with surgery reserved for salvage," *The American Journal of Otolaryngology—Head and Neck Medicine and Surgery*, vol. 22, no. 6, pp. 387–390, 2001.

[3] T. Y. Seiwert, J. K. Salama, and E. E. Vokes, "The concurrent chemoradiation paradigm—general principles," *Nature Clinical Practice Oncology*, vol. 4, no. 2, pp. 86–100, 2007.

[4] N. Normanno, A. de Luca, C. Bianco et al., "Epidermal growth factor receptor (EGFR) signaling in cancer," *Gene*, vol. 366, no. 1, pp. 2–16, 2006.

[5] G. B. Fogarty, N. M. Conus, J. Chu, and G. McArthur, "Characterization of the expression and activation of the epidermal growth factor receptor in squamous cell carcinoma of the skin," *British Journal of Dermatology*, vol. 156, no. 1, pp. 92–98, 2007.

[6] P. Uribe and S. Gonzalez, "Epidermal growth factor receptor (EGFR) and squamous cell carcinoma of the skin: molecular bases for EGFR-targeted therapy," *Pathology Research and Practice*, vol. 207, no. 6, pp. 337–342, 2011.

[7] A. Toll, R. Salgado, M. Yébenes et al., "Epidermal growth factor receptor gene numerical aberrations are frequent events in actinic keratoses and invasive cutaneous squamous cell carcinomas," *Experimental Dermatology*, vol. 19, no. 2, pp. 151–153, 2010.

[8] E. Maubec, P. Duvillard, V. Velasco, B. Crickx, and M. F. Avril, "Immunohistochemical analysis of EGFR and HER-2 in

patients with metastatic squamous cell carcinoma of the skin," *Anticancer Research*, vol. 25, no. 2, pp. 1205–1210, 2005.

[9] S. Ch'ng, I. Low, D. Ng et al., "Epidermal growth factor receptor: a novel biomarker for aggressive head and neck cutaneous squamous cell carcinoma," *Human Pathology*, vol. 39, no. 3, pp. 344–349, 2008.

[10] E. Maubec, P. Petrow, I. Scheer-Senyarich et al., "Phase II study of cetuximab as first-line single-drug therapy in patients with unresectable squamous cell carcinoma of the skin," *Journal of Clinical Oncology*, vol. 29, no. 25, pp. 3419–3426, 2011.

[11] S. Preneau, E. Rio, A. Brocard et al., "Efficacy of cetuximab in the treatment of squamous cell carcinoma," *The Journal of Dermatological Treatment*, vol. 25, no. 5, pp. 424–427, 2014.

[12] J. A. Bonner, P. M. Harari, J. Giralt et al., "Radiotherapy plus cetuximab for squamous-cell carcinoma of the head and neck," *The New England Journal of Medicine*, vol. 354, no. 6, pp. 567–578, 2006.

[13] J. A. Bonner, P. M. Harari, J. Giralt et al., "Radiotherapy plus cetuximab for locoregionally advanced head and neck cancer: 5-year survival data from a phase 3 randomised trial, and relation between cetuximab-induced rash and survival," *The Lancet Oncology*, vol. 11, no. 1, pp. 21–28, 2010.

[14] S. Huang, J. M. Bock, and P. M. Harari, "Epidermal growth factor receptor blockade with C225 modulates proliferation, apoptosis, and radiosensitivity in squamous cell carcinomas of the head and neck," *Cancer Research*, vol. 59, no. 8, pp. 1935–1940, 1999.

[15] G. R. Blumenschein Jr., R. Paulus, W. J. Curran et al., "Phase II study of cetuximab in combination with chemoradiation in patients with stage IIIA/B non-small-cell lung cancer: RTOG 0324," *Journal of Clinical Oncology*, vol. 29, no. 17, pp. 2312–2318, 2011.

[16] L. O. Olivatto, F. M. Vieira, B. V. Pereira et al., "Phase 1 study of cetuximab in combination with 5-fluorouracil, cisplatin, and radiotherapy in patients with locally advanced anal canal carcinoma," *Cancer*, vol. 119, no. 16, pp. 2973–2980, 2013.

[17] H. Safran, M. Suntharalingam, T. Dipetrillo et al., "Cetuximab with concurrent chemoradiation for esophagogastric cancer: assessment of toxicity," *International Journal of Radiation Oncology Biology Physics*, vol. 70, no. 2, pp. 391–395, 2008.

[18] K. N. Moore, M. W. Sill, D. S. Miller et al., "A phase i trial of tailored radiation therapy with concomitant cetuximab and cisplatin in the treatment of patients with cervical cancer: a gynecologic oncology group study," *Gynecologic Oncology*, vol. 127, no. 3, pp. 456–461, 2012.

[19] W. L. Read, R. M. Tierney, N. C. Page et al., "Differential prognostic impact of comorbidity," *Journal of Clinical Oncology*, vol. 22, no. 15, pp. 3099–3103, 2004.

[20] S. B. Edge and American Joint Committee on Cancer, *AJCC Cancer Staging Manual*, Springer, New York, NY, USA, 2010.

[21] National Cancer Institute (U.S.), *Common Terminology Criteria for Adverse Events (CTCAE)*, U.S. Deptartment of Health and Human Services, National Institutes of Health, National Cancer Institute, Bethesda, Md, USA, 2009.

[22] M. R. Kanakamedala, S. Packianathan, and S. Vijayakumar, "Lack of Cetuximab induced skin toxicity in a previously irradiated field: case report and review of the literature," *Radiation Oncology*, vol. 5, no. 1, article 38, 2010.

[23] D. Göppner, S. Nekwasil, I. Franke, H. Gollnick, and M. Leverkus, "Successful combination therapy of a locally advanced squamous cell carcinoma of the skin with cetuximab and γ-irradiation," *JDDG - Journal of the German Society of Dermatology*, vol. 8, no. 10, pp. 826–828, 2010.

[24] U. Wollina, A. Schreiber, K. Merla, and G. Haroske, "Combined cetuximab and volumetric modulated arc-radiotherapy in advanced recurrent squamous cell carcinoma of the scalp," *Dermatology Reports*, vol. 3, no. 3, article e57, 2011.

[25] D. Giacchero, J. Barrière, K. Benezery et al., "Efficacy of cetuximab for unresectable or advanced cutaneous squamous cell carcinoma—a report of eight cases," *Clinical Oncology*, vol. 23, no. 10, pp. 716–718, 2011.

[26] M. Alter, I. Satzger, A. Mattern, A. Kapp, and R. Gutzmer, "Treatment of advanced cutaneous squamous cell carcinomas with epidermal growth factor receptor inhibitors," *Dermatology*, vol. 227, no. 4, pp. 289–294, 2013.

[27] S. J. Kalapurakal, J. Malone, K. T. Robbins, L. Buescher, J. Godwin, and K. Rao, "Cetuximab in refractory skin cancer treatment," *Journal of Cancer*, vol. 3, no. 1, pp. 257–261, 2012.

[28] K. O'Bryan, W. Sherman, G. W. Niedt et al., "An evolving paradigm for the workup and management of high-risk cutaneous squamous cell carcinoma," *Journal of the American Academy of Dermatology*, vol. 69, no. 4, pp. 595.e1–602.e1, 2013.

8

The Experience of Melanoma Follow-Up Care: An Online Survey of Patients in Australia

Janine Mitchell,[1] Peta Callaghan,[1] Jackie Street,[1] Susan Neuhaus,[1,2] and Taryn Bessen[1,2]

[1] School of Population Health, Level 11 Terrace Towers, 178 North Terrace, The University of Adelaide, P.O. Box DX 650 205, Adelaide, SA 5005, Australia

[2] Royal Adelaide Hospital, North Terrace, Adelaide, SA 5000, Australia

Correspondence should be addressed to Janine Mitchell; janine.mitchell@live.com.au

Academic Editor: Mark Lebwohl

Investigating patients' reports on the quality and consistency of melanoma follow-up care in Australia would assist in evaluating if this care is effective and meeting patients' needs. The objective of this study was to obtain and explore the patients' account of the technical and interpersonal aspects of melanoma follow-up care received. An online survey was conducted to acquire details of patients' experience. Participants were patients treated in Australia for primary melanoma. Qualitative and quantitative data about patient perceptions of the nature and quality of their follow-up care were collected, including provision of melanoma specific information, psychosocial support, and imaging tests received. Inconsistencies were reported in the provision and quality of care received. Patient satisfaction was generally low and provision of reassurance from health professionals was construed as an essential element of quality of care. "Gaps" in follow-up care for melanoma patients were identified, particularly provision of adequate psychosocial support and patient education. Focus on strategies for greater consistency in the provision of support, information, and investigations received, may generate a cost dividend which could be reinvested in preventive and supportive care and benefit patient well-being.

1. Introduction

Globally, Australia has the highest incidence of melanoma, with annual rates continuing to rise [1]. Individuals with a primary melanoma have 8–12% risk of developing a second primary melanoma and an increased risk of developing a nonmelanoma skin cancer [2–5], and therefore posttreatment monitoring for recurrence and new primary melanomas is important. The purpose of follow-up is to detect recurrence and/or progression at an early treatable stage, identify treatment-related morbidity (e.g., lymphoedema), identify new melanoma or nonmelanoma skin cancers, and provide reassurance and education [6]. Good practice in follow-up includes effective coordination of care, consistency in care provision [7, 8], evidence-based testing, and psychosocial support [6–9]. Patient perceptions can provide valuable insight into the quality of melanoma follow-up care and identify potential areas for improvement.

Quality of patient care can be defined in both technical and interpersonal terms [10]. Here, "technical" refers to best practice based on current evidence coupled with care providers' knowledge, judgment, and skill in implementation [10]. The 2008 Australian Cancer Network Melanoma Guidelines publication describes best practice guidelines for melanoma follow-up, including judicious use of imaging and blood tests, patient education for detection of recurrence and new primary melanomas, and scheduling follow-up visits with health professionals, on the basis of stage of the cancer, familial history, and patient ability to perform self-examination [6].

The success of technical care depends, in part, on the management of interpersonal care [10], including factors such as communication, empathy, and trust. The subjective nature of interpersonal care makes it a difficult construct to measure; therefore, "best practice guidelines" in this area can be difficult to formulate and implement [10]. Patient satisfaction can be one measure, with self-reported measures of satisfaction helping to determine the values patients themselves associate with quality of care [11]. Measures of patient satisfaction consist of both cognitive evaluation and emotional response to the structure and process and outcome of health services received [12]. The amount and clarity of information received correspond with the cognitive evaluation, whilst the emotional responses encompass psychosocial factors such as receiving adequate support. The psychosocial interventions advocated by the 2008 Australia and New Zealand clinical practice guidelines include cognitive-behavioural group therapy and psychoeducation and access to support groups.

Previous research on melanoma patients' experiences in Australia at follow-up consults recommended a tailored approach to follow-up care with adequate provision of information enabling patients to participate in shared decision-making [9]. Overall high levels of satisfaction with follow-up care were reported by Morton et al. [9]; however, the sample was restricted to patients adhering to follow-up schedules in specialist melanoma centres, potentially targeting only those patients who had a positive experience. Similarly, a systematic review of 15 studies examining the psychosocial aspects of melanoma follow-up care reported high levels of patient satisfaction although none of the studies were Australian [13]. Carter et al. argue that effective delivery of follow-up in Australia and elsewhere is challenging [14]. In particular, the guidelines are based on low-level evidence leading to variation in practice. This study was conducted to investigate if new knowledge in follow-up care in Australia was essential towards fulfilling the health needs of melanoma patients.

We used an online survey distributed across a variety of settings, including nonmetropolitan and multistate, for participant recruitment. Our study aimed to collect the views of patients with a broad base of experience in melanoma follow-up care in Australia, investigating patient perceptions of both the technical and interpersonal aspects of the quality of their follow-up care.

2. Materials and Methods

2.1. Participants. Purposive sampling ensured that only patients with experience of melanoma follow-up care participated. Participants were patients treated in Australia for a primary melanoma since 1 January 2007. Selection criteria excluded patients diagnosed in the previous year, as such patients were deemed to be in "treatment phase" and not in follow-up care.

One hundred and fifty patients accessed the questionnaire with 33 incomplete surveys and 53 surveys that were excluded as the participants were diagnosed before 2007. The remaining 64 participants were included ensuring that only current data on follow-up care was used for this analysis. Patient characteristics are listed in Table 1.

2.2. Materials. Responses were collected using a web-survey through SurveyMonkey. An online information sheet preceded the questionnaire to inform participants about the study and obtain consent. Anonymity was assured and no payment was offered. The 40-question survey, predominantly with "tick box" format, collected information about patient demographics, nature of the melanoma, treatment details, and nature of follow-up care, including the Assessment of

TABLE 1: Characteristics of patients ($n = 64$).

Characteristics		Number of patients
Median age in years (range)	50 (21–78)	64
Sex	Male	25
	Female	39
Highest education level	Year 11 or lower	10
	Year 12/HSC	6
	Certificate/trade/apprenticeship	9
	Diploma	11
	Degree or higher	27
	(missing)	1
Employment status	Full-time employee	33
	Part-time employee	14
	Unemployed	1
	Home duties	4
	Retired	12
Breslow thickness	<1 mm	13
	1–3 mm	23
	>3 mm	15
	Not sure	11
	(missing)	2
Lymph nodes involved	Yes, at time of diagnosis	7
	Yes, at a later time	14
	No	34
	Not sure	5
	(missing)	4
Patients with metastatic disease	Yes	7
	No	54
	Not sure	3
Treatment	Completed	40
	Ongoing	15
	Unsure	8
Secondary disease	Secondary melanoma	9
	Secondary nonmelanoma	18
Follow-up physician	General practitioner	31
	Dermatologist	29
	Skin clinic	13
	Surgeon	32
	Oncologist	12
	Radiotherapist	5
	Other	2
BRaf	Yes	7
	No	50

Survivor Concerns, as developed by Gotay and Pagano [15]. A pilot study with 5 melanoma patients recruited through a surgical oncologist tested the survey before dissemination.

Pilot study participants emphasised the emotional aspects of melanoma follow-up care. As a result, additional questions to assess this factor were included. Free-boxes permitted participants the opportunity to elaborate on their survey responses and contribute further comments. These open-ended comments comprise the study's qualitative data.

2.3. Procedure. Australian state and national organisations involved in melanoma care were approached to support the project ensuring a range of patient experiences, unrestricted by a single specialist centre. The following organisations supported advertisement and recruitment through their websites and networks: Melanoma Patients Australia, the Cancer Council of South Australia and the Cancer Council of Australian Capital Territory, the Australia and New Zealand Melanoma Trials Group, the Melanoma Institute Australia, the National Melanoma Symposium (Melbourne, 2012), Melanoma WA, and Sunbedban. An additional media release in a major South Australian newspaper was also conducted.

Ethics approval was obtained from the University of Adelaide Human Research Ethics Committee (number H-2012-037). Data collection occurred for the period of June-September, 2012. Analysis was supported by IBM SPSS version 19, Armonk, NY, USA (quantitative analysis) and NVivo 10.1 (qualitative analysis) [16].

2.4. Qualitative Analysis. In thematic analysis, as detailed by Braun and Clarke [17], the data were independently coded by two authors (Peta Callaghan and Jackie Street) with iterative discussion to determine concurrence and resolve discrepancies. After open coding, overarching themes were derived, condensing smaller categories: for example, categories relating to mental health and emotional issues, including counselling, fear, stress, and need for reassurance were grouped to form the overarching theme and psychosocial factors.

We were interested in exploring patients' experiences of their care, including information needs, degree of anxiety, experience of follow-up care, and perspectives on potential benefit of a follow-up care coordinator. Our analysis therefore focused on patient experience of melanoma follow-up care.

3. Results

3.1. Patient Satisfaction. Patient satisfaction was determined by three questions that assessed patient experiences of adequate support during follow-up care, patient satisfaction with the amount of information received, and patient preferences for a coordinator to manage follow-up care. Many participants reported that they did not receive adequate support during follow-up (51.6%), that they would have liked to receive more information from their health professionals (64.1%), and that they would like a coordinator to organise their melanoma follow-up care (62.5%).

Whilst the categorical nature of our data restricted multivariate analysis, general response patterns were identified. Participants not supporting the use of follow-up care coordinators also generally reported receiving adequate support

and being satisfied with information provision from their health professionals. This trend was also found in the opposite direction: participants supporting the use of a coordinator generally described inadequate support and information provision during follow-up care.

3.2. Technical Aspects of Quality of Care

3.2.1. Health Professionals Seen and Frequency of Visits. Surgeons were the most frequently reported health professional seen (32 participants), followed by dermatologists (30 participants), although 8 patients saw both. Intervals between visits varied considerably across the patient group; for example, patients with <1 mm melanomas reported being seen 3 monthly. Although 31 patients reported that they regularly saw a general practitioner, it is possible that the reason for these visits may not have specifically related to melanoma follow-up. A minority of participants (22%) reported regular consults with three or more melanoma specialists.

3.2.2. Diagnostic Tests. In follow-up care (after the initial 12-month treatment phase), the most common diagnostic test described was a computed tomography (CT) scan (41 participants), followed by positron emission tomography (PET) scans (17 participants) and chest X-rays (CXR) (11 participants). Several patients indicated a preference to have more scans during follow-up care. Patients constructed the provision of more scans as a means of reassurance (Box 1). Patient awareness of the superiority of self-examination to monitor future risk was not reflected strongly in our data with only one participant explicitly reporting conducting their own skin checks. Comments from many participants indicated that they were unaware of the benefits of skin checks or how to perform adequate self-examination.

3.3. Interpersonal Aspects of Quality of Care. In line with previous research, the most common type of dissatisfaction expressed was with the type of communication and information offered [11]. Sixty-four percent of participants reported they would have liked more information about melanoma, and comments about the quantity and quality of communication dominated the qualitative data.

3.3.1. Information Received. For many participants (40.6%) websites were the main sources of information on melanoma, with the second main source being surgeons (25%). Nearly half of the participants (46.9%) reported not receiving written information, and around 70% reported receiving no information on cancer services, patient support websites, or generic sun protection measures (e.g., avoidance of solariums, use of sunscreens). Thirty-eight participants (59.4%) received a copy of their melanoma pathology report, but only 3 (4.7%) received a written follow-up plan. Box 1 provides examples of participants' comments about information provision. Lack of information was the most commonly reported theme in this category; however, conflicting information and the need for ongoing information due to "forgetting" were also reported.

3.3.2. Communication. Communication was constructed in 2 primary ways: communication between professionals

A preference for monitoring through imaging
...I had heard that there are scanners that they run over your body and somehow it lights up to see if there are any melanoma, I have asked about this and was told that I would have to go to a private clinic that would cost way too much, I just can't afford it at all. Why can't the hospital have equipment like that? [female, 21 yrs]

Regarding the provision of information
Lack of information
...I was not given information... all information I was given in written form was something I had to request... I never received anything from my dermatologist or surgeon. [female, 33 yrs]
...no support or any information... [male, 45 yrs]
I was not given information about metastatic melanoma—I had to google this. I was not told about survival rates. I was not told about recurrence rates. [female, mother of three young children, 33 yrs]
Conflicting information
I've been given conflicting information about what treatment is available to me. [female, 39 yrs]
...it seems to me that cancer information and resources are quite disjointed nationally. If I were to move interstate I'd have no idea where to go for a scan. [female, 45 yrs]
Forgotten information
Telling me things at the time of diagnosis, (and even for my husband who was with me) it was hard to remember exactly what was being communicated beyond dates and times and requirements for surgery and so forth... There were a million details and it seemed the things we would need to know later were the things we forgot in the explosion of activity and emotion surrounding the initial treatment... [female, 45 yrs]

Communication
Poor communication
...there is poor communication between the surgeon and my GP as to how to treat and care for my problem [female, 25 yrs]
...hospitals seem to have a silo mentality, that is, they do not share information. [male, 43 yrs]
Ideal communication
I would probably be reassured if there was a single person who was coordinating my care and who I could communicate with as a single point of contact. [female, 42 yrs]
GPs and medical surgeons and specialists have a duty of care to their patients, and that includes communicating with their patient regarding follow up care, and communicating with one another as health care professionals. [female, 52 yrs]
Good communication
My doctors and surgeons have been very supportive and accommodating with their time and explanations. [female, 39 yrs]
My oncologist and [I] have excellent communication channels. However, when I have been referred to the public system that standard of communication deteriorates. The public system is obviously stretched and personal follow-up and communication is lost. [male, 52 yrs]

A change in health professional
I go to a different clinic from the original one that removed the melanoma. I am scarred mentally and physically as the wound came open after stitches were removed and they did not care or offer treatment... Am happy with new clinic and they are appalled at my scar and lack of treatment I received. [female, 47 yrs]
...the doctors at the ... Clinic show little inclination to want to answer questions at all. I have now switched treatment centres and find that the approach by the oncologists there is much better. [male, 43 yrs]

Preferences for follow-up care coordination
Coordination is a good thing
To ensure all options and information is presented... [male, 36 yrs]
...to have a point of contact as to what I should be doing and who to follow up with would be extremely valuable. [male, 45 yrs]
I can manage, however coordination may be helpful for others
I am confident enough to coordinate my own appointments and tests, however this would be an excellent idea for patients without the same confidence. [female, 63 yrs]
Maybe for aged patients with other challenges. I prefer to self-manage. [male, 47 yrs]

Psychosocial factors
Emotional aspects
I was offered no follow up care... I was afraid and didn't have a lot of knowledge as to what was happening [female, 21 yrs]
Emotional stress was worse than physical symptoms. [female, 46 yrs]
Just waiting for it to come back, not keen on that. [male, 46 yrs]
Therapy/counselling
...If after initial melanoma removed and so forth an actual face to face appointment is made with a counsellor/support service by the surgeon/doctor... Sometimes you just need to talk to someone... [female, 42 yrs]
...lack of mental health care surrounding the diagnosis. [female, 38 yrs]

Box 1: Examples of participant comments.

and communication with professionals. Within these categories, three themes were expressed: poor communication, ideal communication, and good communication with poor communication reported as the most common experience (Box 1). Many participants described the type of communication they felt *should* happen. Ideal communication was frequently constructed in terms of "reassurance" for patients. The lack of information (received or perceived) meant many participants accessed information themselves via the Internet; however, participants also indicated that poor communication with their health care professional meant they often did not know what to look for or which information applied to them.

3.3.3. Changed Professionals. Four participants voluntarily reported having changed health professionals due to dissatisfaction with quality of care, a finding in accord with previous research [11, 18]. Interestingly, each of these participants also reported satisfaction with the care provided by their subsequent health professional.

3.3.4. Psychosocial Factors. With respect to patients' fears and concerns, 29 (45.3%) participants reported that they received inadequate support. Concern was highest in relation to cancer recurrence and the impact on their children's health. Having a coordinator (defined as a person to assist in organising follow-up care) was valued by 40 (62.5%) participants. The qualitative analysis supports this finding with many participants equating coordination with improved support and information provision. Whilst some participants felt that they themselves did not require a coordinator, for a few participants this was constructed as entirely due to personal characteristics: these participants reported that they were organised and were confident. Strong support for a care coordinator in concert with concerns about gaps in care and communication (Box 1) indicates that, for these participants, structural support for melanoma follow-up care within the health care system was inadequate. In addition, participants indicated (Box 1) that lack of consistent support and information compounded the stress and fear associated with melanoma follow-up. Moreover, provision of reassurance from health professionals was constructed as an essential element of quality of care.

4. Discussion

4.1. Patient Satisfaction with Quality of Care. Unlike previous research into patient perceptions of the quality of melanoma follow-up care in Australia [9], our findings indicate considerable dissatisfaction with the quality of care received. The sampling of patients via websites and online support groups provides a cohort of melanoma patients including more nonmetropolitan participants and participants from multiple states than those reported in Morton et al., where participants were recruited from a specialist follow-up centre [9].

The findings suggest that there was considerable variability in perceived quality of care, and for many participants in our study, psychosocial support and information provision

were inadequate. Both factors appeared to affect patients' sense of control, a finding mirrored in previous research [13].

4.2. Technical Aspects of Care. This study also identified considerable variance in follow-up practice in our participants' group with variation in the types of doctors seen and frequency of visits and indications of duplication of care. This finding mirrors a 2011 Netherlands study, where patients were reportedly receiving more follow-up visits than being clinically indicated [7]. In addition, Australian and New Zealand guidelines recommend that patients themselves should play a central role in monitoring for recurrence or new primary melanomas. Our findings suggest that essential education for self-examination, to support such monitoring, may be lacking.

The Australian and New Zealand guidelines do not recommend radiological tests (CXR, CT, and PET) in early stage melanoma [6] with the evidence indicating that routine imaging has minimal value in follow-up, and the additional cost cannot be justified [6, 19]. Some participants reported they would like more testing, and others reported excessive testing across the spectrum of disease. However, our findings must be interpreted with caution, as assessing the "appropriateness" of imaging for each patient (e.g., based on patient, tumour, and treatment characteristics) was beyond the scope of this study.

4.3. Interpersonal Aspects of Care. Our findings indicate that adequate provision of information was lacking for many patients. Lack of information and poor communication were associated with seeking information online, but this did not always provide an adequate alternative. High internet usage for unmet needs has been reported elsewhere [20] and attests to the desire of patients to be fully informed.

Participants reporting they had forgotten information used the terms "explosion" and "shock" (Box 1), suggesting intense emotional reaction to diagnosis of melanoma, may make it difficult to retain information provided. Patients may not recall information received during this time. Previous studies have indicated the need for ongoing tailored discussions with patients about their care throughout the "cancer journey" [21, 22].

Patient fears for their children's health and their own cancer recurring are reasonable given the evidence of recurrence risk and familial predisposition [6, 23]. Despite evidence that such concerns may be decreased with education and support [23, 24], our study suggests that many patients with melanoma receive inadequate support for psychosocial issues. Oliveria et al. showed that patient perceptions of inadequate support through the health care system could lead to suboptimal health outcomes [25]. Provision of a care coordinator, expressed as being of value by over half of the study participants, has been demonstrated to improve health outcomes in breast cancer patients [26] and may go some way to providing mental and emotional support.

5. Limitations

The online nature of the study presents selection bias and although potentially widely accessible across Australia, the number of participants was small. Therefore, the findings may not be representative of national experience of patients undergoing melanoma follow-up. As a retrospective study, the possibility of recall bias is also acknowledged. Reliance on categorical data limited analysis, making it difficult to assess relationships amongst variables.

6. Conclusion

This study provides insights into the nature of melanoma follow-up care in Australia. We identify perceived gaps in patient care, perceptions of inadequate support and information, and variance in patterns of care, all of which suggest that the quality and consistency of melanoma follow-up care in Australia can be improved. Moreover, follow-up care is iterative and the needs of patients, including information, emotional support, and medical care, may be very different from their needs during the treatment phase. According to our data, it appears that these changing needs are not being widely addressed. Moreover, the variation in patterns of care suggests the Australian and New Zealand clinical practice guidelines are not being consistently followed. Our data suggest that provision of targeted support and information from health professionals may improve long-term patient self-care. Whilst this finding deserves greater attention in future research, we also suggest that a focus on developing strategies for generating greater adherence to the clinical guidelines, including the stringent use of investigations as recommended, may generate a cost dividend which could be reinvested in preventive and supportive care. We suggest that greater consistency in the provision of emotional support and information throughout treatment and follow-up phases of melanoma follow-up care could enhance patient well-being.

Acknowledgments

The authors would like to thank the online survey participants; Michelle Lorimer for statistical support; Nino Marciano for editorial support; Melanoma Patients Australia; Cancer Council South Australia; Cancer Council Australian Capital Territory; Australia and New Zealand Melanoma Trials Group; Melanoma Institute Australia; Melanoma WA; Sunbedban; National Melanoma Symposium; David Ellis; and the advertiser for assistance in recruitment of participants.

References

[1] "Cancer. Cat. no . CAN 38; Cancer series no.42," Australian Institute of Health and Welfare, 2012, http://www.aihw.gov.au/cancer/.

[2] A. Uliasz and M. Lebwohl, "Patient education and regular surveillance results in earlier diagnosis of second primary melanoma," *International Journal of Dermatology*, vol. 46, no. 6, pp. 575–577, 2007.

[3] L. Titus-Ernstoff, A. E. Perry, S. K. Spencer et al., "Multiple primary melanoma: two-year results from a population-based study," *Archives of Dermatology*, vol. 142, no. 4, pp. 433–438, 2006.

[4] P. T. Bradford, D. M. Freedman, A. M. Goldstein, and M. A. Tucker, "Increased risk of second primary cancers after a diagnosis of melanoma," *Archives of Dermatology*, vol. 146, no. 3, pp. 265–272, 2010.

[5] G. B. Yang, J. S. Barnholtz-Sloan, Y. Chen, and J. S. Bordeaux, "Risk and survival of cutaneous melanoma diagnosed subsequent to a previous cancer," *Archives of Dermatology*, vol. 147, no. 12, pp. 1395–1402, 2011.

[6] *Clinical Practice Guidelines for the Management of Melanoma in Australia and New Zealand*, Australian Cancer Network Melanoma Guidelines Revision Working Party, 2008, http://www.nhmrc.gov.au/_files_nhmrc/publications/attachments/cp111.pdf.

[7] C. Holterhues, L. V. van de Poll-Franse, E. de Vries, H. A. M. Neumann, and T. E. C. Nijsten, "Melanoma patients receive more follow-up care than current guideline recommendations: a study of 546 patients from the general Dutch population," *Journal of the European Academy of Dermatology and Venereology*, vol. 26, no. 11, pp. 1389–1395, 2012.

[8] U. Leiter, A. A. Marghoob, K. Lasithiotakis et al., "Costs of the detection of metastases and follow-up examinations in cutaneous melanoma," *Melanoma Research*, vol. 19, no. 1, pp. 50–57, 2009.

[9] R. L. Morton, L. Rychetnik, K. McCaffery, J. F. Thompson, and L. Irwig, "Patients' perspectives of long-term follow-up for localised cutaneous melanoma," *European Journal of Surgical Oncology*, vol. 39, no. 3, pp. 297–303, 2013.

[10] A. Donabedian, "The quality of care. How can it be assessed?" *Journal of the American Medical Association*, vol. 260, no. 12, pp. 1743–1748, 1988.

[11] P. D. Cleary and B. J. McNeil, "Patient satisfaction as an indicator of quality care," *Inquiry*, vol. 25, no. 1, pp. 25–36, 1988.

[12] G. C. Pascoe, "Patient satisfaction in primary health care: a literature review and analysis," *Evaluation and Program Planning*, vol. 6, no. 3-4, pp. 185–210, 1983.

[13] L. Rychetnik, K. McCaffery, R. Morton, and L. Irwig, "Psychosocial aspects of post-treatment follow-up for stage I/II melanoma: a systematic review of the literature," *Psycho-Oncology*, vol. 22, no. 4, pp. 721–736, 2013.

[14] D. Carter, H. H. A. Afzali, J. Street, T. Bessen, and S. Neuhaus, "Melanoma follow up: time to generate the evidence," *Australian Health Review*, vol. 37, no. 4, pp. 501–503, 2013.

[15] C. C. Gotay and I. S. Pagano, "Assessment of Survivor Concerns (ASC): a newly proposed brief questionnaire," *Health and Quality of Life Outcomes*, vol. 5, article 15, 2007.

[16] QSR International Pty, *NVivo Qualitative Analysis Software. Version 9*, [computer program], QSR International Pty, 2010.

[17] V. Braun and V. Clarke, "Using thematic analysis in psychology," *Qualitative Research in Psychology*, vol. 3, no. 2, pp. 77–101, 2006.

[18] N. K. Choudhry, R. H. Fletcher, and S. B. Soumerai, "Systematic review: the relationship between clinical experience and quality of health care," *Annals of Internal Medicine*, vol. 142, no. 4, pp. 260–273, 2005.

[19] A. L. Dancey, B. S. Mahon, and S. S. Rayatt, "A review of diagnostic imaging in melanoma," *Journal of Plastic, Reconstructive and Aesthetic Surgery*, vol. 61, no. 11, pp. 1275–1283, 2008.

[20] M. W. Ludgate, M. S. Sabel, D. R. Fullen et al., "Internet use and anxiety in people with melanoma and nonmelanoma skin cancer," *Dermatologic Surgery*, vol. 37, no. 9, pp. 1252–1259, 2011.

[21] P. N. Butow, M. Maclean, S. M. Dunn, M. H. N. Tattersall, and M. J. Boyer, "The dynamics of change: cancer patients' preferences for information, involvement and support," *Annals of Oncology*, vol. 8, no. 9, pp. 857–863, 1997.

[22] G. M. Leydon, M. Boulton, C. Moynihan et al., "Cancer patients' information needs and information seeking behaviour: in depth interview study," *British Medical Journal*, vol. 320, no. 7239, pp. 909–913, 2000.

[23] L. J. Loescher, J. D. Crist, and L. A. C. L. Siaki, "Perceived intrafamily melanoma risk communication," *Cancer Nursing*, vol. 32, no. 3, pp. 203–210, 2009.

[24] L. J. Loescher, J. D. Crist, L. Cranmer, C. Curiel-Lewandrowski, and J. A. Warneke, "Melanoma high-risk families' perceived health care provider risk communication," *Journal of Cancer Education*, vol. 24, no. 4, pp. 301–307, 2009.

[25] S. A. Oliveria, J. L. Hay, A. C. Geller, M. K. Heneghan, M. S. McCabe, and A. C. Halpern, "Melanoma survivorship: research opportunities," *Journal of Cancer Survivorship*, vol. 1, no. 1, pp. 87–97, 2007.

[26] P. Yates, "Cancer care coordinators: realising the potential for improving the patient journey," *Cancer Forum*, vol. 28, no. 3, pp. 128–132, 2004.

9

Protein Kinase Cε, Which Is Linked to Ultraviolet Radiation-Induced Development of Squamous Cell Carcinomas, Stimulates Rapid Turnover of Adult Hair Follicle Stem Cells

Ashok Singh,[1] Anupama Singh,[1] Jordan M. Sand,[1,2] Erika Heninger,[3] Bilal Bin Hafeez,[1] and Ajit K. Verma[1]

[1] *Department of Human Oncology, Wisconsin Institutes for Medical Research, School of Medicine and Public Health, 1111 Highland Avenue, University of Wisconsin, Madison, WI 53705, USA*
[2] *Molecular and Environmental Toxicology Center, Wisconsin Institutes for Medical Research, Paul P. Carbone Comprehensive Cancer Center, School of Medicine and Public Health, University of Wisconsin, Madison, WI 53705, USA*
[3] *UWCCC Flow Cytometry Core Facility, School of Medicine and Public Health, University of Wisconsin, Madison, WI 53705, USA*

Correspondence should be addressed to Ajit K. Verma; akverma@wisc.edu

Academic Editor: Deric L. Wheeler

To find clues about the mechanism by which kinase C epsilon (PKCε) may impart susceptibility to ultraviolet radiation (UVR)-induced development of cutaneous squamous cell carcinomas (SCC), we compared PKCε transgenic (TG) mice and their wild-type (WT) littermates for (1) the effects of UVR exposures on percent of putative hair follicle stem cells (HSCs) and (2) HSCs proliferation. The percent of double HSCs (CD34+ and α6-integrin or CD34+/CD49f+) in the isolated keratinocytes were determined by flow cytometric analysis. Both single and chronic UVR treatments ($1.8 \, \text{kJ/m}^2$) resulted in an increase in the frequency of double positive HSCs in PKCε TG mice as compared to their WT littermates. To determine the rate of proliferation of bulge region stem cells, a 5-bromo-2′-deoxyuridine labeling (BrdU) experiment was performed. In the WT mice, the percent of double positive HSCs retaining BrdU label was 28.4 ± 0.6% compared to 4.0 ± 0.06% for the TG mice, an approximately 7-fold decrease. A comparison of gene expression profiles of FACS sorted double positive HSCs showed increased expression of Pes1, Rad21, Tfdp1 and Cks1b genes in TG mice compared to WT mice. Also, PKCε over expression in mice increased the clonogenicity of isolated keratinocytes, a property commonly ascribed to stem cells.

1. Introduction

The multistage model of mouse skin carcinogenesis is a useful system in which biochemical events unique to initiation, promotion, or progression steps of carcinogenesis can be studied and related to cancer formation. 12-O-Tetradecanoylphorbol-13-acetate (TPA), a component of croton oil, is a potent mouse skin tumor promoter [1, 2]. A major breakthrough in understanding the mechanism of TPA tumor promotion has been the identification of protein kinase C (PKC), as its major intracellular receptor [3]. PKC forms part of the signal transduction system involving the turnover of inositol phospholipids and is activated by DAG, which is produced

as a consequence of this turnover [3]. PKC represents a family of phospholipid-dependent serine/threonine kinases [3–6]. PKCε is among the six PKC isoforms (α, δ, ε, η, μ, and ξ) expressed in both mouse and human skin [7]. We have reported that epidermal PKCε levels dictate the susceptibility of PKCε transgenic (TG) mice to the development of squamous cell carcinomas (SCC) elicited either by repeated exposures to ultraviolet radiation (UVR) [8] or initiation with 7, 12-dimethylbenz[a]anthracene (DMBA) and tumor promotion with 12-O-tetradecanoylphorbol-13-acetate (TPA) [9]. Histologically, SCC in TG mice, like human SCC, is poorly differentiated and metastatic [10].

SCC developed in PKCε transgenic mice is metastatic and originates from the hair follicle [10]. The papilloma-independent carcinomas which develop in PKCε transgenic mice arise from the hair follicle and have increased metastatic potential [10]. The difference in metastatic potential and the different origin of malignancy when compared to WT provided support for the hypothesis that papilloma-independent carcinomas in PKCε TG mice were pathologically distinct from WT mouse carcinomas. Although the papilloma-independent carcinomas appeared to originate from the hair follicle, it was possible that the origin of the tumor was not within the hair follicle. The hair follicle might have been the easiest pathway for invasion. However, this did not appear to be the case because we observed neoplastic cells arising only from the hair follicle and not the epidermis. By harvesting PKCε TG and WT mice after 8 weeks of DMBA + TPA or DMBA + acetone treatments, we identified possible premalignant areas in PKCε transgenic mice as early as 8 weeks after DMBA + TPA treatment. The premalignant lesions originated within the hair follicle [10].

The metastatic potential of a transformed keratinocyte appeared to inversely correlate with the differentiation potential of that keratinocyte in the limited number of tumors studied to date. This conclusion was based on the location of invasion and pathological categorization of PKCε TG mouse carcinomas compared with WT mouse carcinomas. Bulge keratinocytes are located near the sebaceous gland within the hair follicle. Evidence suggests that these cells appear to be the stem or progenitor cells for both the hair follicle and epidermis and, therefore, would be in a less-differentiated state than other epidermal cells [10]. These properties may increase the metastatic potential of these cells. The carcinomas of PKCε TG mice that led to metastases were also less differentiated than carcinomas from WT mice. Evidence suggests that malignant cells invading from the hair follicle were less differentiated and had a higher metastatic potential than cells that invaded from the epidermis. PKCε, when activated either via direct binding to TPA or indirectly by UVR treatment, mediates two potential signals leading to inhibition of apoptosis [11, 12] and induction of cell proliferation.

Epidermal stem cells in the mouse hair follicle are known to be the precursor cells for SCC in the mouse skin [13–17]. Evidence suggests that epithelial stem cells reside in the bulge region [18, 19]. Stem cells, unlike transit amplifying cells, are slowly cycling and thus seem probable target cells. Moreover, stem cells may retain those mutations and pass them on to their progeny [14]. Morris et al. [20] demonstrated that label retaining cells (LRCs) have another property characteristic of potential initiated cells: they could retain carcinogen-DNA adducts. The contribution of follicular and interfollicular stem cells to the induction of skin papillomas and carcinomas was also determined [20]. Both follicular and interfollicular stem cells contributed to the development of papillomas. However, only follicular stem cells were linked to the development of carcinomas.

As a prelude to determine the SCC lineage from HSCs in PKCε TG mice, we compared the responses of PKCε TG and their WT littermates to UVR treatment. We examined the effects on proliferation, turnover, and gene expression profile of HSCs. In this communication, we present for the first time that (1) UVR exposures increased the number of double positive HSCs in TG mice, (2) the percent of double positive HSCs retaining BrdU label in the WT mice was 7-fold more than the TG mice, indicating that the double positive cells in the TG mice cycle at a faster rate, (3) the keratinocytes from PKCε TG mice have higher proliferating potential compared to their WT littermates, and (4) a comparison of gene expression profile of FACS-sorted HSCs showed an increase expression of Pes1, Rad21, Tfdp1, and Cks1b genes in TG mice compared to their WT littermates.

2. Materials and Methods

2.1. Chemicals and Antibodies. BrdU was purchased from Sigma Aldrich (St. Louis, MO, USA). BrdU antibody was purchased from Santa Cruz Biotechnologies (Santa Cruz, CA, USA). Antibodies used for FACS such as α6-integrin PE-conjugated, CD34 FITC-conjugated antibodies, APC BrdU labeling kit, and propidium iodide were purchased from BD Biosciences (San Jose, CA, USA). BrdU antibody conjugated with Alexa Fluor 647 was procured from Biosciences (Frederick, MD, USA). PCR gene array focused to cell cycle was purchased from SA Biosciences (Frederick, MD, USA).

2.2. Keratinocyte Isolation and Flow Cytometric Analysis. Keratinocytes were harvested as described elsewhere [21]. In each experiment an equal size of skin is excised from the WT and TG mice. Viable cell counts were determined using 0.4% Trypan Blue. Keratinocytes were incubated for 1 hr in the dark at 4°C with PE-conjugated Rat Anti-Human α6-integrin antibody at 10 μL per 10^6 cells and FITC-conjugated rat antimouse CD34 antibody at 2 μg per 10^6 cells (PE-α6-integrin and FITC-CD34 antibodies; BD Biosciences). Keratinocyte preparations were sorted based on α6-integrin+ and CD34 status using a FACS Aria cell sorter (BD Biosciences). Cells were stained with PE-conjugated anti-α6-integrin and FITC-conjugated anti-CD34 antibodies for flow cytometry. A 488 nm laser was used to detect FITC with a 530/30 filter and a 532 nm laser for PE with a 575/25 filter. The nozzle size was 130 nm and the pressure used was 14 p.s.i. The live cell population gate was estimated using forward and side scatter positioning and confirmed with 7AAD staining.

2.3. Keratinocyte Colony Forming Assay. Keratinocytes were harvested from the dorsal skin of 7-8 weeks old PKCε overexpressing mice (TG224 and TG215) and their WT littermates. The skin hairs were clipped and the skin pieces trypsinized for 2 hrs at 32°C. Epidermis was scraped in keratinocyte medium (SMEM) to isolate keratinocyte cells. Three thousand cells per dish were seeded onto irradiated 3T3 cells in 60 mm dishes and cultured for 2 weeks in high calcium medium. For feeder layer, 3T3 cells were cultured in EMEM medium with 10% FBS and 1% Penicillin-streptomycin and irradiated in Cesium Gamma Irradiator at 5000 rad. Irradiated 3T3 cells seeded 10^6 cells/dish to the 60 mm dishes a day before seeding keratinocytes. The clonal culture was grown in William's E media with 10% FBS and supplements. For counting and measurement of colonies, dishes were fixed with 10% formalin for overnight. After fixation, the cultures were stained with 0.5% rhodamine B for 30 min to visualize colonies. The dishes were rinsed in cold tap water and dried before counting. The colonies were counted and colony size measured using vernier caliper.

2.4. Mice and UVR Treatment. WT and PKCε TG 224 and 215 mice lines (FVB background) described elsewhere [9, 10] were housed in groups of two to three in plastic bottom cages in light-, humidity-, and temperature-controlled rooms; food and water were available *ad libitum*. The animals were kept in a normal rhythm of 12 h light and 12 h dark periods. The UVR source was Kodacel-filtered FS-40 sun lamps (approximately 60% UVB and 40% UVA). UVR dose was measured using UVX-radiometer. Mice were used for experimentation starting at 5 to 6 weeks of age. For 24 hr, 48 hr, and 72 hr time points, the mice were treated for 10 min ($2 \, kJ/m^2$) and skin was harvested for keratinocyte isolation after UV exposure. However, for multiple or chronic UVR exposures, mice were exposed to UVR ($2 \, kJ/m^2$) three times weekly (Monday, Wednesday, and Friday) or a total of 8 times.

2.5. Detection of BrdU-Labeled Cells in the Hair Follicle Using Flow Cytometric Analysis. To identify the label retaining cells (LRCs), newborn mice (3 days old) were injected subcutaneously with BrdU (50 mg/kg body weight) twice daily for 3 days. There were three mice per group. Mice were sacrificed 3 to 8 weeks after BrdU injection (3, 4, 5, 6, and 8 weeks). Keratinocytes from the epidermis were harvested as described elsewhere [21]. Freshly harvested keratinocytes were incubated with PE-conjugated anti-α6-integrin and FITC-conjugated anti-CD34 antibodies, fixed and stained using the APC BrdU Flow Kit, following the manufacturer's instructions (BD Biosciences, San Jose, CA, USA). To prepare BrdU positive control samples for FACS, 5-week-old female mice were injected BrdU (50 mg/kg body weight) intraperitoneally for two days (2 times each). After two days, the spleen and thymus were harvested for BrdU positive cells and used as a positive control.

For cell cycle analysis, freshly harvested keratinocytes were isolated from mouse dorsal skin and stained with PE-conjugated α6-integrin and FITC-conjugated anti-CD34 antibodies. After surface staining, the cells were fixed and then stained overnight with DAPI for cell cycle analysis. Flow cytometric analysis based on α6-integrin, CD34, and BrdU was performed on a LSRII benchtop flow cytometer (BD Biosciences). A multilength ultraviolet laser along with a 450/50 bandpass filter was used to detect DAPI. DAPI was used for DNA staining for live/dead determinations along with cell cycle. For the detection of APC-conjugated anti-BrdU antibody, a 640 nm laser and a 660/20 filter was used.

2.6. Phenotyping and Estimation of the Frequency of CD34+/α6-Integrin+ Stem Cells. The phenotyping assays were acquired on a BD FACSCalibur (BD Biosciences), and

BrdU assays were acquired on an LSR II (BD Biosciences) benchtop flow cytometer. Both instruments were calibrated daily by the University of Wisconsin Carbone Cancer Center Flow Cytometry Laboratory staff using the manufacturer's Cytometer Settings and Tracking calibration software. Data were analyzed using FlowJo software version 9.4.3 (Treestar, Ashland, OR, USA). Positive staining and gating strategy were determined by comparison to isotype controls. Dead cells were excluded using 7-aminoactinomycin D (7AAD) staining on FACS Calibur assays or Invitrogen Live/Dead Fixable Violet (FLVD) staining for BrdU assays acquired on the BD LSR II. Data demonstrate frequency of cells in a parent population of live intact cells for α6-integrin and CD34 expression and of α6-integrin+/CD34+/live intact cells for BrdU incorporation.

The frequency of CD34+/α6-integrin+ stem cells represents the percent of CD34+/α6-integrin+/7AAD- cells ("cells" determined by FSC/SSC morphologic gate) in the total 7AAD population. The absolute number of CD34+/α6-integrin+ cells in individual samples was calculated by multiplying frequency of CD34+/α6-integrin+ stem cells by the total number of Trypan-Blue excluding cells in the single cell keratinocyte preparation. The data represent absolute number of CD34+/α6-integrin+ stem cells from the equal size of dorsal skin from WT and TG mice used in the study.

Similarly, for calculation for the absolute count of CD34+/α6-integrin+/BrdU+ cells, the total frequency of CD34+/α6-integrin+/BrdU+/FLDV-cells in total FLVD- was multiplied by the total counts of Trypan-Blue excluding cells in the single cell keratinocyte preparation.

2.7. Immunofluorescence Analysis. To identify the LRCs, newborn mice (3 days old) were injected subcutaneously with BrdU (50 mg/kg body weight) twice daily for 3 days. Mice were sacrificed at 3, 4, 5, 6, and 8 weeks after BrdU injection. Mouse skin was then excised promptly after euthanasia and immediately placed in 10% neutral-buffered formalin for fixation and then embedded in paraffin. Four to five μm sections were cut for immunohistochemistry of BrdU and K15.

For immunofluorescence study extra paraffin was removed using three xylene gradient washes followed by alcohol gradient (95%, 90%, 70%, 50%, and 30%) for 10 min each. The slides were washed with Milli-Q water, and then 1XPBS. The antigen retrieval was done using antigen unmasking solution as per the protocol (Vector Laboratories). The blocking process was done in normal goat and normal horse serum for 1 hr at room temperature (RT). After blocking, primary antibodies (Keratin-15 monoclonal from Neomarkers, CA, dilution 1:30) and BrdU (Santa Cruz, dilution 1:50) were incubated to tissue section on the slides for overnight. Tissue sections were incubated with their secondary antibodies for 1 hr at RT such as Alexa-Fluor 488-Donkey antimouse IgG (H + L) and Alexa-Fluor 594-Donley antirat IgG (H + L) for k15 and BrdU from Invitrogen, respectively. After incubation with secondary antibody slides were washed three times with 1XPBS, mounted with DAPI, and observed under the fluorescent microscope (Vectra).

2.8. PCR Array and Real-Time PCR. TG mice and their WT littermates were exposed to UV once (2kJ/m^2), and 24 hrs after UV treatment mice were sacrificed and the dorsal skin removed for keratinocyte isolation. The cells were stained with fluorescent conjugated CD34 and α6-integrin antibodies and sorted. The cells were sorted into 5 mL tubes containing 0.5 mL of heat inactivated, chelated, fetal bovine serum. The collected cells were then spun down and placed into 300 mL of RNAprotect Cell Reagent (Qiagen; Valencia, CA, USA). RNA was isolated from double positive HSCs using SA Biosciences RT^2 qPCR grade isolation Kit (SA Biosciences, Frederick, MD, USA). 250 ng RNA was used for first-strand cDNA synthesis with the SA Biosciences RT^2 FirstStrand Kit. The resulting cDNA was used in the SA Biosciences Cell Cycle Gene Array according to the manufacturer's instructions.

The real-time expression primers of PKCε in the study were selected from Origene website and further checked in NCBI primer blast for their primer-specific details such as proper target binding and amplification product (http://www.ncbi.nlm.nih.gov/tools/primer-blast/index.cgi?LINK_LOC=BlastHome). The RNA was isolated from FACS-sorted keratinocytes using Qiagen RNeasy mini kit. The samples were treated with DNAse to remove the DNA contamination using Qiagen RNase-free DNase set (Qiagen). For cDNA synthesis SuperScript First-Strand Synthesis Kit (Invitrogen) was used as per the manufacturer' protocol.

Briefly a total of $50 \mu L$ reaction mixture consisted of $25 \mu L$; 2X FastStart Universal SYBR Green master (ROX) mix, $30.0 \mu M$ ($1 \mu L$) forward and reverse primers, and PCR grade water, and 50–100 ng of cDNA ($5–10 \mu L$) was used. Final volume of the reaction was adjusted with RNase-free water provided with the kit. The PCR was set up as per instrument protocol in MyiQ Biorad machine. A cycle to threshold (Ct) value was assigned automatically at the beginning of the logarithmic phase of real-time PCR. Finally, differences in Ct value of control (mouse Gapdh) and stem cell samples were used to determine the relative gene expression or fold changes of the PKCε.

3. Results

3.1. Hair Follicle Stem Cells and Clonogenicity of Epidermal Keratinocytes Isolated from PKCε Overexpressing Mice and Wild-Type Littermates. To determine the basal levels of double positive HSCs (CD34+/α6-integrin+) in untreated WT, TG224, and TG215 mice, freshly harvested keratinocytes were labeled with CD34 and α6-integrin antibodies and analyzed by flow cytometry for their total frequency. We observed higher frequency and absolute count of total HSCs in TG215 mice compared to WT and TG224 mice (Figures 1(a) and 1(b)). Furthermore, we determined the effects of PKCε on the clonogenicity of keratinocytes. Clonogenicity is an intrinsic property of adult stem cells. In this experiment (Figures 1(c) and 1(d)), an equal number of isolated keratinocytes from WT, TG224, and TG215 mice were seeded onto the irradiated 3T3 (fibroblast) cells and left for two weeks. We observed increased colony formation in keratinocytes isolated from TG224 and TG215 mice compared with their WT littermates

indicating more proliferative potential (Figures 1(c) and 1(d)). Notably, the colonies greater than 2 mm and total numbers of colonies were higher in TG215 mice compared to their WT littermates (Figure 1(d)).

3.2. UVR Treatment Stimulates Putative Hair Follicle Stem Cell Proliferation. The cell surface markers CD34 and α6-integrin mark mouse hair follicle bulge cells, which have attributes of stem cells, including quiescence and multipotency. We determined the effects of UV treatment on total number of HSCs. In this experiment, PKCε TG and WT mice were exposed to a single or chronic UV doses (1.8kJ/m^2, Monday, Wednesday, and Friday). At the indicated times after last UV exposure, mice were sacrificed and the number of putative HSCs was determined by flow cytometric analysis. The total frequency as well as absolute count of double positive HSCs were increased at 48 and 72 hr in TG224 after-UV exposure (Figures 2(a) and 2(b)) and 24, 48, and 72 hr in TG215 (Figures 2(c) and 2(d)) compared to their WT littermates. As shown in Figures 3(a) and 3(b), chronic UV exposures also showed an increase in total double positive HSCs in both TG224 and TG215 mice compared to their WT littermates.

3.3. PKCε TG Mice Have Increased Turnover of Putative HSCs. To determine the proliferation rates of bulge region stem cells in WT and TG mice, a 5-bromo-2$'$-deoxyuridine labeling (BrdU) experiment was performed. In this experiment, three-day-old neonatal mice were injected with 50 mg/kg of BrdU in PBS twice daily for three days. At 3, 4, 5, 6, and 8 weeks after BrdU injections, mice were sacrificed and the dorsal skin excised for keratinocyte isolation. Immunohistochemistry results revealed that, at 3-week time point, BrdU labeling was prominent in bulge region of hair follicle, interfollicular epidermis, and sebaceous glands of TG 224, 215, and their WT littermates (Figures 4(a)–4(c)). However, at later time points (6 and 8 weeks), BrdU labeling was decreased in TG mice compared to WT mice and localized to bulge region only (Figures 4(d)–4(h)). It is interesting to note that even after 3 weeks, some cells of interfollicular epidermis are able to retain the BrdU label (Figures 4(a)–4(c)). Moreover, dual immunofluorescence staining of BrdU and k15 indicates the colocalization of BrdU with k15 expressing cells in the stem cell-specific compartment, that is, bulge (Figures 4(i)–4(k)).

We further evaluated the cell cycle pattern in sorted double positive HSCs in TG 215 and their WT littermates at 8 weeks after-BrdU injection. The percent of BrdU-labeled cells was different in WT and TG215 mice. In the WT mice, the percent of double positive cells maintaining BrdU label was $28.4 \pm 0.6\%$ compared to $4.0 \pm 0.06\%$ for the TG, an approximately 7-fold decrease (Figure 5(a)).

We further determined the turnover of HSCs in WT and TG 224 mice. In this experiment, we analyzed the BrdU retaining double positive HSCs in isolated keratinocytes from WT and TG mice. BrdU retaining cells were analyzed at 4, 5, and 8 weeks after-BrdU injections. The frequency of BrdU retaining double positive HSCs was at 4 weeks (WT = 0.246%, TG = 0.0807%), 5 weeks (WT = 0.0364%, TG = 0.00337%), and 8 weeks (WT = 0.167%, TG = 0.008%).

(a)

(b)

(c)

(d)

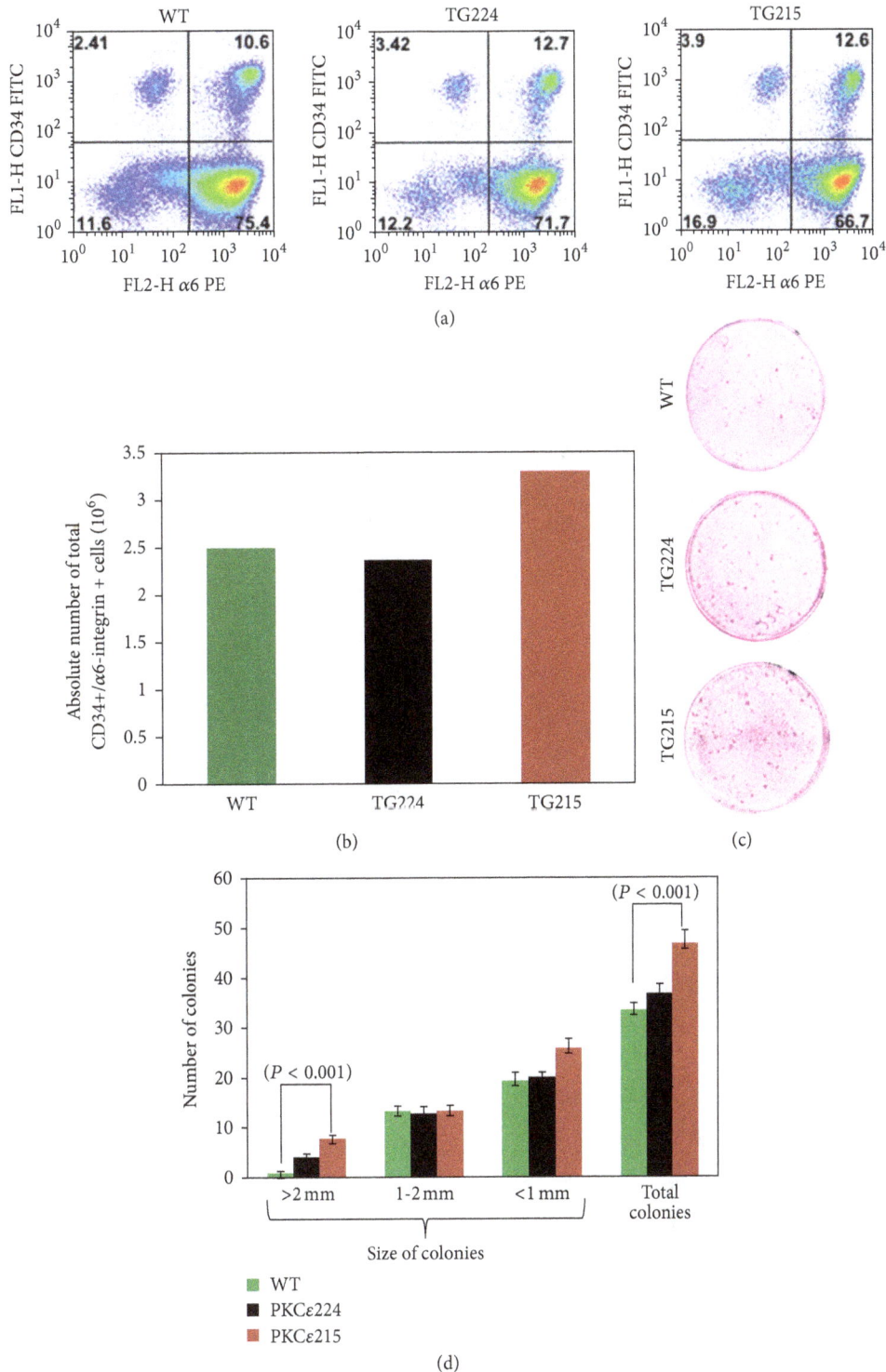

FIGURE 1: Hair follicle stem cells and clonogenicity of epidermal keratinocytes isolated from PKCε overexpressing mice and wild-type littermates. (a) is showing the representative gating of epidermal stem cell population in a dot plot from untreated WT, TG224, and TG215 mice. In each dot plot, the upper right quadrant is representing the CD34+/α6-integrin+ (double positive HSCs) stem cell population. Each value in the histogram is an average of FACS analysis of triplicate samples from keratinocytes pooled from two mice. (b) represents the total frequency of CD34+/α6-integrin+ keratinocytes in untreated indicated mice. (c) and (d) Clonogenicity of epidermal keratinocytes. Briefly, the keratinocytes from 7-8 weeks old indicated that mice were harvested using SMEM harvesting medium. Irradiated 3T3 cells seeded at density 10^6 cells/dish to the 60 mm dishes a day before seeding keratinocytes. For feeder layer, irradiated 3T3 cells were cultured in EMEM medium with 10% FBS and 1% penicillin-streptomycin. Equal numbers of keratinocyte cells (3000 cells/dish) were seeded for each type of mice and cultured with William's E media for 2 weeks. For counting and measurement of colonies, dishes were fixed with 10% formalin and stained with 0.5% rhodamine B. (c) Keratinocyte colonies. Shown are the representative dishes of adult keratinocyte colonies from PKCε TG mice and their WT littermates. (d) Quantitation of colonies. The colonies were counted and colony size measured by using vernier caliper (Figure 1(c)). Each value is the mean ±SE of colonies from 4–7 dishes.

(a)

(b)

(c)

(d)

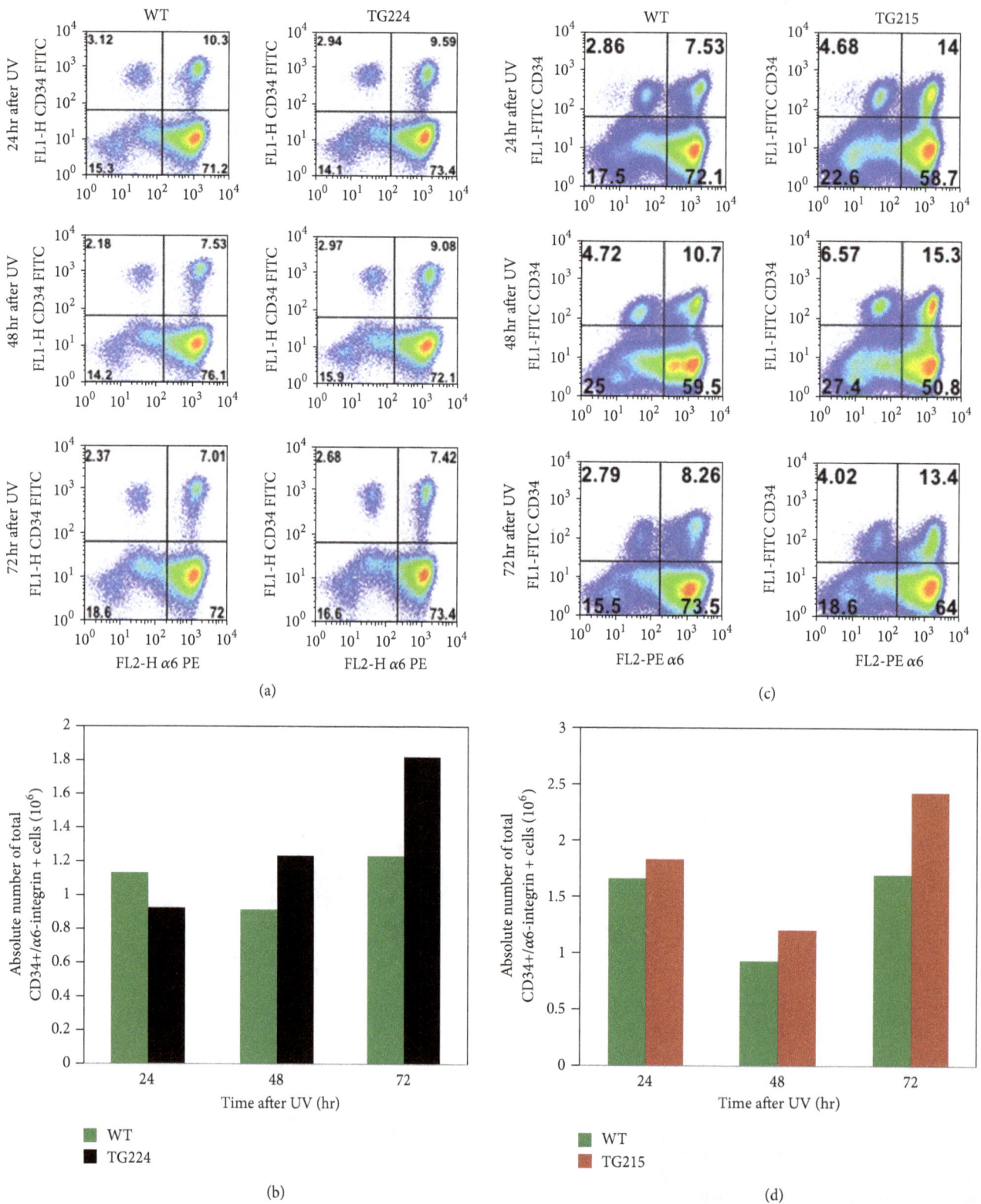

FIGURE 2: Effects of single UV exposure on live epidermal stem cell population determined by flow cytometric analysis. PKCε overexpressing TG and their WT littermates were exposed once to UV (1.8 kJ/m^2). At the indicated times after UV, mice were sacrificed and the dorsal skin removed for keratinocyte isolation as previously described [21]. (a) and (c) Percent distribution of FACS-sorted keratinocytes following UV exposure of the indicated mice at the indicated times after UV exposure. (b) and (d) Frequency of total double positive HSCs (CD34+/α6-integrin+) in TG224, TG215, and their WT littermates at the indicated times after single UV exposure.

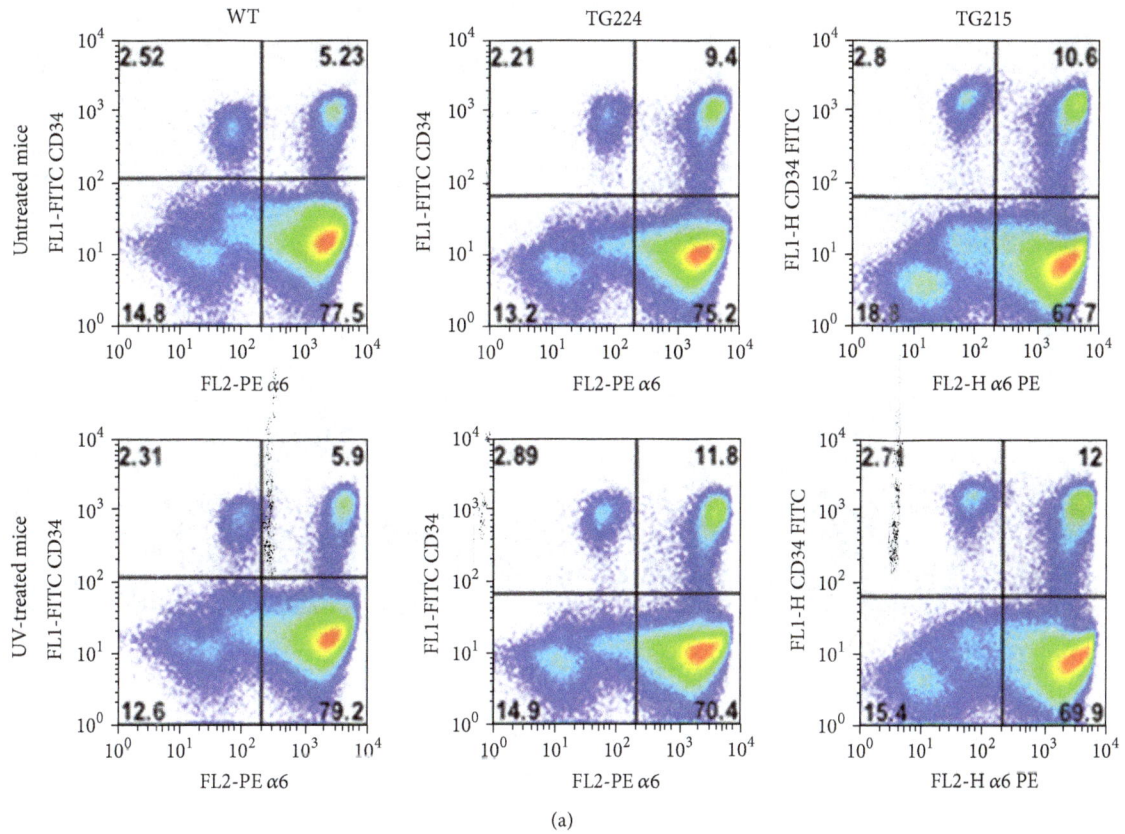

(a)

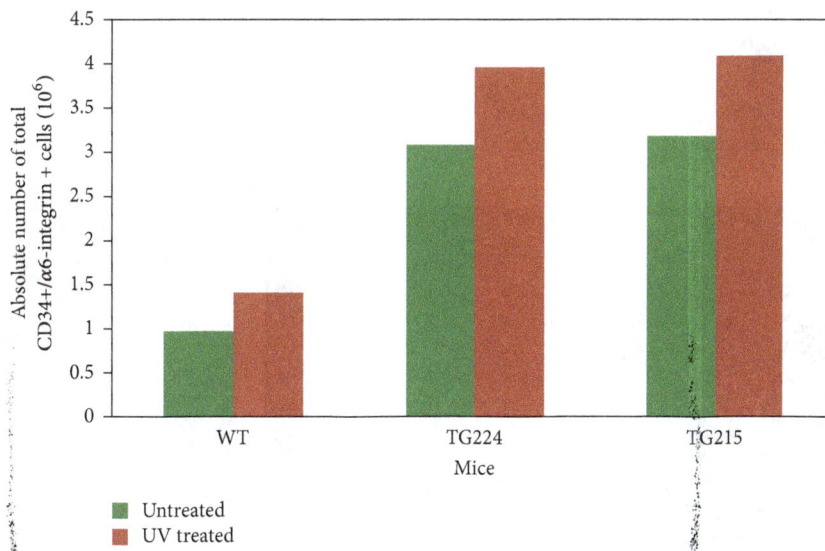

(b)

FIGURE 3: Effects of chronic UV exposures on live epidermal stem cell population determined by flow cytometric analysis. PKCε overexpressing TG and their WT littermates were given total eight UV exposures ($1.8\,kJ/m^2$, Monday, Wednesday, and Friday). At 24 hr after the last UV exposure, mice were sacrificed and the dorsal skin removed for keratinocyte isolation. (a) Percent distribution of FACS-sorted keratinocytes following UV exposures of the indicated mice. (b) Frequency of total double positive HSCs (CD34+/α6-integrin+) keratinocytes in UV-treated mice.

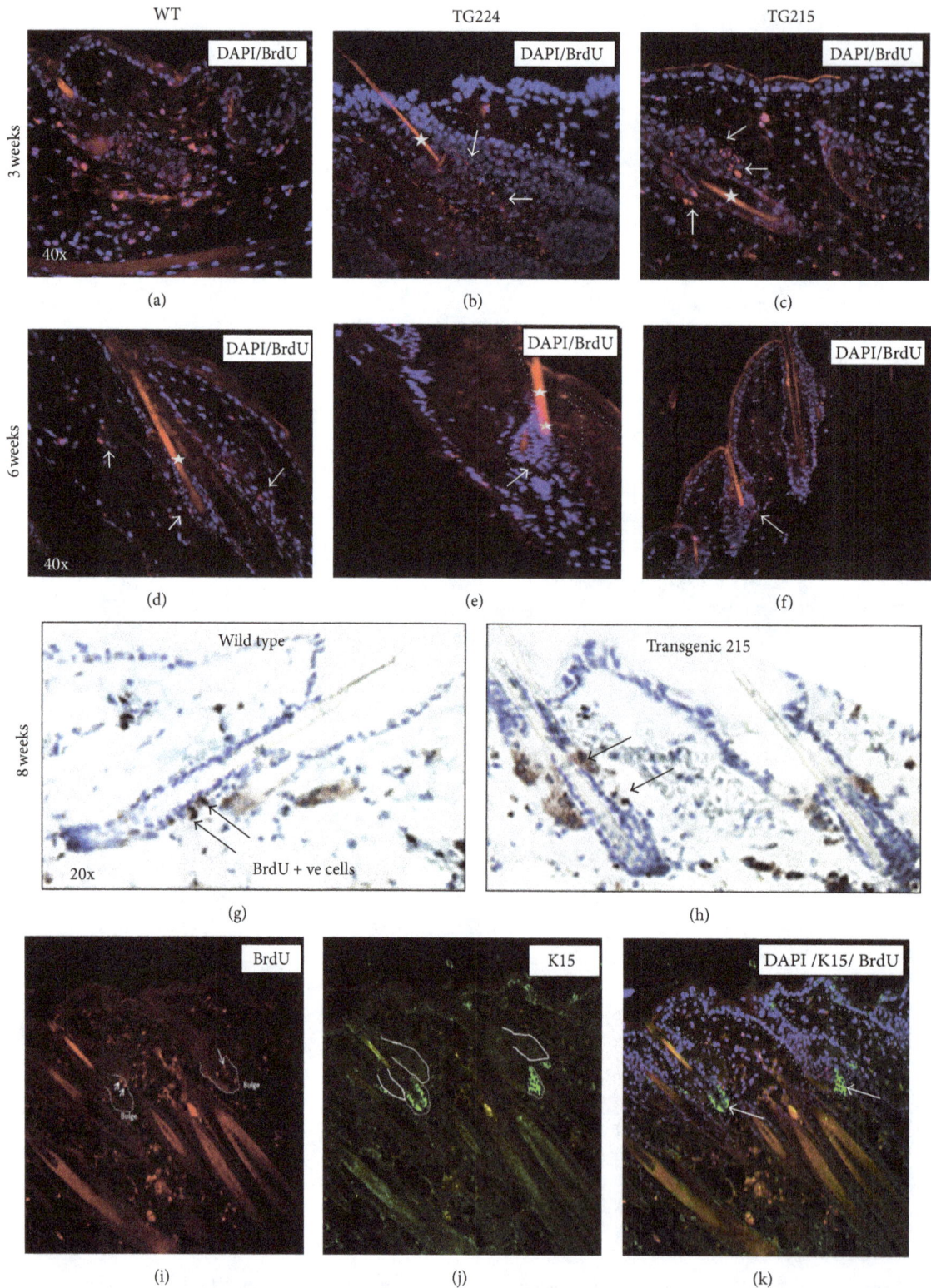

FIGURE 4: Detection of label retaining cells (LRC) by immunostaining using antibody to BrdU: to identify the LRCs, newborn mice (3 days old) were injected subcutaneously with BrdU (50 mg/kg body weight) twice daily for 3 days. Mice were sacrificed at 3, 6, and 8 weeks after BrdU injection. Shown are the representative photographs of BrdU-labeled cells from paraffin-fixed skin sections from WT and TG mice. The white arrow points to BrdU positive cells in the bulge region of hair follicle. In all the figures, the asterisk is the autofluorescence of the hair shaft. The incorporation and retention of BrdU are shown in the various parts of hair follicle at 3, 6, and 8 weeks in the indicated mice (a)–(h). (i)–(k) are showing the dual labeling of BrdU and k15 expressing cells in the bulge region of hair follicle.

(a)

(b)

(c)

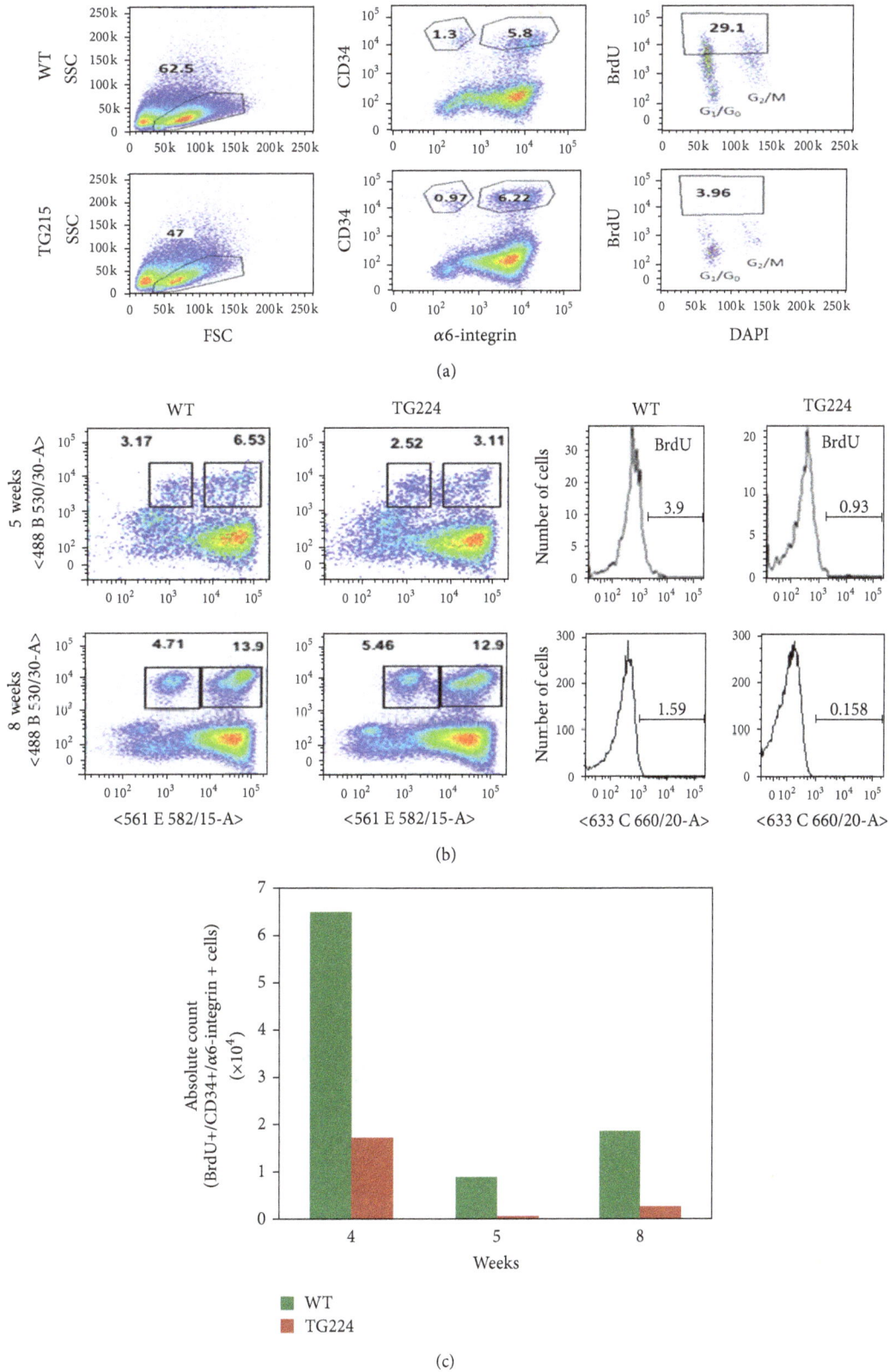

FIGURE 5: PKCε overexpressing transgenic mice have increased turnover of HSCs as determined by BrdU retaining double positive HSCs (CD34+/α6-integrin+). To identify LRCs, newborn mice (3 days old) were injected subcutaneously with BrdU (50 mg/Kg body weight) twice daily for 3 days. Mice were then sacrificed at 8 weeks after the last BrdU injection. There were four mice per group. (a) Representative gating of cell populations for side scatter (SSC) versus forward scatter (FSC). (b) Representative gating of cell populations at 5 and 8 weeks in the indicated mice. (c) Frequency of total BrdU-labeled double positive (CD34+/α6-integrin+) keratinocytes in TG 224 and their WT littermates at 4, 5, and 8 weeks.

TABLE 1: List of differentially expressed genes in CD34+/α6-integrin+ stem cells from PKCε TG mice. Overexpression of PKCε in the epidermis results in increased expression of genes linked to cell transformation, invasion, and metastasis.

Serial number	Gene name	Upregulated (↑) genes/fold change	Serial number	Gene name	Downregulated (↓) genes/fold change
(1)	Pescadillo	(3.2) ↑	(8)	Ccnf	(0.06) ↓
(2)	Tfdp-1 (Transcriptional factor)	(2.2) ↑	(9)	Cdkn1a (p21)	(0.5) ↓
(3)	Rad21	(1.8) ↑	(10)	Pkd-1	(0.5) ↓
(4)	Nfatc1	(1.7) ↑	(11)	Taf10 (TafII30)	(0.5) ↓
(5)	Cks1b	(1.6) ↑	(12)	Sfn	(0.6) ↓
(6)	Ak1	(1.3) ↑	(13)	Sumo1	(0.7) ↓
(7)	Itgb1	(1.2) ↑	(14)	RAN	(0.8) ↓

There was also a decrease in total frequency as well as absolute count of BrdU retaining double positive HSCs in TG224 mice compared to WT littermates (Figures 5(b) and 5(c)).

3.4. PKCε mRNA Levels in FACS-Sorted Keratinocytes.

We first analyzed the percent distribution of CD34+, CD34+/α6-integrin+ (double positive HSCs), α6-integrin+, and CD34−/α6-integrin- (double negative) in TG224, TG215, and their WT littermates. The α6-integrin+ cells were 70.9%, 62.7%, and 54.8% in WT, TG224, and TG215 mice, respectively. The CD34+ cells were 2.8%, 4.0%, and 3.1% in WT, TG224, and TG215 mice, respectively (Figure 6(a)). We analyzed the PKCε mRNA expression levels in FACS-sorted keratinocytes (Figure 6(b)). The higher expression of PKCε was recorded in double positive HSCs of TG215 mice compared to WT and TG224 (Figure 6(b)).

3.5. PKCε Transgenic Mice Have Increased Expression of Genes Linked to Cell Transformation, Invasion, and Metastasis.

A possibility explored that an increased turnover of HSCs in TG mice may be the result of changes in specific genes. In this experiment (Table 1), the effect of UV on cell cycle-related genes in double positive HSCs of TG and WT was determined using a focused cell cycle PCR array. Double positive HSCs of TG215 and their WT littermates were sorted out. A comparison of gene expression profiles of double positive HSCs is shown in Table 1. A 1.7- to 3.2-fold increase in the expression of Pes1, Rad21, Tfdp1, and Cks1b genes was observed in TG215 mice compared to their WT littermates. However, downregulation of Ccnf, Cdkn1a (p21), pkd-1, and Taf10 was observed in TG215 mice as compared to WT littermates.

4. Discussion

Chronic exposure of Sun's UV radiation is linked to the development of human SCC, a metastatic nonmelanoma skin cancer [22]. We found using a novel PKCε TG mouse model that the PKCε levels in epidermis dictate the susceptibility of transgenic mice to the induction of SCC by UV [8]. PKCε TG mice, when exposed to UV ($2 \, \text{kJ/m}^2$ thrice weekly), elicited 3-fold increased SCC multiplicity and decreased tumor latency by 12 weeks. PKCε overexpression in mice suppressed UV-induced sunburn (apoptotic) cell formation and enhanced both UV-induced hyperplasia and levels of specific cytokines (tumor necrosis factor α (TNFα), granulocyte colony-stimulating factor (G-CSF), granulocyte macrophage colony-stimulating factor, and interleukin six (IL-6)), implying inhibition of apoptosis and promotion of preneoplastic cell survival [8, 23]. Additionally, PKCε may impart sensitivity to UVR carcinogenesis via its association with Stat3, a transcriptional factor that is constitutively activated in both mouse and human SCC [24]. We now present that PKCε-mediated susceptibility to UV carcinogenesis may involve stimulation of putative HSCs proliferation possibly mediated by PKCε and other specific genes linked to the cell cycle regulation.

The epidermis undergoes a continual renewal throughout life, and the process is facilitated by various stem cell localized in both interfollicular epidermis and other specialized stem cell niches such as bulge. The skin stem cells present in different compartment of hair follicles respond differently to various signals mediated by their microenvironment [25]. Interestingly, multiple skin stem cell populations exist in the epidermis and play an important role during the process of controlled proliferation and differentiation (reviewed in [26]). The major stem cell population of hair follicle includes interfollicular label retaining cells (LRCs), double positive HSCs (CD34+/α6-integrin+), Mts24+ cells, Blimp1, Nestin, Lgr5+, and Lgr6+ cells (reviewed in [26]). However, the bulge region of hair follicle is considered as the major niche for keratinocyte stem cells [27, 28]. Particularly, the CD34+/α6-integrin+ cells are slow cycling and colocalize with LRCs and confined to bulge region of hair follicles. In terms of their colony forming ability (clonogenicity), CD34+ cells make larger colonies compared to CD34− cells [16, 29]. Keratinocytes isolated from PKCε overexpressing TG have higher frequency of double positive HSCs (CD34+/α6-integrin+) and clonogenicity than their WT littermates (Figure 1).

UV treatment resulted in a modest increase in total double positive HSCs in both TG224 and TG215 mice compared to their WT littermates (Figure 2). UV treatment in TG mice as compared to WT mice leads to constitutive activation of Stat3, increased Stat3-DNA binding [24], and increased

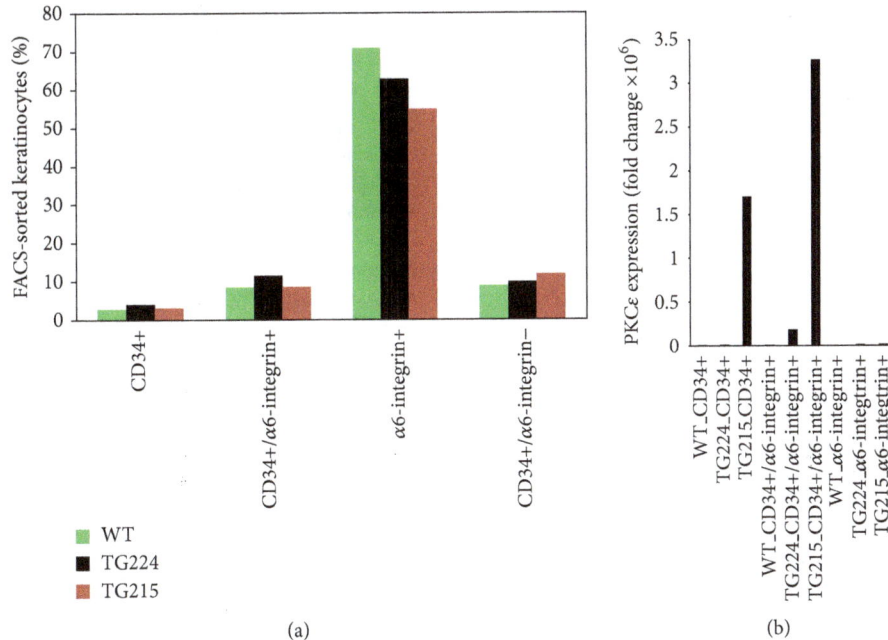

FIGURE 6: Distribution and expression of PKCε in FACS-sorted keratinocytes from WT, TG224, and TG215 mice. (a) FACS-sorted keratinocytes. The keratinocytes were harvested from 5 weeks old wild-type and TG mice and incubated with the CD34 and α6-integrin florescent antibodies. After labeling, the cells were washed twice, filtered, and sorted for CD34+, α6-integrin+ cells, CD34+/α6-integrin+, and CD34−/α6-integrin-cells. (b) PKCε expression. The RNA was isolated from the sorted cell, followed by cDNA preparation, and then real-time PCR using SYBR Green double-strand DNA binding dye. After real-time PCR Ct values were calculated and analyzed for expression. All the expression values shown in the figures are relative to their mouse Gapdh internal control.

expression of TNFα and G-CSF [8]. Results from genetic experiments indicate that both Stat3 and TNFα are linked to UV-induced development of SCC. It yet remains to be proven that PKCε downstream components Stat3 and TNFα directly affect the proliferation of putative HSCs.

We observed less BrdU retaining double positive HSCs cells in TG mice compared to WT (Figure 3). These results indicate rapid turnover of double positive HSCs cells in TG mice. Evidence indicates that at least two types of cell population exist: the slow cycling designated as stem cells and rapidly cycling cells as transit amplifying cells [30–32]. Rapid turnover of double positive HSCs cells in TG mice may be the effect of overexpression of PKCε in TG mice and its associated cytokines such as TNFα and G-CSF [33]. Additionally, the level or percentage of BrdU retention in the stem cell populations is not consistently uniform. BrdU retention is influenced by mice age, time of labeling, and site of labeling [34]. This may be the possible explanation that the amount of BrdU retained varies in different repeat experiments (Figure 3). However, BrdU retaining double positive HSCs cells were consistently less in TG mice compared to WT.

An analysis of focused cell cycle cDNA array revealed up- and downregulation of specific genes. The genes found to be overexpressed in double positive HSCs in TG215 were Pescadillo, Tfdp-1, Rad21, Nfatc1, Cks1b, AK1, and Itgb1. The gene Tfdp-1 is found to be overexpressed in SCC [35–38]. Interestingly, Nfatc1 gene is found to be overexpressed in many cancers, and its loss is linked with constant hair cycling

and no quiescence [39]. Nfatc1 is also responsible for the balance between the quiescence and proliferation stage of skin stem cells [40]. Other overexpressed genes, Pescadillo, Rad21, Cks1b, Ak1, and Itgb1, are also linked with the process of carcinogenesis (Table 1).

5. Conclusion

In summary, we present for the first time an association of PKCε with HSCs, the SCC precursors [20]. PKCε overexpression in mice increased the clonogenicity of isolated keratinocytes, a property commonly ascribed to stem cells. Both single and chronic UV-treatments resulted in an increase in the frequency of double positive HSCs in PKCε TG mice as compared to their WT littermates. In TG mice, HSCs cycle at a faster rate as compared to wild-type mice. A comparison of gene expression profiles of FACS-sorted double positive keratinocytes isolated from UV-treated WT and TG mice indicated increased expression of Pes1, Rad21, Tfdp1, and Cks1b genes in TG mice linked to cell transformation, invasion, and metastasis of cancer cells.

It is believed that the skin stem cells are the major targets of carcinogen [15, 41]. However, the identification and the precise location of cancer initiating cells in cutaneous SCC is not clear. Furthermore, the role of nonstem cell cannot be overlooked during the process of carcinogenesis. It has been observed that the differentiated, nondividing epidermal cells with activated MAPK kinase 1 and inflammatory infiltrate can initiate benign tumor formation [42]. Interestingly, the differentiated keratinocytes can reenter into active cell cycling, dedifferentiating, and acquiring the stemness [43]. In future it will be interesting to study the link of double positive HSCs and other skin stem cell populations, along with other inflammatory signals in UV-induced Squamous cell carcinoma.

Abbreviations

BrdU: 5-Bromo-2′-deoxyuridine
DAG: Diacylglycerol
DMBA: 7,12-Dimethylbenz[a]anthracene
FACS: Fluorescence assisted cell sorting
G-CSF: Granulocyte colony-stimulating factor
GM-CSF: Granulocyte macrophage
            colony-stimulating factor
HSCs: Hair follicle stem cells
LRCs: Label retaining cells
PKCε: Protein Kinase C epsilon
SCC: Squamous cell carcinoma
TNFα: Tumor necrosis factor alpha
TPA: 12-O-Tetradecanoylphorbol-13-acetate
UVR: Ultraviolet radiation.

Acknowledgments

The authors are thankful to Nancy E. Dreckschmidt for her technical support. The study was supported by NIH Grant (CA102431) to Ajit K. Verma and Molecular and Environmental Toxicology Center predoctoral training Grant (T32ES007015) to Jordan M. Sand. The authors are also thankful to UWCC Cancer Center core facility.

References

[1] R. K. Boutwell, "The function and mechanism of promoters of carcinogenesis," *CRC Critical Reviews in Toxicology*, vol. 2, no. 4, pp. 419–443, 1974.

[2] S. H. Yuspa, A. A. Dlugosz, M. F. Denning, and A. B. Click, "Multistage carcinogenesis in the skin," *Journal of Investigative Dermatology*, vol. 1, no. 2, pp. 147–150, 1996.

[3] E. M. Griner and M. G. Kazanietz, "Protein kinase C and other diacylglycerol effectors in cancer," *Nature Reviews Cancer*, vol. 7, no. 4, pp. 281–294, 2007.

[4] H. Mellor and P. J. Parker, "The extended protein kinase C superfamily," *The Biochemical Journal*, vol. 332, no. 2, pp. 281–292, 1998.

[5] A. C. Newton, "Protein kinase C: structural and spatial regulation by phosphorylation, cofactors, and macromolecular interactions," *Chemical Reviews*, vol. 101, no. 8, pp. 2353–2364, 2001.

[6] D. Mochly-Rosen and L. M. Kauvar, "Modulating protein kinase C signal transduction," *Advances in Pharmacology*, vol. 44, pp. 91–145, 1998.

[7] M. F. Denning, "Epidermal keratinocytes: regulation of multiple cell phenotypes by multiple protein kinase C isoforms," *The International Journal of Biochemistry and Cell Biology*, vol. 36, no. 7, pp. 1141–1146, 2004.

[8] D. L. Wheeler, K. E. Martin, K. J. Ness et al., "Protein kinase C ε is an endogenous photosensitizer that enhances ultraviolet radiation-induced cutaneous damage and development of squamous cell carcinomas," *Cancer Research*, vol. 64, no. 21, pp. 7756–7765, 2004.

[9] P. J. Reddig, N. E. Dreckschmidt, J. Zou, S. E. Bourguignon, T. D. Oberley, and A. K. Verma, "Transgenic mice overexpressing protein kinase Cε in their epidermis exhibit reduced papilloma burden but enhanced carcinoma formation after tumor promotion," *Cancer Research*, vol. 60, no. 3, pp. 595–602, 2000.

[10] A. P. Jansen, E. G. Verwiebe, N. E. Dreckschmidt, D. L. Wheeler, T. D. Oberley, and A. K. Verma, "Protein kinase C-ε transgenic mice: a unique model for metastatic squamous cell carcinoma," *Cancer Research*, vol. 61, no. 3, pp. 808–812, 2001.

[11] A. Basu and U. Sivaprasad, "Protein kinase Cε makes the life and death decision," *Cellular Signalling*, vol. 19, no. 8, pp. 1633–1642, 2007.

[12] A. K. Verma, D. L. Wheeler, M. H. Aziz, and H. Manoharan, "Protein kinase Cε and development of squamous cell carcinoma, the nonmelanoma human skin cancer," *Molecular Carcinogenesis*, vol. 45, no. 6, pp. 381–388, 2006.

[13] C. Blanpain, "Tracing the cellular origin of cancer," *Nature Cell Biology*, vol. 15, no. 2, pp. 126–134, 2013.

[14] T. Tumbar, G. Guasch, V. Greco et al., "Defining the epithelial stem cell niche in skin," *Science*, vol. 303, no. 5656, pp. 359–363, 2004.

[15] T. Kangsamaksin, H. J. Park, C. S. Trempus, and R. J. Morris, "A perspective on murine keratinocyte stem cells as targets of chemically induced skin cancer," *Molecular Carcinogenesis*, vol. 46, no. 8, pp. 579–584, 2007.

[16] C. S. Trempus, R. J. Morris, C. D. Bortner et al., "Enrichment for living murine keratinocytes from the hair follicle bulge with the cell surface marker CD34," *Journal of Investigative Dermatology*, vol. 120, no. 4, pp. 501–511, 2003.

[17] A. Faurschou, M. Haedersdal, T. Poulsen, and H. C. Wulf, "Squamous cell carcinoma induced by ultraviolet radiation originates from cells of the hair follicle in mice," *Experimental Dermatology*, vol. 16, no. 6, pp. 485–489, 2007.

[18] R. J. Morris, Y. Liu, L. Marles et al., "Capturing and profiling adult hair follicle stem cells," *Nature Biotechnology*, vol. 22, no. 4, pp. 411–417, 2004.

[19] C. S. Trempus, R. J. Morris, M. Ehinger et al., "CD34 expression by hair follicle stem cells is required for skin tumor development in mice," *Cancer Research*, vol. 67, no. 9, pp. 4173–4181, 2007.

[20] R. J. Morris, K. A. Tryson, and K. Q. Wu, "Evidence that the epidermal targets of carcinogen action are found in the interfollicular epidermis or infundibulum as well as in the hair follicles," *Cancer Research*, vol. 60, no. 2, pp. 226–229, 2000.

[21] W. Y. Wu and R. J. Morris, "Method for the harvest and assay of in vitro clonogenic keratinocytes stem cells from mice," *Methods in Molecular Biology*, vol. 289, pp. 79–86, 2005.

[22] J. Schmitt, A. Seidler, T. L. Diepgen, and A. Bauer, "Occupational ultraviolet light exposure increases the risk for the development of cutaneous squamous cell carcinoma: a systematic review and meta-analysis," *British Journal of Dermatology*, vol. 164, no. 2, pp. 291–307, 2011.

[23] D. L. Wheeler, K. J. Ness, T. D. Oberley, and A. K. Verma, "Protein kinase Cε is linked to 12-O-tetradecanoylphorbol-13-acetate-induced tumor necrosis factor-α ectodomain shedding and the development of metastatic squamous cell carcinoma in protein kinase Cε transgenic mice," *Cancer Research*, vol. 63, no. 19, pp. 6547–6555, 2003.

[24] M. H. Aziz, H. T. Manoharan, J. M. Sand, and A. K. Verma, "Protein kinase Cε interacts with Stat3 and regulates its activation that is essential for the development of skin cancer," *Molecular Carcinogenesis*, vol. 46, no. 8, pp. 646–653, 2007.

[25] M. Petersson and C. Niemann, "Stem cell dynamics and heterogeneity: implications for epidermal regeneration and skin cancer," *Current Medicinal Chemistry*, vol. 19, no. 35, pp. 5984–5992, 2012.

[26] A. Singh, H. Park, T. Kangsamaksin, N. Readio, and R. J. Morris, "Keratinocyte stem cells and the targets for nonmelanoma skin cancer," *Photochemistry and Photobiology*, vol. 88, no. 5, pp. 1099–1110, 2012.

[27] G. Cotsarelis, T. T. Sun, and R. M. Lavker, "Label-retaining cells reside in the bulge area of pilosebaceous unit: implications for follicular stem cells, hair cycle, and skin carcinogenesis," *Cell*, vol. 61, no. 7, pp. 1329–1337, 1990.

[28] R. J. Morris and C. S. Potten, "Slowly cycling (label-retaining) epidermal cells behave like clonogenic stem cells in vitro," *Cell Proliferation*, vol. 27, no. 5, pp. 279–289, 1994.

[29] C. Blanpain, W. E. Lowry, A. Geoghegan, L. Polak, and E. Fuchs, "Self-renewal, multipotency, and the existence of two cell populations within an epithelial stem cell niche," *Cell*, vol. 118, no. 5, pp. 635–648, 2004.

[30] K. M. Braun and F. M. Watt, "Epidermal label-retaining cells: background and recent applications," *Journal of Investigative Dermatology*, vol. 9, no. 3, pp. 196–201, 2004.

[31] R. J. Morris, S. M. Fischer, and T. J. Slaga, "Evidence that the centrally and peripherally located cells in the murine epidermal proliferative unit are two distinct cell populations," *Journal of Investigative Dermatology*, vol. 84, no. 4, pp. 277–281, 1985.

[32] J. R. Bickenbach, "Identification and behavior of label-retaining cells in oral mucosa and skin," *Journal of Dental Research*, vol. 60, pp. 1611–1620, 1981.

[33] D. L. Wheeler, Y. Li, and A. K. Verma, "Protein kinase C epsilon signals ultraviolet light-induced cutaneous damage and development of squamous cell carcinoma possibly through induction of specific cytokines in a paracrine mechanism," *Photochemistry and Photobiology*, vol. 81, no. 1, pp. 9–18, 2005.

[34] J. R. Bickenbach, J. McCutecheon, and I. C. Mackenzie, "Rate of loss of tritiated thymidine label in basal cells in mouse epithelial tissues," *Cell and Tissue Kinetics*, vol. 19, no. 3, pp. 325–333, 1986.

[35] L. R. Bandara, V. M. Buck, M. Zamanian, L. H. Johnston, and N. B. La Thangue, "Functional synergy between DP-1 and E2F-1 in the cell cycle-regulating transcription factor DRTF1/E2F," *The EMBO Journal*, vol. 12, no. 11, pp. 4317–4324, 1993.

[36] K. Yasui, H. Okamoto, S. Arii, and J. Inazawa, "Association of over-expressed TFDP1 with progression of hepatocellular carcinomas," *Journal of Human Genetics*, vol. 48, no. 12, pp. 609–613, 2003.

[37] T. Shinomiya, T. Mori, Y. Ariyama et al., "Comparative genomic hybridization of squamous cell carcinoma of the esophagus: the possible involvement of the DP1 gene in the 13q34 amplicon," *Genes, Chromosomes & Cancer*, vol. 24, no. 4, pp. 337–344, 1999.

[38] L. Melchor, L. P. Saucedo-Cuevas, I. Muñoz-Repeto et al., "Comprehensive characterization of the DNA amplification at 13q34 in human breast cancer reveals TFDP1 and CUL4A as likely candidate target genes," *Breast Cancer Research*, vol. 11, no. 6, article R86, 2009.

[39] F. M. Watt and K. B. Jensen, "Epidermal stem cell diversity and quiescence," *EMBO Molecular Medicine*, vol. 1, no. 5, pp. 260–267, 2009.

[40] V. Horsley, A. O. Aliprantis, L. Polak, L. H. Glimcher, and E. Fuchs, "NFATc1 balances quiescence and proliferation of skin stem cells," *Cell*, vol. 132, no. 2, pp. 299–310, 2008.

[41] J. Perez-Losada and A. Balmain, "Stem-cell hierarchy in skin cancer," *Nature Reviews Cancer*, vol. 3, no. 6, pp. 434–443, 2003.

[42] E. N. Arwert, R. Lal, S. Quist, I. Rosewell, N. Van Rooijen, and F. M. Watt, "Tumor formation initiated by nondividing epidermal cells via an inflammatory infiltrate," *Proceedings of the National Academy of Sciences of the United States of America*, vol. 107, no. 46, pp. 19903–19908, 2010.

[43] J. Mannik, K. Alzayady, and S. Ghazizadeh, "Regeneration of multilineage skin epithelia by differentiated keratinocytes," *Journal of Investigative Dermatology*, vol. 130, no. 2, pp. 388–397, 2010.

10

Sociodemographic and Psychological Correlates of Sun Protection Behaviors among Outdoor Workers

Vinayak K. Nahar,[1] M. Allison Ford,[1] Jeffrey S. Hallam,[2] Martha A. Bass,[1] and Michael A. Vice[1]

[1] *Department of Health, Exercise Science & Recreation Management, The University of Mississippi, 215 Turner Center, P.O. Box 1848, University, MS 38677, USA*

[2] *Department of Social and Behavioral Sciences, College of Public Health, Kent State University, 750 Hilltop Drive, Kent, OH 44242, USA*

Correspondence should be addressed to Vinayak K. Nahar; vknahar@go.olemiss.edu

Academic Editor: Giuseppe Argenziano

Outdoor workers are at a higher risk for developing skin cancer due to their increased sun exposure. The primary objective of this review was to synthesize the current research literature that addresses sociodemographic and psychological factors related to sun protection behaviors in outdoor workers. Two additional purposes were to provide an overview of sun exposure and describe sun protection behaviors of outdoor workers. To identify the studies for this review, a methodical search was performed in the PubMed, PsycInfo, MEDLINE, and ERIC databases. Fifteen studies met the review criteria. Despite regular and prolonged sun exposure, many outdoor workers fail to engage in sufficient sun protection behaviors. Correlates of outdoor workers' sun protection behaviors include being female, older age, being white, personal skin cancer history, time (hours/years) spent at work, sun safety training, perceived prioritization of sun protection, concern about sun exposure, workplace support, families' expectations, and familial information giving. However, limited attention is given to designing theoretically grounded studies to identify factors to inform future research. There is a need to conduct research based on solid theoretical foundations that explains the relationships among the factors in this domain.

1. Introduction

Skin cancer is a significant public health problem in the US [1, 2]. Each year over 3.5 million cases of skin cancer are diagnosed, resulting in nearly 12,000 deaths [3]. Since sun exposure is the primary risk factor for all forms of skin cancer, nearly 90% of skin cancers are considered preventable [4, 5]. Recommended sun protection behaviors include using the shade, avoiding being outdoors during the hours of highest sun intensity (between 10:00 a.m. and 4:00 p.m.), and using sun protective clothing, hats, sunglasses, and sunscreen, preferably a sunscreen with a sun protection factor (SPF) not less than 30 [3].

All individuals are at risk for developing skin cancer; however, there are groups, most notably outdoor workers, who are more vulnerable to skin cancer compared to other populations [6, 7]. This is quite obvious considering the regular and considerable amount of time they spend exposed to solar ultraviolet radiation (UVR) during work—at least two to eight hours per day [8, 9]. In addition, it is documented that outdoor workers exposure to UVR is much higher than the recommended guidelines [8].

There is substantial evidence to support the significant association between skin cancer and cumulative, as well as, intermittent sun exposure in outdoor workers [7, 10–13]. In addition, solar UVR dose received by outdoor workers is about six to eight times higher than indoor workers, and outdoor workers have a greater chance of being diagnosed with skin cancer [8, 14–17]. In addition, high incidence and mortality rates of skin cancer are found in occupational groups that work outdoors [18–20].

Outdoor workers make up a sizable proportion of the work population that spreads across a wide range of jobs.

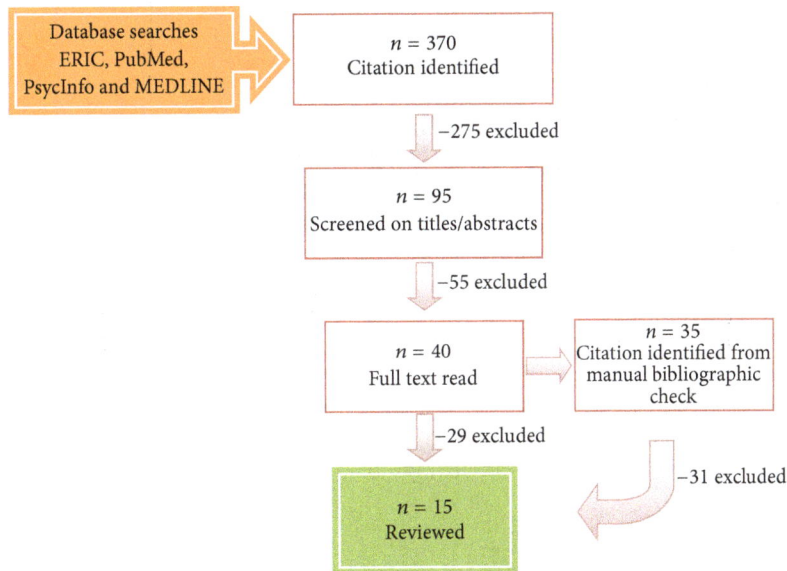

FIGURE 1: Flow chart of the literature search.

According to the US Census Bureau, occupational groups that work outdoors represent more than eight percent of the total US national work force (over 9 million workers) [21]. These groups tend to have an ethnoracial majority of fair skinned individuals which is strongly linked with an elevated risk for skin cancer, primarily due to inherently low amounts of melanin present in the skin, the pigment responsible for skin color and protection against harmful UVR [21–24].

Furthermore, several epidemiological studies note that men are at a significantly higher skin cancer risk than women [25–27]. Existence of skin cancer development disparity between men and women is not a natural phenomenon but is due to greater percentage of men in outdoor occupations and the differences between men and women in skin protection behaviors and lifestyle choices [24, 26–31].

Despite the fact that sun protection behaviors are promoted, incidence rates of skin cancer in outdoor workers continue to be high. Prior research has addressed personal and behavioral factors, but no review published to date has examined the sociodemographic and psychological correlates of skin cancer and the sun protection practices of outdoor workers. Therefore, the primary objective of this review is to provide an overview of the available research that addresses sociodemographic and psychological factors associated with sun protection behaviors in outdoor workers. In addition, this review includes a description of sun exposure and sun protection practices of outdoor workers.

2. Methods

To identify the studies for the review, a methodical comprehensive computerized search was performed using PubMed, PsycInfo, MEDLINE, and ERIC databases. The terms "skin cancer," "melanoma," "sun protection," "sun exposure," "sun behavior," and "skin cancer prevention in outdoor workers," were searched as keywords or phrases. Additional searches

were performed in the websites of the following organizations: the Centers for Disease Control and Prevention (CDC), the American Cancer Society (ACS), the American Academy of Dermatology (AAD), the Skin Cancer Foundation, and the Melanoma Foundation of Australia. Bibliographies of articles were also manually searched to identify pertinent articles that were not identified in the initial search.

The search was limited to studies published in English. In the last two decades, there was a surge in interest and research on the topic of skin cancer; therefore, the decision to review articles published from 1990 to the present was made to include seminal research conducted within the last 20 years.

Research studies specifically emphasizing outdoor workers' skin cancer or sun-protection-related knowledge, beliefs, behaviors, and attitudes towards sun safety were considered eligible for inclusion in the review. Articles were excluded if (1) the results of the article were not relevant to the aims of the review; (2) the article examined clinical issues or the effect of specific treatments or settings; (3) the article described sun protection behavior of different population groups along with outdoor workers; (4) the article was a duplicate, a conference abstract, an editorial, a case report, a letter, or commentary; or (5) the article was published in an online newspapers that is not peer reviewed.

The electronic search identified 370 citations, with 275 citations being excluded on the basis of the inclusion criteria. Titles and abstracts of the remaining 95 citations were screened, and 55 more articles were eliminated. The remaining 40 articles were read to determine if they met the inclusion criteria. We identified 35 additional articles from the reference lists of the 40 articles. Of these 75 articles, 15 fully met the inclusion criteria and were included in this review. The summary of reviewed studies is provided in Table 1, and the process of the literature search is illustrated in Figure 1.

TABLE 1: A Summary of the reviewed studies.

Author, date	Study design, methods	Population, sample size (n)	Average sun exposure and occupational years	Sun protection behaviors	Barriers to sun protection	Correlates of sun protection behavior	Limitations
Marlenga [36]	Cross-sectional Self-administered mail surveys	Dairy farmers, 100% male, n = 202	4.15 hours/day 42.95 years	Long pants (90%), wide-brimmed hat (13%), sunscreen (8%), and long-sleeved shirts (7%)	Too hot to wear long-sleeved shirt (88%), tan looks attractive (>50%), and I forgot to wear sunscreen (45%)	*Psychological:* perceived barriers	Results were not generalizable to all farmers
Rosenman et al. [32]	Cross-sectional Self-administered mail survey	Farmers, n = 1,342	Not reported	65% of the women and 43% of the men were very likely to practice some type of sun protection	Not reported	*Demographic:* female gender, increased age, higher personal history of skin cancer, and greater income among females	Results were not generalizable to all rural populations Superficial data on potential confounders
Parrott et al. [37]	Cross-sectional pilot Intercept survey, field observations, and in-depth interviews	Intercept survey: 155 farmers, 100% White. Fields observations: 49 farmers, 41 construction workers, 39 road workers, and 15 other outdoor workers In-depth interview: 9 farmers	Not reported	65% did not wear long-sleeved shirts, 49% did not apply sunscreen, and 43% did not wear wide-brimmed hats	Amount of time needed to put on long-sleeved shirt (30%), wide-brimmed hats are uncomfortable (21%), and sunscreen is messy to apply (11%)	*Demographic:* increased age	Not reported
Stepanski and Mayer [35]	Cross-sectional field observation, and self-administered survey	Construction workers, Caltrans workers, and mail carriers 80.1% males and 61.0% White, n = 240 (survey data) n = 312 (observation data)	5.11–7.94 hours/work day	50.4% reported sufficient use of sun protection (observational data)	Not reported	Not found	Observational data did not represent typical sun protection behavior Convenience sample Recall, social desirability, and self-selection bias Study design
Shoveller et al. [38]	Cross-sectional Telephone survey	General outdoor workers, 80% male, n = 546	>2 hours/work day (70%)	Sun protective clothing (60%), hat (58%), sunscreen on face (23%), and sunscreen on body (18%)	I forgot (61%), inconvenient (54%), liked tanned skin (38%), and not worried about UVR exposure (34%)	Not reported	No information was provided about types of hats worn and lengths of sleeves on shirts
Cioffi et al. [39]	Cross-sectional Self-administered survey	Construction workers, 97.8% males, n = 142	Not reported	Sunglasses (61%), wide-brimmed hat (54%), sunscreen (34%), long-sleeved shirt (11%), and use of shade (5%)	Perceived tan is attractive (72%) and healthy (44%)	Not reported	Validity and reliability of instrument was not tested Convenience sample
Woolley et al. [29]	Cross-sectional Self-administered mail survey	General outdoor workers, 100% males, n = 300	>50% of mainly outdoor workers spent >6 hours/work day	Wide-brimmed hat (77.2%) and long-sleeved shirts (43.6%)	Not get around to putting it on (24%), inconvenience (22%), and forget to bring it along (21%)	*Demographic:* sun sensitive skin type and personal history of skin cancer	Recall bias Self-selection bias Low response rate
Parrott and Lemieux [40]	Cross-sectional Telephone survey	Farmers, 100% males, n = 448	37.5 years	Not reported	Not reported	*Psychological:* knowledge about skin cancer *Social:* families' expectations and familial information giving	Not reported

TABLE 1: Continued.

Author, date	Study design, methods	Population, sample size (n)	Average sun exposure and occupational years	Sun protection behaviors	Barriers to sun protection	Correlates of sun protection behavior	Limitations
Pichon et al. [6]	Cross-sectional Self-administered survey	Postal workers, 68% males, 53.63% White, n = 2,543	4 hours/day 12 years	Sunscreen (14–30%), wide-brim hat (20–34%), and sunglasses use (44%–63%)	Not reported	*Demographic*: ethnicity, sensitive skin type, female gender (sunscreen), and male gender (hat)	Self-identified race Social desirability bias
Salas et al. [41]	Cross-sectional Interview and observation Self-administered survey	Farmworkers, 100% males, 100% Latino, n = 326	14.23 years	Long-sleeved shirt (89.7%), wide-brimmed hat (6%), sunglasses (2.5%), and sunscreen (1.6%)	Not reported	*Demographic*: longer years of work	Design of the study Convenience sample Social desirability bias
Lewis et al. [33]	Cross-sectional Field observation Self-administered survey	Postal workers, 69% males, 51.3% White, n = 2,600	3.9 hours/work day 3.3 hours/nonwork day	Sunscreen during work (25%) Sunscreen during leisure time (12%) Hat during work (24%) Hat during leisure time (4%)	Not reported	*Demographic*: ethnicity, sun sensitive skin type, hours spent outdoors, female gender with sunscreen use, male gender with hat use, and family history of skin cancer	Design of the study Differences in time period for reporting work days (5 days) and nonworking days (2 days) sun safety behavior
Hammond et al. [42]	Cross-sectional Self-administered survey Sun protection chart diary	Horticulture, roading, and building, 82% males, n = 74	Not reported	Not reported	Not reported	*Psychological*: suntan attitude and perceived risk of skin cancer *Social*: workplace support	Validity and reliability was not checked Small sample size Convenience sample Low response rate
Gies et al. [43]	Cross-sectional Field observation Self-administered survey 4-day diary	Lifeguards, 59.3% females, n = 168	4.29 hours/day	Phoenix: sunglasses (90.4%) and sunscreen (76.4%) Austin: hat (57%) and shade (31.2%) Portland: shirt (31.3%)	Not reported	Not reported	2-day UVR exposure measurements Difference in availability of natural shade at each pool site
McCool et al. [34]	Cross-sectional Self-administered survey	General outdoor workers, n = 1,283	Not reported	Not reported	Not reported	*Demographic*: female gender, increased age, and higher education *Psychological*: knowledge, perceived priority of sun protection, and higher concern about sun exposure *Social*: workplace support	Use of other sun protection measures (e.g., clothing and hat) were not investigated Self-selection bias
Madgwick et al. [44]	Cross-sectional Self-administered survey	Construction workers, 100% male, n = 360	6.6 hours/day	Sunscreen (≤0%), wearing long-sleeved loose fitted tops and trousers (51%), sunglasses (≤4%), and wide-brimmed hat (23%)	Not reported	*Demographic*: age, personal history of skin cancer, family history of skin cancer, hours spent outdoors, and receipt of sun safety training *Psychological*: desire for suntan	Self-selection bias Response bias

3. Results

3.1. Demographic

3.1.1. Disparity between Men and Women.
Of the five studies which reported sun protection behavior of both male and female outdoor workers, four studies documented differences between men and women in sun-related behaviors. Rosenman et al. (1995) found that female farmers in Michigan were more likely to practice some type of sun protection behaviors than male farmers [32]. Further support for gender differences was found in studies on postal workers. Results showed that female postal workers were more likely to wear sunscreen, whereas their male counterparts were more likely to wear a hat [6, 33]. Another important finding noted by Lewis et al. (2006) was that being female was the only common predictor of sunscreen use for both working and nonworking days [33]. Moreover, in a New Zealand study with a large sample of outdoor workers ($n = 1,283$), consistent with the previous studies, McCool et al. (2009) found that females were significantly more likely to wear sunscreen than males [34]. On the other hand, Stepanski and Mayer (1998) did not find a difference in UVR protection behaviors between male and female outdoor workers although this similarity in sun protective behaviors may result from clothing policies enforced by the companies [35].

3.1.2. Age.
There is evidence showing the relationship between age of outdoor workers and skin cancer prevention behaviors, although the study by Stepanski and Mayer (1998) demonstrates no correlation between age and sun protection behaviors [35]. However, Rosenman et al. (1995) show that increasing age influenced individuals to use protective measures against sun exposure [32]. Moreover, in-depth interviews conducted by Parrott et al. (1996) reveal that older participants were more willing to engage in sun protection practices than younger counterparts [37]. Supporting this, McCool and colleagues (2009) note that a greater likelihood of sunscreen use was related to being older [34]. In addition, Madgwick et al. (2011) find that age was positively correlated with wearing long-sleeved, loose fitting tops and trousers [44].

3.1.3. Ethnicity.
Ethnic background was recognized in the following studies as one of the factors related to outdoor workers sun protection behavior. Pichon et al. (2005) surveyed 2,660 participants (non-Latino White, Latino, Asian American, African American, and Pacific Islander) to compare sun-safety behaviors across ethnoracial groups employed as letters carriers at United States Postal Service (USPS) [6]. Results show that ethnicity was significantly associated with the use of sunscreen and sunglasses. Also, rates of sunscreen and sunglasses use in non-Latino White are significantly higher than the other four groups. Similar results for sunscreen use are echoed in a Lewis and colleagues (2006) study conducted one year later (i.e., sunscreen use at work is significantly associated with ethnicity and sunscreen use in non-Latino White postal workers was significantly higher than in Asians and African Americans postal workers) [33].

Therefore, ethnicity correlates with particular sun protection behaviors.

3.1.4. Skin Type.
Influence of skin type on sun protection behavior is investigated in many studies. Woolley et al. (2002) report a positive relationship between skin type and sun protective clothing use [29]. An encouraging result emerging from this study is that outdoor workers with more vulnerable skin types avoided the sun between 10:00 a.m. and 2:00 p.m.. Pichon et al. (2005) and Lewis et al. (2006) show increased sunscreen use and hat use with greater sun sensitivity [6, 33]. On the contrary, there are studies that yield no significant association between skin type and sun protection clothing use [34, 41]. However, Salas et al. (2005) speculate that there is no relationship because the use of sun protection clothing by outdoor workers is not to protect their skin but to protect themselves from occupational hazards such as handling pesticides or thorny branches [41]. Additionally, in McCool et al.'s (2009) study, researchers examined only sunscreen use behavior, whereas studies that show an association investigate more than one sun protection behavior [34]. After taking all the results and limitations of these studies into consideration, it is concluded that sensitive skin type plays a role in the sun protection behavior of outdoor workers.

3.1.5. Education.
Two studies were found that examined the relationship between education and sun protection behavior. The results are equivocal. Rosenman et al. (1995) report that increased education in farmers did not affect the likelihood of using sun protection [32]. Moreover, findings from a more recent study indicate that outdoor workers with higher education were significantly more likely to use sunscreen than outdoor workers with lower education [34]. The scarcity and ambiguity of data on the impact of education in outdoor workers makes it difficult to draw any firm conclusion.

3.1.6. Income.
To our knowledge, only one study documents the influence of income on sun protection behaviors [32]. Results show that increased income in female farmers appeared to increase the likelihood of using sun protection presumably because money is required for the purchase of sun protection modalities; whereas, male farmers show no increase in the likelihood of using sun protection with an increased income.

3.1.7. Time (Hours/Years) Spent at Work.
The amount of time (hours/years) that outdoor workers spend at work is found to be related to sun protection behavior. Lewis et al. (2006) show that the use of occupational sunscreen and hats in postal carriers is positively associated with hours worked outdoors [33]. Also, Madgwick et al. (2011) report that the more time construction workers spend outdoors, the more likely those construction workers will wear wide-brimmed hats [44]. In terms of years, Salas and colleagues (2005) note that participants who use higher levels of sun protective clothing worked as farm workers a significantly longer period of time than the participants who reported lower levels of protection [41].

3.1.8. Personal History of Skin Cancer. The evidence of the relationship between personal history of skin cancer and sun protection behaviors in outdoor workers is clearly seen in the study of Woolley et al. (2002) in which solar protection (77.4% wore wide-brimmed hats, 52% wore long-sleeved shirts, and 50% wore sunscreen when out for significant amount of time) of male outdoor workers with previously removed nonmelanoma skin cancer was considerably higher than solar protection of outdoor workers in other studies [29]. This reflects the finding of a prior study that documented personal history of skin cancer increased the likelihood of sun protective measures use in farmers and their spouses [32].

3.1.9. Family History of Skin Cancer. There is not sufficient evidence to support the influence of family history of skin cancer on sun protection behavior amongst outdoor workers. Participants of Rosenman et al.'s (1995) study did not show increased use of sun protection measure against sun if they had a family member or friend with skin cancer history [32]. Also, Stepanski and Mayer (1998) noted that UVR behavior score did not vary between participants with and without a family history of skin cancer [35]. Lewis et al. (2006) report having a family history of skin cancer as being significantly associated with engaging in sunscreen use, whereas no association was reported with occupational hats use [33]. Unfortunately, with only one study that somewhat supports the association between family history of skin cancer and outdoor workers sun protection behavior, any conclusion is speculative at best.

3.1.10. Sun Safety Training. The results of Madgwick et al.'s (2011) study show a positive association between receipt of sun safety training and sun protective behaviors including use of sunscreen [44].

3.2. Psychological

3.2.1. Knowledge. Of the research reviewed on sun protection behavior, one factor assessed in several studies is knowledge related to skin cancer or melanoma. A large number of studies reported that there appears to be a reasonable level of knowledge about the skin cancer. Wisconsin dairy farm workers report an average score of 70% correct on knowledge questions about skin cancer [36]. Also, 83% of Georgia farmers report having knowledge that the level of SPF in sun block or sunscreen should be 15 or higher and 90% indicate that melanoma is the most dangerous type of skin cancer [37]. In an Australian study, most of the outdoor construction workers report a high level of knowledge about skin cancer risk (94%), common areas of body to cover with sunscreen (82%), and use of sunglasses (85%) [39]. Moreover, the researchers of these studies report that this knowledge is not translated into sun protection behaviors; therefore, actual engagement in skin cancer prevention practices was poor. These findings further support the finding of Hammond et al. (2008) who show that sun protection practices are related to personal factors such as perceived susceptibility of developing skin cancer and perceived workplace support but not to

knowledge about skin cancer and prevention [42]. However, there is an inconsistency in the literature with regard to association between knowledge and skin cancer prevention. Studies yielded conflicting data, for example, Parrott and Lemieux (2003) find skin cancer knowledge of farmers positively associated with use of sunscreen, long-sleeved shirts, and sun protective hats [40]. Another example is McCool et al.'s (2009) who describe sunscreen use as strongly related to perceived knowledge about skin cancer [34].

3.2.2. Perceived Susceptibility. Of the research studies reviewed, only two studies examined the role of perceived susceptibility to skin cancer in determining sun protection behavior. Marlenga (1995) indicates that participants perceived a susceptibility to skin cancer; however, they did not use sun protection methods [36]. In contrast, Hammond and coworkers (2008) report that increased perceived susceptibility to skin cancer is one of the factors that increased the likelihood of using sun protection in outdoor workers [42]. Based on contradictory findings, it is not possible to suggest that sun protection behavior is associated with perceived susceptibility.

3.2.3. Perceived Barriers. A considerable amount of perceived barriers to sun protection are recognized in the reviewed studies. These include difficulty in remembering to use [29, 36, 38], amount of time [37], inconvenience or uncomfort to use [29, 36–38], not worrying about sun exposure [38], and perceived physical attractiveness of suntan [36, 38, 39, 44]. Furthermore, results of a study conducted by Marlenga (1995) reveal that, of all the addressed Health Belief Model (HBM) variables (except self-efficacy), perceived barriers was the only important predictor of whether farmers protect their skin from sun exposure [36].

3.2.4. Suntan Attitude. Two studies report an association between suntan attitudes and sun protection behaviors although findings were inconsistent. Hammond et al.'s (2008) study results suggested that positive suntan attitude in outdoor workers tended to reduce sun protection use [42], although findings from McCool et al.'s (2009) study suggest no significant association [34].

3.2.5. Perceived Priority. McCool et al. (2009) suggest that perceived priority of sun protection at work was significantly associated with use of sunscreen [34].

3.2.6. Concern. The results of McCool et al.'s (2009) study also suggested significant association between higher concern about sun exposure at work and sunscreen use [34].

3.3. Social

3.3.1. Workplace Support. In the recent years, researchers have investigated the association between workplace support and sun protection behavior in outdoor workers. McCool et al. (2009) report a positive association between workplace support and sun protection practice [34]. The findings of this study corroborate the results of a previous study [42]. This association is strong and persistent.

3.3.2. Familial Expectations and Information Giving. Parrott and Lemieux (2003) report that familial expectations and information giving was positively correlated with sun protection behaviors [40].

3.4. Sun Exposure. A Canadian national survey on sun exposure and protective behaviors reports that 70% of participants who worked outdoors experienced more than two hours of sun exposure during an average working day [38]. Sun exposure of construction workers in Britain was estimated at 6.6 hours per day [44]. In the US, construction workers, transportation workers, and letter carriers spent an average of 7.94, 6.95, and 5.11 hours, respectively, working outdoors [35]. Moreover, surveys of larger samples of postal workers in Southern California report receiving an average of 4 hours of sun exposure on workday [6]. Similarly, Wisconsin dairy farmers report being outdoors 4.15 hours daily [36]. Lifeguards in Austin, Phoenix, Omaha, and Portland recount spending an average of 4.29 hours a day in the sun [43].

Additionally, farmers report an average of between 14 and 43 years of farming experience [36, 40, 41]. Postal workers indicate an average of 12 years of prolonged occupational sun exposure history [6].

3.5. Sun Protection Behaviors. Most of the studies examined the use of at least two of the following sun protection measures in combination: wearing a hat, sunscreen application, wearing sunglasses, wearing protective clothing, and staying in the shade or otherwise limiting exposure to sun during the midday hour. Field observations studies conducted on transportation workers, construction workers, and postal workers revealed that 50.4% of the workers adequately protected their skin from the sun [35]. However, among Wisconsin dairy farmers, only 7% report that they frequently or always wore long-sleeved shirts, 13% report frequently or always wearing wide-brimmed hat, and 8% report frequently or always using sunscreen [36]. Among Californian farmworkers, few report frequently or always wearing a wide-brimmed hat (6%), using sunscreen (1.6%), and wearing sunglasses (2.6%) when working outside in the sun for more than 15 minutes. On the other hand, a considerable number of California farmworkers report frequently or always wearing a shirt with long sleeves (89.7%) [41]. Farmers, road workers, construction workers, and other outdoor workers in Georgia describe less use of adequate sun protection. Although 86% wore long pants and 74% wore sunglasses, only 5% report wearing wide-brimmed hats or caps with flaps and 5% report wearing long-sleeved shirts [37].

The sun protection behavior patterns of outdoor workers observed in the US are similar to those in other countries. Studies note that many outdoor workers fail to adequately engage in sun protective practices. Participants in Canadian research on outdoor workers conclude the following sun safety practices: wearing protective clothing (60%), wearing hats (58%), avoiding the sun (38%), and using sunscreen

(between 18% and 23%) [38]. In Britain, the most commonly used primary prevention strategies include using sunscreen (60%), wearing long-sleeved tops or trousers (51%), and wearing sunglasses (44%), with fewer participants reporting that they wore wide-brimmed hats (23%), and were using shade or otherwise limiting exposure to sun (between 19% and 23%) [44]. Likewise, construction workers in a study carried out in Australia report frequently or always wearing sunglasses (61%), using wide-brimmed hats (54%), using sunscreen (34%), wearing long-sleeved shirts (11%), and using shade (5%) [39].

Furthermore, studies identify the UVR exposure pattern of outdoor workers during workdays and days off. Among male outdoor workers in Australia, 51% of the participants experience over six hours of sun exposure on an average working day and 76% spent over two hours in the sun on the average weekend day or day off [29]. With regard to sun protection behavior, 43.6% and 77.2% usually wear long-sleeved shirts and wear a wide-brimmed hat, respectively. Mail carriers report reasonably similar amounts of sun exposure for working (3.9 hours) when compared to nonworking (3.3 hours) days, although reported use of protective measures for nonworking days was considerably lower [33]. On working days, 24% of mail carriers recount wearing a hat versus only 4% wearing a hat on nonworking days and 25% recount using sunscreen on working days and 12% on nonworking days [33].

4. Discussion

Outdoor workers constitute an important target group, who are susceptible to developing skin cancer, given the considerable amount of hours they spend outdoors on workdays and days off. This intense UVR exposure is experienced by outdoor workers for prolonged periods throughout their lives, since they tend to spend several years in outdoor occupations. Although receiving high UVR exposure on regular basis, overall data show that a majority of outdoor workers did not adequately protect themselves from sun exposure.

The findings of this review suggest that there are several factors that correlate with outdoor workers' sun protection behaviors. These correlates include being female, older age, being White, a personal history of skin cancer, time (hours/years) spent at work, sun safety training, perceived priority of sun protection, concern about sun exposure, workplace support, families' expectations, and familial information giving. On the other hand, factors that appear to be related to lower levels of sun protection behavior include being male, younger age, and reporting perceived barriers.

With regard to sun protection behavior, findings were sparse and inconsistent regarding the relationship of factors such as skin type, education, income, perceived susceptibility, and suntan attitude. Therefore, considerably more research work is required to determine potential importance of these factors and before any conclusion is drawn regarding the relationship of these factors to engaging in sun protection practices.

The relationship of family history of skin cancer with sun protection behavior is likewise difficult to assess because in the research reviewed, this item was assessed through use of a single dichotomous question that did not define first-degree relatives (i.e., parent, sibling, or child). Additional research that explores this issue through a more specifically worded question might provide more accurate and useful results.

Knowledge of skin cancer is widely studied for its relationship to sun protection behavior, and research on this construct continues to yield inconsistent results. This may be accounted for by differences in measures, methods, and analysis. However, in general, outdoor workers report that they are knowledgeable about skin cancer, but many do not engage in adequate sun protection behaviors. Therefore, it may be that knowledge alone is not enough to lead to sun protection behaviors. It is possible that other cognitive factors or combinations of factors are influencing the adoption of sun protective behaviors. At this time, however, little is known about psychological factors that explain why outdoor workers, despite a high level of knowledge about skin cancer, choose not to practice sun protection.

Only two of the identified articles described research that had a theoretical foundation. One study was based on constructs of the HBM [36, 45]. Perceived barriers were found to be the single predictor that explained why farmers did not engage in sun protection practice which led the author to suggest that the utility of HBM with Wisconsin dairy farmers is questionable. It should be noted, however, that this research did not utilize the revised version of HBM which includes the construct of self-efficacy [46]. This leads one to the following question: what would the results be if the author had included self-efficacy in the study?

The other theoretically grounded study was based on social cognitive theory (SCT) [37]. The purpose of the study was to assess use of constructs of SCT to identify personal determinants of farmers' skin cancer and prevention behavior and environmental influences that might either facilitate or inhibit the impact of skin cancer prevention campaigns directed at farmers. Unfortunately this research was conducted as a pilot study with an instrument that had no established psychometric properties, so both reliability and validity of these findings are uncertain.

No study focused exclusively on the relationship between sun protection self-efficacy and sun protection behaviors among outdoor workers. Self-efficacy reflects the confidence an individual has in his or her ability to successfully perform a behavior in order to achieve a desired outcome [47]. A self-efficacy-based intervention demonstrated some success in improving the responsiveness of young females to health information regarding skin cancer and aging effects of the sun [48]. Therefore, this construct merits further study in the context of outdoor workers.

Generalizing the results of these multiple studies is made difficult due to the range of occupations that comprise outdoor workers. Farmers, construction workers, and postal workers are the most frequent targets of research on sun protection behaviors. However, specific behaviors may differ among outdoor workers due to specific job types, proportion of males or females in occupations, and ethnicity/race [21, 41]. In addition, few studies investigated participants in a variety of occupations, and most of the studies did not examine

the differences in sun protection behaviors between the subgroups of the samples. Assessing sun protection behaviors of subgroups in an outdoor worker population will be useful in designing or tailoring effective and specific group-focused sun protection intervention which addresses the specific sun protection needs of each specific group.

5. Limitations

This review has several shortcomings that need to be addressed. First, this review is subject to publication bias because the authors limited their review to studies published in English. Second, reviewed studies had cross-sectional designs, and therefore causation cannot be determined. Third, since the data gathered in the studies were collected through self-report, the influence of social desirability and recall bias in the results cannot be discounted. Finally, the majority of the reviewed studies did not report the validity and reliability of the survey instruments used to collect the data, and therefore the results are suspect.

6. Conclusion

This literature review provides an assessment on a variety of sociodemographic and psychological factors that are related to the likelihood of outdoor workers adopting sun protection behaviors. Unfortunately, few theoretically grounded studies, which may have greater potential to identify factors or to generate predictions, have been published. The studies identified for this review that had greater theoretical emphasis were weakened by methodological issues. Without further assessment, it is difficult to determine whether the existing health behavior theories are useful in predicting sun protection behavior in outdoor workers. There is a need to conduct a study based on solid theoretical foundations that attempts to provide a potential and systematic explanation of relationships of factors in this domain. A deeper understanding of factors influencing sun protection practices could serve as a base for future studies and preventive interventions.

References

[1] S. J. Balk, H. J. Binns, H. L. Brumberg et al., "Ultraviolet radiation: a hazard to children and adolescents," *Pediatrics*, vol. 127, no. 3, pp. e791–e817, 2011.

[2] K. Glanz, E. Carbone, and V. Song, "Formative research for developing targeted skin cancer prevention programs for children in multiethnic Hawaii," *Health Education Research*, vol. 14, no. 2, pp. 155–166, 1999.

[3] American Cancer Society, 2012, http://www.cancer.org/cancer/cancercauses/sunanduvexposure/skin-cancer-facts.

[4] K. Glanz, R. A. Lew, V. Song, and L. Murakami-Akatsuka, "Skin cancer prevention in outdoor recreation settings: effects of the Hawaii SunSmart Program," *Effective Clinical Practice*, vol. 3, no. 2, pp. 53–61, 2000.

[5] International Agency for Research on Cancer, *Solar and Ultraviolet Radiation*, vol. 55 of *IARC Monographs on the Evaluation of Carcinogenic Risks to Humans*, International Agency for

Research on Cancer, World Health Organization, Lyon, France, 1992.

[6] L. C. Pichon, J. A. Mayer, D. J. Slymen, J. P. Elder, E. C. Lewis, and G. R. Galindo, "Ethnoracial differences among outdoor workers in key sun-safety behaviors," *American Journal of Preventive Medicine*, vol. 28, no. 4, pp. 374–378, 2005.

[7] M. Saraiya, K. Glanz, P. A. Briss et al., "Interventions to prevent skin cancer by reducing exposure to ultraviolet radiation: a systematic review," *American Journal of Preventive Medicine*, vol. 27, no. 5, pp. 422–466, 2004.

[8] P. Gies and J. Wright, "Measured solar ultraviolet radiation exposures of outdoor workers in Queensland in the building and construction industry," *Journal of Photochemical Photobiology*, vol. 78, pp. 342–348, 2003.

[9] T. Batra, "The invisible risk of Ultraviolet rays at outdoor workplaces," *International Journal of Environmental Sciences*, vol. 2, no. 1, pp. 73–78, 2010.

[10] N. Håkansson, B. Floderus, P. Gustavsson, M. Feychting, and N. Hallin, "Occupational sunlight exposure and cancer incidence among Swedish construction workers," *Epidemiology*, vol. 12, no. 5, pp. 552–557, 2001.

[11] B. Perez-Gomez, M. Pollán, P. Gustavsson, N. Plato, N. Aragonés, and G. López-Abente, "Cutaneous melanoma: hints from occupational risks by anatomic site in Swedish men," *Occupational and Environmental Medicine*, vol. 61, no. 2, pp. 117–126, 2004.

[12] B. C. Vitasa, H. R. Taylor, P. T. Strickland et al., "Association of nonmelanoma skin cancer and actinic keratosis with cumulative solar ultraviolet exposure in Maryland watermen," *Cancer*, vol. 65, no. 12, pp. 2811–2817, 1990.

[13] G. Severi and D. R. English, "Descriptive epidemiology of skin cancer," in *Prevention of Skin Cancer*, D. J. Hill, J. M. Elwood, and D. R. English, Eds., Kluwer Academic, Dordrecht, The Netherlands, 2004.

[14] B. K. Armstrong and A. Kricker, "The epidemiology of UV induced skin cancer," *Journal of Photochemistry and Photobiology B*, vol. 63, no. 1–3, pp. 8–18, 2001.

[15] L. Fritschi and J. Siemiatycki, "Melanoma and occupation: results of a case-control study," *Occupational and Environmental Medicine*, vol. 53, no. 3, pp. 168–173, 1996.

[16] J. A. Mayer, D. J. Slymen, E. J. Clapp et al., "Promoting sun safety among US postal service letter carriers: impact of a 2-year intervention," *American Journal of Public Health*, vol. 97, no. 3, pp. 559–565, 2007.

[17] M. Radespiel-Tröger, M. Meyer, A. Pfahlberg, B. Lausen, W. Uter, and O. Gefeller, "Outdoor work and skin cancer incidence: a registry-based study in Bavaria," *International Archives of Occupational and Environmental Health*, vol. 82, no. 3, pp. 357–363, 2009.

[18] S. Gruber and B. K. Armstrong, "Cutaneous malignant melanoma," in *Cancer Epidemiology and Prevention*, D. Schottenfeld and J. F. Fraumeni, Eds., pp. 1230–1250, Oxford University Press, New York, NY, USA, 3rd edition, 2006.

[19] C. Young, "Solar ultraviolet radiation and skin cancer," *Occupational Medicine*, vol. 59, no. 2, pp. 82–88, 2009.

[20] J. Scotto, T. R. Fears, and J. F. Fraumeni, "Incidence of non-melanoma skin cancer in the United States," 1983.

[21] K. Glanz, D. B. Buller, and M. Saraiya, "Reducing ultraviolet radiation exposure among outdoor workers: state of the evidence and recommendations," *Environmental Health*, vol. 6, article 22, 2007.

[22] M. Brenner and V. J. Hearing, "The protective role of melanin against UV damage in human skin," *Photochemistry and Photobiology*, vol. 84, no. 3, pp. 539–549, 2008.

[23] P. Callister, J. Galtry, and R. Didham, "The risks and benefits of sun exposure: should skin colour or ethnicity be the main variable for communicating health promotion messages in New Zealand?" *Ethnicity and Health*, vol. 16, no. 1, pp. 57–71, 2011.

[24] M. L. Stock, M. Gerrard, F. X. Gibbons et al., "Sun protection intervention for highway workers: long-term efficacy of UV photography and skin cancer information on men's protective cognitions and behavior," *Annals of Behavioral Medicine*, vol. 38, no. 3, pp. 225–236, 2009.

[25] P. G. Buettner and B. A. Raasch, "Incidence rates of skin cancer in Townsville, Australia," *International Journal of Cancer*, vol. 78, pp. 587–593, 1998.

[26] H. I. Hall, D. S. May, R. A. Lew, H. K. Koh, and M. Nadel, "Sun protection behaviors of the U.S. white population," *Preventive Medicine*, vol. 26, no. 4, pp. 401–407, 1997.

[27] E. M. McCarthy, K. P. Ethridge, and R. F. Wagner Jr., "Beach holiday sunburn: the sunscreen paradox and gender differences," *Cutis*, vol. 64, no. 1, pp. 37–42, 1999.

[28] G. G. Giles, B. K. Armstrong, R. C. Burton, M. P. Staples, and V. J. Thursfield, "Has mortality from melanoma stopped rising in Australia? Analysis of trends between 1931 and 1994," *British Medical Journal*, vol. 312, no. 7039, pp. 1121–1125, 1996.

[29] T. Woolley, P. G. Buettner, and J. Lowe, "Sun-related behaviors of outdoor working men with a history of non-melanoma skin cancer," *Journal of Occupational and Environmental Medicine*, vol. 44, no. 9, pp. 847–854, 2002.

[30] T. Woolley, J. Lowe, B. Raasch, M. Glasby, and P. G. Buettner, "Workplace sun protection policies and employees' sun-related skin damage," *American Journal of Health Behavior*, vol. 32, no. 2, pp. 201–208, 2008.

[31] Skin Cancer Foundation, 2012, http://www.skincancer.org/prevention/are-you-at-risk/men-and-skin-cancer-solving-the-knowledge-gap .

[32] K. D. Rosenman, J. Gardiner, G. M. Swanson, P. Mullan, and Z. Zhu, "Use of skin-cancer prevention strategies among farmers and their spouses," *American Journal of Preventive Medicine*, vol. 11, no. 5, pp. 342–347, 1995.

[33] E. C. Lewis, J. A. Mayer, and D. Slymen, "Postal workers' occupational and leisure-time sun safety behaviors (United States)," *Cancer Causes and Control*, vol. 17, no. 2, pp. 181–186, 2006.

[34] J. P. McCool, A. I. Reeder, E. M. Robinson, K. J. Petrie, and D. F. Gorman, "Outdoor workers' perceptions of the risks of excess sun-exposure," *Journal of Occupational Health*, vol. 51, no. 5, pp. 404–411, 2009.

[35] B. M. Stepanski and J. A. Mayer, "Solar protection behaviors among outdoor workers," *Journal of Occupational and Environmental Medicine*, vol. 40, no. 1, pp. 43–48, 1998.

[36] B. Marlenga, "The health beliefs and skin cancer prevention practices of Wisconsin dairy farmers," *Oncology Nursing Forum*, vol. 22, no. 4, pp. 681–686, 1995.

[37] R. Parrott, C. Steiner, and L. Coldenhar, "Georgia's harvesting healthy habits: a formative evaluation," *Journal of Rural Health*, vol. 12, no. 4, pp. 291–300, 1996.

[38] J. A. Shoveller, C. Y. Lovato, L. Peters, and J. K. Rivers, "Canadian national survey on sun exposure and protective behaviours: outdoor workers," *Canadian Journal of Public Health*, vol. 91, no. 1, pp. 34–35, 2000.

[39] J. Cioffi, L. Wilkes, and J. Hartcher-O'Brien, "Outdoor workers and sun protection: knowledge and behavior," *The Australian Journal of Construction Economics and Building*, vol. 2, no. 2, pp. 10–14, 2002.

[40] R. L. Parrott and R. Lemieux, "When the worlds of work and wellness collide: the role of familial support on skin cancer control," *Journal of Family Communication*, vol. 3, no. 2, pp. 95–106, 2003.

[41] R. Salas, J. A. Mayer, and K. D. Hoerster, "Sun-protective behaviors of California farmworkers," *Journal of Occupational and Environmental Medicine*, vol. 47, no. 12, pp. 1244–1249, 2005.

[42] V. Hammond, A. I. Reeder, A. R. Gray, and M. L. Bell, "Are workers or their workplaces the key to occupational sun protection?" *Health Promotion Journal of Australia*, vol. 19, no. 2, pp. 97–101, 2008.

[43] P. Gies, K. Glanz, D. O'Riordan, T. Elliott, and E. Nehl, "Measured occupational solar UVR exposures of lifeguards in pool settings," *American Journal of Industrial Medicine*, vol. 52, no. 8, pp. 645–653, 2009.

[44] P. Madgwick, J. Houdmont, and R. Randall, "Sun safety measures among construction workers in Britain," *Occupational Medicine*, vol. 61, no. 6, pp. 430–433, 2011.

[45] I. Rosenstock, "Historical origins of the health beliefs model," *Health Education Monographs*, vol. 2, no. 4, pp. 328–335, 1974.

[46] I. M. Rosenstock, V. J. Strecher, and M. H. Becker, "Social learning theory and the Health Belief Model," *Health Education Quarterly*, vol. 15, no. 2, pp. 175–183, 1988.

[47] A. Bandura, "Self-efficacy: toward a unifying theory of behavioral change," *Psychological Review*, vol. 84, no. 2, pp. 191–215, 1977.

[48] A. Good and C. Abraham, "Can the effectiveness of health promotion campaigns be improved using self-efficacy and self-affirmation interventions? an analysis of sun protection messages," *Psychology and Health*, vol. 26, no. 7, pp. 799–818, 2011.

11

The Influence of the Coexpression of CD4 and CD8 in Cutaneous Lesions on Prognosis of Mycosis Fungoides: A Preliminary Study

Sergio Umberto De Marchi,[1] **Giuseppe Stinco,**[2] **Enzo Errichetti,**[2] **Serena Bonin,**[1] **Nicola di Meo,**[1] **and Giusto Trevisan**[1]

[1] *Institute of Dermatology and Venereology, University of Trieste, Ospedale Maggiore, Piazza Ospedale 1, 34100 Trieste, Italy*
[2] *Institute of Dermatology, Department of Experimental and Clinical Medicine, University of Udine, Ospedale San Michele, Piazza Rodolone 1, 33013 Gemona del Friuli, Italy*

Correspondence should be addressed to Nicola di Meo; nickdimeo@libero.it

Academic Editor: Iris Zalaudek

Background. Although techniques of immunophenotyping have been successful in characterizing the cells in the cutaneous infiltrates of mycosis fungoides little evidence suggests that variations in the phenotypic characterization correlate with prognosis. *Objectives.* In a preliminary prospective, single-centre, study we correlated the T-cell phenotype in cutaneous biopsies with the progression of the disease to determine whether the coexpression of CD4 and CD8 has an impact on prognosis. *Methods.* Skin biopsy specimens from 30 newly diagnosed patients were stained with immunoperoxidase techniques to determine their phenotypic characteristics. After a median followup of 42 months patients were divided into two groups with stable and progressive disease. *Results.* Eighteen patients had the conventional CD4+CD8− T-cell phenotype. Ten patients showed the coexpression of CD4 and CD8 and had a slightly lower rate of progressive disease. *Conclusions.* The coexpression of CD4 and CD8 in cutaneous lesions is not rare and is associated with a slightly lower rate of progressive disease. Since double positive CD4/CD8 phenotype is rarely reported in mycosis fungoides the presence on conventional immunophenotyping of both CD may be due to a "mixture" of neoplastic cells and inflammatory CD8+ tumor infiltrating lymphocytes. Immunohistochemical study combined with confocal microscopy could clarify this issue.

1. Introduction

Mycosis fungoides (MF) represents the prototype of cutaneous T-cell lymphoma, which is defined as clonal expansion of skin-homing T lymphocytes [1]. The natural history of MF is characterized by an indolent progression through four stages: patch, plaque, tumor, and visceral involvement. The disease begins with lightly erythematous patches that subsequently evolve into well-demarcated scaling plaques. These plaques may then progress to tumor lesions and subsequently spread to the viscera, but this progression is not necessarily seen in all patients [2]. MF is classified into clinical stages using the TNM classification. Previous studies of prognostic indicators have shown that the skin (T) stage and the presence or absence of extracutaneous disease are the most important determinants of outcome. Patients with limited skin involvement (T1) have a favorable prognosis, whereas patients with tumor (T3) or erythrodermic MF (T4) have an unfavorable prognosis [3, 4]. The diagnosis of MF relies on histopathological examination of skin biopsies [5]. Usually, MF is characterized by an infiltrate of α/β T helper memory lymphocytes (βF1+, CD3+, CD4+, CD5+, CD8−, and CD45RO+) [1]. However, in a minority of cases the neoplastic cells exhibit a T-cytotoxic (CD4−CD8+), γ/δ (βF1−, CD3+, CD4−, CD5+, and CD8+) or a CD4/CD8 double-negative phenotype, that show no clinical and/or prognostic differences [6]. Recently, a previously unrecognized phenotype characterized by coexpression of CD4 and

CD8 has been described [7, 8], but the influence of such a phenotype on prognosis of MF has not been evaluated. Therefore, although techniques of immunophenotyping have been successful in characterizing the cells in the cutaneous infiltrates of MF little evidence suggests that variations in the phenotypic characterization correlate with prognosis.

In this preliminary prospective, single-centre study on a limited number of patients with MF we correlated the T-cell phenotype in cutaneous lesions with the progression of the disease to determine whether the coexpression of CD4 and CD8, compared to conventional CD4+CD8− phenotype, has an impact on prognosis.

2. Patients and Methods

Patients with MF were prospectively included in this study between January 2005 and December 2012, after giving informed consent according to the declaration of Helsinki. The diagnosis of MF was made according to the criteria of the WHO-EORTC classification for cutaneous lymphomas [1]. The clinical stage at presentation was determined using the TNM classification adapted for MF [9]. Patients received a comprehensive history and physical examination, complete blood cell count including peripheral smear for Sézary cells, and general chemistry panel. Lesional cutaneous biopsies were obtained in all patients upon admission into the study before the start of therapy. Patients with clinically significant adenopathy had their nodes evaluated by fine needle aspiration or lymph node biopsy. When indicated, patient had an extensive staging evaluation, including bone marrow aspirate and biopsy, and appropriate radiologic studies to determine visceral involvement.

We included in the study only newly diagnosed patients who had not previously received topical therapies (corticosteroids, topical nitrogen mustard, carmustine, and psoralen with ultraviolet A), interferon, chlorambucil, methotrexate, or polychemotherapy.

After initial evaluation, the patients were included into a program of visits that were made every three months throughout the period of followup. According to the course of the disease and, more specifically, to their clinical status at the time of the last clinical update, patients were classified into two groups. The first group was formed by patients with a progressive disease defined as the change to a more advanced stage. In the second group patients who underwent complete or partial remission and patients with stable disease defined as presence of MF without progression were included. Factors associated with disease progression were studied with special emphasis to T-cell phenotype. The study did not consider the therapy received by the patients. Indeed treatments were administered according to clinical stage and were relatively homogeneous within each study group for most of the patients, but no prospective therapeutic trial was simultaneously performed. At early stages (I-IIa), most of the patients were treated by topical therapies (corticosteroids, topical nitrogen mustard, carmustine, and psoralen with ultraviolet A). At advanced stages, radiotherapy was performed on tumors, and interferon, chlorambucil, methotrexate, or polychemotherapy was administered as needed.

3. Histopathologic and Immunohistologic Analysis

Formalin fixed and paraffin-embedded tissues of lesional cutaneous biopsies were obtained from all patients. Specimens were fixed in 10% buffered formalin and subsequently embedded in paraffin. Sections were stained with haematoxylin and eosin for routine histopathological evaluation. The diagnosis of MF was established according to the criteria proposed by Guitart et al. [10].

Immunostaining was performed on fixed, paraffin-embedded tissue sections as previously described [11] using monoclonal antibodies specific for T-cell associated antigens (CD3, CD4, and CD8) and for B cell-associated antigens (CD20).

4. Statistical Analysis

Statistical analysis was performed with dedicated STATA SE 12 (Stata Corporation, TX, USA). The Fisher's exact test and the Pearson χ^2-test were used to identify the differences between the variables. A multivariate logistic regression was used to evaluate the relationship among variables. Logistic regression is a variation of ordinary regression which predicts the probability of the occurrence of a specific event as a function of two or more independent variables. The results obtained were expressed in terms of the odds ratio (OR) associated with each predictor value, defined as the probability of the event occurring divided by the probability of the event not occurring. In all analyses, the cut-off level of statistical significance was set at 0.05.

5. Results

Thirty patients (17 men and 13 women) with clinical and histologic diagnosis of MF were included in the study. The mean age at diagnosis was 64.5 years (range 49–78 years). According to the TNM classification 8 patients were in stage I, 13 in stage II, 6 in stage III, and 3 in stage IV. The thirteen patients in stage II were classified as 6 stage IIa and 7 stage IIb. Stages I-IIa were considered as early stages and stages IIb–IV as advanced stages. At the time of diagnosis, MF was in a more advanced stage in women than men. Indeed, 52.9% of men (versus 38.4% of women) were in early stages whereas 61.6% of women (versus 47.1% of men) were in advanced stages.

Immunophenotypic analysis demonstrated that 93.3% (28 out 30) of the patients with MF were CD4 positive. CD20 was negative in all patients. Eighteen out 30 patients had the mature CD4+/CD8− T-cell phenotype. The cytotoxic T-cell phenotype CD4−/CD8+ was present in only one patient as well as the CD4/CD8 double-negative phenotype. Ten out of 30 patients (33.3%) had an immunophenotypic profile characterized by the coexpression of CD4 and CD8. When we compared the distribution of patients with the coexpression and those with the conventional CD4+/CD8− phenotype according to the TNM staging we could not find any association between phenotypes and clinical stage. Indeed the percentages of the patients with advanced stage,

TABLE 1: Factors associated with the disease progression in patients with mycosis fungoides.

Disease progression	Odds ratio	Standard error	z	P value	95% confidence interval	
Phenotype	17,03	28,79	1,68	0,09	0,62	467,7
TNM stage	2,07	1,19	1,26	0,21	0,67	6,39
Duration of followup	1,19	0,16	1,31	0,19	0,91	1,55
Age at diagnosis	0,29	0,38	0,94	0,35	0,02	3,82

In the logistic regression model the dependent variable was the disease progression defined as the change to a more advanced stage; the independent variables were T-cell phenotype (CD4+CD8+ vs CD4+CD8−), TNM stage at presentation, duration of followup, and age at diagnosis.

as compared with those in early stage, were not significantly different in both groups (group CD4+/CD8− 50% versus 50%; group CD4+/CD8+ 40% versus 60%).

The median follow-up time in the study was 42 months (ranging from 12 to 70 months) and was comparable among the different clinical stages and phenotypes. None of the patients died during the study period. At the end of the followup 23 of 30 patients underwent complete or partial remission or presented a stable disease without extension of the lesions or increase of the number of lesions. Seven patients showed a progressive disease defined as the change to a more advanced stage. The age of patient at diagnosis (<65 years versus >65 years), the sex, the duration of symptoms before diagnosis of MF (<60 months versus >60 months), and the TNM stage at presentation (early stages versus advanced stages) were not associated with disease progression in univariate as in multivariate analysis. The results of the logistic regression analysis are reported in Table 1. None of the independent variables introduced in the logistic regression model was associated with disease progression defined as the change to a more advanced stage. However, by analyzing the distribution of T-cell phenotypes within the progressing and nonprogressing groups we found that patients with the coexpression CD4 and CD8 had a slightly lower rate of progressive disease as compared to patients with conventional phenotype (10.0% versus 27.8%). In the logistic regression model the value obtained by the independent variable phenotype has almost reached the statistical significance (odds ratio 17.03, $P = 0.09$, 95% confidence interval 0.62–467.7).

6. Discussion

In this preliminary prospective, single-centre study, we found by conventional immunophenotyping a profile characterized by the coexpression of CD4 and CD8 in one-third of patients with MF. These patients showed a slightly lower rate of progressive disease, compared to patients with conventional CD4+/CD8− phenotype. These findings raise the possibility that the coexpression of CD4 and CD8 in cutaneous lesions may confer a better prognosis in MF.

In our patients the conventional T-helper phenotype (CD4+/CD8−) was the most common (60% of patients), thus confirming previous studies [1, 12]. Twelve patients had a different phenotype. Two patients showed, respectively, the cytotoxic phenotype (CD4−/CD8+) and the double negative phenotype (CD4−/CD8−). The conventional immunostaining in the remaining 10 patients (33.3%) showed the coexpression of CD4 and CD8.

The coexpression of CD4 and CD8 is an expected event on common thymocytes, but it is fairly infrequent on normal peripheral T lymphocytes. There is evidence that in certain situations the normal CD4+ cells may coexpress CD8 and interleukin-4 is able to induce the expression of CD8 on T CD4+ clones [13]. Peripheral T lymphocytes with CD4+/CD8+ phenotype have been described in some solid and hematologic malignancies [14, 15]. However the double positive CD4/CD8 phenotype is extremely rare in mycosis fungoides [7, 8]. The findings of our patients may not be due to the coexpression of both CD in the same neoplastic cell but to the presence in the cutaneous lesions of a "mixture" of neoplastic cells and inflammatory CD8+ tumor infiltrating lymphocytes as previously demonstrated by Hoppe et al. [16]. Immunohistochemical study combined with confocal microscopy might clarify this issue as recently reported by Tournier and coworkers [8] in a 31-year-old woman. In their patient this technique revealed in lesional cutaneous biopsies the coexpression of CD4 and CD8 in a subset of atypical T lymphocytes.

In typical lesional biopsy specimens of MF other non-neoplastic mononuclear cells are present including CD8+ tumor-infiltrating lymphocytes. The role that these cells play in etiopathogenesis and natural history of MF is still unclear [17].

In our patients with MF the subgroup with the coexpression of CD4 and CD8 has a slightly lower rate of progressive disease in comparison to patients with conventional CD4+/CD8− phenotype (10.0% versus 27.8%), and in the logistic regression model the value obtained by the independent variable T-cell phenotype has almost reached the statistical significance.

This data might be of interest taking into account that the limited number of patients and the median follow-up period of just 3.5 years, although similar to those of other investigations, may not allow adequate time for this indolent lymphoma to progress.

The lower tendency to progression of disease in our patients with the coexpression of CD4 and CD8 might be related to increased activity of antitumor CD8+ lymphocytes infiltrating the lesions. Our results may be consistent with previous findings by Hoppe et al. [16] who demonstrated that CD8+ tumor-infiltrating lymphocytes influenced the long-term survival of patients with MF.

Another problem is the possibility that CD8+ inflammatory cells can appear in the course of treatment. This is not the case of our patients because we have included in the present study only newly diagnosed patients who had not previously received topical therapies (corticosteroids, topical nitrogen mustard, carmustine, and psoralen with ultraviolet A), interferon, chlorambucil, methotrexate, or polychemotherapy.

Finally, in this preliminary prospective, single-centre study, conventional immunophenotyping demonstrates the coexpression of CD4 and CD8 in lesional cutaneous biopsies of one-third of patients with MF. These patients show a slightly lower rate of progressive disease, compared to patients with conventional CD4+/CD8− phenotype. A prospective multicenter study on a larger population of patients with a longer followup might be useful to confirm if the coexpression of CD4 and CD8 may confer a better prognosis in patients with MF.

References

[1] R. Willemze, E. S. Jaffe, G. Burg et al., "WHO-EORTC classification for cutaneous lymphomas," *Blood*, vol. 105, no. 10, pp. 3768–3785, 2005.

[2] A. L. Lorincz, "Cutaneous T-cell lymphoma (mycosis fungoides)," *The Lancet*, vol. 347, no. 9005, pp. 871–876, 1996.

[3] H. S. Zackheim, S. Amin, M. Kashani-Sabet, and A. McMillan, "Prognosis in cutaneous T-cell lymphoma by skin stage: long-term survival in 489 patients," *Journal of the American Academy of Dermatology*, vol. 40, no. 3, pp. 418–425, 1999.

[4] Y. H. Kim, H. L. Liu, S. Mraz-Gernhard, A. Varghese, and R. T. Hoppe, "Long-term outcome of 525 patients with mycosis fungoides and Sézary syndrome: clinical prognostic factors and risk for disease progression," *Archives of Dermatology*, vol. 139, no. 7, pp. 857–866, 2003.

[5] E. A. Sausville, J. L. Eddy, R. W. Makuch et al., "Histopathologic staging at initial diagnosis of mycosis fungoides and the Sezary syndrome. Definition of three distinctive prognostic groups," *Annals of Internal Medicine*, vol. 109, no. 5, pp. 372–382, 1988.

[6] A. D. Tosca, A. G. Varelzidis, J. Economidou, and J. D. Stratigos, "Mycosis fungoides: evaluation of immunohistochemical criteria for the early diagnosis of the disease and differentiation between stages," *Journal of the American Academy of Dermatology*, vol. 15, no. 2, pp. 237–245, 1986.

[7] C. F. Knapp, R. Mathew, J. L. Messina, and M. H. Lien, "CD4/CD8 dual-positive mycosis fungoides: a previously unrecognized variant," *The American Journal of Dermatopathology*, vol. 34, no. 3, pp. e37–e39, 2012.

[8] E. Tournier, C. Laurent, M. Thomas et al., "Double-positive CD4/CD8 mycosis fungoides: a rarely reported immunohistochemical profile," *Journal of Cutaneous Pathology*, vol. 41, pp. 58–62, 2014.

[9] S. I. Lamberg, S. B. Green, D. P. Byar et al., "Clinical staging for cutaneous T cell lymphoma," *Annals of Internal Medicine*, vol. 100, no. 2, pp. 187–192, 1984.

[10] J. Guitart, J. Kennedy, S. Ronan, J. S. Chmiel, Y. Hsiegh, and D. Variakojis, "Histologic criteria for the diagnosis of mycosis fungoides: proposal for a grading system to standardize pathology reporting," *Journal of Cutaneous Pathology*, vol. 28, no. 4, pp. 174–183, 2001.

[11] S. Miertusova Tothova, S. Bonin, G. Trevisan, and G. Stanta, "Mycosis fungoides: is it a Borrelia burgdorferi-associated disease?" *British Journal of Cancer*, vol. 94, no. 6, pp. 879–883, 2006.

[12] C. Massone, G. Crisman, H. Kerl, and L. Cerroni, "The prognosis of early mycosis fungoides is not influenced by phenotype and T-cell clonality," *British Journal of Dermatology*, vol. 159, no. 4, pp. 881–886, 2008.

[13] C. Ortolani, *Flow Cytometry of Hematological Malignancies*, Wiley-Blackwell, Hoboken, NJ, USA, 2011.

[14] E. T. Yanagihara, J. W. Parker, P. R. Meyer, M. J. Cain, F. Hofman, and R. J. Lukes, "Mycosis fungoides, Sezary's syndrome progressing to immunoblastic sarcoma: a T-cell lymphoproliferation with both helper and suppressor phenotypes," *The American Journal of Clinical Pathology*, vol. 81, no. 2, pp. 249–257, 1984.

[15] T. Nagatani, S. Kim, N. Baba et al., "Phenotypic heterogeneity of lymphoma of the skin," *The Journal of Dermatology*, vol. 16, no. 6, pp. 443–452, 1989.

[16] R. T. Hoppe, L. J. Medeiros, R. A. Warnke, and G. S. Wood, "CD8-positive tumor-infiltrating lymphocytes influence the long-term survival of patients with mycosis fungoides," *Journal of the American Academy of Dermatology*, vol. 32, no. 3, pp. 448–453, 1995.

[17] G. S. Wood, A. Edinger, R. T. Hoppe, and R. A. Warnke, "Mycosis fungoides skin lesions contain CD8+ tumor-infiltrating lymphocytes expressing an activated, MHC-restricted cytotoxic T-lymphocyte phenotype," *Journal of Cutaneous Pathology*, vol. 21, no. 2, pp. 151–156, 1994.

12

Saphenous Vein Sparing Superficial Inguinal Dissection in Lower Extremity Melanoma

Muhammed Beşir Öztürk,[1] Arzu Akan,[2] Özay Özkaya,[3] Onur Egemen,[3] Ali Rıza Öreroğlu,[4] Turgut Kayadibi,[3] and Mithat Akan[5]

[1] Department of Plastic Reconstructive and Aesthetic Surgery, Tekirdag Government Hospital, 59020 Tekirdag, Turkey
[2] Department of General Surgery, Okmeydani Training and Research Hospital, 34445 Istanbul, Turkey
[3] Department of Plastic Reconstructive and Aesthetic Surgery, Okmeydani Training and Research Hospital, 34445 Istanbul, Turkey
[4] Department of Plastic Reconstructive and Aesthetic Surgery, Prof. Dr. A. Ilhan Ozdemir State Hospital, 28000 Giresun, Turkey
[5] Department of Plastic Reconstructive and Aesthetic Surgery, Medipol University Hospital, 34200 Istanbul, Turkey

Correspondence should be addressed to Muhammed Beşir Öztürk; muhammedozturk@msn.com

Academic Editor: Iris Zalaudek

Aim. The classic inguinal lymph node dissection is the main step for the regional control of the lower extremity melanoma, but this surgical procedure is associated with significant postoperative morbidity. The permanent lymphedema is the most devastating long-term complication leading to a significant decrease in the patient's quality of life. In this study we present our experience with modified, saphenous vein sparing, inguinal lymph node dissections for patients with melanoma of the lower extremity. *Methods.* Twenty one patients (10 women, 11 men) who underwent saphenous vein sparing superficial inguinal lymph node dissection for the melanoma of lower extremity were included in this study. The effects of saphenous vein sparing on postoperative complications were evaluated. *Results.* We have observed the decreased rate of long-term lymphedema in patients undergoing inguinal lymphadenectomy for the lower extremity melanoma. *Conclusion.* The inguinal lymphadenectomy with saphenous vein preservation in lower extremity melanoma patients seems to be an oncologically safe procedure and it may offer reduced long-term morbidity.

1. Introduction

Regional lymph node dissection is the standard treatment regimen for patients with sentinel lymph node biopsy (SLNB) positive melanoma or clinically evident palpable lymph node metastasis of the disease. Inguinal lymph node dissection is the main step for the regional control of the lower extremity melanoma, but this surgical procedure is associated with significant postoperative morbidity. Wound complication rates up to 71% have been reported, including hematoma, seroma, skin necrosis, wound infection, and wound dehiscence [1]. The permanent lymphedema is the most devastating long-term complication leading to a significant decrease in the patient's quality of life [2].

Many techniques have been reported to reduce postoperative lymphedema, such as preserving the muscle fascia [3],

pedicled omentoplasty [4], sartorius transposition [5], and saphenous vein sparing inguinal lymphadenectomy [6]. The reported studies on sparing the saphenous vein in inguinal node dissection suggest a reduced rate of lymphedema and other postoperative complications [6, 7]. Randomized controlled trials are needed to prove the benefits of various technical modifications.

The classic inguinal lymphadenectomy includes en bloc removal of all lymph node bearing fibrofatty tissue and the saphenous vein within the femoral triangle. Catalona defined the saphenous vein sparing inguinal lymphadenectomy, postulating a decrease in the postoperative complication rates in vulvar and penile malignancies [6].

In this study, we present our experience with sparing the saphenous vein during inguinal lymph node dissections for

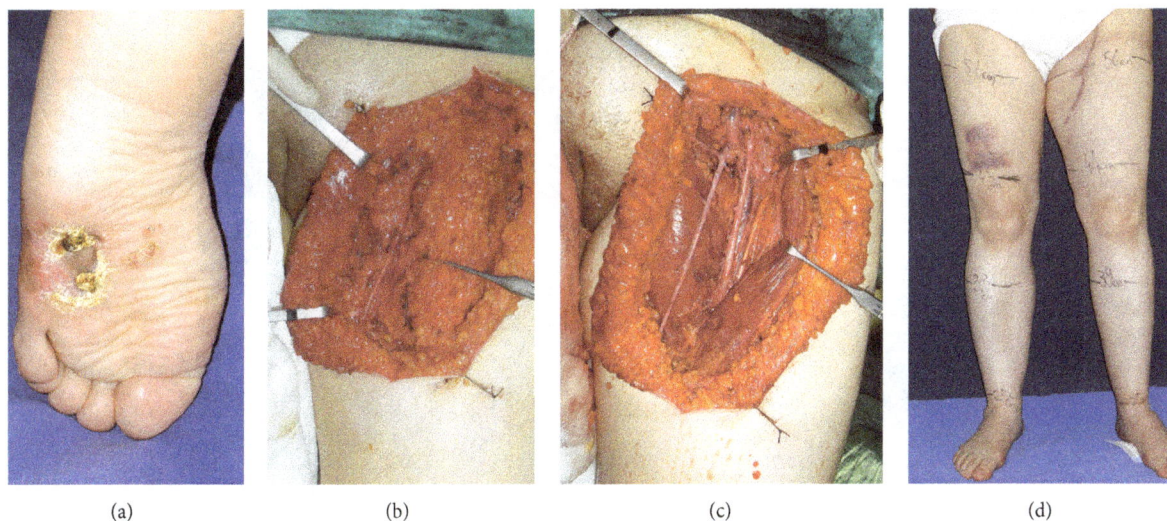

| (a) | (b) | (c) | (d) |

FIGURE 1: (a) 45-year-old female patient having T4 (4 mm) melanoma of the left plantar foot. (b) Intraoperative view of the sparing long saphenous vein. (c) En block removal of lymph node bearing fibrofatty tissue. (d) The 12th month follow-up of the patient without any sign of lymphedema.

patients with melanoma of the lower extremity. The effects of saphenous vein sparing on postoperative complications were evaluated.

2. Patients and Methods

Twenty-one patients (10 women, 11 men) who underwent saphenous vein sparing superficial inguinal lymph node dissection for the melanoma of lower extremity between February 2011 and April 2013 were included in this study.

Melanoma diagnoses were based on pathologic investigations and all patients were histologically diagnosed prior to surgery. All patients were staged clinically.

Lymph node dissection was performed on patients with clinically detectable inguinal lymph node metastases, for SLNB positive patients and for patients with thick (>4 mm) primary melanomas.

Inguinal lymph node dissection was performed through a standard 12 cm incision extending from 2 cm below the inguinal ligament to the apex of the femoral triangle. All the fibrofatty tissue, extending from the external oblique aponeurosis 2 cm above the inguinal ligament to the medial border of the adductor longus muscle medially and sartorius muscle laterally, was removed. According to the saphenous vein preserving inguinal lymph node dissection technique described by Catalona, the main truncus of the saphenous vein was found at the level of femoral artery entry point and was preserved during the dissection (Figure 1) [6].

After completion of the dissection, all the vascular compromised skin was excised. Suction drains were used routinely. All the patients were administered with low molecular weight heparin 6 hours postoperatively for deep vein thrombosis prophylaxis and prophylactic antibiotics. The patients were observed for any short-term complications and were

discharged when the suction drainage was less than 40 cc in 24 hours.

All patients were called for regular visits at the postoperative 1st week, postoperative 2nd week, postoperative 6th week, postoperative 6th month, postoperative 1st year, and postoperative 18th month at the outpatient clinic. Patients were asked to wear compressive garments for 3–6 months during the postoperative period. The day before the visit they were asked to take off the compressive garments.

Patient's demographic characteristics and associated comorbidities were analyzed. During observations, prospective assessment of the wound complications including wound dehiscence, skin necrosis, wound infection, seroma, and hematoma as well as palpable inguinal lymph nodes and locoregional recurrences was noted. Pathologic information included Breslow thickness, ulceration of the primary tumor, total number of the excised nodes, and the number of the positive nodes.

A short-term complication was defined as an occurrence within the first 6 months of the operation and a long-term complication was any complication occurring after that period.

Wound infection was defined by the use of antibiotics for culture-proven infected drainage postoperatively and wound dehiscence was described as wound healing problem with a measured defect of at least 1 cm in length. Seroma was defined as a palpable subcutaneous fluid collection at the operation area requiring percutaneous drainage.

Lymphedema was determined as a change equal to or greater than 7% of the sum of all the circumferences (of the predetermined 4 circumference measurement points) between the two legs [8]. Patients were followed up for the development of lymphedema and limb circumference measurements were performed for both legs preoperatively and during the regular visits. Measurements were done at

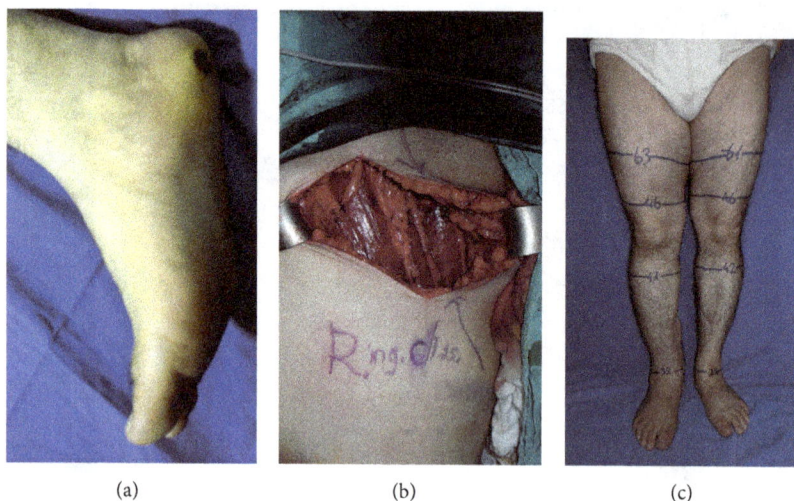

(a)   (b)   (c)

FIGURE 2: (a) Preoperative view of the 43-year-old male patient having T4 (4,8 mm) melanoma located to the right heel. (b) Right-sided saphenous vein superficial inguinal dissection, intraoperative view. (c) Postoperative 16th month picture, showing no sign of lymphedema (note that the right ankle is thick because of the use of posterior tibial artery perforator flap in the right heel reconstruction).

the points of the medial malleolus, 10 centimeters below the medial tibial condyle (MTC), 10 centimeters above the MTC, and the midpoint between anterior superior iliac spine and MTC (Figure 2).

3. Results

Twenty-one patients (10 women, 11 men) were included in this study. The median age at diagnosis of the melanoma was 48 years (range 39–68 years).

The average Breslow depth of the primary melanomas was 4,2 mm (1,2 mm–8 mm). Five patients underwent inguinal dissection after groin lymphadenopathy was noted on physical examination at the time of primary lower extremity melanoma diagnosis, 3 patients had positive SLNB, one patient had wide spread in-transit metastasis, and the other 12 patients underwent dissection for primary thick melanomas (≥4 mm).

The mean follow-up period was 14.8 months. The follow-up period was 18 months for 12 patients, 12 months for 7 patients, and 6 months for 2 patients.

Twenty patients did not show any local or regional recurrences or systemic metastasis during the follow-up period. Only one patient (who had widespread in-transit metastasis at the first admission) developed pulmonary metastasis 6 months after the operation and he was lost during the follow-up.

Five short-term complications (23.8%) were observed related to the inguinal area. Seroma formation was noted in 3 patients (14.3%) and hematoma formation was noted in 2 patients (9.5%). There was no noted occurrence of wound infection or wound dehiscence.

Short-term lymphedema formation was observed in 3 patients (3/21, 14.2%) at the 2nd week, in 8 patients (8/21, 38%) at the 6th week, and in 6 patients (6/21, 28,5%) at the 6th month. Long-term lymphedema was noted in 2 patients

(2/19, 10.5%) at the 12th month. There was not any persistent lymphedema formation at the 18th month follow-up of 12 patients (0/12).

4. Discussion

Inguinal lymph node dissection is associated with significant morbidity despite the refinements in surgical techniques. Complications with inguinal dissections are significantly more common than the other regional lymph node dissections and tend to be a rule rather than exception [1].

Complications following inguinal dissection can be classified into short-term/wound complications and long-term/lymphedema formation. The most frequent wound complications are wound infections, wound dehiscence, seroma formation, and hematoma formation. Serpell et al. reported an overall incidence of wound complication rate as high as 71% after inguinal lymph node dissection for melanoma with a 25% incidence of infection, 25% incidence of delayed wound healing, 46% incidence of seroma, and 29% incidence of lymphedema [1]. Similarly, Chang et al. found 77% wound complication rate after inguinal dissection for melanoma in a prospective study with 55% incidence of infection, 53% incidence of wound dehiscence, 28% incidence of seroma, and 45% incidence of lymphedema [9].

Wound infections/necrosis were frequently observed after inguinal dissections with the prevalence rates 7–55% reported in the literature [1, 9–11]. The wide discrepancies in the incidence of reported complication rates may be attributed to the retrospective design of the studies [8]. Also, there is no universally accepted description of these complications. In our study, wound infection was defined by the use of antibiotics for culture-proven infected drainage postoperatively and wound dehiscence was described as wound healing problem with a measured defect of at least 1 cm. Wound infections/necrosis were not observed in our prospective study [9]. These clear definitions for the complications in our study contribute the low reported incidence. A second explanation for the low incidence of complications is that our patients were relatively young (mean 48 years) with minimal associated comorbidities. Aseptic surgical technique and removal of the vascular compromised skin during the procedure may further help the low complication rate.

Seroma formation was observed in 3 patients (14.3%) and hematoma formation was noted in 2 patients (9.5%) in our study. Seromas were managed with sterile aspirations in outpatient clinic and no additional treatment was needed for these patients. Studies show that the incidence of hematoma/seroma formation ranges from 2 percent to 42 percent and our complication rates were similar to the literature [10–15].

The most debilitating long-term morbidity after inguinal dissection is chronic lymphedema. Lymphedema is a progressive pathological condition in which there is an accumulation of a protein rich fluid and subsequent inflammation, adipose tissue hypertrophy, and fibrosis. Physicosocial morbidity, decreased extremity function, cellulitis, epidermal lymph leak (lymphorrhea), and lymphangiosarcoma development are observed in lymphedema patients. These conditions further diminish the patients' quality of life [16].

The reported incidence of lymphedema after inguinal dissection for melanoma varies widely, ranging from 9 percent to 64 percent [1, 10–14, 16]. Wide range of reported difference is related to the problem that there is no universally accepted definition of the lymphedema also. Some authors define lymphedema as the patients self-complaint about the presence of lymphedema [1], a greater than 2 cm circumference increase compared to the contralateral limb [17], and a volume difference of more than 20% between limbs [18]. All these definitions have their limitations. For example, the effect of the same volume increase in a small person's limb is more prominent than in a larger person's limb. Also, the use of >2 cm circumference difference for the definition of lymphedema does not comprise the severity of the impairment. Spillane et al. studied the definition of lymphedema and suggested 2 alternative equally appropriate definitions of lymphedema, the whole perometer percentage change ≥15% and the sum of circumferences (of the predetermined measurement points) percentage change ≥7 [8]. The optoelectric perometer is not readily available at our clinic and so we used the sum of circumferences percentage change in this study.

We have noticed that lower limb lymphedema was the worst in the first six months and it gradually improved. This is a previously reported pattern [19], but it was striking that, at the 12th month measurements, the lymphedema incidence was found to be 10.5% and lymphedema disappeared completely after 18 months. Review of the literature reveals high prevalence of long-term lymphedema in inguinal dissections ranging from 9 percent to 64 percent and it can be concluded that the procedure of saphenous vein preserving inguinal dissection has been associated with a lower incidence of lymphedema in lower extremity melanoma patients.

Majority of our patients had primary thick (≥4 mm) melanomas. Melanomas thicker than 4.00 mm have a high risk of systemic disease and approximately 40% of them have clinically unapparent nodal involvement at the time of primary diagnosis [20]. Although sentinel lymph node biopsy has gained wide spread acceptance for its safety and minimal morbidity, it is widely used for the intermediate thickness melanomas (1 mm–4 mm) and its use in thick melanomas (≥4 mm) is unclear [21]. With a follow-up period ranging from 6 to 18 months, no patient experienced local or regional recurrence of the primary lesion. All patients, except for one who developed systemic metastasis and was lost during the follow up, continue to do well with no evidence of recurrence, and they are free from the disease. Although the time period for the follow-up is relatively short and the number of patients is relatively low, this technique seems to be an oncologically safe procedure for lower extremity melanoma patients.

During the past century, the original destructive lymph node dissections have been improved with preserving the nonlymphatic structures to limit the surgery related morbidity [22]. In radical neck dissections, the dissections of the internal and external jugular veins often cause maxillofacial edema due to the poor face venous reflux or cause intracranial hypertension and subsequently dizziness and headache [23]. To prevent such complications, modified radical neck dissection, which preserves important structures, such as the internal jugular vein, sternocleidomastoid muscle, and accessory nerve, was described by Suárez, in 1963 [24]. This technique was refined and popularized by various authors in the literature [22, 25, 26]. Modified or "functional" neck dissection avoids much of the morbidity of radical neck dissection while achieving equivalent degrees of control of regional disease in properly selected cases [22].

Also, in inguinal dissections, saphenous vein sparing dissections were described for vulvar and penile malignancies in the literature to avoid postoperative complications such as lymphedema [13, 15]. It is suggested that saphenous vein sparing is associated with a decreased risk of postoperative morbidity without compromising outcomes [6, 13, 15].

Although the exact mechanism of the preserving of a nonlymphatic tissue, the saphenous vein, and the decreased rate of the lymphedema is not clear, it is suggested that the increased venous reflux and subsequent decreased pressure in the venous end and lymphaticovenous connections within the saphenous vein territory may play a role [23, 27, 28].

In conclusion, the inguinal lymphadenectomy with saphenous vein preservation in lower extremity melanoma patients seems to be an oncologically safe procedure and it may offer reduced long-term morbidity.

References

[1] J. W. Serpell, P. W. G. Carne, and M. Bailey, "Radical lymph node dissection for melanoma," *Journal of Surgery*, vol. 73, no. 5, pp. 294–299, 2003.

[2] J. Ul-Mulk and L. R. Hölmich, "Lymph node dissection in patients with malignant melanoma is associated with high risk

of morbidity," *Danish Medical Journal*, vol. 59, no. 6, p. A4441, 2012.

[3] G. Lawton, H. Rasque, and S. Ariyan, "Preservation of muscle fascia to decrease lymphedema after complete axillary and ilio-inguinofemoral lymphadenectomy for melanoma," *Journal of the American College of Surgeons*, vol. 195, no. 3, pp. 339–351, 2002.

[4] L. Benoit, C. Boichot, N. Cheynel et al., "Preventing lymphedema and morbidity with an omentum flap after ilioinguinal lymph node dissection," *Annals of Surgical Oncology*, vol. 12, no. 10, pp. 793–799, 2005.

[5] P. L. Judson, A. L. Jonson, P. J. Paley et al., "A prospective, randomized study analyzing sartorius transposition following inguinal-femoral lymphadenectomy," *Gynecologic Oncology*, vol. 95, no. 1, pp. 226–230, 2004.

[6] W. J. Catalona, "Modified inguinal lymphadenectomy for carcinoma of the penis with preservation of saphenous veins: technique and preliminary results," *Journal of Urology*, vol. 140, no. 2, pp. 306–310, 1988.

[7] S. Abbas and M. Seitz, "Systematic review and meta-analysis of the used surgical techniques to reduce leg lymphedema following radical inguinal nodes dissection," *Surgical Oncology*, vol. 20, no. 2, pp. 88–96, 2011.

[8] A. J. Spillane, R. P. M. Saw, M. Tucker, K. Byth, and J. F. Thompson, "Defining lower limb lymphedema after inguinal or ilio-inguinal dissection in patients with melanoma using classification and regression tree analysis," *Annals of Surgery*, vol. 248, no. 2, pp. 286–293, 2008.

[9] S. B. Chang, R. L. Askew, Y. Xing et al., "Prospective assessment of postoperative complications and associated costs following inguinal lymph node dissection (ILND) in melanoma patients," *Annals of Surgical Oncology*, vol. 17, no. 10, pp. 2764–2772, 2010.

[10] T. M. D. Hughes, R. P. A'Hern, and J. M. Thomas, "Prognosis and surgical mananagement of patients with palpable inguinal lymph node metastases from melanoma," *British Journal of Surgery*, vol. 87, no. 7, pp. 892–901, 2000.

[11] C. P. Karakousis and D. L. Driscoll, "Groin dissection in malignant melanoma," *British Journal of Surgery*, vol. 81, no. 12, pp. 1771–1774, 1994.

[12] M. de Vries, W. G. Vonkeman, R. J. van Ginkel, and H. J. Hoekstra, "Morbidity after inguinal sentinel lymph node biopsy and completion lymph node dissection in patients with cutaneous melanoma," *European Journal of Surgical Oncology*, vol. 32, no. 7, pp. 785–789, 2006.

[13] R. Rouzier, B. Haddad, G. Dubernard, P. Dubois, and B. Paniel, "Inguinofemoral dissection for carcinoma of the vulva: effect of modifications of extent and technique on morbidity and survival," *Journal of the American College of Surgeons*, vol. 196, no. 3, pp. 442–450, 2003.

[14] M. M. Guggenheim, U. Hug, F. J. Jung et al., "Morbidity and recurrence after completion lymph node dissection following sentinel lymph node biopsy in cutaneous malignant melanoma," *Annals of Surgery*, vol. 247, no. 4, pp. 687–693, 2008.

[15] R. Ravi, "Morbidity following groin dissection for penile carcinoma," *British Journal of Urology*, vol. 72, no. 6, pp. 941–945, 1993.

[16] A. G. Warren, H. Brorson, L. J. Borud, and S. A. Slavin, "Lymphedema: a comprehensive review," *Annals of Plastic Surgery*, vol. 59, no. 4, pp. 464–472, 2007.

[17] E. C. Holmes, H. S. Moseley, D. L. Morton, W. Clark, D. Robinson, and M. M. Urist, "A rational approach to the surgical management of melanoma," *Annals of Surgery*, vol. 186, no. 4, pp. 481–490, 1977.

[18] P. C. Baas, H. S. Koops, H. J. Hoekstra, J. J. Van Bruggen, L. T. Van der Weele, and J. Oldhoff, "Groin dissection in the treatment of lower-extremity melanoma: Short-term and long-term morbidity," *Archives of Surgery*, vol. 127, no. 3, pp. 281–286, 1992.

[19] J. H. James, "Lymphoedema following ilio-inguinal lymph node dissection," *Scandinavian Journal of Plastic and Reconstructive Surgery*, vol. 16, no. 2, pp. 167–171, 1982.

[20] *The Clinical Practice Guidelines for the Management of Melanoma in Australia and New Zealand*, Cancer Council Australia; Australian Cancer Network; Ministry of Health, New Zealand, Sydney, Australia, 2008.

[21] G. Landi, M. Polverelli, G. Moscatelli et al., "Sentinel lymph node biopsy in patients with primary cutaneous melanoma: Study of 455 cases," *Journal of the European Academy of Dermatology and Venereology*, vol. 14, no. 1, pp. 35–45, 2000.

[22] A. Ferlito, A. Rinaldo, C. E. Silver et al., "Neck dissection: then and now," *Auris Nasus Larynx*, vol. 33, no. 4, pp. 365–374, 2006.

[23] Y. Li, J. Zhang, and K. Yang, "Evaluation of the efficacy of a novel radical neck dissection preserving the external jugular vein, greater auricular nerve, and deep branches of the cervical nerve," *OncoTargets and Therapy*, vol. 6, pp. 361–367, 2013.

[24] O. Suárez, "El problema de las metastasis linfáticas y alejadas del cáncer de laringe e hipofaringe," *Revista de Otorrinolaringología*, vol. 23, pp. 83–99, 1963.

[25] A. Ferlito, A. Rinaldo, K. T. Robbins, and C. E. Silver, "Neck dissection: past, present and future?" *Journal of Laryngology and Otology*, vol. 120, no. 2, pp. 87–92, 2006.

[26] S. Samant and K. T. Robbins, "Evolution of neck dissection for improved functional outcome," *World Journal of Surgery*, vol. 27, no. 7, pp. 805–810, 2003.

[27] W. Pan, H. Suami, and G. I. Taylor, "Lymphatic drainage of the superficial tissues of the head and neck: anatomical study and clinical implications," *Plastic and Reconstructive Surgery*, vol. 121, no. 5, pp. 1614–1624, 2008.

[28] C. Lin, R. Ali, S. Chen et al., "Vascularized groin lymph node transfer using the wrist as a recipient site for management of postmastectomy upper extremity lymphedema," *Plastic and Reconstructive Surgery*, vol. 123, no. 4, pp. 1265–1275, 2009.

13

Ambulatory Melanoma Care Patterns in the United States

**Andrew L. Ji,[1] Michael R. Baze,[2] Scott A. Davis,[1]
Steven R. Feldman,[1,3,4] and Alan B. Fleischer Jr.[1,5]**

[1] Galderma Center for Dermatology Research, Department of Dermatology, Wake Forest School of Medicine,
  Winston-Salem, NC 27157-1071, USA

[2] Nova Southeastern University/Broward Health Medical Center, Department of Dermatology, Fort Lauderdale, FL 33315, USA

[3] Galderma Center for Dermatology Research, Department of Pathology, Wake Forest School of Medicine,
  Winston-Salem, NC 27157-1071, USA

[4] Galderma Center for Dermatology Research, Department of Public Health Sciences, Wake Forest School of Medicine,
  Winston-Salem, NC 27157-1071, USA

[5] Wake Forest University School of Medicine, Department of Dermatology, Medical Center Boulevard,
  Winston-Salem, NC 27157-1071, USA

Correspondence should be addressed to Alan B. Fleischer Jr.; afleisch@wfubmc.edu

Academic Editor: Mark Lebwohl

Objective. To examine trends in melanoma visits in the ambulatory care setting. *Methods.* Data from the National Ambulatory Medical Care Survey (NAMCS) from 1979 to 2010 were used to analyze melanoma visit characteristics including number of visits, age and gender of patients, and physician specialty. These data were compared to US Census population estimates during the same time period. *Results.* The overall rate of melanoma visits increased ($P < 0.0001$) at an apparently higher rate than the increase in population over this time. The age of patients with melanoma visits increased at approximately double the rate (0.47 year per interval year, $P < 0.0001$) of the population increase in age (0.23 year per interval year). There was a nonsignificant ($P = 0.19$) decline in the proportion of female patients seen over the study interval. Lastly, ambulatory care has shifted towards dermatologists and other specialties managing melanoma patients and away from family/internal medicine physicians and general/plastic surgeons. *Conclusions.* The number and age of melanoma visits has increased over time with respect to the overall population, mirroring the increase in melanoma incidence over the past three decades. These trends highlight the need for further studies regarding melanoma management efficiency.

1. Introduction

In 2013, the American Cancer Society estimates that there will be 76,690 new cases of melanoma diagnosed, with 61,300 being melanoma *in situ* [1]. Melanoma management costs the US billions of dollars in direct annual expenses [2]. Worldwide, during the past several decades, there has been a substantial increase in the incidence of melanoma, particularly among white populations [3, 4]. In the US, the incidence of melanoma also continues to rise. From 1973 to 1994, US melanoma incidence rates increased 154.4% in males (from 6.8 to 17.3 per 100,000) and 90.2% in females (from 6.1 to 11.6 per 100,000) [5]. The melanoma incidence rates during 2006 to 2010 reveal a similar trend in males (27.4 per 100,000) and

females (16.7 per 100,000), nearly quadrupling in men and tripling in women over the past three to four decades [6]. More specifically, during this period, the incidence rates per 100,000 persons were 31.9 and 20.0 in white men and women, respectively; 4.7 and 4.4 in Hispanic men and women, respectively; 1.6 and 1.1 in Asian men and women, respectively; and 1.1 and 1.0 in black men and woman, respectively [6].

According to the National Cancer Institute Surveillance Epidemiology End Results data, from 2006 to 2010, the median age at diagnosis for melanoma was 61 years, with approximately 65% of cases occurring in those 55 years and older [6]. Current estimates of lifetime risk for Americans experiencing melanoma are 1 in 37 for men and 1 in 56 for women, which contrasts with the lifetime risk of 1 in 1,500 for Americans born in 1935 [7, 8]. With increasing incidence, an understanding of the ambulatory management patterns of melanoma care has national significance. We sought to characterize how office visits for melanoma are changing.

2. Methods

The number of melanoma visits in physician office based settings was estimated using data from the National Ambulatory Medical Care Survey (NAMCS). The NAMCS is conducted by the Division of Health Care Statistics of the National Center for Health Statistics to provide data on a representative sample of ambulatory physician office visits in USA. The complex sampling frame examines nonhospital-based physician office visits, and the primary unit of analysis is the visit. These data are weighted to produce national estimates that describe the utilization of ambulatory medical care services in USA. The number of visits was obtained by identifying melanoma visits (ICD-9-CM diagnosis code of 172.0 to 172.9) for all patients for the interval years 1979 to 2010. Tumor staging information is not included in diagnosis coding. A total of 872,197 records estimating the experience of 26 billion office visits were searched to identify 819 unique melanoma visit records which estimate the experience of 17.4 million visits to USA physicians. Data extracted contain information about patient demographics and specialty of treating physicians. All analysis was performed using the survey procedures (SURVEYFREQ, SURVEYREG, and SURVEYMEANS) contained within SAS 9.1.3 (Cary, NC, USA).

Population data were derived from the US Census Bureau (http://www.census.gov/) over the representative period using both historical data (http://www.census.gov/popest/data/historical/index.html) and current estimate data (http://www.census.gov/popest/data/index.html).

3. Results

To test the hypothesis that ambulatory melanoma visit rates have changed in relation to the population, we compared NAMCS melanoma visits to US Census population estimates. Estimates of the numbers of melanoma visits demonstrated a significant increase in the interval from 1979 to 2010 ($P < 0.0001$). These data, as well as US population data from the Census Bureau, are plotted in Figure 1. The rate of increase in number of melanoma visits appears to be higher than the rate of increase in US population. Because the estimates are derived using widely disparate methods, direct comparison of the two datasets cannot be performed.

The age of patients with melanoma visits appears to be rising at approximately double the rate of the rise in the population increase in age (Figure 2). We estimated that the age of patients with melanoma visits increased by 0.47 year per interval year from 1979 to 2010, whereas the aging rate of the population was 0.23 year per interval year for the general population. Note that population means were obtained for the NAMCS melanoma visits, whereas only population medians from the census data were available.

To test the hypothesis that the gender distribution of melanoma visits has changed over time, Figure 3 shows

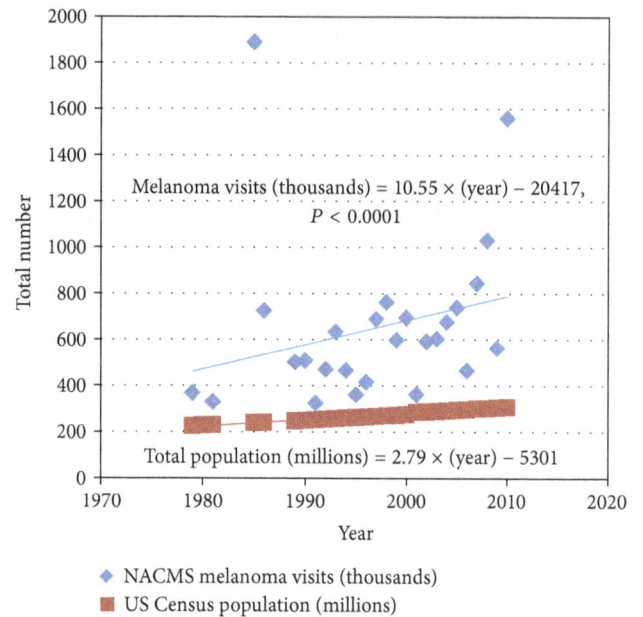

FIGURE 1: Estimated number of melanoma visits (thousands) from the US National Ambulatory Medical Care Survey (NACMS) from 1979 to 2010 compared to total US population (millions).

the proportion of the visits by female patients over the study interval, which demonstrates a nonsignificant ($P = 0.19$) decline in the proportion of female patients seen over the study interval.

Ambulatory care by different specialties appears to be changing over time, with a significant increase in the proportion of visits to dermatologists ($P = 0.0003$) and a corresponding decrease in the proportion of visits to family/internal medicine physicians ($P = 0.0056$) and general/plastic surgeons ($P < 0.0001$) (Figures 4(a), 4(b), and 4(c)). There was also an increasing trend in melanoma management by all other specialties ($P < 0.0001$) (Figure 4(d)).

4. Discussion

Our findings show that the overall rate of melanoma visits has increase in comparison to the baseline increase in population (Figure 1). Given that the melanoma visits sampled in this study could be either initial visits or follow-up visits for a previously diagnosed melanoma, we are unable to comment on melanoma incidence from these data. However, other studies indicate that the incidence of melanoma has been on the rise over the past several decades [5, 6], which would help explain why the number of visits has significantly increased. The increase in number of visits also suggests that management in the ambulatory care setting has accommodated the rising number of melanoma patients. There are a few explanations for this trend. Partly contributing to the increasing melanoma incidence are better detection practices and earlier detection of melanoma [9], which both occur most often in the ambulatory care setting. It has also been shown that the rise in incidence is mainly attributable to thin melanomas,

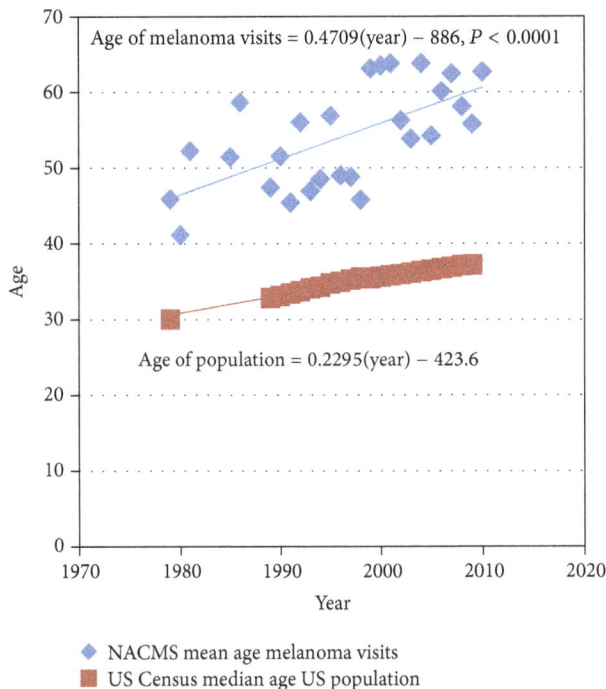

FIGURE 2: Mean age of melanoma visits from the US National Ambulatory Medical Care Survey (NAMCS) from 1979 to 2010 compared to median age of US population.

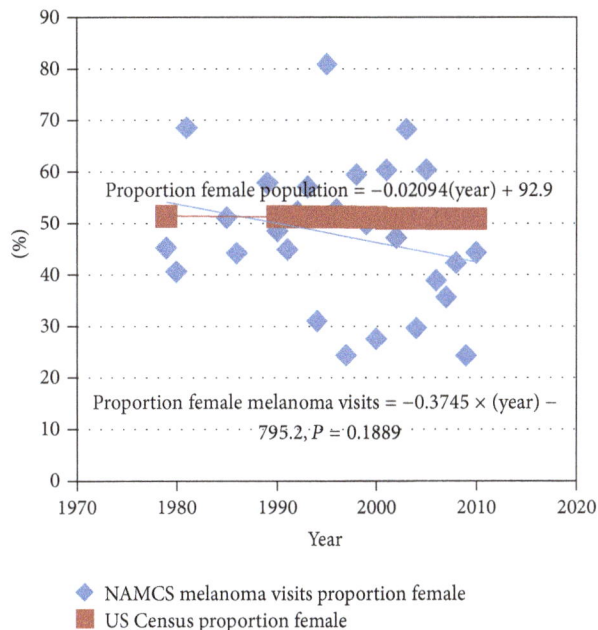

FIGURE 3: Proportion of female melanoma visits from the US National Ambulatory Medical Care Survey (NAMCS) from 1979 to 2010 compared to proportion female in population.

while the number of intermediate or thick melanomas has remained stable [10, 11]. Recent data show that dermatologists are diagnosing more melanomas and are doing so at earlier stages than any other specialty [12, 13]. They are now managing cases previously referred to surgical specialties. With dermatologists increasingly handling more diagnosis responsibilities, these factors could easily contribute to the observed increase in number of visits in the ambulatory care setting. It would be important to discern whether ambulatory care visits by these patients are the most efficient way to manage their disease. Efficiency in this context could be described as the least number of patient visits necessary in the appropriate management of a given melanoma.

Our study also reveals that the age of patients with melanoma visits increasing at approximately twice the rate of the population age increase (Figure 2). The mean age of patients with melanoma visits was about 45 years in 1979 and about 60 years in 2010. This suggests that the age at which people are diagnosed with melanoma is advancing over time. An analysis of the crude and birth-cohort adjusted age-specific rates of melanoma suggests that rates will continue to increase as earlier cohorts age [14]. However, it seems likely that this trend is due to more than just an aging population; otherwise the mean age of melanoma visits would track more closely with the mean age of the population. A reasonable explanation could include the changing solar exposure practices over the past decades and the long latency to the development of melanoma. If preventative practices were being appropriately employed, we would expect to see fewer young people developing melanoma, thereby contributing to the

higher age at diagnosis. In recent years, however, adolescents and young adults have been reported to be at increased risk of skin cancer due to suboptimal sunscreen use, high rates of sunburning, and tanning bed use [15]. Time will tell if these practices will lead to a higher incidence of melanoma in the younger populations. Further concerning evidence is that in US females, melanoma is reported to be the most common cancer in the 25 to 29 age group, and the second most common cancer in women aged 30 to 34 years [16]. As mentioned previously, better detection practices over the years could also explain an older age at diagnosis given the long latency period of the disease, especially if a diagnosis was missed at an earlier age.

During the time period examined by our study, the proportion of melanoma visits by women appears to closely correlate with the proportion of females in the population (Figure 3). However, albeit small, there is still a decline in the proportion of melanoma visits by females. This contrasts the fairly constant proportion of females in the population. In a study of melanoma incidence and mortality in US whites from 1969 to 1999, Geller et al. demonstrated increased melanoma incidence in men and women (aged 20 to 65 years or older), with greater increases noted in the older male population [17]. Other studies support these findings [18, 19]. With evidence demonstrating a greater incidence in males, we would expect to see a greater proportion of male melanoma visits. Possibly explaining this trend is that men may be less likely to visit a physician or maintain compliance with follow-up visits. Studies have demonstrated that while women have higher medical care service utilization and are more likely to use outpatient medical services, men are less likely to have physician office visits or preventative care visits

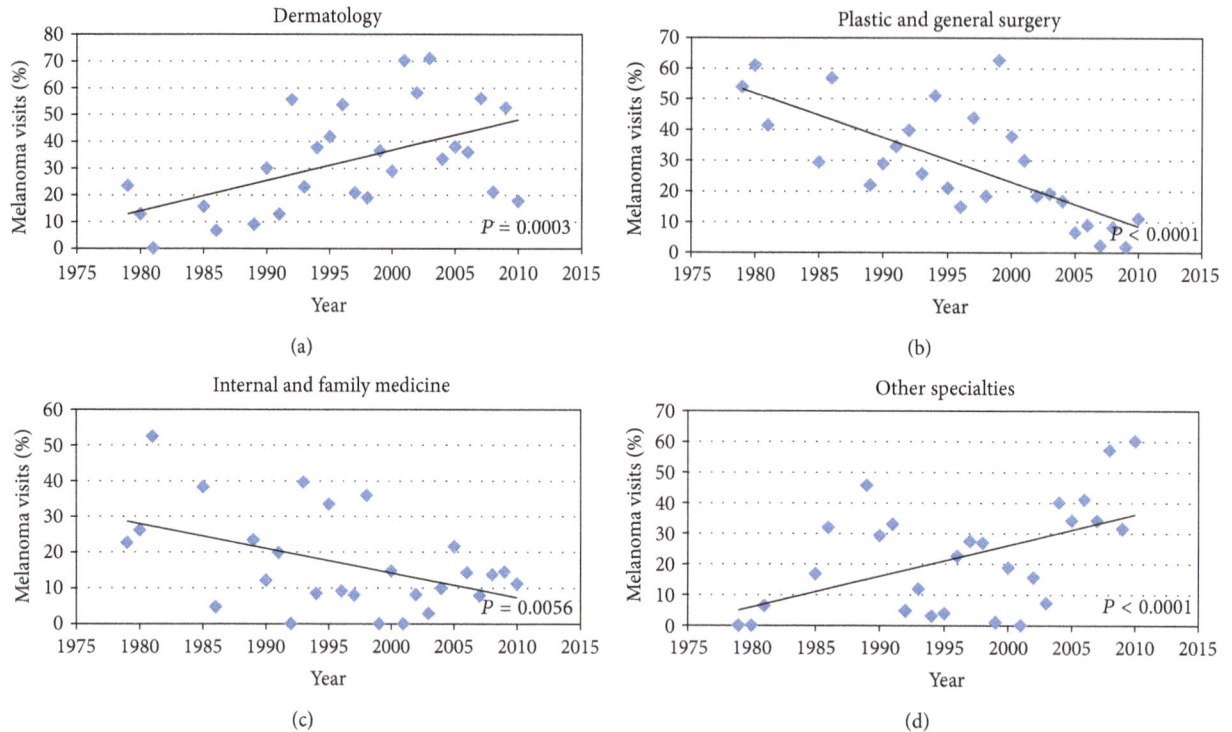

FIGURE 4: Proportion of melanoma visits by specialty from the US National Ambulatory National Care Survey (NAMCS) from 1979 to 2010 in (a) dermatology, (b) plastic and general surgery, (c) internal and family medicine, and (d) other specialties.

[20–22]. Further, men are presenting to the physician with thicker melanomas than women, possibly necessitating inpatient treatment, which is not accounted for by the NAMCS data [23]. Women living longer and having lower melanoma mortality can also influence this trend. While men and women aged 20 to 44 had a melanoma mortality decrease of 29% and 39%, respectively, men 65 years and older had a 157% mortality increase [17]. This was a 3-fold greater increase than for women of the same age.

In an effort to contain healthcare expenditures, greater emphasis has been placed on primary care physicians (PCPs) providing healthcare, as specialists, including dermatologists, are assumed to be more costly. In terms of management of skin conditions, this positions PCPs in a difficult situation, as much of their practice involves management of chronic conditions like hypertension and diabetes mellitus, and relatively little time diagnosing and treating skin disease. Fleischer Jr. et al. found that some of the most common cutaneous diagnoses made by family physicians were diagnosed at least 10 times more frequently by dermatologists [12]. Smith et al. demonstrated the large disparity in experience between dermatologists and other physicians with outpatient management of skin cancer [24]. The authors found that the majority of skin cancer visits (81%) were managed by dermatologists, with the remaining visits being managed by nondermatologists. Consistent with this, our data shows that over a few decades, dermatologists received more melanoma visits, while melanoma visits to family and internal medicine physicians have significantly decreased over this time period (Figures 4(a)–4(c)). Given that the majority of melanoma

visits have been going to dermatologists, nondermatologists may have relatively little clinical exposure to melanoma. Studies show that most PCPs referred patients presenting with suspicious appearing pigmented lesions to a dermatologist, as many PCPs did not feel confident in their ability to recognize melanoma and thought their training was not adequate to prepare them to diagnose and manage pigmented lesions [25, 26]. In surveys of US medical students and residents, the majority reported little to no training in skin care examinations and felt a lack of competency and confidence in performing these [27–29]. With a declining proportion of melanoma visits going to PCPs, this lack of confidence may only worsen. Conversely, for dermatologists, the increase in melanoma clinical experience has likely led to an increased level of confidence and expertise in melanoma management. The effect of greater physician experience on improved quality of care and medical cost reduction has been demonstrated [30, 31].

The rise in melanoma visits to dermatologists over the past three decades has also corresponded with a decline in visits to surgeons (Figure 4), a finding that is also reflected in other studies. In a study looking at the surgical management of melanoma by dermatologists and surgeons, the percentage of the total patients treated by dermatologists rose from 18% in 1979–84 to 57% in 1991–97, while those treated by general surgeons decreased from 58% to 15% and from 23% to 13% for plastic surgeons over the same period [32]. Many factors could contribute to this trend, including public recognition of dermatologists as skin care experts, and dermatology residencies providing more surgical and procedural training than in the past, allowing graduates to offer more comprehensive skin care than before [33].

As NAMCS data is derived from office-based physician practices in USA, one of the limitations of this study is the lack of data from hospital inpatient and military medical facilities. In the case of advanced melanomas managed by the general or plastic surgeons, this could underestimate both the overall total number of melanoma visits and the number of melanoma visits seen by these providers. With the NAMCS database limited to physicians primarily involved in outpatient care outside the federal system, this could lead to potential selection bias or sampling error. Another limitation of this study is that the melanoma visits could represent either new diagnosis or followups on previously diagnosed melanoma. To better estimate the new cases of melanoma, perhaps visits associated with excisions would provide a more accurate assessment. Lastly, the NAMCS data reflect the ability of the various practitioners to make an accurate diagnosis. For those with less experience in dealing with pigmented lesions, misdiagnosis could occur. For example, it is not uncommon for a seborrheic keratosis to masquerade as melanoma, which could lead to an overestimation of melanoma visits. Likewise, if a practitioner is using a particular system for diagnosis, such as the Asymmetry, Borders, Color, and Diameter (ABCD) system, they potentially could misdiagnose a melanoma that did not fit this system. This could lead to either an underestimation or overestimation of melanoma visits.

5. Conclusion

The trends demonstrated in our study offer insight into characteristics of ambulatory melanoma visits over three decades. Specifically, our investigation revealed that both the number and age of melanoma visits has risen over time, mirroring the increase in incidence of melanoma. Further, no gender differences were identified over time. Primary care physicians and surgeons have decreased their contribution to care, while dermatologists and other specialties have increased their contribution of care. While these findings allow for the possible exploration and understanding of contributing factors, they also highlight the need for further studies. For example, a study looking at the number of visits associated with a given type and stage of melanoma could provide information that would allow for a more accurate assessment of melanoma management efficiency. Not only would this have the potential of raising the standard of care but also lower healthcare expenditures. With dermatologists expanding their scope of practice to include more surgical and procedural dermatology, along with the general recognition of dermatologists as the skin cancer experts, the disparities in melanoma visits between dermatologists and nondermatologists will likely continue to grow.

Authors' Contribution

Andrew L. Ji and Michael R. Baze contributed equally to this work.

References

[1] American Cancer Society, *Cancer Facts and Figures 2013*, American Cancer Society, Atlanta, Ga, USA, 2013.

[2] D. R. Bickers, H. W. Lim, D. Margolis et al., "The burden of skin diseases: 2004," *Journal of the American Academy of Dermatology*, vol. 55, no. 3, pp. 490–500, 2006.

[3] T. L. Diepgen and V. Mahler, "The epidemiology of skin cancer," *British Journal of Dermatology*, vol. 146, 61, pp. 1–6, 2002.

[4] J. V. Schaffer, D. S. Rigel, A. W. Kopf, and J. L. Bolognia, "Cutaneous melanoma—past, present, and future," *Journal of the American Academy of Dermatology*, vol. 51, supplement 1, pp. S65–S69, 2004.

[5] H. I. Hall, D. R. Miller, J. D. Rogers, and B. Bewerse, "Update on the incidence and mortality from melanoma in the United States," *Journal of the American Academy of Dermatology*, vol. 40, no. 1, pp. 35–42, 1999.

[6] N. Howlader, A. M. Noone, M. Krapcho et al., Eds., *SEER Cancer Statistics Review, 1975–2010*, National Cancer Institute, Bethesda, MD, USA.

[7] A. Jemal, R. Siegel, J. Xu, and E. Ward, "Cancer statistics," *CA: A Cancer Journal for Clinicians*, vol. 60, no. 5, p. 277, 2010.

[8] D. S. Rigel and J. A. Carucci, "Malignant melanoma: prevention, early detection, and treatment in the 21st century," *Ca: A Cancer Journal for Clinicians*, vol. 50, no. 4, pp. 215–236, 2000.

[9] K. C. Lee and M. A. Weinstock, "Melanoma is up: are we up to this challenge?" *Journal of Investigative Dermatology*, vol. 129, no. 7, pp. 1604–1606, 2009.

[10] D. M. Lipsker, G. Hedelin, E. Heid, E. M. Grosshans, and B. J. Cribier, "Striking increase of thin melanomas contrasts with stable incidence of thick melanomas," *Archives of Dermatology*, vol. 135, no. 12, pp. 1451–1456, 1999.

[11] M. Demierre, C. Chung, D. R. Miller, and A. C. Geller, "Early detection of thick melanomas in the United States: beware of the nodular subtype," *Archives of Dermatology*, vol. 141, no. 6, pp. 745–750, 2005.

[12] A. B. Fleischer Jr., C. Herbert, S. R. Feldman, and F. O'Brien, "Diagnosis of skin disease by nondermatologists," *American Journal of Managed Care*, vol. 6, no. 10, pp. 1149–1156, 2000.

[13] S. C. Chen, M. L. Pennie, P. Kolm et al., "Diagnosing and managing cutaneous pigmented lesions: primary care physicians versus dermatologists," *Journal of General Internal Medicine*, vol. 21, no. 7, pp. 678–682, 2006.

[14] L. K. Dennis, "Melanoma incidence by body site: effects of birth-cohort adjustment," *Archives of Dermatology*, vol. 135, no. 12, pp. 1553–1554, 1999.

[15] A. C. Geller, G. Colditz, S. Oliveria et al., "Use of sunscreen, sunburning rates, and tanning bed use among more than 10,000 US children and adolescents," *Pediatrics*, vol. 109, no. 6, pp. 1009–1014, 2002.

[16] L. Brochez and J.-M. Naeyaert, "Understanding the trends in melanoma incidence and mortality: where do we stand?" *European Journal of Dermatology*, vol. 10, no. 1, pp. 71–76, 2000.

[17] A. C. Geller, D. R. Miller, G. D. Annas, M. Demierre, B. A. Gilchrest, and H. K. Koh, "Melanoma incidence and mortality among US whites, 1969–1999," *Journal of the American Medical Association*, vol. 288, no. 14, pp. 1719–1720, 2002.

[18] R. A. Desmond and S. Soong, "Epidemiology of malignant melanoma," *Surgical Clinics of North America*, vol. 83, no. 1, pp. 1–29, 2003.

[19] A. Jemal, S. S. Devesa, P. Hartge, and M. A. Tucker, "Recent trends in cutaneous melanoma incidence among whites in the United States," *Journal of the National Cancer Institute*, vol. 93, no. 9, pp. 678–683, 2001.

[20] R. M. Pinkhasov, J. Wong, J. Kashanian et al., "Are men short-changed on health? Perspective on health care utilization and health risk behavior in men and women in the United States," *International Journal of Clinical Practice*, vol. 64, no. 4, pp. 475–487, 2010.

[21] K. D. Bertakis, R. Azari, L. J. Helms, E. J. Callahan, and J. A. Robbins, "Gender differences in the utilization of health care services," *Journal of Family Practice*, vol. 49, no. 2, pp. 147–152, 2000.

[22] P. D. Cleary, D. Mechanic, and J. R. Greenley, "Sex differences in medical care utilization: an empirical investigation," *Journal of Health and Social Behavior*, vol. 23, no. 2, pp. 106–119, 1982.

[23] J. L. Schwartz, T. S. Wang, T. A. Hamilton, L. Lowe, V. K. Sondak, and T. M. Johnson, "Thin primary cutaneous melanomas: associated detection patterns, lesion characteristics, and patient characteristics," *Cancer*, vol. 95, no. 7, pp. 1562–1568, 2002.

[24] E. S. Smith, S. R. Feldman, A. B. Fleischer Jr., B. Leshin, and A. McMichael, "Characteristics of office-based visits for skin cancer: dermatologists have more experience than other physicians in managing malignant and premalignant skin conditions," *Dermatologic Surgery*, vol. 24, no. 9, pp. 981–985, 1998.

[25] K. P. Friedman, D. L. Whitaker-Worth, C. Grin, and J. M. Grant-Kels, "Melanoma screening behavior among primary care physicians," *Cutis*, vol. 74, no. 5, pp. 305–311, 2004.

[26] R. S. Kirsner, S. Muhkerjee, and D. G. Federman, "Skin cancer screening in primary care: prevalence and barriers," *Journal of the American Academy of Dermatology*, vol. 41, no. 4, pp. 564–566, 1999.

[27] M. Lee, C. S. Hodgson, and L. Wilkerson, "Predictors of self-perceived competency in cancer screening examinations," *Journal of Cancer Education*, vol. 17, no. 4, pp. 180–182, 2002.

[28] M. M. Moore, A. C. Geller, Z. Zhang et al., "Skin cancer examination teaching in US medical education," *Archives of Dermatology*, vol. 142, no. 4, pp. 439–444, 2006.

[29] E. Wise, D. Singh, M. Moore et al., "Rates of skin cancer screening and prevention counseling by US medical residents," *Archives of Dermatology*, vol. 145, no. 10, pp. 1131–1136, 2009.

[30] W. Chang, T. Li, and C. Lin, "The effect of physician experience on costs and clinical outcomes of laparoscopic-assisted vaginal hysterectomy: a multivariate analysis," *Journal of the American Association of Gynecologic Laparoscopists*, vol. 10, no. 3, pp. 356–359, 2003.

[31] J. A. Sosa, H. M. Bowman, J. M. Tielsch, N. R. Powe, T. A. Gordon, and R. Udelsman, "The importance of surgeon experience for clinical and economic outcomes from thyroidectomy," *Annals of Surgery*, vol. 228, no. 3, pp. 320–330, 1998.

[32] D. B. Mckenna, J. C. Marioni, R. J. Lee, R. J. Prescott, and V. R. Doherty, "A comparison of dermatologists', surgeons' and general practitioners' surgical management of cutaneous melanoma," *British Journal of Dermatology*, vol. 151, no. 3, pp. 636–644, 2004.

[33] M. M. Todd, J. J. Miller, and C. T. Ammirati, "Dermatologic surgery training in residency," *Dermatologic Surgery*, vol. 28, no. 7, pp. 547–550, 2002.

14

Melanoma-Targeted Chemothermotherapy and *In Situ* Peptide Immunotherapy through HSP Production by Using Melanogenesis Substrate, NPrCAP, and Magnetite Nanoparticles

Kowichi Jimbow,[1,2] Yasue Ishii-Osai,[2] Shosuke Ito,[3] Yasuaki Tamura,[4] Akira Ito,[5]
Akihiro Yoneta,[2] Takafumi Kamiya,[2] Toshiharu Yamashita,[2] Hiroyuki Honda,[6]
Kazumasa Wakamatsu,[3] Katsutoshi Murase,[7] Satoshi Nohara,[7] Eiichi Nakayama,[8]
Takeo Hasegawa,[9] Itsuo Yamamoto,[10] and Takeshi Kobayashi[11]

[1] Institute of Dermatology & Cutaneous Sciences, 1-27 Odori West 17, Chuo-ku, Sapporo 060-0042, Japan
[2] Department of Dermatology, School of Medicine, Sapporo Medical University, South 1 West 16, Chuo-ku, Sapporo 060-8556, Japan
[3] Department of Chemistry, School of Health Sciences, Fujita Health University, 1-98 Dengakugakubo,
   Kutsukake-cho, Toyoake, Aichi 470-1192, Japan
[4] Department of Pathology 1, School of Medicine, Sapporo Medical University, South 1 West 16, Chuo-ku, Sapporo 060-8556, Japan
[5] Department of Chemical Engineering, Faculty of Engineering, Kyushu University, 744 Motooka, Nishi-ku, Fukuoka 819-0395, Japan
[6] Department of Biotechnology, School of Engineering, Nagoya University, Furo-cho, Chikusa-ku, Nagoya 464-8603, Japan
[7] Meito Sangyo Co., Ltd., 25-5 Kaechi, Nishibiwajima-cho, Kiyosu, Aichi 452-0067, Japan
[8] Faculty of Health and Welfare, Kawasaki University of Medical Welfare, 288 Matsushimai, Kurashiki, Okayama 701-0193, Japan
[9] Department of Hyperthermia Medical Research Laboratory, Louis Pasteur Center for Medical Research, 103-5,
   Tanakamonzen-cho, Sakyo-ku, Kyoto 606-8225, Japan
[10] Yamamoto Vinita Co., Ltd., 3-12 ueshio 6, Tennoji-ku, Osaka 543-0002, Japan
[11] Department of Biological Chemistry, College of Bioscience and Biotechnology, Chubu University,
   1200 Matsumoto-cho, Kasugai, Aichi 487-8501, Japan

Correspondence should be addressed to Kowichi Jimbow; jimbow@sapmed.ac.jp

Academic Editor: Mohammed Kashani-Sabet

Exploitation of biological properties unique to cancer cells may provide a novel approach to overcome difficult challenges to the treatment of advanced melanoma. In order to develop melanoma-targeted chemothermoimmunotherapy, a melanogenesis substrate, N-propionyl-4-S-cysteaminylphenol (NPrCAP), sulfur-amine analogue of tyrosine, was conjugated with magnetite nanoparticles. NPrCAP was exploited from melanogenesis substrates, which are expected to be selectively incorporated into melanoma cells and produce highly reactive free radicals through reacting with tyrosinase, resulting in chemotherapeutic and immunotherapeutic effects by oxidative stress and apoptotic cell death. Magnetite nanoparticles were conjugated with NPrCAP to introduce thermotherapeutic and immunotherapeutic effects through nonapoptotic cell death and generation of heat shock protein (HSP) upon exposure to alternating magnetic field (AMF). During these therapeutic processes, NPrCAP was also expected to provide melanoma-targeted drug delivery system.

1. Introduction

The incidence of melanoma is increasing worldwide at an alarming rate [1, 2]. As yet, management of metastatic melanoma is an extremely difficult challenge. Less than 10% with metastatic melanoma patients survive currently for five years because of the lack of effective therapies [3]. There is, therefore, an emerging need to develop innovative therapies for the control of metastatic melanoma.

The major advance of drug discovery for targeted therapy to cancer cells can be achieved by exploiting their unique biological property. The biological property unique to the melanoma cell resides in the biosynthesis of melanin pigments, that is, melanogenesis occuring within specific compartments, melanosomes. Melanogenesis begins with the conversion of amino acid, tyrosine to dopa and subsequently to dopaquinone in the presence of tyrosinase. This pathway is uniquely expressed by all melanoma cells. It is well known that the clinically "amelanotic" melanoma tissues always have tyrosinase activity to some extent, and that "in vitro amelanotic" melanoma cells become "melanotic" ones when they are regrown in the in vivo condition. Melanin precursors are inherently cytotoxic through reacting with tyrosinase to form unstable quinone derivatives [4]. Thus, tyrosine analogues that are tyrosinase substrates can be good candidates for developing drugs to melanoma-targeting therapies [5]. N-propionyl and N-acetyl derivatives (NPr- and NAcCAP) of 4-S-cysteaminylphenol, that is, sulfur-amine analogue of tyrosine, were synthesized as possible melanoma-targeted drugs (Figure 1) and found to possess selective cytotoxic effects on in vivo and in vitro melanomas through the oxidative stress that derives from production of cytotoxic free radicals by interacting with tyrosinase within melanogenesis cascade [6–10].

Intracellular hyperthermia using magnetite nanoparticles (10–100 nm-sized Fe_3O_4) may be another choice to overcome the difficult challenges for melanoma treatment. It has been shown to be effective for treating cancers in not only primary but also metastatic lesions [11, 12]. Incorporated magnetite nanoparticles generate heat (thermotherapy) within the cells after exposure to AMF due to hysteresis loss [13]. In this treatment, there is not only the heat-mediated cell death but also immune reaction due to the generation of heat shock proteins (HSPs) [14–23]. HSP expression induced by hyperthermia has been shown to be involved in tumor immunity, providing the basis for developing a cancer thermoimmunotherapy.

Based upon these rationales, we now provide evidence that melanoma-targeted chemothermotherapy can be achieved by conjugating a chemically modified melanogenesis substrate, NPrCAP with magnetite nanoparticles, which then produce apoptotic and non-apoptotic cell death through interacting with tyrosinase and heat-mediated oxidative stress; hence, immunotherapy with production of in situ peptides is being established (Figure 2).

2. Melanogenesis Substrate as a Potential Candidate for Development of Selective Drug Delivery System and Cytotoxicity to Melanoma

2.1. Synthesis of Sulfur-Amine Analogues of Tyrosine, Cysteaminylphenols, and Their Selective Incorporation into Melanogenesis Cascade.
With the interaction of melanocyte-stimulating hormone (MSH)/melanocortin 1 receptor (MC1R), the melanogenesis cascade begins from activation

of microphthalmia transcription factor (MITF) for induction of either eu- or pheomelanin biosynthesis. Tyrosinase is the major player in this cascade. Tyrosinase is a glycoprotein, and its glycosylation process is regulated by a number of molecular chaperons, including calnexin in the endoplasmic reticulum [24, 25]. Vesicular transport then occurs to carry tyrosinase and its related proteins (TRPs) from trans-Golgi network to melanosomal compartments, which appear to derive from early and late endosomal compartments. In this process a number of transporters, such as small GTP-binding protein, adaptor proteins, and PI3-kinase, play important roles. Once melanin biosynthesis is completed to conduct either eu- or pheomelanogenesis within melanosomes, they then move along dendritic processes and are transferred to surrounding keratinocytes in normal skin [26–28]. In metastatic melanoma cells, however, there will be practically no melanosome transfer inasmuch as there will be no receptor cells such as keratinocytes. Thus melanosomes synthesized by melanoma cells are aggregated within autophagic vacuoles in which melanogenesis-targeted drugs will be retained. In order to utilize this unique melanogenesis pathway for developing melanoma-targeted drugs, N-acetyl and N-propionyl derivatives of cysteaminylphenols (NAc- and NPrCAPs) have been synthesized [8, 29] (Figure 1).

2.2. In Vivo and In Vitro Melanocyte Toxicity and Anti-Melanoma Effects of Cysteaminylphenols (CAPs).
Both NPrCAP and NAcCAP were found to selectively disintegrate follicular melanocytes after single or multiple ip administration to newborn or adult C57 black mice, respectively [12, 30]. In the case of adult mice after repeated ip administration of NPrCAP, white follicles with 100% success rate can be seen at the site where hair follicles were plucked to stimulate new melanocyte growth and to activate new tyrosinase synthesis. A single ip administration of NPrCAP into a new born mouse resulted in the development of silver follicles in the entire body coat. The selective disintegration of melanocytes which is mediated by apoptotic cell death can be seen as early as in 12 hr after a single ip administration. None of surrounding keratinocytes or fibroblasts showed such membrane degeneration and cell death [31, 32] (Figure 3).

A high, specific uptake of NAcCAP was seen in vitro by melanoma cell lines compared to nonmelanoma cells [9]. A melanoma-bearing mouse showed, on the whole body autoradiogram, the selective uptake and covalent binding of NAcCAP in melanoma tissues of lung and skin [6]. The specific cytotoxicity of NPrCAP and NAcCAP was examined on various types of culture cells by MTT assay, showing that only melanocytic cells except HeLa cells possessed the low IC50 [8, 9]. The cytotoxicity on DNA synthesis inhibition was timedependent and irreversible on melanoma cells but was transient on HeLa cells [10].

The in vitro culture and in vivo lung metastasis assays showed the melanoma growth can be blocked by administration of NAcCAP combined with buthionine sulfoximide (BSO), which blocked the effect of antioxidants through reducing glutathione levels. There was a marked growth inhibition of cultured melanoma cells in the presence of BSO

	Km (μM)	V_{max} (μmole/min/mg)
Tyrosine	0.3	1.8
N-acetyl-4-S-CAP (NAcCAP)	375	9.28
N-propionyl-4-S-CAP (NPrCAP)	340.9	5.43

FIGURE 1: Synthesis and chemical structures of NAcCAP and NPrCAP and their tyrosinase kinetics.

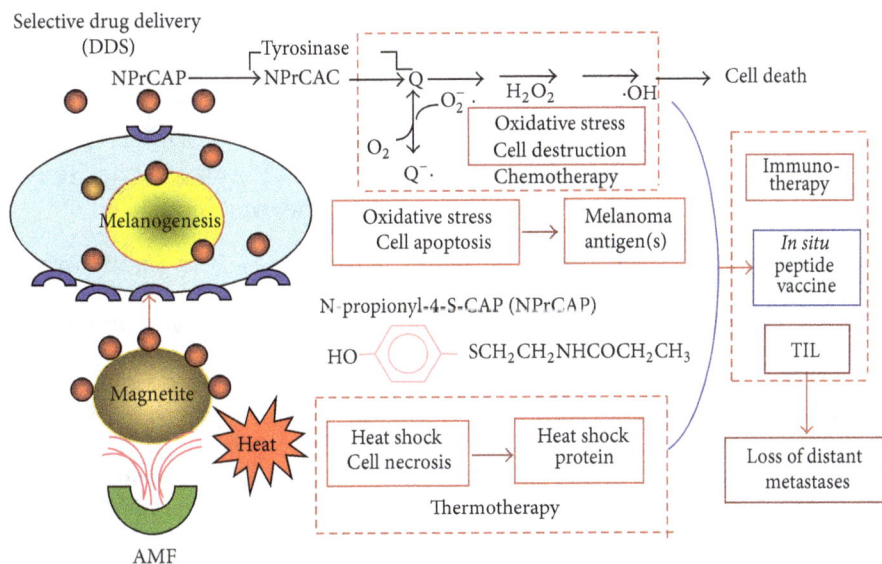

FIGURE 2: Strategy for melanogenesis-targeted CTI and *in situ* peptide vaccine therapy by conjugates of NPrCAP and magnetite nanoparticles with AMF exposure.

indicating that the selective cytotoxicity by CAP is mediated by the production of cytotoxic free radicals. The *in vivo* lung metastasis experiment also showed the decreased number of lung melanoma colonies [6]. The problem was, however, that a fairly large number of amelanotic melanoma lesions were seen to grow in the lung [6]. NPrCAP has been developed and conjugated with magnetite nanoparticles in the hope of increasing the cytotoxicity and overcoming the problem.

3. Conjugation of NPrCAP with Magnetite Nanoparticles and *In Vivo* Evaluation of Melanoma Growth Inhibition with/without Thermotherapy

3.1. Synthesis for Conjugates of NPrCAP with Magnetite Nanoparticles and Their Selective Aggregation in Melanoma for

Development of Chemo-Thermo-Immunotherapy. Magnetite nanoparticles have been employed for thermotherapy in a number of cancer treatments including human gliomas and prostate cancers [33–35]. They consist of 10–100 nm-sized iron oxide (Fe_3O_4) with a surrounding polymer coating and generate heat when exposed to AMF [12]. We expected the combination of NPrCAP and magnetite nanoparticles to be a potential source for developing not only antimelanoma pharmacologic but also immunogenic agent. Based upon the melanogenesis-targeted drug delivery system (DDS) of NPrCAP, NPrCAP/magnetite nanoparticles complex was expected to be selectively incorporated into melanoma cells. It was also hypothesized that the degradation of melanoma tissues may occur from oxidative and heat stresses by exposure of NPrCAP to tyrosinase and by exposure of magnetite nanoparticles to AMF. These two stress processes may then produce the synergistic or additive effect for generating tumor-infiltrating lymphocytes (TIL) by *in situ* formation of peptides that will kill melanoma cells in distant metastases (Figure 2).

In order to develop effective melanoma-targeted chemotherapy (by NPrCAP) and thermo-immunotherapy (by magnetite nanoparticles with HSP), hence providing a basis for chemo-thermo-immunotherapy (CTI therapy), we synthesized conjugates of NPrCAP and magnetite nanoparticles, on which NPrCAP is bound directly or indirectly on the surface of magnetite nanoparticles or magnetite-containing liposomes (Figure 4). Among these NPrCAP and magnetite complexes listed in Figure 4, NPrCAP/M and NPrCAP/PEG/M were chemically stable, did not lose biological property, and could be filtered as well as easily produced in large quantities. Most of the experiments described below were carried out by employing the direct conjugate of NPrCAP and magnetite nanoparticles, NPrCAP/M. A preliminary clinical trial, however, used NPrCAP/PEG/M to which polyethylene glycol (PEG) was employed to conjugate NPrCAP and magnetite nanoparticles.

In our studies, we found that NPrCAP/M nanoparticle conjugates were selectively aggregated in melanoma cells compared to non-melanoma cells [36]. The conjugates of NPrCAP and magnetite nanoparticles would be selectively aggregated on the cell surface of melanoma cells through still unknown surface receptor and then incorporated into melanoma cells by early and late endosomes. The conjugates were then incorporated into melanosomal compartment as the stage I melanosomes derive from late endosome-related organelles, to which tyrosinase was transported from the trans-Golgi network by vesicular transport [26].

3.2. In Vivo Growth Inhibition of Mouse Melanoma by Conjugates of NPrCAP and Magnetite Nanoparticles with/without Thermotherapy. The intracellular hyperthermia using magnetic nanoparticles is effective for treating certain types of primary and metastatic cancers [11, 12, 35–39]. Incorporated magnetic nanoparticles generate heat within the cells after exposure to the AMF due to hysteresis loss or relaxational loss [13, 40]. In our study of B16 melanoma cells using B16F1, B16F10, and B16OVA cells, we compared the thermo-therapeutic protocols in detail by evaluating the growth of the rechallenge melanoma transplants as well as the duration and rates of survival of melanoma-bearing mice.

By employing B16F1 and F10 cells, we first evaluated the chemotherapeutic effect of NPrCAP/M with or without AMF exposure which generates heat. NPrCAP/M without heat inhibited growth of primary transplants to the same degree as did NPrCAP/M with heat, indicating that NPrCAP/M alone has a chemotherapeutic effect. However, there was a significant difference in the melanoma growth inhibition of re-challenge transplants between the groups of NPrCAP/M with and without heat. NPrCAP/M with AMF exposure showed the most significant growth inhibition in re-challenge melanoma transplants and increased life span of the host animals, that is, almost complete rejection of re-challenge melanoma growth, whereas NPrCAP/M without heat was

much less, indicating that NPrCAP/M with heat possesses a thermo-immunotherapeutic effect (Figures 5(a), 5(b), and 5(c)).

Specifically our study indicated that the most effective thermoimmunotherapy for re-challenge B16F1 and F10 melanoma cells can be obtained at a temperature of 43°C for 30 min with the treatment repeated three times on every other day intervals without complete degradation of the primary melanoma [37]. This therapeutic approach and its biologic effects differ from those of magnetically mediated hyperthermia on the transplanted melanomas reported previously. In previous studies by Suzuki et al. [38] and Yanase et al. [39], cationic magnetoliposomes were used for B16 melanoma. They showed that hyperthermia at 46°C once or twice led to regression of 40–90% of primary tumors and to 30–60% survival of mice, whereas their hyperthermia at 43°C failed to induce regression of the secondary tumors and any increase of survival in mice [38, 39].

4. Production of Heat Shock Protein, Nonapoptotic Cell Death, and Tumor-Infiltrating Lymphocytes by Conjugates of NPrCAP and Magnetite Nanoparticles with Thermotherapy

4.1. Production of Heat Shock Protein and Non-Apoptotic Melanoma Cell Death by NPrCAP/Magnetite Nanoparticle Conjugates with Thermotherapy. It has been shown that hyperthermia treatment using magnetite cationic liposomes (MCLs), which are cationic liposomes containing 10-nm magnetite nanoparticles, induced antitumor immunity through HSP expression [12, 22, 41, 42]. In our studies using B16F1, F10, and OVA melanoma cells [43], the hyperthermia using NPrCAP/M with AMF exposure also showed antitumor immune responses via HSP-chaperoned antigen (Figure 6) [43]. It may be speculated that the HSPs-antigen peptide complex released from melanoma cells treated with this intracellular hyperthermia is taken up by dendritic cells (DCs) and cross-presented HSP-chaperoned peptide in the context of MHC class I molecules [44]. In our CTI therapy with AMF exposure, the heat-mediated melanoma cell necrosis was induced to NPrCAP/M-incorporated cells. In this group, we also found that repeated hyperthermia (3 cycles of NPrCAP/M administration and AMF irradiation) was required to induce the maximal antitumor immune response [37].

If melanoma cells escaped from this necrotic cell death, repeated hyperthermia should produce further necrotic cell death to the previously heat-shocked melanoma cells in which HSPs were induced. Our CTI therapy with AMF exposure using B16OVA cells showed that Hsp72/Hsc73, Hsp90, and ER-resident HSPs participated in the induction of CD8$^+$ T-cell response [43]. Different from the results of B16F1 and F10 cells, Hsp72 was largely responsible for the augmented antigen presentation to CD8$^+$ T cells. As Hsp72 is known to upregulate in response to hyperthermia or heat shock treatment [41], newly synthesized Hsp72 has a chance to bind to the heat-denatured melanoma-associated antigen.

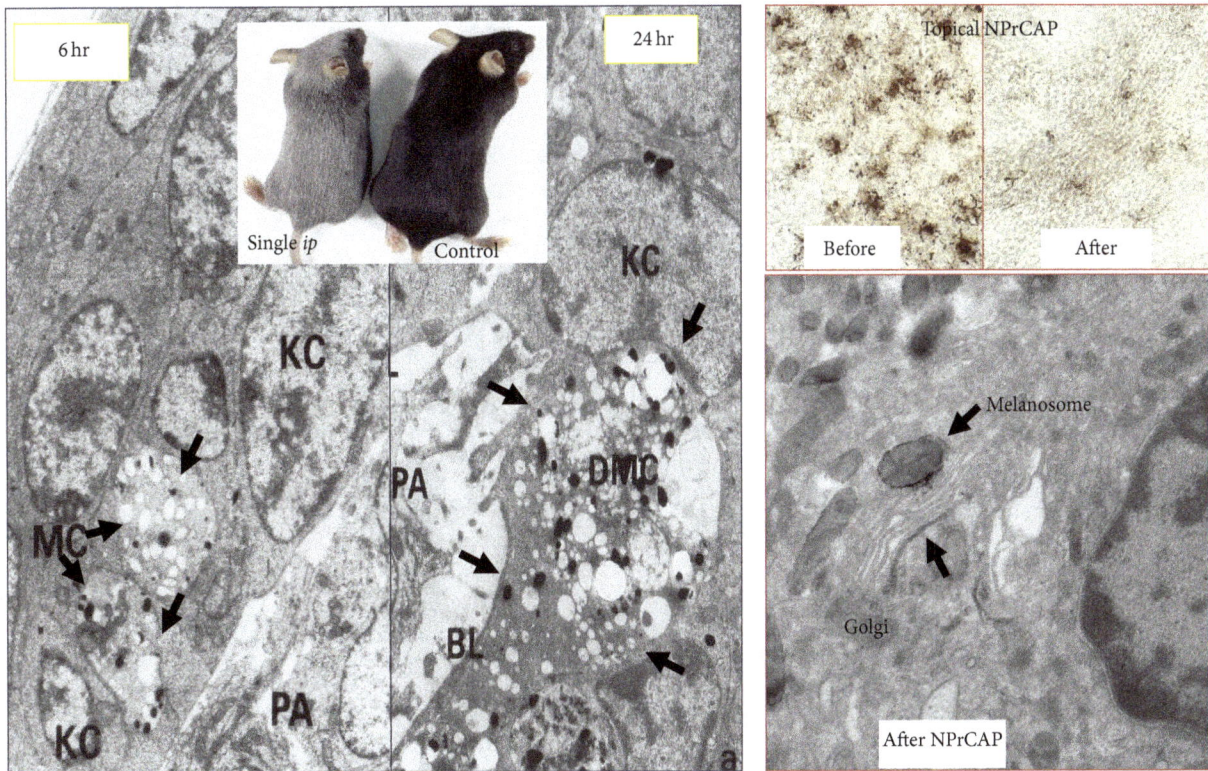

(a) Depigmentation of C57 black mouse hair by a single *ip* administration of NPrCAP or NAcCAP

(b) Depigmentation of black skin by topical NPrCAP

FIGURE 3: Depigmenting effect of NPrCAP. (a) Depigmentation of C57 black mouse hair follicles by a single *ip* administration of NPrCAP or NAcCAP results in complete loss of melanin pigmentation. Entire coat color changes to silver from black. Electron microscopic observation reveals selective degradation of melanocytes and melanogenic organelles such as early-stage melanosomes at 6 hr after administration. At 24 hr after administration, these melanocytes reveal total degradation. (b) Depigmentation of black skin after topical application of NPrCAP. There is a marked decrease of melanocyte populations after topical application. Electron microscopic observation indicates selective accumulation of NPrCAP in the tyrosinase areas such as in melanosomes and Golgi apparatus as indicated by the deposition of electron dense materials (see arrows).

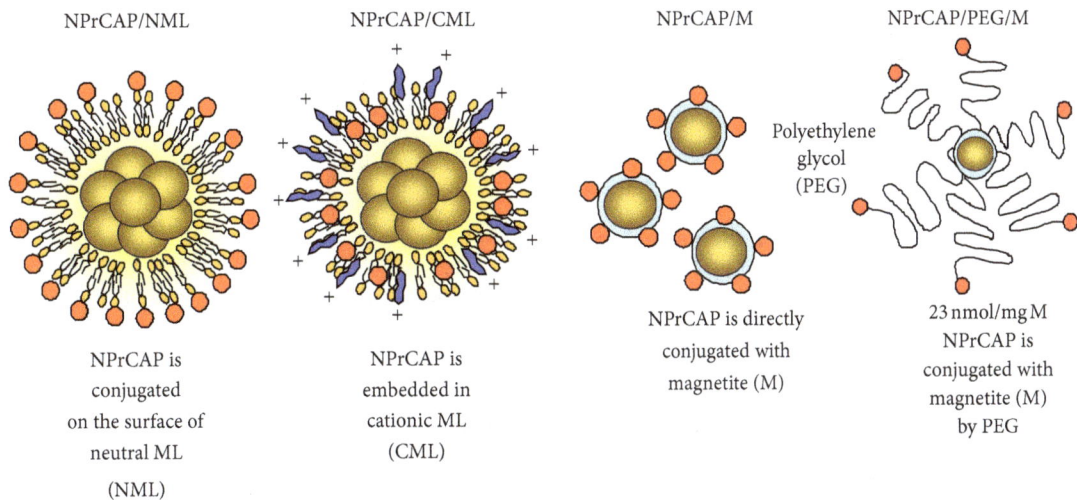

FIGURE 4: Conjugates of NPrCAP/magnetite nanoparticles for developing melanogenesis-targeted melanoma nanomedicine.

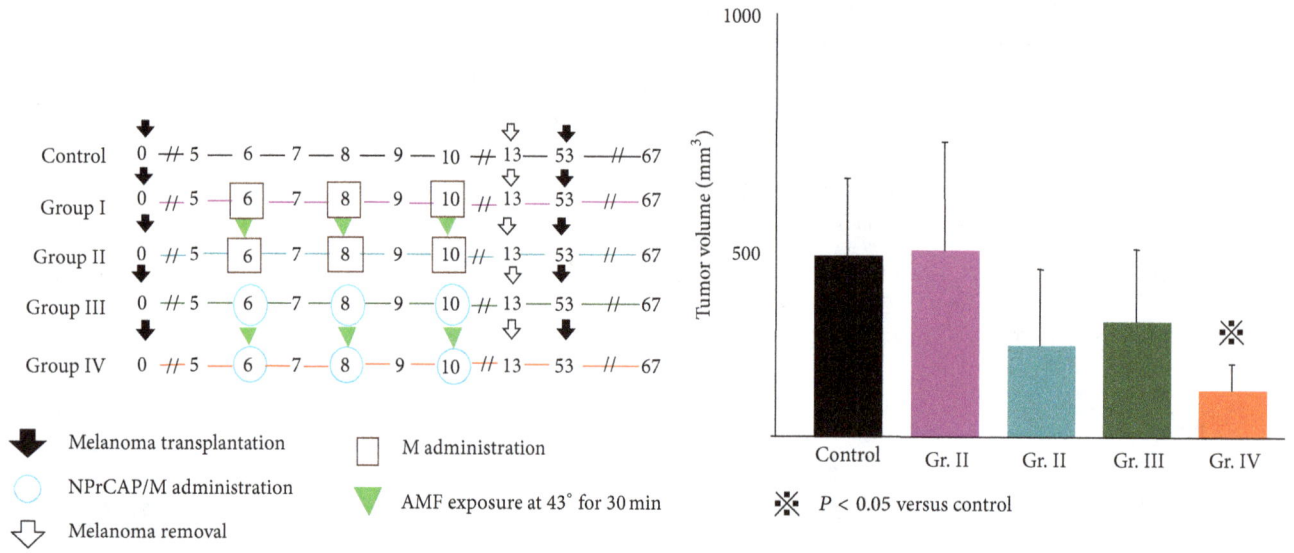

(a) Protocols of Groups I, II, III, and IV of experimental mice

(b) Tumor volumes of rechallenge B16F1 melanoma transplants

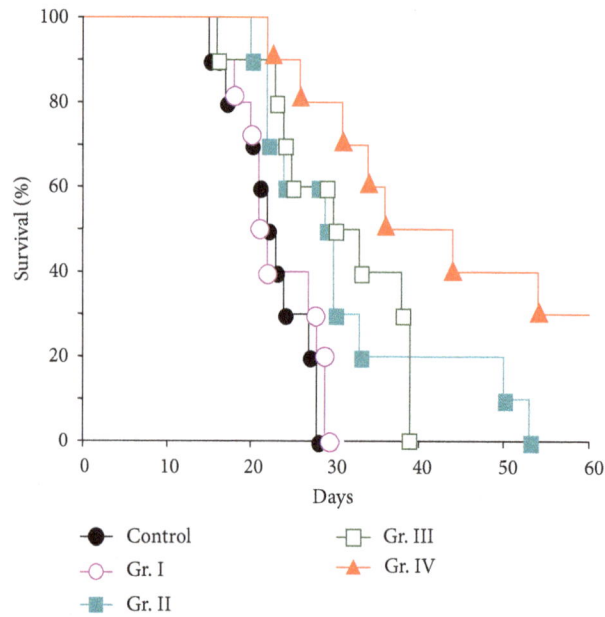

(c) Kaplan-Meier survival after tumor rechallenge

FIGURE 5: Melanoma growth and survival of melanoma-bearing mice by CTI therapy using NPrCAP/M with and without AMF exposure. (a) Experimental protocols. (b) Tumor volumes of rechallenge melanoma transplants on day 13 of after transplantation. (c) Kaplan-Meier survival of melanoma-bearing mice after treatment following experimental protocols of Figure 5(a).

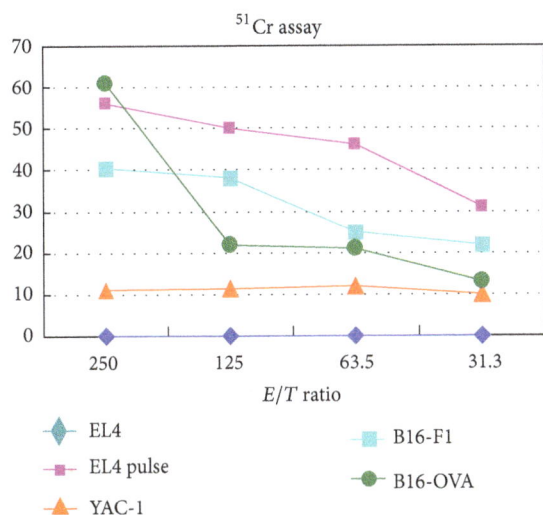

FIGURE 6: Hyperthermia of melanoma cells using B16OVA cells for induction of CTL in CTI therapy. Cytotoxic activity of spleen cells after CTI therapy against B16OVA cells, B16F1 cells, EL4 cells, EL4 cells pulsed with SL8 peptide (OVA-immunodominant peptide), or YAC-1 cells was determined by standard ^{51}Cr-release assay. B16OVA cells were subjected to hyperthermia using NPrCAP/M with AMF exposure *in vitro*.

4.2. T-Cell Receptor Repertoires of Tumor-Infiltrating Lymphocytes by Conjugates of NPrCAP and Magnetite Nanoparticles with Heat Exposure (Hyperthermia). It is clear now from our previous studies [22, 41] that conjugates of NPrCAP/magnetite nanoparticles (NPrCAP/M) with heat treatment (hyperthermia) can successfully induce the growth inhibition of primary and secondary melanoma transplants. It is also found that NPrCAP/M with hyperthermia elicited the response of cytotoxic T lymphocyte (CTL) via the release of HSP-peptide complex from degraded tumor cells [43] (Figure 6). In addition, CD8$^+$ T cells were observed within B16 melanoma nodules after hyperthermia using NPrCAP/M [37]. TIL reactivity to antigen is mediated via T-cell receptors (TCRs) consisting of α and β chains. We studied the TCR repertoire after hyperthermia using NPrCAP/M in order to further understand the T-cell response to melanoma after hyperthermia using NPrCAP/M [45]. We found that TCR repertoire was restricted in TILs, and the expansion of Vβ11$^+$ T cells was preferentially found. DNA sequences of the third complementarity determining regions were identified. This approach is based on subcutaneous melanoma transplantation in the hind foot pad, which confines the DLN to the inguinal and popliteal lymph nodes. Melanoma growth was significantly suppressed by the treatment of NPrCAP/M-mediated hyperthermia. CD8$^+$ T cells were observed substantially around the tumor and slightly within the tumor, while few and no CD8$^+$ T cells were observed around and within the tumor of nontreated mice.

In addition, significant enlargement of inguinal DLNs was observed in all of tumor-bearing mice including nontreated mice and NPrCAP/M-injected mice. The number of

CD8$^+$ T cells in inguinal DLNs increased significantly in the mice treated with NPrCAP/M-mediated hyperthermia.

5. Melanocytotoxic and Immunogenic Properties of NPrCAP without Hyperthermia

5.1. Induction of Apoptosis, Reactive Oxygen Species (ROS), and Tumor-Specific Immune Response by NPrCAP Administration Alone. In our animal study, those animals bearing B16F1 and B16F10 melanoma cells showed, to certain degree, rejection of second re-challenge melanoma transplantation by administration of both NPrCAP alone and NPrCAP/M minus AMF exposure [46]. Our working hypothesis for this finding is that there is a difference in the cytotoxic mechanism and immunogenic property of NPrCAP/M between experimental groups with and without hyperthermia by AMF exposure. The animals with NPrCAP/M without AMF exposure resulted in non-necrotic, apoptotic cell death. The animals with NPrCAP/M plus AMF exposure, on the other hand, resulted in nonapoptotic, necrotic cell death with immune complex production of melanoma peptide as well as Hsp70 and a small amount of Hsp 90.

To further examine the mechanism of the cell death induced by NPrCAP, those cells treated with NPrCAP alone were subjected to flow cytometric analysis, caspase 3 assay, and TUNEL staining [46]. The sub-G1 fraction was increased in the NPrCAP-treated B16F1 cells, comparable to TRAIL-exposed B16F1, but not in the NPrCAP-treated non-melanoma cells (NIH3T3, RMA) or nonpigmented melanoma cells (TXM18) (Figure 7). The luminescent assay detected caspase 3/7 activity in the NPrCAP-treated B16F1 cells remarkably increased (35.8-fold) compared to that in the nontreated cells. NIH3T3, RMA, and TXM18 cells treated with TRAIL showed 10.6-, 7.1-, and 5.8-fold increases of caspase 3/7 activation compared to the control, respectively, whereas those with NPr-4-S-CAP showed increases of 4.1-, 1.4-, and 1.8-fold, respectively. The number of TUNEL-positive cells was significantly increased only in the B16F1 tumor treated with NPrCAP. This increase was not observed in the B16F1 tumor without NPrCAP or in the RMA tumors with or without NPrCAP. The findings indicate that NPrCAP induces apoptotic cell death selectively in melanoma cells.

5.2. Melanocytotoxic and Immunogenic Properties of NPrCAP Compared to Monobenzyl Ether Hydroquinone. Monobenzyl ether of hydroquinone has long been known to produce the skin depigmentation at both the drug-applied area by direct chemical reaction with tyrosinase and the non-applied distant area by immune reaction with still unknown mechanism [43, 48–50]. The melanogenesis-related cytotoxicity primarily derives from tyrosinase-mediated formation of dopaquinone and other quinone intermediates, which produce ROSs such as superoxide and H_2O_2 [4, 31, 32, 51]. This unique biological property of melanin intermediates not only causes cell death, but also may produce immunogenic properties. We postulated that the cytotoxic action of NPrCAP appears to involve two major biological processes. One is

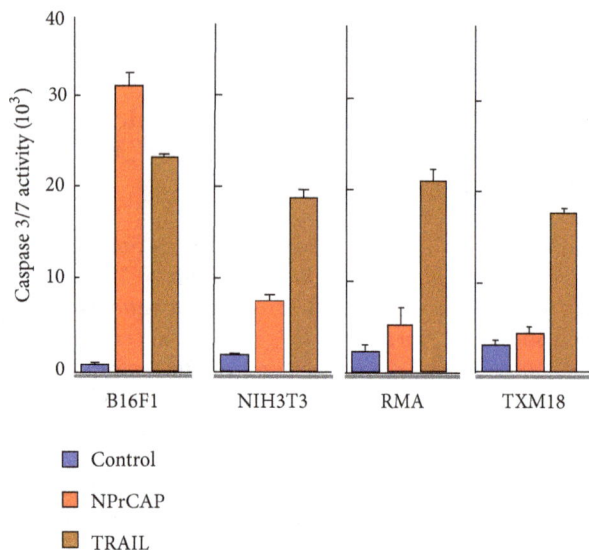

FIGURE 7: NPrCAP-mediated apoptotic cell death of B16F1 melanoma cells. Assay of caspase 3/7 in cells treated with NPrCAP or TRAIL. Cells were cultured in the presence of NPrCAP, TRAIL, or propylene glycol in 96-well plates and then processed for measurement of caspases 3 and 7 using a Caspase-Glo3/7 assay kit. From Ishii-Osai et al. [46].

cytostatic process which derives from the DNA synthesis inhibition through the interaction of quinone and free radicals with SH enzymes and thymidine synthase. Another is the cytocidal process by damage of DNA and mitochondrial ATP through oxidative stress and interaction with SH-enzyme [10]. They bind protein disulphide isomerase [52].

Monobenzyl ether form of hydroquinone was shown to produce a reactive *ortho*-quinone generated by tyrosinase-catalyzed oxidation and self-coupling and thiol conjugation reactions [53]. It was also shown to induce cell death without activating the caspase cascade or DNA fragmentation, indicating that the death pathway is non-apoptotic [53, 54]. It was further suggested that monobenzyl ether hydroquinone induced the immunogenicity to melanocytes and melanoma cells by forming quinone-haptens to tyrosinase protein and by inducing the release of tyrosinase and melanoma antigen recognized by T cells-1 (MART-1) containing CD63+ exosomes following melanosome oxidative stress induction. The drug further augmented the processing and shedding of melanocyte differentiation antigens by inducing melanosome autophagy and enhanced tyrosinase ubiquitination, ultimately activating dendritic cells, which induced cytotoxic melanoma-reactive cells. These T cells eradicated melanoma *in vivo* [54, 55].

5.3. Development of Vitiligo during Melanoma Immunotherapy and Activation of NPrCAP by Tyrosinase to Form Possible Antigen Peptides.
Advanced melanoma patients and melanoma patients treated by vaccine immunotherapy often reveal vitiligo-like changes of the skin. Interestingly, this vitiligo development is associated with a superior prognosis in melanoma patients [56]. Although there have been

several separate theories for the pathogenesis of vitiligo, the haptenation theory has recently been put forth to explain the molecular mechanism of monobenzone-induced skin depigmentation [54, 57, 58]. Westerhof et al. proposed the haptenation theory in which increased intracellular H_2O_2 could trigger the increased turnover of elevated levels of surrogate substrates of tyrosinase, resulting in melanocyte-specific T-cell responses [57, 59]. According to this hypothesis, tyrosinase could be recognized as a melanoma-specific tumor antigen in relation to the systemic immune responses.

Phenolic substrates as prohaptens are oxidized by tyrosinase to produce *ortho*-quinones, which act as haptens that covalently bind to tyrosinase or other melanosomal proteins to generate possible neoantigens [44, 53, 54]. These neo-antigens, in turn, trigger an immunological response cascade that results in a melanocyte-specific delayed-type hypersensitivity reaction leading to melanocyte elimination to produce depigmentation in vitiligo and melanoma rejection. We examined the tyrosinase-mediated oxidation of NPrCAP and its subsequent binding to sulfhydryl compounds (thiols) in NPrCAP-treated melanoma tissues and demonstrated that NPrCAP is oxidized by tyrosinase to form a highly reactive *ortho*-quinone, (N-propionyl-4-S-cysteaminylcatechol, NPrCAQ; Figure 8), which then binds covalently to biologically relevant thiols including proteins through the cysteine residues. *In vitro* and *in vivo* studies were also conducted to prove the binding of the quinone-hapten NPrCAQ to proteins. The thiol adducts were analyzed after acid hydrolysis as 5-S-cysteaminyl-3-S-cysteinylcatechol (CA-CysC) (Figure 8). Our results specifically provided evidence that NPrCAP is oxidized by tyrosinase to an *ortho*-quinone, NPrCAQ, which is highly reactive yet stable enough to survive and then interact with biologically relevant thiols to form covalent adducts. The activation of NPrCAP to NPrCAQ by tyrosinase and the subsequent binding to proteins through cysteine residues were also demonstrated in the *in vitro* and *in vivo* experiments. Our finding was the first demonstration that the quinone-protein adduct formation actually takes place in melanoma cells and melanoma tissues through the tyrosinase-mediated mechanism. Furthermore, 60–80% of the NPrCAQ-thiol adducts were found in the protein fraction in melanoma cells and in the tumors. This is surprising when we consider the much lower reactivity of protein sulfhydryl groups compared with those in small thiols such as cysteine [60, 61]. The remaining nonprotein SH adducts were produced by the reaction of NPrCAQ with free cysteine or glutathione as a detoxifying mechanism. In this connection, it was previously shown that the depletion of glutathione augmented the melanocytotoxicity and antimelanoma effects of NAcCAP [62].

According to the potent melanoma immunotherapy theory using monobenzone [54, 55, 57–59], tyrosinase appears to trigger melanoma regression. Tyrosinase oxidation of monobenzone produces a highly reactive quinone-hapten [44, 54] and ROS concurrently [54]. The quinone-hapten binds to cysteine residues in tyrosinase or other melanosomal proteins thereby generating possible neoantigen, which activate hapten-reactive CD8+ T-cells. The latter cells kill monobenzone-exposed melanocytes expressing haptenated

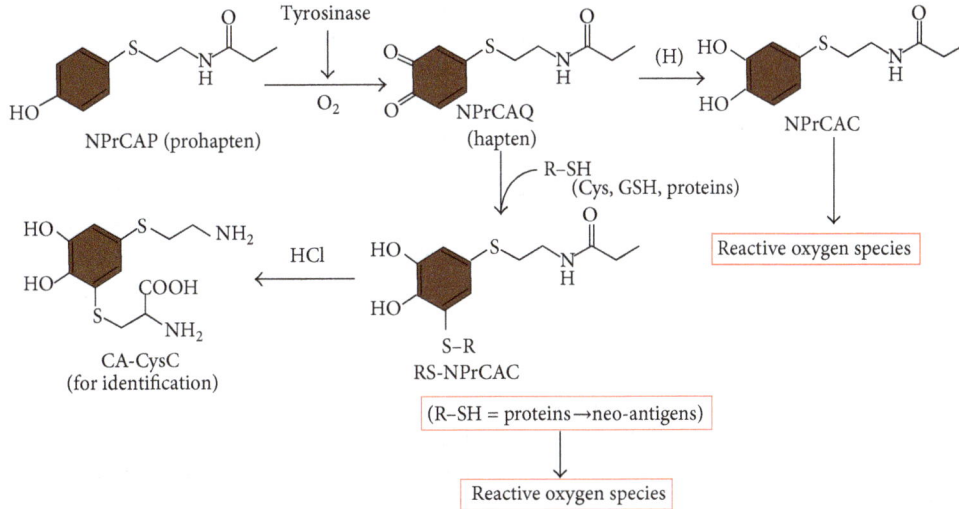

Figure 8: Tyrosinase activation of NPrCAP (prohapten) and binding of the quinone-hapten NPrCAQ with proteins thorough cysteine residues. Oxidation of NPrCAP with tyrosinase produces the quinone NPrCAQ, which is reduced to the catechol NPrCAC or binds to thiols (cysteine, glutathione, melanosomal proteins). The production of NPrCAQ-thiol adducts can be confirmed by the detection of CA-CysC after acid hydrolysis. NAcCys-NPrCAC is produced by the addition reaction of NAcCys (R-SH) with NPrCAQ. From Ito et al. [47].

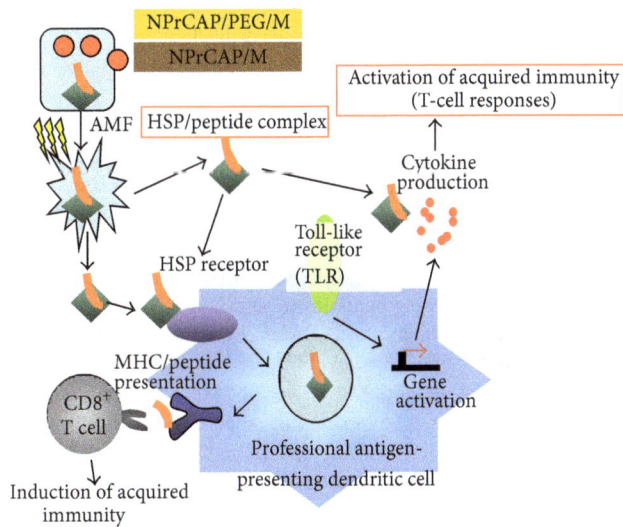

Figure 9: Scheme of intracellular hyperthermia using NPrCAP /PEG/M or NPrCAP/M with AMF exposure. NPrCAP/PEG/M nanoparticles are selectively incorporated in melanoma cells. Intracellular hyperthermia can induce necrotic cell death, and adjacent live melanoma cells suffer heat shock, resulting in increased level of intracellular HSP-peptide complexes. Repeated hyperthermia turns heat-shocked cells to necrotic cells, leading to the release of HSP-peptide complexes into extracellular milieu. The released HSPs-peptide complexes are taken up by dendritic cells (DCs). Then, DCs migrate into regional lymph nodes and cross-present HSP chaperoned antigenic peptides to CD8+ T cells in the context of MHC class I molecules, thereby inducing antimelanoma cytotoxic CD8+ T cells.

antigens on their surface, further liberating melanocyte antigens for presentation by dendritic cells. Finally, the antigen-specific T-cell response is induced and propagated [54, 57–59]. The ROS generated also causes damage to melanosomes

leading to the presentation of melanosome-derived antigens and the induction of antigen-specific T-cell responses [58].

These immunological events can also be expected to occur for our NPrCAP because the involvement of CD8+ T cells and the production of ROS in NPrCAP-treated melanoma cells were demonstrated in our previous study [46]. We expect the production of NPrCAC through redox exchange in melanoma cells and the subsequent production of ROS from the catechol because the closely related catechol, 4-S-cysteaminylcatechol, was shown to produce superoxide radicals (which are rapidly converted to hydrogen peroxide) [63]. The thiol adduct RS-NPrCAC, as a catechol, may also contribute to the production of ROS.

6. Summary and Conclusion

Several clinical trials using melanoma peptides or an antibody that blocks cytotoxic T-lymphocyte-associated antigen on lymphocytes have been shown to improve overall melanoma survival [64–66]. Promising oncogene-targeted melanoma therapy has also been successfully introduced recently [67].

Our study may however indicate that exploitation of a specific biological property to cancer cells can be another approach for developing novel melanoma-targeted drugs which can also trigger the production of melanoma-targeted in situ vaccine. Our approach using melanogenesis substrate and magnetite nanoparticles is based upon the expectation of (i) direct killing of melanoma cells by chemotherapeutic and thermo-therapeutic effect of melanogenesis-targeted drug (NPrCAP/M) and (ii) indirect killing by immune reaction (in situ peptide vaccine) after exposure to AMF. It is hoped from these rationales that a tumor-specific DDS is developed by NPrCAP, and selective cell death can be achieved by exposure of conjugates of NPrCAP/M nanoparticles to AMF. Hyperthermia increases the expression of intracellular HSPs which is important in and necessary for the induction of antitumor immunity [41, 68]. Overexpression of HSPs increases tumor immunogenicity by augmenting the chaperoning ability of antigenic peptides and presentation of antigenic peptides in MHC class I molecules [39, 69]. In this process professional antigen-presenting dendritic cells play unique and important roles in taking up, processing, and presenting exogenous antigens in association with MHC class I molecules. Our study indicated that combination of melanogenesis substrate, NPrCAP, and local magnetite nanoparticles with hyperthermia could induce *in situ* a form of vaccine against tumor cells and may be effective not only for primary melanoma but also for distant secondary metastases (Figure 9).

Interestingly we found that NPrCAP by itself has potent chemotherapeutic and immune-adjuvant effects. It was demonstrated that the phenol NPrCAP, as a prohapten, can be activated in melanoma cells by tyrosinase to the reactive quinone-hapten NPrCAQ which binds to melanosomal proteins through their cysteine residues to form possible neo-antigens, thus triggering the immunological response (Figure 8).

Abbreviations

AMF:	Alternating magnetic field
BSA:	Bovine serum albumin
BSO:	Buthionine sulfoximide
CA-CysC:	5-*S*-cysteaminyl-3-*S*-cysteinylcatechol
CAP:	Cysteaminylphenol
CDR3:	Third complementarity determining region
CML:	Cationic magneto-liposome
CTI therapy:	Chemothermoimmunotherapy
CTL:	Cytotoxic T lymphocyte
DCs:	Dendritic cells
DDS:	Drug delivery system
DLNs:	Draining lymph nodes
HSP/Hsp:	Heat shock protein
IL:	Interleukin
M:	Magnetite nanoparticle
mAb:	Monoclonal antibody
MART-1:	Melanoma antigen recognized by T cells-1
MCLs:	Magnetite cationic liposomes
MC1R:	Melanocortin 1 receptor
MHC:	Major histocompatibility complex
MITF:	Microphthalmia transcription factor
ML:	Noncationic magnetoliposome
MSH:	Melanocyte stimulating hormone
NAcCAP:	N-acetyl-4-S cysteaminylphenol
NDLN:	Nondraining lymph node
NPrCAC:	N-propionyl-4-S cysteaminylcatechol
NPrCAP:	N-propionyl-4-S cysteaminylphenol
NPrCAQ:	N-propionyl-4-S-cysteaminylquinine
Nrf2:	NF-E2-related factor 2
OVA:	Ovu-albumin
PEG:	Polyethylene glycol
ROS:	Reactive oxygen species
RT-PCR:	Reverse transcription polymerase chain reaction

TILs:	Tumor-infiltrating lymphocytes
TCRs:	T-cell receptors
TRP-2:	Tyrosinase-related protein-2.

Acknowledgments

This work was supported by a Health and Labor Sciences Research Grant-in-Aid for Research on Advanced Medical Technology from the Ministry of Health, Labor, and Welfare of Japan. The authors express their sincere appreciation to Mr. Noboru Minowa, Toray Industries, Inc., Tokyo, Japan, and Drs. Akiko Sato, Makito Sato, Tomoaki Takada, and Ichiro Ono, Sapporo Medical University, Sapporo, Japan, who have supported to carry out basic experiments and clinical trials of this study. The authors also express thier sincere appreciation to Ms. Makiko Jizou and Ms. Ikuko Ichimura for their secretarial help.

References

[1] E. de Vries, L. V. van de Poll-Franse, W. J. Louwman, F. R. de Gruijl, and J. W. W. Coebergh, "Predictions of skin cancer incidence in the Netherlands up to 2015," *The British Journal of Dermatology*, vol. 152, no. 3, pp. 481–488, 2005.

[2] C. M. Balch, J. E. Gershenwald, S. J. Soong et al., "Final version of 2009 AJCC melanoma staging and classification," *Journal of Clinical Oncology*, vol. 27, no. 36, pp. 6199–6206, 2009.

[3] C. M. Balch, A. C. Buzaid, S. J. Soong et al., "Final version of the American joint committee on cancer staging system for cutaneous melanoma," *Journal of Clinical Oncology*, vol. 19, no. 16, pp. 3635–3648, 2001.

[4] K. Reszka and K. Jimbow, "Electron donor and acceptor properties of melanin pigments in the skin," in *Oxidative Stress in Dermatology*, J. Fuchs and L. Packer, Eds., pp. 287–320, Marcel Dekker, New York, NY, USA, 1993.

[5] K. Jimbow, T. Iwashina, F. Alena, K. Yamada, J. Pankovich, and T. Umemura, "Exploitation of pigment biosynthesis pathway as a selective chemotherapeutic approach for malignant melanoma," *Journal of Investigative Dermatology*, vol. 100, no. 2, pp. s231–s238, 1993.

[6] F. Alena, T. Iwashina, A. Gili, and K. Jimbow, "Selective *in vivo* accumulation of N-acetyl-4-S-cysteaminylphenol in B16F10 murine melanoma and enhancement of its *in vitro* and *in vivo* antimelanoma effect by combination of buthionine sulfoximine," *Cancer Research*, vol. 54, no. 10, pp. 2661–2666, 1994.

[7] J. M. Pankovich and K. Jimbow, "Tyrosine transport in a human melanoma cell line as a basis for selective transport of cytotoxic analogues," *Biochemical Journal*, vol. 280, no. 3, pp. 721–725, 1991.

[8] M. Tandon, P. D. Thomas, M. Shokravi et al., "Synthesis and antitumour effect of the melanogenesis-based antimelanoma agent N-Propionyl-4-S-cysteaminylphenol," *Biochemical Pharmacology*, vol. 55, no. 12, pp. 2023–2029, 1998.

[9] A. Gili, P. D. Thomas, M. Ota, and K. Jimbow, "Comparison of *in vitro* cytotoxicity of N-acetyl and N-propionyl derivatives of phenolic thioether amines in melanoma and neuroblastoma cells and the relationship to tyrosinase and tyrosine hydroxylase enzyme activity," *Melanoma Research*, vol. 10, no. 1, pp. 9–15, 2000.

[10] P. D. Thomas, H. Kishi, H. Cao et al., "Selective incorporation and specific cytocidal effect as the cellular basis for the antimelanoma action of sulphur containing tyrosine analogs," *Journal of Investigative Dermatology*, vol. 113, no. 6, pp. 928–934, 1999.

[11] A. Ito, M. Shinkai, H. Honda, and T. Kobayashi, "Medical application of functionalized magnetic nanoparticles," *Journal of Bioscience and Bioengineering*, vol. 100, no. 1, pp. 1–11, 2005.

[12] N. Kawai, A. Ito, Y. Nakahara et al., "Anticancer effect of hyperthermia on prostate cancer mediated by magnetite cationic liposomes and immune-response induction in transplanted syngeneic rats," *Prostate*, vol. 64, no. 4, pp. 373–381, 2005.

[13] M. Shinkai, M. Yanase, H. Honda, T. Wakabayashi, J. Yoshida, and T. Kobayashi, "Intracellular hyperthermia for cancer using magnetite cationic liposomes: *in vitro* study," *Japanese Journal of Cancer Research*, vol. 87, no. 11, pp. 1179–1183, 1996.

[14] A. Ménoret and R. Chandawarkar, "Heat-shock protein-based anticancer immunotherapy: an idea whose time has come," *Seminars in Oncology*, vol. 25, no. 6, pp. 654–660, 1998.

[15] P. K. Srivastava, A. Ménoret, S. Basu, R. Binder, and K. Quade, "Heat shock proteins come of age: primitive functions acquired new roles in an adaptive world," *Immunity*, vol. 8, no. 6, pp. 657–665, 1998.

[16] Y. Tamura, N. Tsuboi, N. Sato, and K. Kikuchi, "70 kDa heat shock cognate protein is a transformation-associated antigen and a possible target for the host's anti-tumor immunity," *Journal of Immunology*, vol. 151, no. 10, pp. 5516–5524, 1993.

[17] Y. Tamura, P. Peng, K. Liu, M. Daou, and P. K. Srivastava, "Immunotherapy of tumors with autologous tumor-derived heat shock protein preparations," *Science*, vol. 278, no. 5335, pp. 117–120, 1997.

[18] Y. Tamura and N. Sato, "Heat shock proteins: chaperoning of innate and adaptive immunities," *Japanese Journal of Hyperthermic Oncology*, vol. 19, pp. 131–139, 2003.

[19] P. K. Srivastava, "Immunotherapy for human cancer using heat shock protein-peptide complexes," *Current Oncology Reports*, vol. 7, no. 2, pp. 104–108, 2005.

[20] Y. Tamura, S. Takashima, J. M. Cho et al., "Inhibition of natural killer cell cytotoxicity by cell growth-related molecules," *Japanese Journal of Cancer Research*, vol. 87, no. 6, pp. 623–630, 1996.

[21] G. Ueda, Y. Tamura, I. Hirai et al., "Tumor-derived heat shock protein 70-pulsed dendritic cells elicit-tumor-specific cytotoxic T lymphocytes (CTLs) and tumor immunity," *Cancer Science*, vol. 95, no. 3, pp. 248–253, 2004.

[22] A. Ito, H. Honda, and T. Kobayashi, "Cancer immunotherapy based on intracellular hyperthermia using magnetite nanoparticles: a novel concept of "heat-controlled necrosis" with heat shock protein expression," *Cancer Immunology, Immunotherapy*, vol. 55, no. 3, pp. 320–328, 2006.

[23] H. Shi, T. Cao, J. E. Connolly et al., "Hyperthermia enhances CTL cross-priming," *Journal of Immunology*, vol. 176, no. 4, pp. 2134–2141, 2006.

[24] J. Dakour, T. Vinayagamoorthy, K. Jimbow et al., "Identification of a cDNA coding for a Ca^{2+}-binding phosphoprotein (p90) calnexin, on melanosomes in normal and malignant human melanocytes," *Experimental Cell Research*, vol. 209, no. 2, pp. 288–300, 1993.

[25] K. Toyofuku, I. Wada, K. Hirosaki, J. S. Park, Y. Hori, and K. Jimbow, "Promotion of tyrosinase folding in Cos 7 cells by calnexin," *Journal of Biochemistry*, vol. 125, no. 1, pp. 82–89, 1999.

[26] K. Jimbow, P. F. Gomez, K. Toyofuku et al., "Biological role of tyrosinase related protein and its biosynthesis and transport from TGN to stage I melanosome, late endosome, through gene transfection study," *Pigment Cell Research*, vol. 10, no. 4, pp. 206–213, 1997.

[27] K. Jimbow, J. S. Park, F. Kato et al., "Assembly, target-signaling and intracellular transport of tyrosinase gene family proteins in the initial stage of melanosome biogenesis," *Pigment Cell Research*, vol. 13, no. 4, pp. 222–229, 2000.

[28] K. Jimbow, C. Hua, P. F. Gomez et al., "Intracellular vesicular trafficking of tyrosinase gene family protein in Eu- and pheomelanosome biogenesis," *Pigment Cell Research*, vol. 13, no. 8, pp. 110–117, 2000.

[29] T. Miura, K. Jimbow, and S. Ito, "The *in vivo* antimelanoma effect of 4-S-cysteaminylphenol and its N-acetyl derivative," *International Journal of Cancer*, vol. 46, no. 5, pp. 931–934, 1990.

[30] S. Ito, T. Kato, K. Ishikawa, T. Kasuga, and K. Jimbow, "Mechanism of selective toxicity of 4-S-cysteinylphenol and 4-S-cysteaminylphenol to melanocytes," *Biochemical Pharmacology*, vol. 36, no. 12, pp. 2007–2011, 1987.

[31] Y. Minamitsuji, K. Toyofuku, S. Sugiyama, K. Yamada, and K. Jimbow, "Sulfur containing tyrosine analogs can cause selective melanocytotoxicity involving tyrosinase-mediated apoptosis," *Journal of Investigative Dermatology Symposium Proceedings*, vol. 4, no. 2, pp. 130–136, 1999.

[32] K. Jimbow, Y. Miyake, K. Homma et al., "Characterization of melanogenesis and morphogenesis of melanosomes by physico-chemical properties of melanin and melanosomes in malignant melanoma," *Cancer Research*, vol. 44, no. 3, pp. 1128–1134, 1984.

[33] B. Thiesen and A. Jordan, "Clinical applications of magnetic nanoparticles for hyperthermia," *International Journal of Hyperthermia*, vol. 24, no. 6, pp. 467–474, 2008.

[34] M. Johannsen, U. Gneveckow, L. Eckelt et al., "Clinical hyperthermia of prostate cancer using magnetic nanoparticles: presentation of a new interstitial technique," *International Journal of Hyperthermia*, vol. 21, no. 7, pp. 637–647, 2005.

[35] A. Ito, M. Fujioka, T. Yoshida et al., "4-S-Cysteaminylphenol-loaded magnetite cationic liposomes for combination therapy of hyperthermia with chemotherapy against malignant melanoma," *Cancer Science*, vol. 98, no. 3, pp. 424–430, 2007.

[36] M. Sato, T. Yamashita, M. Ohkura et al., "N-propionyl-cysteaminylphenol-magnetite conjugate (NPrCAP/M) Is a nanoparticle for the targeted growth suppression of melanoma cells," *Journal of Investigative Dermatology*, vol. 129, no. 9, pp. 2233–2241, 2009.

[37] T. Takada, T. Yamashita, M. Sato et al., "Growth inhibition of re-challenge B16 melanoma transplant by conjugates of melanogenesis substrate and magnetite nanoparticles as the basis for developing melanoma-targeted chemo-thermo-immunotherapy," *Journal of Biomedicine and Biotechnology*, vol. 2009, Article ID 457936, 13 pages, 2009.

[38] M. Suzuki, M. Shinkai, H. Honda, and T. Kobayashi, "Anticancer effect and immune induction by hyperthermia of malignant melanoma using magnetite cationic liposomes," *Melanoma Research*, vol. 13, no. 2, pp. 129–135, 2003.

[39] M. Yanase, M. Shinkai, H. Honda, T. Wakabayashi, J. Yoshida, and T. Kobayashi, "Intracellular hyperthermia for cancer using magnetite cationic liposomes: an *in vivo* study," *Japanese Journal of Cancer Research*, vol. 89, no. 4, pp. 463–469, 1998.

[40] R. Hergt, S. Dutz, R. Müller, and M. Zeisberger, "Magnetic particle hyperthermia: nanoparticle magnetism and materials

development for cancer therapy," *Journal of Physics Condensed Matter*, vol. 18, no. 38, pp. S2919–S2934, 2006.

[41] A. Ito, M. Shinkai, H. Honda et al., "Heat shock protein 70 expression induces antitumor immunity during intracellular hyperthermia using magnetite nanoparticles," *Cancer Immunology, Immunotherapy*, vol. 52, no. 2, pp. 80–88, 2003.

[42] A. Ito, F. Matsuoka, H. Honda, and T. Kobayashi, "Antitumor effects of combined therapy of recombinant heat shock protein 70 and hyperthermia using magnetic nanoparticles in an experimental subcutaneous murine melanoma," *Cancer Immunology, Immunotherapy*, vol. 53, no. 1, pp. 26–32, 2004.

[43] A. Sato, Y. Tamura, N. Sato et al., "Melanoma-targeted chemo-thermo-immuno (CTI)-therapy using N-propionyl-4-S-cysteaminylphenol-magnetite nanoparticles elicits CTL response via heat shock protein-peptide complex release," *Cancer Science*, vol. 101, no. 9, pp. 1939–1946, 2010.

[44] P. Manini, A. Napolitano, W. Westerhof, P. A. Riley, and M. D'Ischia, "A reactive ortho-quinone generated by tyrosinase-catalyzed oxidation of the skin depigmenting agent monobenzone: self-coupling and thiol-conjugation reactions and possible implications for melanocyte toxicity," *Chemical Research in Toxicology*, vol. 22, no. 8, pp. 1398–1405, 2009.

[45] A. Ito, M. Yamaguchi, N. Okamoto et al., "T-cell receptor repertoires of tumor-infiltrating lymphocytes after hyperthermia using functionalized magnetite nanoparticles," *Nanomedicine*, 2012.

[46] Y. Ishii-Osai, T. Yamashita, Y. Tamura et al., "N-Propionyl-4-S-cysteaminylphenol induces apoptosis in B16F1 cells and mediates tumor-specific T-cell immune responses in a mouse melanoma model," *Journal of Dermatological Science*, vol. 67, no. 1, pp. 51–60, 2012.

[47] S. Ito, A. Nishigaki, Y. Ishii-Osai et al., "Mechanism of putative neo-antigen formation from N-propionyl-4-S-cysteaminylphenol, a tyrosinase substrate, in melanoma models," *Biochemical Pharmacology*, vol. 84, no. 5, pp. 646–653, 2012.

[48] K. Jimbow, H. Obata, M. A. Pathak, and T. B. Fitzpatrick, "Mechanism of depigmentation by hydroquinone," *Journal of Investigative Dermatology*, vol. 62, no. 4, pp. 436–449, 1974.

[49] J. J. Nordlund, B. Forget, J. Kirkwood, and A. B. Lerner, "Dermatitis produced by applications of monobenzone in patients with active vitiligo," *Archives of Dermatology*, vol. 121, no. 9, pp. 1141–1144, 1985.

[50] R. E. Boissy and P. Manga, "On the etiology of contact/occupational vitiligo," *Pigment Cell Research*, vol. 17, no. 3, pp. 208–214, 2004.

[51] C. J. Cooksey, K. Jimbow, E. J. Land, and P. A. Riley, "Reactivity of orthoquinones involved in tyrosinase-dependent cytotoxicity: differences between alkylthio- and alkoxy-substituents," *Melanoma Research*, vol. 2, no. 5-6, pp. 283–293, 1993.

[52] P. G. Parsons, D. Favier, M. McEwan, H. Takahashi, K. Jimbow, and S. Ito, "Action of cysteaminylphenols on human melanoma cells *in vivo* and *in vitro*: 4-S-cysteaminylphenol binds protein disulphide isomerase," *Melanoma research*, vol. 1, no. 2, pp. 97–104, 1991.

[53] V. Hariharan, J. Klarquist, M. J. Reust et al., "Monobenzyl ether of hydroquinone and 4-tertiary butyl phenol activate markedly different physiological responses in melanocytes: relevance to skin depigmentation," *Journal of Investigative Dermatology*, vol. 130, no. 1, pp. 211–220, 2010.

[54] J. G. van den Boorn, D. I. Picavet, P. F. van Swieten et al., "Skin-depigmenting agent monobenzone induces potent T-cell autoimmunity toward pigmented cells by tyrosinase haptenation and melanosome autophagy," *Journal of Investigative Dermatology*, vol. 131, no. 6, pp. 1240–1251, 2011.

[55] J. G. van den Boorn, D. Konijnenberg, E. P. Tjin et al., "Effective melanoma immunotherapy in mice by the skin-depigmenting agent monobenzone and the adjuvants imiquimod and CpG," *PloS ONE*, vol. 5, no. 5, Article ID e10626, 2010.

[56] P. Quaglino, F. Marenco, S. Osella-Abate et al., "Vitiligo is an independent favourable prognostic factor in stage III and IV metastatic melanoma patients: results from a single-institution hospital-based observational cohort study," *Annals of Oncology*, vol. 21, no. 2, pp. 409–414, 2010.

[57] W. Westerhof, P. Manini, A. Napolitano, and M. d'Ischia, "The haptenation theory of vitiligo and melanoma rejection: a close-up," *Experimental Dermatology*, vol. 20, no. 2, pp. 92–96, 2011.

[58] J. G. van den Boorn, C. J. Melief, and R. M. Luiten, "Monobenzone-induced depigmentation: from enzymatic blockage to autoimmunity," *Pigment Cell and Melanoma Research*, vol. 24, no. 4, pp. 673–679, 2011.

[59] W. Westerhof and M. D'Ischia, "Vitiligo puzzle: the pieces fall in place," *Pigment Cell Research*, vol. 20, no. 5, pp. 345–359, 2007.

[60] T. Kato, S. Ito, and K. Fujita, "Tyrosinase-catalyzed binding of 3,4-dihydroxyphenylalanine with proteins through the sulfhydryl group," *Biochimica et Biophysica Acta*, vol. 881, no. 3, pp. 415–421, 1986.

[61] S. Ito, T. Kato, and K. Fujita, "Covalent binding of catechols to proteins through the sulphydryl group," *Biochemical Pharmacology*, vol. 37, no. 9, pp. 1707–1710, 1988.

[62] F. Alena, K. Jimbow, and S. Ito, "Melanocytotoxicity and antimelanoma effects of phenolic amine compounds in mice *in vivo*," *Cancer Research*, vol. 50, no. 12, pp. 3743–3747, 1990.

[63] K. Hasegawa, S. Ito, S. Inoue, K. Wakamatsu, H. Ozeki, and I. Ishiguro, "Dihydro-1,4-benzothiazine-6,7-dione, the ultimate toxic metabolite of 4-S-cysteaminylphenol and 4-S-cysteaminylcatechol," *Biochemical Pharmacology*, vol. 53, no. 10, pp. 1435–1444, 1997.

[64] F. S. Hodi, S. J. O'Day, D. F. McDermott et al., "Improved survival with ipilimumab in patients with metastatic melanoma," *The New England Journal of Medicine*, vol. 363, no. 8, pp. 711–723, 2010.

[65] D. J. Schwartzentruber, D. H. Lawson, J. M. Richards et al., "gp100 peptide vaccine and interleukin-2 in patients with advanced melanoma," *The New England Journal of Medicine*, vol. 364, no. 22, pp. 2119–2127, 2011.

[66] C. Robert, L. Thomas, I. Bondarenko et al., "Ipilimumab plus dacarbazine for previously untreated metastatic melanoma," *The New England Journal of Medicine*, vol. 364, pp. 2517–2526, 2011.

[67] P. B. Chapman, A. Hauschild, C. Robert et al., "Improved survival with vemurafenib in melanoma with BRAF V600E mutation," *The New England Journal of Medicine*, vol. 364, no. 26, pp. 2507–2516, 2011.

[68] K. Mise, N. Kan, T. Okino et al., "Effect of heat treatment on tumor cells and antitumor effector cells," *Cancer Research*, vol. 50, no. 19, pp. 6199–6202, 1990.

[69] A. Ito, F. Matsuoka, H. Honda, and T. Kobayashi, "Heat shock protein 70 gene therapy combined with hyperthermia using magnetic nanoparticles," *Cancer Gene Therapy*, vol. 10, no. 12, pp. 918–925, 2003.

15

A Clinicopathological and Immunohistochemical Correlation in Cutaneous Metastases from Internal Malignancies: A Five-Year Study

Sarita Nibhoria,[1] Kanwardeep Kaur Tiwana,[1] Manmeet Kaur,[1] and Sumir Kumar[2]

[1] *Department of Pathology, G.G.S. Medical College & Hospital BFUHS, Faridkot, Punjab 151203, India*
[2] *Department of Skin and VD, G.G.S. Medical College & Hospital BFUHS, Faridkot, Punjab 151203, India*

Correspondence should be addressed to Kanwardeep Kaur Tiwana; kanwardeepjhajj@gmail.com

Academic Editor: Günther Hofbauer

Cutaneous metastases from internal malignancies are uncommon and occur in 0.6%–10.4% of all patients with cancer. In most cases, cutaneous metastases develop after the initial diagnosis of the primary internal malignancy and late in the course of the disease. Skin tumors are infrequent in Asian population and cutaneous metastases are quite rare. Cutaneous metastases carry a poor prognosis with average survival of few months. In the present five-year study 1924 malignant tumors were screened which included only nine cases of cutaneous metastatic deposits. A wide range of site and clinical presentations including nodules, plaques, and ulcers was noted. Histopathological findings were significant and corresponded with the primary internal malignancy. Cutaneous metastases from breast carcinoma (44.4%) were the most common finding followed by non-Hodgkin lymphoma and renal cell carcinoma (22.2% each) and carcinoma cervix (11.1%). The aim of our study is to classify the cutaneous metastases and to evaluate their clinicopathologic and immunohistochemical correlation with the primary tumor.

1. Introduction

Cutaneous metastasis can be defined as the spread of a tumor from the site of its primary origin to the skin [1]. Skin metastasis may be the first sign of an advanced cancer or an indicator of cancer recurrence [2, 3]. Up to 9% of patients with cancer may develop skin metastases, while metastasis may develop more than 10 years after initial cancer diagnosis [3]. A wide morphologic spectrum of clinical appearances has been described in cutaneous metastases including nodules, plaques, papules, tumors, and ulcers [4]. While carcinomas are the most common type of cancer to metastasize, sarcomas, lymphomas, and leukemias also represent a substantial percentage of all skin metastases [5]. The relative frequencies of metastatic skin disease in each sex correlate with the frequency of different types of primary cancer. Thus women with the skin metastases have the following distribution in decreasing order of primary malignancies: breast, ovary, oral cavity, lung, and large intestine. In men, the distribution is as follows: lung, large intestine, oral cavity, kidney, breast, esophagus, pancreas, stomach, and liver [4]. Generally, cutaneous metastases herald a poor prognosis with average survival time of a few months.

2. Materials and Method

In the present five-year study, patients diagnosed with an internal malignancy including hematolymphoid neoplasms, registered between March 2009 and March 2014 in the Pathology Department, were consecutively screened. The H&E stained histopathological sections of skin biopsies received in the Pathology Department were reevaluated. The inclusion criteria were cases of cutaneous metastatic deposits with or without known primary malignant tumor. Cases with direct extension of primary malignancy into the overlying skin were excluded. Physical and dermatologic examination details were obtained from the patient files and histopathology requisition forms. The clinical presentation, site, and histopathological details, especially those suggesting the primary tumor site, were evaluated

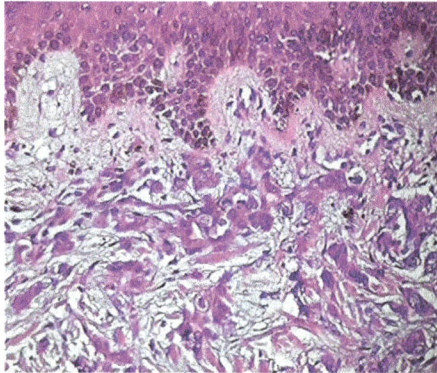

FIGURE 1: Sections show deposits of metastatic breast carcinoma (H&E ×100).

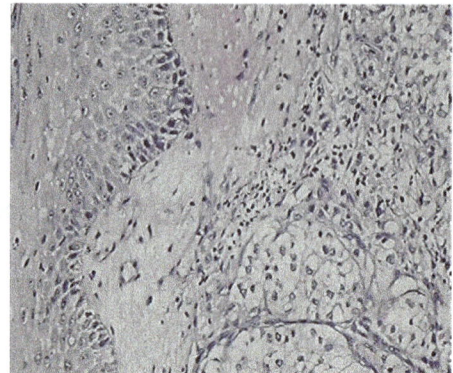

FIGURE 2: Sections show islands of clear tumour cells in dermis suggesting metastatic renal cell carcinoma (H&E ×100).

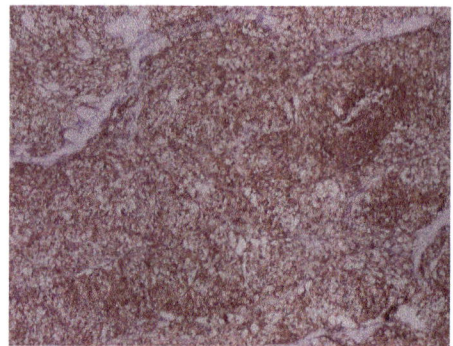

FIGURE 3: On IHC showing diffuse CD10 positivity confirming metastatic renal cell carcinoma (×40).

along with the secondary morphological changes in the skin tissue. Immunohistochemistry was performed on all except for one case of cutaneous metastases and correlation with the primary internal malignancy was done.

3. Results

In the present five-year study, a total of 1924 malignant tumors were screened which included nine cases of cutaneous metastatic deposits. The cutaneous metastases were seen more in females (5 out of 9 patients). The four male patients had skin metastases from renal cell carcinoma and from non-Hodgkin lymphoma (2 cases each). The age range was found to be 30–72 with mean age 60 years.

A wide range of clinical presentations and regional localizations was noted. Plaque and nodule were the most frequent clinical presentation (4 cases each out of 9) followed by ulcer (1 case out of 9). The size of the skin lesions varied from 0.25 cm to 5.0 cm.

The regional localization in cases of breast carcinoma included chest (2 cases), chest and abdomen (1 case), and face, scalp, and trunk (1 case). Both cases of renal cell carcinoma showed deposits on abdomen. A case of non-Hodgkin lymphoma showed widespread skin deposits on face, scalp, and trunk while another case showed localized deposits on abdomen only. A single case of carcinoma cervix showed skin deposits on thigh (Table 1).

The duration of time after which the cutaneous metastases developed was variable and ranged from 10 months to five years. In majority of the cases, patients had prior history of a primary internal malignancy.

The histopathologic examination revealed significant findings. The morphological patterns and microscopic appearances suggested the likely tissue of origin. In cases of cutaneous metastases from carcinoma breast, the histologic examination revealed invasion of dermis and subcutis by groups, cords, and nests of tumor cells. The tumor cells were large with large pleomorphic nuclei. Fibrosis was evident in one case only (Figure 1). ER/PR positivity was seen in 3 out of 4 cases of cutaneous metastases from carcinoma breast. The metastatic deposits which were negative for ER/PR had

previous reports of ER/PR negativity in the primary tumor too. The deposits of renal cell carcinoma showed presence of tumor cells in glandular configuration or in nests. The tumor cells showed oval nuclei with abundant, clear cytoplasm. IHC (CD-10) was applied and confirmed the diagnosis in both cases (Figures 2 and 3).

The deposits of non-Hodgkin lymphoma showed diffuse presence of atypical lymphoid cells in the dermis and subcutis. The atypical lymphoid cells showed finely stippled chromatin, inconspicuous nucleoli, and sparse cytoplasm. There was no evidence of epidermotropism which ruled out the possibility of primary cutaneous lymphoma. Leucocyte common antigen (CD 45) was positive in both of the cases (Figures 4 and 5).

The deposits of carcinoma cervix showed presence of tumor cells arranged in groups and nests. The tumor cells were large and showed vesicular nuclei and moderate amount of eosinophilic cytoplasm. As the epidermis was not involved, the differentiation of cutaneous metastatic deposits from primary squamous cell carcinoma was possible. Moreover, a prior history of squamous cell carcinoma of cervix three years back also suggested metastatic skin deposits.

In all the cases of cutaneous metastatic deposits, the main challenge for the pathologist is to exclude the possibility of

TABLE 1: Table depicting the summary of the study.

Sample number	Age (years)	Sex	Primary internal malignancy	Site of cutaneous metastasis	Clinical presentation	Duration of appearance of cutaneous metastasis
Case number 1	65 years	Female	Carcinoma cervix	Left thigh	Nodules	3 years
Case number 2	72 years	Male	Renal cell carcinoma	Abdomen	Nodules	5 years
Case number 3	70 years	Male	Non-Hodgkin lymphoma	Abdomen	Plaque	1 year
Case number 4	55 years	Female	Carcinoma breast	Chest	Plaque	2 years
Case number 5	50 years	Female	Carcinoma breast	Chest	Ulcers	3 years
Case number 6	30 years	Male	Non-Hodgkin lymphoma	Scalp, face, trunk	Plaques	10-11 months
Case number 7	60 years	Female	Carcinoma breast	Scalp, face, trunk	Nodules	3 years
Case number 8	72 years	Male	Renal cell carcinoma	Abdomen	Plaque	3 years
Case number 9	66 years	Female	Carcinoma breast	Chest, abdomen	Nodules	2.5 years

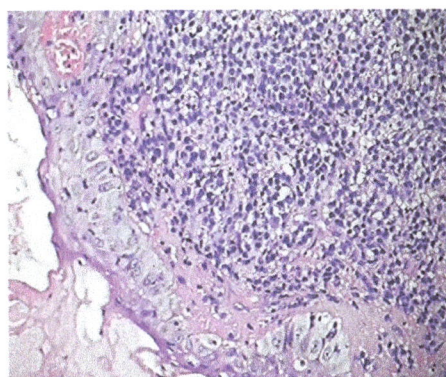

FIGURE 4: Sections show monomorphic sheets of non-Hodgkin lymphoma cells with spared epidermis (H&E ×100).

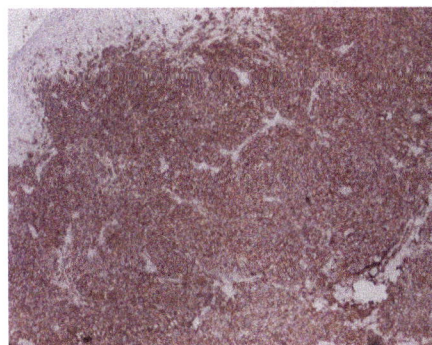

FIGURE 5: On IHC showing diffuse CD45 positivity confirming metastatic non-Hodgkin lymphoma (×40).

primary skin neoplasms (including benign and malignant adnexal tumors) and inflammatory conditions of skin especially in cases of skin deposits of NHL. Immunohistochemistry supported the histologic diagnosis and correlated well with the primary internal malignancy.

4. Discussion

Cutaneous metastases occur infrequently and are rarely present at the time the cancer is initially diagnosed [6]. Cutaneous metastases occur in 0.6%–10.4% of all patients with cancer and represent 2% of all skin tumors [4]. In the present five-year study, only 9 cases out of a total of 1924 patients with internal malignancies presented with cutaneous metastases, thus showing a prevalence rate of approximately 0.5% which is near to the lower limit of the reported range.

Cutaneous metastases may either be the initial manifestation of an internal malignancy or represent recurrent neoplastic disease [7]. In the present study, all the nine patients had prior history of primary internal malignancy, thus representing the recurrence of the primary tumor.. A landmark study by Brownstein and Helwig from 1972 found the most common tumors to metastasizing to the skin were breast, lung, colorectal, and melanoma [8]. While Gul et al. in their study found that most common cancer types metastasizing to skin were breast, colon, and ovary in females and lung and colon cancers in males. In the present study, the order of cutaneous metastases from internal malignancy was carcinoma breast (4/9 cases) and carcinoma cervix (1/9 case) in females while it was renal cell carcinoma and non-Hodgkin lymphoma (2/9 cases each) in males. Cutaneous metastases from carcinoma breast were the most common finding which is in concordance with the above mentioned studies.

According to Basu and Mukherjee, gynecological malignancies rarely give rise to metastatic deposits on the skin [9]. Skin metastasis from uterine cervical carcinoma is a rare event with the reported incidence ranging from 0.1 to 2% [10]. Our study also included a single case of cutaneous metastasis from carcinoma cervix which is quite rare.

Skin metastases of renal cell carcinoma are not easily identified because of the low suspicion index for these skin lesions, which usually mimic common dermatologic disorders. Skin metastases of renal cell carcinoma have been reported to occur in around 3% of renal tumors and are more common in males [11]. In our study we reported two cases of cutaneous metastases from renal cell carcinoma and both the patients were males.

Cutaneous metastases were most frequently (2.6%) seen in cases with hematological malignancies in a study done by Gul et al. [7], while in the present study cutaneous metastases from NHL and RCC were the most common tumors in males.

It has been observed that many carcinomas spread through the lymphatic route to areas having common lymphatic drainage as that of the primary site [12]. In the present study as well, the skin deposits from breast carcinoma were mainly localized to the chest wall. Other cutaneous deposits have also shown corresponding patterns of skin localization. Scalp is relatively a rare site for the localization of skin metastases [8]. In our study, two out of nine cases showed cutaneous metastases on scalp. According to Lookingbill et al., the most common presentation of cutaneous metastatic deposits is multiple nodular lesions [6]. Contrary to that nodules and plaque were the most common clinical presentation in our study.

Metastatic carcinomas are usually differentiated from primary skin carcinomas because of the latter's typical histological patterns, the epidermal connection, intraepidermal/intraadnexal (in situ component) tumor, or the presence of a benign counterpart [3, 6]. In cases where distinction between metastatic and primary skin tumor is difficult, a variety of immunohistochemical staining panels can be helpful [13–17]. In our study too, IHC applied in eight out of nine cases correlated well with the primary tumor. Tumor markers are becoming increasingly important in breast cancer research because of their impact on prognosis, treatment, and survival [18]. The ER and PR markers used in skin deposits from breast carcinoma confirmed the primary tumor.. According Bauer et al., ER, PR, and HER-2 neu negative breast cancers affect younger women and were more aggressive and these women had poorer survival regardless of stage [18]. In two cases, histopathological diagnosis was clear cell carcinoma which on immunostaining with CD 10 was confirmed as metastatic renal cell carcinoma. Similarly, LCA positivity confirmed the metastatic deposits of NHL in other two cases.

To conclude, cutaneous metastases occur infrequently and that internal malignancy rarely presents with skin involvement. However, early diagnosis is necessary which may have profound effect on patient management and survival. Immunohistochemistry is an important ancillary aid in the diagnosis of cutaneous metastases.

References

[1] C. Y. B. Wong, M. A. Helm, T. N. Helm, and N. Zeitouni, "Patterns of skin metastases: a review of 25 years, experience at a single cancer center," International Journal of Dermatology, vol. 53, pp. 55–60, 2014.

[2] P. S. Spencer and T. N. Helm, "Skin metastases in cancer patients," Cutis, vol. 39, no. 2, pp. 119–121, 1987.

[3] R. A. Schwartz, Skin Cancer: Recognition and Management, Blackwell, Malden, Mass, USA, 2nd edition, 2008.

[4] I. Alcaraz, L. Cerroni, A. Rütten, H. Kutzner, and L. Requena, "Cutaneous metastases from internal malignancies: a clinicopathologic and immunohistochemical review," The American Journal of Dermatopathology, vol. 34, no. 4, pp. 347–393, 2012.

[5] R. A. Schwartz, "Cutaneous metastatic disease," Journal of the American Academy of Dermatology, vol. 33, no. 2, pp. 161–182, 1995.

[6] D. P. Lookingbill, N. Spangler, and K. F. Helm, "Cutaneous metastases in patients with metastatic carcinoma: a retrospective study of 4020 patients," Journal of the American Academy of Dermatology, vol. 29, no. 2, pp. 228–236, 1993.

[7] U. Gul, A. Kihc, M. Gonul et al., "Spectrum of cutaneous metastases in 1287 cases of internal malignancies: a study from Turkey," Acta Dermato-Venereologica, vol. 87, pp. 160–162, 2007.

[8] M. H. Brownstein and E. B. Helwig, "Patterns of cutaneous metastasis," Archives of Dermatology, vol. 105, no. 6, pp. 862–868, 1972.

[9] B. Basu and S. Mukherjee, "Cutaneous metastasis in cancer of the uterine cervix: a case report and review of the literature," Journal of the Turkish German Gynecology Association, vol. 14, no. 3, pp. 174–177, 2013.

[10] L. W. Brady, E. A. O'Neill, and S. H. Farber, "Unusual sites of metastases," Seminars in Oncology, vol. 4, no. 1, pp. 59–64, 1977.

[11] P. Sountoulides, L. Metaxa, and L. Cindolo, "Atypical presentations and rare metastatic sites of renal cell carcinoma: a review of case reports," Journal of Medical Case Reports, vol. 5, article 429, 2011.

[12] R. Bansal and R. Naik, "A study of 70 cases of cutaneous metastases from internal carcinoma," Journal of the Indian Medical Association, vol. 96, no. 1, pp. 10–12, 1998.

[13] M. R. Wick, P. E. Swanson, J. H. Ritter, and J. F. Fitzgibbon, "The immunohistology of cutaneous neoplasia: a practical perspective," Journal of Cutaneous Pathology, vol. 20, no. 6, pp. 481–497, 1993.

[14] S. Saeed, C. A. Keehn, and M. B. Morgan, "Cutaneous metastasis: a clinical, pathological, and immunohistochemical appraisal," Journal of Cutaneous Pathology, vol. 31, no. 6, pp. 419–430, 2004.

[15] H. S. Qureshi, A. H. Ormsby, M. W. Lee, R. J. Zarbo, and C. K. Ma, "The diagnostic utility of p63, CK5/6, CK 7, and CK 20 in distinguishing primary cutaneous adnexal neoplasms from metastatic carcinomas," Journal of Cutaneous Pathology, vol. 31, no. 2, pp. 145–152, 2004.

[16] D. Ivan, A. H. Diwan, and V. G. Prieto, "Expression of p63 in primary cutaneous adnexal neoplasms and adenocarcinoma metastatic to the skin," Modern Pathology, vol. 18, no. 1, pp. 137–142, 2005.

[17] D. Ivan, J. W. Nash, V. G. Prieto et al., "Use of p63 expression in distinguishing primary and metastatic cutaneous adnexal neoplasms from metastatic adenocarcinoma to skin," Journal of Cutaneous Pathology, vol. 34, no. 6, pp. 474–480, 2007.

16

Decrease in Self-Reported Tanning Frequency among Utah Teens following the Passage of Utah Senate Bill 41: An Analysis of the Effects of Youth-Access Restriction Laws on Tanning Behaviors

Rebecca G. Simmons, Kristi Smith, Meghan Balough, and Michael Friedrichs

Utah Department of Health, Salt Lake City, UT 84116, USA

Correspondence should be addressed to Rebecca G. Simmons; rebeccasimmons@utah.gov

Academic Editor: Mark Lebwohl

Introduction. Adolescent use of indoor tanning facilities is associated with an increased risk in later development of melanoma skin cancers. States that have imposed age restrictions on access to indoor tanning generally show lower self-reported rates of indoor tanning than states with no restrictions, but currently no studies have assessed indoor tanning use before and after such restrictions. *Methods.* In 2013, we compared self-reported indoor tanning data collected in the Prevention Needs Assessment (PNA) survey in 2011 to PNA 2013 data. We also assessed predictors of continued tanning after passage of the bill. *Results.* Prior to the passage of Senate Bill 41, 12% of students reported at least one incident of indoor tanning in the past 12 months. After passage, only 7% of students reported indoor tanning in the past 12 months ($P < 0.0001$). Students who continued indoor tanning were more likely to be older and female and to engage in other risk behaviors, including smoking and alcohol use. Lower parental education levels were also associated with continued tanning. *Conclusion.* Indoor tanning restrictions showed beneficial impact on tanning rates in adolescents in Utah. Stricter restrictions may show even greater impact than restrictions that allow for parental waivers. Stronger enforcement of bans is needed to further reduce youth access.

1. Introduction

Unlike many cancers which have seen a decrease in incidence and mortality over the past thirty years, incidence of melanoma skin cancer has been steadily increasing in the United States [1]. Incidence rates of melanoma skin cancer in Utah are 61% higher than the national average, with an incidence rate of 31 per 100,000 people, compared to the national rate of 19.3 per 100,000 people between 2006 and 2010 [2, 3]. Utah's melanoma mortality is also 30% higher than the national average (3.5 per 100,000 Utahns compared to 2.7 per 100,000 people nationally) [2, 3].

Melanoma is typically diagnosed later in life, but risks to adolescents and young adults have been increasing and melanoma is currently the third most common cause of cancer in individuals aged 15 to 39 years old [4]. Unlike most types of adolescent cancer, which are largely caused by genetic susceptibility, melanoma is associated with both genetic predisposition and behavioral risk factors, including the use of indoor tanning facilities [4, 5]. Indoor tanning before age 35 has been shown to increase the risk of melanoma and other skin cancers, including squamous and basal cell carcinomas [5–7], yet interventions aimed at reducing indoor tanning have shown mixed results [8–10]. Increasingly, legislative action banning teen access to indoor tanning salons has been seen as a direct way to reduce future cancer [11].

Currently, 34 states have laws in place that restrict teen access to tanning facilities in one way or another [12, 13]. Most of these laws contain exceptions that allow indoor tanning for teens who obtain physician notes or parental waivers, although, by the end of 2014, eight states (California, Illinois, Louisiana, Minnesota, Nevada, Oregon, Texas, and Vermont) will have instituted bans on *any* access to tanning facilities for those under 18. In 2014, a study by Guy et al. suggested that states with indoor tanning restrictions had significantly lower self-reported tanning rates than states without such restrictions [14]. Overall, the study found a 30% decrease in teen self-reported indoor tanning in states with any tanning laws, and a 42% decrease in self-reported indoor tanning in states with systems access, parental permissions, and age restriction laws [14]. To date, however, no study has shown the impact to adolescent indoor tanning rates before and after the passage of legislative restrictions.

The current study assesses changes in self-reported indoor teen tanning behaviors before and after the passage of Utah Senate Bill 41 in 2012, which stipulates that individuals under the age of 18 are forbidden from using indoor tanning facilities unless (1) they obtain a note from a physician or (2) they are accompanied at each tanning visit by a parent or guardian who signs a waiver on their behalf [15]. To our knowledge, this study represents the first study assessing change in teen self-reported indoor tanning behaviors immediately before and after the passage of indoor tanning restriction legislation in the United States.

2. Methods

Our study compares self-reported indoor tanning prevalence among teens in 2011 (prior to legislation) to prevalence in 2013 (after legislation), using Prevention Needs Assessment (PNA) survey data. Due to the deidentified, public nature of our data, no IRB approval was necessary for our study.

2.1. Survey Instrument. The Prevention Needs Assessment (PNA) survey is a biannual cross-sectional behavioral risk survey that is conducted as part of the Student Health and Risk Prevention (SHARP) statewide survey. The PNA survey collects self-reported data from adolescents in grades 6, 8, 10, and 12 on issues such as mental health, suicidality, health and fitness, family life, academic attitudes, drug use, and other behavioral issues. The survey is anonymous and students are informed that the answers they provide will not be traceable back to them. In order to participate in the survey, students had to return signed, parental consent forms. The survey is stratified by school district and weighted to adjust for differential response rates by grade, sex, and school district.

Both the 2011 and the 2013 PNA included the question, "during the past 12 months, how many times did you use an indoor tanning device such as sunlamps, sunbed, or tanning booth (do not include spray tan)?" Answer options included "0 times, 1 or 2 times, 3 to 9 times, 10 to 19 times, 20 to 39 times, and 40 or more times."

2.2. Participants. Participants were all Utah teens in participating school districts and charter schools who were eligible for either the 2011 survey or the 2013 survey. Inclusion criteria for the survey were those adolescents in the appropriate grades, with parental permission, who were in attendance on the survey day. Exclusion criteria were those individuals who did not obtain parental permission to participate, those not in the surveyed grade levels, who were absent during the survey day, or who personally declined participation. At the

end of the survey, teens were asked to report whether or not they had been honest in their survey answers. For our data, teens who reported not being honest or whose data showed high probability of dishonesty (e.g., reporting "Yes" on all questions) were excluded from the analysis. After excluding dishonest students, survey response rates were 65.1% and 69.8% in 2011 and 2013, respectively.

2.3. Statistical Analyses. In order to determine whether self-reported indoor tanning frequency had decreased between the 2011 PNA survey and the 2013 survey, we conducted Wald χ^2 tests comparing self-reported tanning frequencies by demographic factors from 2011 to 2013. We also conducted Wald χ^2 tests to assess whether there were demographic changes to the survey population between 2011 and 2013.

We were interested in examining factors in the 2013 PNA survey associated with continued indoor tanning use after the 2012 legislation. Prior to performing any analyses, we identified variables that were of interest or had previously been showhn to be associated with higher indoor tanning, including age, sex, race, parental education level, risk-seeking behaviors including alcohol and drug use, self-esteem measures, and anxiety measures [4]. Univariate logistic regression analyses were conducted to identify those variables showing significance ($P \leq .05$). Variables meeting significance in the univariate analyses were included into the multivariate model using backward stepwise logistic regression.

All analyses were performed using survey procedures in SAS 9.3.

3. Results

Overall, self-reported indoor tanning frequency significantly decreased in both sexes and across grades between 2011 and 2013 (Table 1). In 2011, 12.0% of students reported indoor tanning at least once in the past 12 months, compared to 7.7% in 2013 ($P < 0.0001$). No significant population differences were found between the years with regard to sex ($P = 0.820$), grade ($P = 0.971$), race ($P = 0.637$), or parental education ($P = 0.394$). Significant decreases ($P \leq 0.05$) in indoor tanning after legislation appeared with relative consistency across demographic groups, with nonsignificant decreases most likely being due to smaller sample sizes for some subpopulations. The exception to this was when stratifying by local health district, wherein sample size did not appear to be a factor.

Table 2 provides odds ratios (OR's) and 95% confidence intervals (CI's) for the full multivariate logistic regression analysis of predictors of continued tanning in 2013. Many predictors of postlegislation indoor tanning use, including sex, grade level, parental education level, race/ethnicity, substance use, and health district remained significant in the full model. Obesity did not remain significant in the full model but emerged as a significant predictor in an all-girls model, with individuals who were obese being less likely to report indoor tanning than those who were not obese (OR: 0.68, 95% CI: 0.47, 0.97).

TABLE 1: Comparisons in self-reported indoor tanning between PNA surveys 2011–2013 before and after passage of SB 41.

	2011 total[a]	2011 indoor tanned	2013 total[a]	2013 indoor tanned	Chi-square	P value
Sex						
Female	8,316	1420 (17.6%)	8004	882 (11.7%)	10.2	0.002
Male	7,293	442 (6.4%)	7180	276 (3.8%)	9.64	0.002
Combined	15,609	1862 (12%)	15,184	1158 (7.7%)	11.37	<0.0001
Grade Level						
8th grade	6,035	332 (5.2%)	6,186	228 (3.3%)	7.8	0.005
10th grade	5,389	669 (11.9%)	5,069	417 (7.4%)	8.9	0.003
12th grade	4,187	861 (19.6%)	3,970	516 (12.6%)	9.1	0.003
Race/ethnicity						
American Indian	512	58 (9.8%)	501	38 (6.7%)	1.8	0.18
Asian	462	31 (5.9%)	517	33 (6.4%)	0.53	0.82
Black	399	39 (8.1%)	422	23 (4.7%)	2.35	0.13
Hispanic	2,061	146 (6.9%)	2,347	114 (4.5%)	5.43	0.02
Pacific Islander	415	33 (7.1%)	424	26 (5.8%)	0.32	0.57
White	12,724	1,657 (13.3%)	12,242	1,009 (8.5%)	11.35	<0.0001
Substance use						
Smoked in past 30 days	823	233 (30.6%)	620	126 (19.7%)	7.53	0.006
Did not smoke in past 30 days	14,701	1,625 (11%)	14,533	1,029 (7.2%)	10.94	0.001
Drank alcohol within past 30 days	1,759	464 (26.4%)	1,387	268 (19.2%)	11.8	<0.0001
Did not drink within the past 30 days	13,746	1,386 (10.2%)	13,704	876 (6.5%)	10.92	0.0010
Body weight status						
Normal weight	12,655	1,620 (12.9%)	11,255	924 (8.3%)	11.03	0.001
Obese (>95th percentile for weight)	1,068	55 (6.1%)	1123	60 (6.3%)	0.015	0.901
Parental education level						
<High school	822	81 (11.3%)	902	60 (7.5%)	2.98	0.09
High school graduate	2,166	311 (14.8%)	2,128	217 (10.5%)	6.17	0.01
Some college	2,657	370 (14%)	2,524	227 (8.4%)	7.36	0.007
Bachelor degree	5,781	642 (11.1%)	5,453	387 (7%)	8.73	0.003
Graduate degree	2,471	301 (12%)	2,457	154 (6.7%)	9.01	0.003
Local health district						
Bear River	1,745	198 (11.7%)	1,773	134 (7.5%)	3.34	0.07
Central	1,007	163 (15.9%)	964	111 (11.5%)	2.51	0.11
Davis	1,678	200 (13.5%)	590	51 (8.2%)	4.51	0.03
Salt Lake	3,984	393 (10.1%)	4,197	263 (6.6%)	7.35	0.007
Southeast	559	54 (8.3%)	597	57 (9.8%)	0.45	0.49
Southwest	1,065	156 (14%)	1,290	140 (9.7%)	2.95	0.09
Summit	424	50 (11.6%)	477	25 (5.3%)	4.02	0.05
Tooele	855	90 (10.8%)	993	74 (7.8%)	1.78	0.18
Tri-County	432	71 (19.7%)	433	45 (12.3%)	1.85	0.17
Utah County	2,177	274 (11.7%)	2,427	135 (6.7%)	5.02	0.03
Wasatch	321	40 (12.9%)	278	24 (9.5%)	0.58	0.44
Weber-Morgan	1,364	173 (14.5%)	1,206	102 (9.7%)	2.36	0.12

PNA: Prevention Needs Assessment survey; SB 41: Senate Bill 41, Utah 2012 [15].
[a]Data provided in the table have been weighted to account for the probability of selection and the distribution of students by sex, grade, and race/ethnicity using iterative proportional fitting.

4. Discussion

In 2011, approximately 12% of all Utah teens reported at least some form of indoor tanning within the past year. Following the passage of the legislative tanning restrictions in 2012, only 7.7% of teens reported indoor tanning within the past year.

Guy et al. reported a national decrease of 42% in states with stricter restriction policies [14]; Utah's law, which allows some leniency with parental consent/waivers, represents a middle ground in restriction policy and shows a smaller effect (36% decrease) than perhaps states such as California, which have implemented complete bans for individuals under 18. To our

TABLE 2: Predictors of adolescent self-reported indoor tanning in the PNA after passage of SB 41.

Variable	Odds ratio	95% confidence interval
Sex		
Male	Referent	Referent
Female	3.72	3.05, 4.55
Grade level		
8th grade	Referent	Referent
10th grade	2.16	1.64, 2.84
12th grade	3.95	3.05, 5.15
Race/ethnicity		
Non-white or Hispanic	0.46	0.34, 0.63
White	Referent	Referent
Parent education level		
Less than college education	Referent	Referent
College graduate	0.78	0.65, 0.94
Alcohol use		
No alcohol within 30 days	Referent	Referent
Drank alcohol within 30 days	2.90	2.23, 3.78
Local health district		
Bear River	1.18	0.87, 1.60
Central	1.76	1.30, 2.39
Davis	1.34	1.01, 1.76
Salt Lake	Referent	Referent
Southeast	1.37	0.98, 1.91
Southwest	1.45	1.03, 2.03
Summit	0.57	0.39, 0.83
Tooele	1.07	0.72, 1.58
Tri-County	1.43	0.79, 2.60
Utah County	1.03	0.74, 1.45
Wasatch	1.24	1.04, 1.49
Weber-Morgan	1.31	1.00, 1.71

PNA: Prevention Needs Assessment survey; SB 41: Utah Senate Bill 41 (2012) [15].

knowledge, this is the first study to demonstrate a significant decrease in risk behavior following the passage of indoor tanning restrictions. Our study also demonstrates a type of policy-related dose-response relationship, consistent with prior research, suggesting that while moderate restrictions do decrease indoor tanning, stricter bans may have larger effect. Such information has important implications for health policy makers, legislators, and other individuals interested in promoting sun safety behaviors in youth.

Policy restrictions on teen indoor tanning have been compared to legal restrictions placed on teen access to tobacco, in that both are legally enforced limitations on youth to known carcinogens. Yet, while both teen smoking and indoor tanning use have been the subject of legislative policy, resulting restrictions have primary differences in how they are enforced. Policy enforcement procedures, such as compliance checks and active enforcement of tobacco sales, have resulted in a sustained decrease in teen tobacco consumption

[16, 17]. Currently, no ban enforcement policies exist in Utah to assure that tanning facilities comply with age-restrictions. A 2007 study conducted by the University of Utah on tanning facility compliance to prior (and less restrictive) age-bans found that only 27% of facilities in Salt Lake County were compliant with parental consent regulations [18]. Similar national studies have found low levels of regulation compliance from tanning facilities in states with some form of teen access bans [19–21]. Enforcement of current indoor tanning bans represents an important component of policy success, nationwide.

Although overall fewer students reported indoor tanning after the legislation, there was variation in the decrease by local health district, which also remained a significant predictor of self-reported indoor tanning after legislation. It is noteworthy that local health districts that did not see a significant decrease in indoor tanning are also districts that tend to be rural. The population of Utah is largely concentrated along the mountain range of the Wasatch Front, with the majority of the total population residing within a few health districts (including Weber-Morgan, Davis, Salt Lake, and Utah County). Continued indoor tanning in more remote areas may be indicative of less oversight or enforcement in these areas or less access to media/education informing about the legislation.

Characteristics of teens who reported indoor tanning in 2013, despite legislative restrictions, mirrored outcomes of previous research. The likelihood of using indoor tanning facilities was higher in teen girls than in teen boys and increased with age, with high school seniors being the most likely to report tanning after the legislation [4, 11, 22, 23]. Teens with parents who were college graduates were less likely to continue indoor tanning in 2013 than those whose parents had not graduated from college, suggesting that parental influence plays a role in indoor tanning behavior. Previous studies have also found the correlation between parental education levels and tanning behaviors, suggesting that parental education about the dangers of indoor tanning use is an important public health component of promoting youth sun safety behavior [11, 23]. Unlike other states, such as California, that restrict any access to indoor tanning facilities in those under 18, the Utah law allows parents to sign a waiver at a tanning facility that allows temporary access to indoor tanning. Future research comparing legislative bans that do not provide parental exceptions to those that do could provide insight into the effect that such exceptions have in furthering risk behaviors.

Teens who reported engaging in risky behaviors like smoking and alcohol use were more likely to report indoor tanning than those who did not engage in other risk behaviors, though smoking fell out in the full regression model (most likely due to interaction with alcohol use). This association has been previously identified in other studies; risk taking behaviors may have some association with self-image [24]. In previous research teens have reported tanning in order to address body image issues, including a desire to look thinner and feel more confident about their bodies [23, 24]. Body image issues, including weight control, are also a primary factor in teenage decisions to smoke [25, 26].

Though underlying issues at play with such risk behaviors may not fully be understood, the association between indoor tanning use and tobacco and alcohol use could present opportunities for partnerships between cancer prevention and tobacco/alcohol cessation partners in interventions aimed at teen risk behavior reduction.

The current study had several limitations. Due to the cross-sectional nature of the PNA survey, it is impossible to say with surety that the decrease in self-reported indoor tanning use in teens was solely the result of the legislative restrictions. Sun safety education campaigns have been an ongoing part of state cancer prevention efforts and it is possible that education on the dangers of indoor tanning or other sun safety activities contributed to the reduction.

Additionally, the legislation did result in a considerable amount of news coverage over the course of the bill's proposal and passage, including at least seven television news stories on prominent news channels and more than a dozen in-depth articles in local newspapers and online. As such, it is possible that teens reporting indoor tanning use in 2013 were aware of the ban and reported tanning less as a result of awareness about the restrictions rather than an actual decrease in use. However, the PNA survey asks many questions that could be considered sensitive, including questions about things like drug use, dating violence, and self-harm behaviors. The survey goes through a rigorous evaluation process to identify students who may not have answered honestly (e.g., answering "no" to questions about alcohol use and then reporting drinking in other questions). Additionally, the PNA survey asks students whether or not they have answered questions honestly, excluding surveys from students who report dishonesty. Given the protocols to identify students who were being dishonest and the anonymity of the survey, it is likely that most students were not dishonest in their report.

To our knowledge, this study provides the first look at the effect of a state-specific legislative restriction to teen indoor tanning in the United States. Although limitations exist, this study does provide evidence to suggest that bans on indoor tanning access do appear to affect teen tanning behaviors within a short period of time. Such findings represent unique feedback for health policy makers, legislators, and others who make decisions regarding cancer prevention. While bans may decrease teen indoor tanning use, more action is needed to support such efforts, including ban enforcement measures and behavioral risk interventions that comprehensively target related risk behaviors, like tanning and alcohol use.

Acknowledgment

The authors would like to acknowledge Lynne Nilson for her oversight and management of the project within the Utah Cancer Control Program.

References

[1] D. E. Fisher and W. D. James, "Indoor tanning—science, behavior, and policy," *The New England Journal of Medicine*, vol. 363, no. 10, pp. 901–903, 2010.

[2] Office of Air and Radiation, "Just the facts: skin cancer in Utah," Environmental Protection Agency, http://www.epa.gov/sunwise/doc/ut_facts_print.pdf.

[3] Surveillance Epidemiology and End Results Program [SEER], *SEER Stat Fact Sheets: Melanoma of the Skin*, National Cancer Institute, 2014, http://seer.cancer.gov/statfacts/html/melan.html.

[4] H. K. Weir, L. D. Marrett, V. Cokkinides et al., "Melanoma in adolescents and young adults (ages 15–39 years): United States, 1999–2006," *Journal of the American Academy of Dermatology*, vol. 65, no. 5, pp. S38–S49, 2011.

[5] International Agency for Research on Cancer [IARC], "Sunbed use in youth unequivocally associated with skin cancer," 2006, http://www.iarc.fr/en/media-centre/pr/2006/pr171.html.

[6] M. R. Wehner, M. L. Shive, M. Chren, J. Han, A. A. Qureshi, and E. Linos, "Indoor tanning and non-melanoma skin cancer: systematic review and meta-analysis," *The British Medical Journal*, vol. 345, no. 7877, Article ID e5909, 2012.

[7] M. Boniol, P. Autier, P. Boyle, and S. Gandini, "Cutaneous melanoma attributable to sunbed use: systematic review and meta-analysis," *BMJ*, vol. 345, no. 7877, Article ID e4757, 2012.

[8] B. W. Abar, R. Turrisi, J. Hillhouse, E. Loken, J. Stapleton, and H. Gunn, "Preventing skin cancer in college females: heterogeneous effects over time," *Health Psychology*, vol. 29, no. 6, pp. 574–582, 2010.

[9] D. Lazovich, K. Choi, C. Rolnick, J. M. Jackson, J. Forster, and B. Southwell, "An intervention to decrease adolescent indoor tanning: a multi-method pilot study," *Journal of Adolescent Health*, vol. 52, no. 5, pp. S76–S82, 2013.

[10] J. Stapleton, R. Turrisi, J. Hillhouse, J. K. Robinson, and B. Abar, "A comparison of the efficacy of an appearance-focused skin cancer intervention within indoor tanner subgroups identified by latent profile analysis," *Journal of Behavioral Medicine*, vol. 33, no. 3, pp. 181–190, 2010.

[11] M. Watson, D. M. Holman, K. A. Fox et al., "Preventing skin cancer through reduction of indoor tanning: current evidence," *American Journal of Preventive Medicine*, vol. 44, no. 6, pp. 682–689, 2013.

[12] M. T. Pawlak, M. Bui, M. Amir, D. L. Burkhardt, A. K. Chen, and R. P. Dellavalle, "Legislation restricting access to indoor tanning throughout the world," *Archives of Dermatology*, vol. 148, no. 9, pp. 1006–1012, 2012.

[13] "National Conference of State Legislators. Indoor tanning restrictions for minors- a state-by-state comparison," 2014, http://www.ncsl.org/research/health/indoor-tanning-restrictions.aspx.

[14] G. P. Guy, Z. Berkowitz, S. E. Jones et al., "State indoor tanning laws and adolescent indoor tanning," *American Journal of Public Health*, vol. 104, no. 4, pp. e69–e74, 2014.

[15] Utah State Legislature, Senate. S.B. 41: Regulation of Tanning Facilities. Jones: The Senate, 2012, http://le.utah.gov/~2012/htmdoc/sbillhtm/SB0041.htm.

[16] M. C. Farrelly, B. R. Loomis, B. Han et al., "A comprehensive examination of the influence of state tobacco control programs and policies on youth smoking," *The American Journal of Public Health*, vol. 103, no. 3, pp. 549–555, 2013.

[17] D. T. Levy, R. G. Boyle, and D. B. Abrams, "The role of public policies in reducing smoking: the minnesota simsmoke tobacco policy model," *American Journal of Preventive Medicine*, vol. 43, no. 5, supplement 3, pp. S179–S186, 2012.

[18] K. Harris, L. Vanderhooft, L. Burt, S. Vanderhooft, and C. Hull, "Tanning business practices in Salt Lake County, Utah," *Journal of the American Academy of Dermatology*, vol. 66, no. 3, pp. 513–514, 2012.

[19] C. A. Culley, J. A. Mayer, L. Eckhardt et al., "Compliance with federal and state legislation by indoor tanning facilities in San Diego," *Journal of the American Academy of Dermatology*, vol. 44, no. 1, pp. 53–60, 2001.

[20] E. J. Hester, L. F. Heilig, R. D'Ambrosia, A. L. Drake, L. M. Schilling, and R. P. Dellavalle, "Compliance with youth access regulations for indoor UV tanning," *Archives of Dermatology*, vol. 141, no. 8, pp. 959–962, 2005.

[21] J. K. Makin, K. Hearne, and S. J. Dobbinson, "Compliance with age and skin type restrictions following the introduction of indoor tanning legislation in Melbourne, Australia," *Photodermatology Photoimmunology and Photomedicine*, vol. 27, no. 6, pp. 286–293, 2011.

[22] S. I. Lee, A. Macherianakis, and L. M. Roberts, "Sunbed use, attitudes, and knowledge after the under-18s ban: a school-based survey of adolescents aged 15 to 17 years in sandwell, United Kingdom," *Journal of Primary Care & Community Health*, vol. 4, no. 4, pp. 265–274, 2013.

[23] J. A. Mayer, S. I. Woodruff, D. J. Slymen et al., "Adolescents' use of indoor tanning: a large-scale evaluation of psychosocial, environmental, and policy-level correlates," *American Journal of Public Health*, vol. 101, no. 5, pp. 930–938, 2011.

[24] L. R. Holman, J. B. Bricker, and B. A. Comstock, "Psychological predictors of male smokeless tobacco use initiation and cessation: a 16-year longitudinal study," *Addiction*, vol. 108, no. 7, pp. 1327–1335, 2013.

[25] G. Cafri, J. K. Thompson, P. B. Jacobsen, and J. Hillhouse, "Investigating the role of appearance-based factors in predicting sunbathing and tanning salon use," *Journal of Behavioral Medicine*, vol. 32, no. 6, pp. 532–544, 2009.

[26] J. J. Koval, L. L. Pederson, X. Zhang, P. Mowery, and M. McKenna, "Can young adult smoking status be predicted from concern about body weight and self-reported BMI among adolescents? Results from a ten-year cohort study," *Nicotine and Tobacco Research*, vol. 10, no. 9, pp. 1449–1455, 2008.

17

Melanoma in Buckinghamshire: Data from the Inception of the Skin Cancer Multidisciplinary Team

J. J. Cubitt,[1,2] A. A. Khan,[1] E. Royston,[1] M. Rughani,[1] M. R. Middleton,[3] and P. G Budny[1]

[1] Stoke Mandeville Hospital, Mandeville Road, Aylesbury HP21 8AL, UK
[2] The Welsh Centre for Burns and Plastic Surgery, Morriston Hospital, Morriston, SA6 6NL, UK
[3] Oxford NIHR Biomedical Research, Churchill Hospital, Old Road, Headington, OX3 7LE, UK

Correspondence should be addressed to J. J. Cubitt; jonathan.cubitt@wales.nhs.uk

Academic Editor: Iris Zalaudek

Background. Melanoma incidence is increasing faster than any other cancer in the UK. The introduction of specialist skin cancer multidisciplinary teams intends to improve the provision of care to patients suffering from melanoma. This study aims to investigate the management and survival of patients diagnosed with melanoma around the time of inception of the regional skin cancer multidisciplinary team both to benchmark the service against published data and to enable future analysis of the impact of the specialisation of skin cancer care. *Methods.* All patients diagnosed with primary cutaneous melanoma between January 1, 2003 and December 3, 2005 were identified. Data on clinical and histopathological features, surgical procedures, complications, disease recurrence and 5-year survival were collected and analysed. *Results.* Two hundred and fourteen patients were included, 134 female and 80 males. Median Breslow thickness was 0.74 mm (0.7 mm female and 0.8 mm male). Overall 5-year survival was 88% (90% female and 85% male). *Discussion.* Melanoma incidence in Buckinghamshire is in keeping with published data. Basic demographics details concur with classic melanoma distribution and more recent trends, with increased percentage of superficial spreading and thin melanomas, leading to improved survival are reflected.

1. Introduction

Melanoma is currently the 6th commonest cancer in the United Kingdom with more than 12,000 new cases diagnosed each year [1]. The incidence of melanoma is increasing faster than any other cancer in the UK with rises of 62% in males and 49% in females in the last decade. Despite this, the rise in mortality has been more modest with increases of 14% in males and 12% in females, and therefore overall survival rates have improved. This disparity between increased incidence and mortality and improved survival is due to the noncongruent increase in the different histological subtypes: superficial spreading, *in situ*, and thin melanoma incidence has increased significantly more than nodular and thicker melanomas [2, 3]. The prognosis of superficial spreading melanoma is considerably better than nodular melanoma, and therefore survival rates are improving with 80% of men and 90% of women now surviving 5 years [1].

The importance of melanoma thickness and depth of invasion for melanoma survival was noted by Clark in 1967 and Breslow in 1970 when they devised their respective staging systems [4]. The thickness of melanoma is still a crucial predictor of melanoma survival and current staging systems, for example, the American Joint Committee on Cancer (AJCC) staging for melanoma, combine the melanoma thickness with pathological information, including ulceration, lymph node metastases, and dermal mitoses (in the most recent edition), to predict the overall survival. The AJCC staging system is recommended by the British Association of dermatologists and the British Association of Plastic and Reconstructive Surgeons and was therefore used in this study. In order to optimise the delivery of skin cancer care in the United Kingdom specialist skin cancer multidisciplinary teams and national melanoma guidelines have been developed [5, 6].

The aim of this study was to investigate the surgical management, pathology, and survival outcomes of all patients diagnosed with melanoma who were referred into our regional centre (Buckinghamshire Healthcare NHS Trust) around the time of inception of the regional Skin Cancer Multidisciplinary Team (2003). This is both to benchmark the service against published data and to subsequently be able to gauge the effects of specialisation in provision of skin cancer care. These aims are in line with recommendations from the recent Melanoma Taskforce publication "Quality in Melanoma Care: A Best Practice Pathway" [7].

2. Patients and Methods

In 2003, melanoma referrals into the unified skin cancer service of Buckinghamshire Healthcare NHS Trust came through 4 NHS hospitals with a patient catchment population of approximately 500,000 people. Stoke Mandeville Hospital provides the surgical tertiary referral care with complex reconstructions and lymphadenectomies. Nonsurgical oncology for the region is provided by the Churchill Hospital in Oxford and all appropriate patients (stage 2A and above) are referred for consideration of adjuvant treatment or research trials. The skin cancer multidisciplinary team is made up of 5 dermatologists, 2 plastic surgeons, and 2 oncologists. Approximately 2400 new patients are referred into our skin cancer service annually via the "two-week wait" cancer referral system and 11.5% of these are diagnosed and treated for skin cancer.

All patients who received a primary diagnosis of cutaneous melanoma between January 1, 2003 and December 3, 2005 were identified through a histopathological database. Patients with ocular or gynaecological melanoma were excluded along with patients whose initial diagnosis occurred prior to 2003 but had new histological specimens: local recurrence, intransit, nodal or distant metastases during the data collection period. Data on clinical and histopathological features, surgical procedures, complications, disease recurrence (nodal and non-nodal), and 5-year survival were collected. Patients were staged using the 2001 AJCC guidelines as these were used at the time of their diagnosis [8]. Statistical analysis, including Log-rank (Mantel-Cox) test for Kaplan Meier curves and Mann-Whitney test for comparison of medians, was performed using Prism (GraphPad) software and statistical significance was accepted at a P value of <0.05.

3. Results

The results are summarised in Table 1 to aid comparison.

3.1. Patient Demographics. Two hundred and twenty-nine patients were identified, and 214 were included in our final analysis: 134 females (63%) and 80 males (37%). The 15 patients who were excluded moved out of area during the follow-up period. The median age was 62 years (61 years in females and 62 years in males) with an age range from 21 to 100 years. Overall 20% of melanomas arose in high-risk anatomical site (as described by Rogers et al. [7]): hands 1%;

TABLE 1: Summary of results.

Variable	Number	Percentage
Total number of patients	214	
Male	80	37%
Female	134	63%
Histology		
In situ	32	15%
Superficial spreading	104	49%
Lentigo maligna	3	1%
Lentigo maligna melanoma	22	5%
Nodular melanoma	36	17%
Acral melanoma	4	2%
Other	2	1%
Not specified	22	10%
Breslow thickness		
In situ	36	17%
<1 mm	96	45%
1-2 mm	40	19%
2–4 mm	22	10%
>4 mm	19	9%
Ulceration		
Present	36	17%
Absent	156	73%
Not Specified	22	10%

scalp 2%, feet 5%, midline trunk 6%, and upper thigh 6% (Figure 1). The commonest site in females was the lower limb (45%) and in men it was the trunk (47%).

The AJCC stage (2001) at presentation can be seen in Figure 2. There was only 1 patient with a stage 3A at time of initial presentation, as sentinel lymph node biopsies were not routinely carried out at this time. Five out of 214 patients presented with nodal disease (3 cervical, 1 inguinal and 1 axillary) and 3 went on to have lymphadenectomies at the time of their first surgery or treatment margin wider excision. Two patients presented with widespread metastatic disease, 1 of whom had palpable lymphadenopathy and is included in the 5 patients presenting with nodal disease above. Both these patients were referred for oncological management and did not undergo any further surgical management. The remaining 1 patient who presented with lymphadenopathy opted not to have any further management.

3.2. Surgical Excision. The first surgery was performed by a general practitioner in 11% of cases, dermatologists in 72%, plastic surgeons in 16% and a general surgeon in 1% (1 patient with an abdominal melanoma). One hundred and eighty-eight patients went on to have treatment margin wider excision, which was performed by dermatologists in 46%, plastic surgeons in 53%, and an orthopaedic surgeon in 1% (1 patient undergoing toe amputation).

In general the excision margins for first surgery of suspicious pigmented lesions were 2 mm however in a number of cases where the clinician felt that the lesion was obviously a melanoma, and in discussion with the patient, wider margins

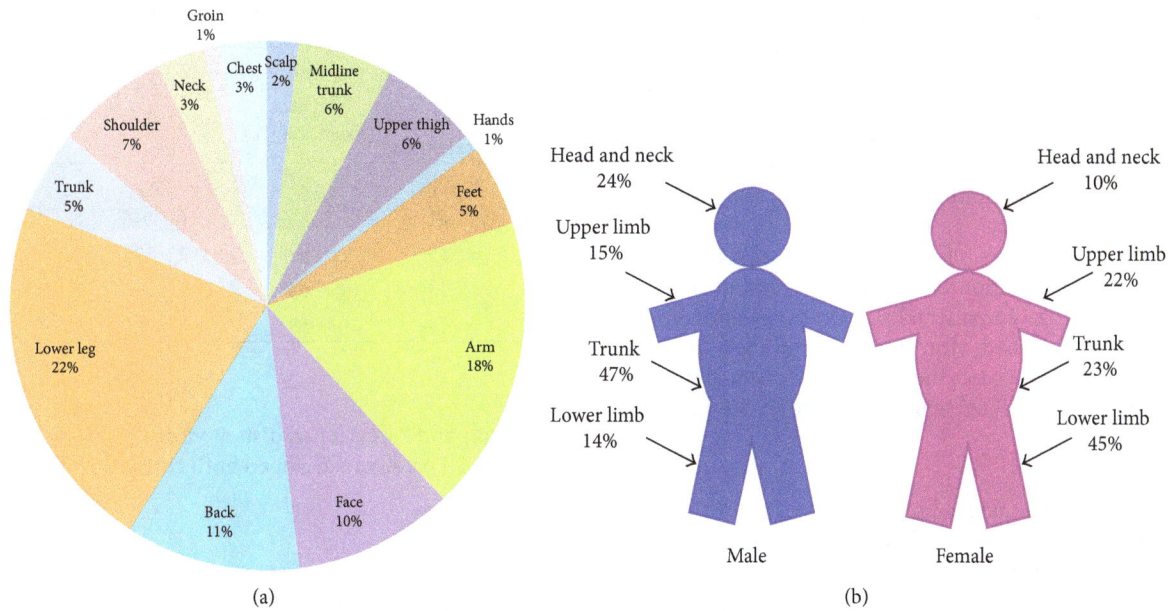

FIGURE 1: Anatomical distribution of melanomas. (a) Overall (b) Male and Female distribution.

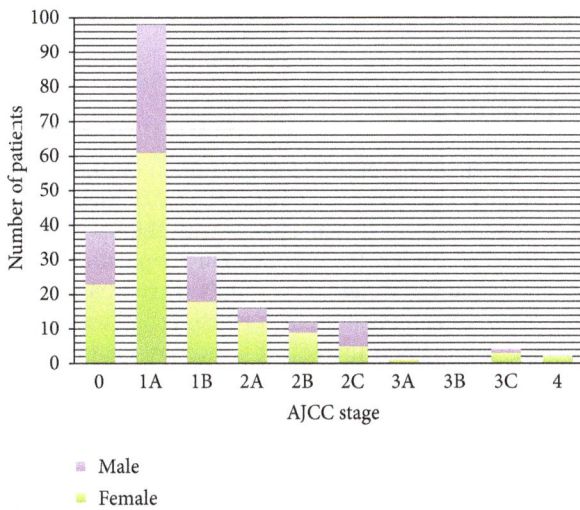

FIGURE 2: AJCC stage at presentation.

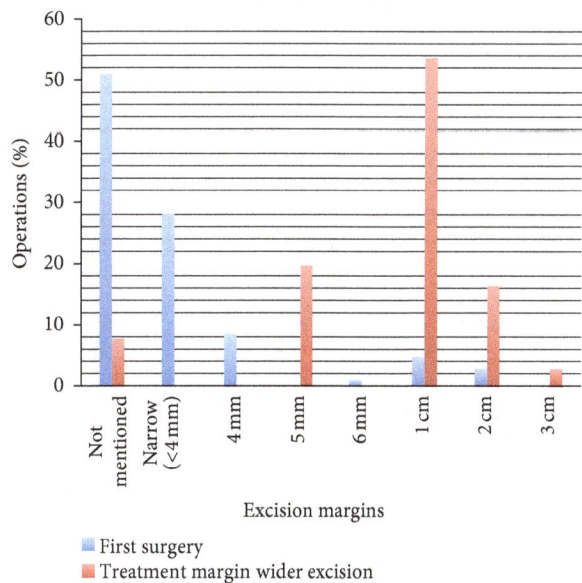

FIGURE 3: Margins of excision for first and treatment margin wider excision operations.

were taken to reduce the need for treatment margin wider excision. These margins ranged from 5 mm to 3 cm and this was the case for 23 of the 26 patients who did not undergo secondary excision (5 nodular melanomas, 9 superficial spreading, 5 in situ, 1 lentigo maligna melanoma, 1 acral and 2 cases where the subtype was not specified). The remaining 3 patients who did not undergo treatment margin wider resection were not fit for further surgery due to comorbidities or widespread disease at the time of presentation. Three patients required more than 1 additional excision.

Fifty-one per cent of first surgery did not have an excision margin documented: 67% of general practitioners, 51% of dermatologists, and 38% of plastic surgeons. Seven percent of treatment margin wider excision also did not

have the excision margin documented: representing 8% of dermatologists, and 6% of plastic surgeons. The excision margins for first surgery and treatment margin wider excision are shown in Figure 3.

Incisional/punch biopsies were carried out in 31 cases, representing 13% of first surgery for general practitioners, 16% of dermatologists and 6% of plastic surgeons. Seven of these lesions were lentigo maligna melanoma, 4 were acral, 10 were superficial spreading, 3 was nodular, 1 in situ and in 6 patients the subtype was not stated.

The incomplete excision rate for the first surgery, excluding incisional or punch biopsies, was 11%, 24 patients (29% general practitioners, 63% dermatologists, 8% plastic surgeons). Ninety-eight percent of first surgery and 71% of treatment margin wider excisions were closed directly and of the remaining wider excisions, 14% were reconstructed with a local flap, 4% with a full thickness skin graft, and 9% with a split thickness skin graft.

Histological analysis of the treatment margin wider excision specimens demonstrated residual tumour in 11.7% of these specimens (22 patients). Of these specimens with residual tumour, 6 had clear margins on their primary histology, and in these cases the presence of residual tumour represented microsatellites which correlate to 3% of specimens overall.

3.3. Histology.

On histological analysis, 96 patients (45%) had a Breslow thickness of <1 mm, 40 (19%) 1-2 mm, 22 (10%) 2–4 mm, 19 (9%) >4 mm, and 35 (17%) were in situ melanomas. The median Breslow thickness for women was 0.7 mm and for men was 0.8 mm (Mann Whitney Test $P = 0.7726$).

Seventeen percent of tumours showed ulceration (20% of female patients and 11% of male), 25% showed regression, 58% showed lymphocytic reaction and 15% showed vascular invasion.

The melanoma histological subtype observed most commonly was the superficial spreading variety (49%) followed by nodular (17%), in situ (including lentigo maligna, (16%)), lentigo maligna melanoma (5%), acral (2%), and intradermal (1%). The melanoma subtype was not specified in (10%). Nodular melanoma was commoner in females, accounting for (20%) of female melanomas and only (11%) of male melanomas.

3.4. Lymphadenectomy.

In our series, a total of 27 patients had nodal disease: 5 at the time of presentation and 22 developing during the follow-up period. Of these, 21 patients went on to have a lymphadenectomy: 5 cervical, 6 axillary and 10 inguinal. The median age of the patients undergoing lymphadenectomy was 69 years and 72 years in the non-operated patients. The average number of nodes harvested was 23 cervical, 9 inguinal and 11 axillary and the mean number of positive melanoma containing nodes were 2 cervical, 3 inguinal and 2 axillary nodes. The 4 patients who presented with lymphadenopathy during follow up but did not have lymphadenectomy included 2 patients with widespread disease and 2 patients who opted not to have any further surgical management.

3.5. Survival

3.5.1. Disease Free.

The 5-year disease-free survival in our series was 87% (86% female and 89% male, $P = 0.6197$) (Figure 4). Twenty-seven out of 214 patients developed nodal metastases and 20 patients developed non-nodal metastases during the follow-up period (9 patients developed both nodal and non-nodal metastases). Of the patients with nonnodal recurrence, 9 developed cutaneous recurrences (7 local and

TABLE 2: Recurrence and survival by AJCC stage. AJCC stage above 3 is not shown due to the small numbers in the study population.

AJCC stage	5-year disease-free survival (%)	5-year survival (%)	AJCC 5-year survival data (%)	CRUK 5-year survival data (%)
1A	96	97	95	95
1B	81	87	89–91	88–92
2A	69	87	77–79	77–79
2B	73	64	63–67	61–70
2C	53	58	45	43–47

2 regional) and 7 developed distant visceral metastases. Four out of the 20 patients developed both cutaneous and visceral metastases.

3.5.2. Survival.

The overall 5-year survival was 88% (90% female and 85% male, $P = 0.3021$) (Figure 4). Of the patients who died, 9 deaths were melanoma related and 10 were due to other, unrelated, causes, and for 7 the cause of death was unknown.

The survival and recurrence data relating to AJCC staging is displayed in Table 2.

4. Discussion

The overall incidence of melanoma found in our population in Buckinghamshire is 14/100,000 (12/100,000 if melanoma in situ is excluded), which is analogous with the national data and other UK studies [1, 3, 9, 10]. Our population is predominantly Caucasian, and these results are comparable with other predominantly Caucasian populations in Europe [2, 11] and significantly lower than other Caucasian Populations in territories with greater ultraviolet exposure, such as the USA, Australia, and New Zealand [12–14].

Our data follows the classical pattern of melanoma data with a female predominance, an average age of 61 years and a higher proportion of lower limb melanoma in women and trunk melanoma in men [10, 15]. The high percentage of superficial spreading melanoma subtype and thin melanoma (lower Breslow thickness) is also in agreement with publications describing the changing trends in histological types and thickness of melanomas being diagnosed globally [4, 16]. This increase in the thin melanoma cohort may reflect screening and increased public awareness of melanoma.

The majority of first surgery was being performed by specialist doctors which reflects the British Association of Dermatologist guidelines [6]; however significant proportions, 11%, were still being performed by general practitioners. This may partly be due to lesions that are not characteristic of melanoma or due to poor adherence to guidelines. The recent introduction of the Improving Outcomes for People with Skin Tumours by NICE in 2010 has meant that this compliance with the guidelines has significantly improved [17]. All treatment margin wider excisions were carried out by specialist doctors.

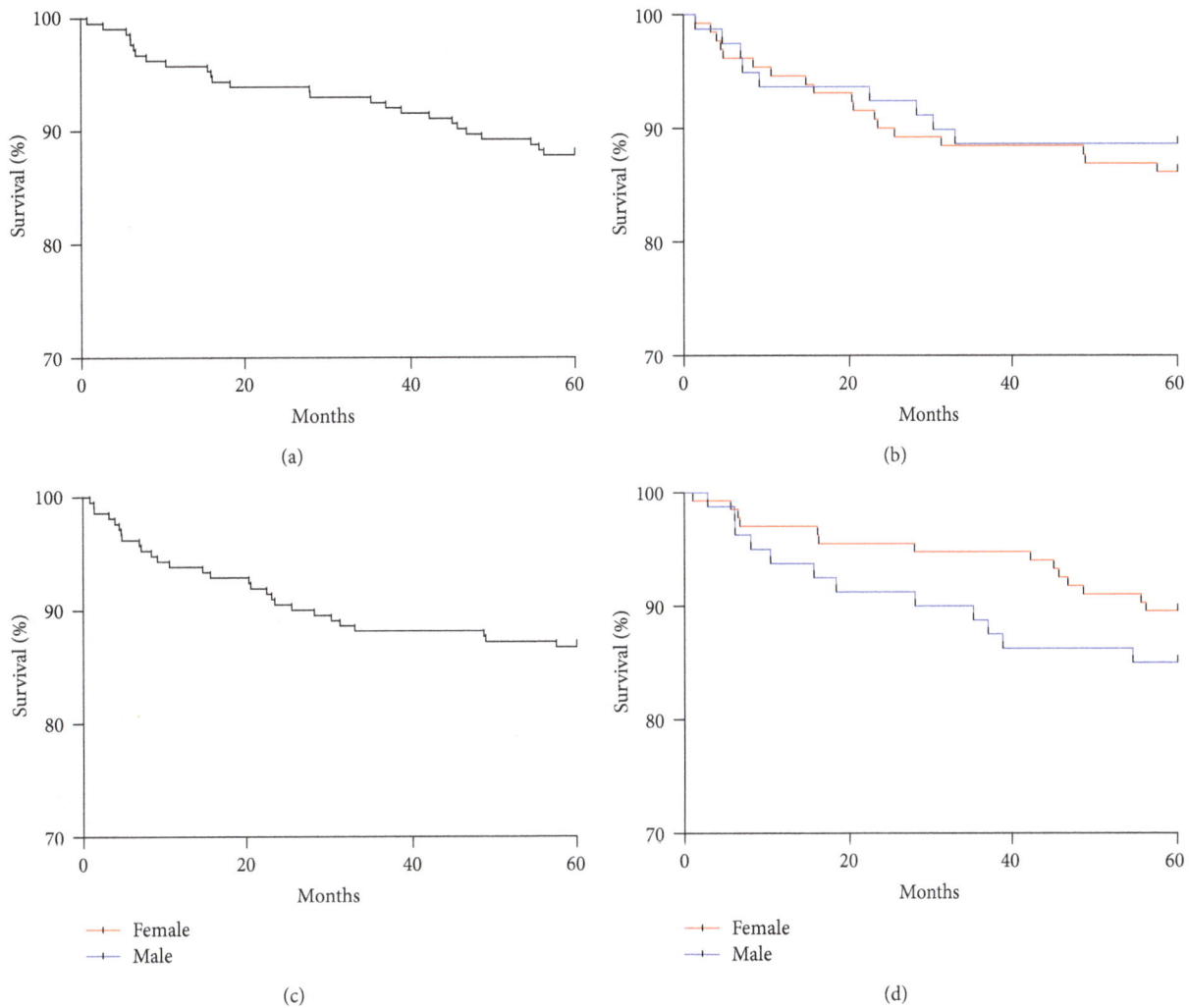

FIGURE 4: Survival plots over 5 years. (a) Disease free survival overall. (b) Disease free survival by gender. (c) Overall survival. (d) Overall survival by gender.

In this cohort we found a high percentage of first surgery and treatment margin wider excisions where the excision margin was not documented. Ideally the excision margin should be documented for all operations so that the width of excision for the wider excision can be planned appropriately.

On examination of the 188 wider excision specimens, 22 contained residual disease. Six of these patients had clear margins on the primary excision therefore the presence of residual tumour represented the presence of microsatellites. This highlights the importance of wider local excision to ensure the clearance of residual local disease and help guide prognosis [18].

Increasing AJCC stage increases the risk of recurrence and melanoma-related mortality. Our overall survival according to AJCC stage compares favourably with the published national data, however, direct comparison should be limited to stage 1 as the numbers in the other groups are not large enough to give statistical significant results (Table 1) [1, 19]. The national and AJCC data will also include patients who have undergone sentinel lymph node biopsies. If our

patients underwent sentinel lymph node biopsies we would expect a number of stage 2 patients to be upgraded to stage 3. This would ultimately improve the outcome of the stage 2 patients.

The 5-year overall survival for male patients was better than expected (85% as opposed to 80%) which reflects the high proportion of thin melanomas (60% with Breslow thickness <1 mm) and low AJCC stage (65% Stage 0 or 1A). The difference between female and male overall survival (90% and 85%) does not achieve statistical significance ($P = 0.3021$) but raises an interesting point: despite a higher incidence of ulceration (20% versus 11%) and nodular tumours (13% versus 4%), with a very similar Breslow thickness (0.7 mm versus 0.8 mm, $P = 0.7088$) and risk of recurrence within 5 years (14% versus 11%, $P = 0.6197$), women have a greater overall 5-year survival.

There are some limitations of our data. Patients living in Buckinghamshire may choose to receive melanoma treatment from neighbouring regions or from further afield, closer to their place of work, for example, London. This to some extent would be counteracted by an influx of patients from neighbouring regions but would no doubt exert some mobility bias. In addition, a small number of patients will have chosen to receive treatment in the private sector; however, from available data these numbers appear to be very small.

We hope that this study acts as a baseline for future comparison of our own service (and others) and will allow evaluation of the impact of specialist skin cancer multidisciplinary teams. Through other studies, we already have an example of early evidence for the value of this development of skin cancer care provision, with the total number of lymph nodes harvested at axillary dissection increasing from a mean of 13.3 in May 2004 to 23.4 in October 2008, reflecting the increasing expertise coming from centralisation of the service.

References

[1] Cancer Research UK, 2012, http://info.cancerresearchuk.org/cancerstats/.

[2] E. Crocetti, A. Caldarella, A. Chiarugi, P. Nardini, and M. Zappa, "The thickness of melanomas has decreased in central Italy, but only for thin melanomas, while thick melanomas are as thick as in the past," *Melanoma Research*, vol. 20, no. 5, pp. 422–426, 2010.

[3] J. Hardwicke, A. M. Brunt, G. Rylands, and S. Rayatt, "Ten-year audit of melanoma in a central England population," *Acta Dermato-Venereologica*, vol. 91, no. 4, pp. 440–443, 2011.

[4] D. E. Elder, "Thin melanoma," *Archives of Pathology & Laboratory Medicine*, vol. 135, no. 3, pp. 342–346, 2011.

[5] National Institute for Health and Clinical Excellence, Improving Outcomes for People with Skin Tumours including Melanoma, 2006, http://www.nice.org.uk/nicemedia/live/10901/28906/28906.pdf.

[6] J. R. Marsden, J. A. Newton-Bishop, L. Burrows et al., "Revised UK guidelines for the management of cutaneous melanoma 2010," *Journal of Plastic, Reconstructive and Aesthetic Surgery*, vol. 63, no. 9, pp. 1401–1419, 2010.

[7] The Melanoma Taskforce, Quality in Melanoma care: A best practice pathway, 2012, http://www.bapras.org.uk/download-doc.asp?id=856.

[8] C. M. Balch, A. C. Buzaid, S. J. Soong et al., "Final version of the American Joint Committee on Cancer staging system for cutaneous melanoma," *Journal of Clinical Oncology*, vol. 19, no. 16, pp. 3635–3648, 2001.

[9] G. S. Rogers, A. W. Kopf, and D. S. Rigel, "Effect of anatomical location on prognosis in patients with clinical stage I melanoma," *Archives of Dermatology*, vol. 119, no. 8, pp. 644–649, 1983.

[10] M. Mowbray, D. L. Stockton, and V. R. Doherty, "Changes in the site distribution of malignant melanoma in South East Scotland (1979–2002)," *British Journal of Cancer*, vol. 96, no. 5, pp. 832–835, 2007.

[11] P. Amerio, L. Manzoli, M. Auriemma et al., "Epidemiology and clinical and pathologic characteristics of cutaneous malignant melanoma in Abruzzo (Italy)," *International Journal of Dermatology*, vol. 48, no. 7, pp. 718–722, 2009.

[12] S. Hu, Y. Parmet, G. Allen et al., "Disparity in melanoma: a trend analysis of melanoma incidence and stage at diagnosis among whites, Hispanics, and blacks in Florida," *Archives of Dermatology*, vol. 145, no. 12, pp. 1369–1374, 2009.

[13] M. J. Sneyd, B. Cox, A. Reeder, and A. Richardson, "European melanoma incidence: a response to Professor Shaw's melanoma editorial," *New Zealand Medical Journal*, vol. 121, no. 1285, pp. 141–142, 2008.

[14] M. Makredes, S. K. Hui, and A. B. Kimball, "Melanoma in Hong Kong between 1983 and 2002: a decreasing trend in incidence observed in a complex socio-political and economic setting," *Melanoma Research*, vol. 20, no. 5, pp. 427–430, 2010.

[15] D. S. Rigel, "Epidemiology of melanoma," *Seminars in Cutaneous Medicine and Surgery*, vol. 29, no. 4, pp. 204–209, 2010.

[16] K. E. Harman, L. C. Fuller, J. R. Salisbury, E. M. Higgins, and A. W. P. du Vivier, "Trends in the presentation of cutaneous malignant melanoma over three decades at King's College Hospital, London," *Clinical and Experimental Dermatology*, vol. 29, no. 5, pp. 563–566, 2004.

[17] National Institute for Health and Clinical Excellence, Improving Outcomes for People with Skin Tumours including Melanoma (update), 2010, http://www.nice.org.uk/nicemedia/live/10901/48878/48878.pdf.

[18] L. Shaikh, R. W. Sagebiel, C. M. M. Ferreira, M. Nosrati, J. R. Miller III, and M. Kashani-Sabet, "The role of microsatellites as a prognostic factor in primary malignant melanoma," *Archives of Dermatology*, vol. 141, no. 6, pp. 739–742, 2005.

[19] J. Lutzky, "New therapeutic options in the medical management of advanced melanoma," *Seminars in Cutaneous Medicine and Surgery*, vol. 29, no. 4, pp. 249–257, 2010.

18

Melanocyte and Melanoma Cell Activation by Calprotectin

Stephanie H. Shirley, Kristine von Maltzan, Paige O. Robbins, and Donna F. Kusewitt

Department of Molecular Carcinogenesis, Science Park, University of Texas MD Anderson Cancer Center, 1808 Park Road 1C, Smithville, TX 78957, USA

Correspondence should be addressed to Donna F. Kusewitt; dkusewitt@mdanderson.org

Academic Editor: Iris Zalaudek

Calprotectin, a heterodimer of S100A8 and S100A9, is a proinflammatory cytokine released from ultraviolet radiation-exposed keratinocytes. Calprotectin binds to Toll-like receptor 4, the receptor for advanced glycation end-products, and extracellular matrix metalloproteinase inducer on target cells to stimulate migration. Melanocytes and melanoma cells produce little if any calprotectin, but they do express receptors for the cytokine. Thus, keratinocyte-derived calprotectin has the potential to activate melanocytes and melanoma cells within the epidermis in a paracrine manner. We examined the ability of calprotectin to stimulate proliferation and migration in normal human melanocytes and melanoma cells *in vitro*. We first showed, by immunofluorescence and quantitative RT-PCR, that the melanocytic cells employed expressed a calprotectin receptor, the receptor for advanced end-products. We then demonstrated that calprotectin significantly enhanced proliferation, migration, and Matrigel invasion in both normal human melanocytes and melanoma cells. Thus, calprotectin is one of the numerous paracrine factors released by ultraviolet radiation-exposed keratinocytes that may promote melanomagenesis and is a potential target for melanoma prevention or therapy.

1. Introduction

In normal human epidermis, each melanocyte associates with approximately 35 keratinocytes to form an "epidermal melanin unit" [1]. The keratinocytes in each unit exert considerable control over the behavior of the associated melanocyte, via interactions of cell-cell adhesion molecules and release of paracrine factors. Ultraviolet radiation (UVR) can substantially alter keratinocyte-melanocyte interactions. UVR exposure enhances keratinocyte production of a wide variety of paracrine factors, including interleukins, growth factors, interferons, and chemokines, that may profoundly affect melanocyte and melanoma cell proliferation, migration, and gene expression [1–4]. Such paracrine modulation of melanocyte behavior may promote melanomagenesis [1, 4].

Within the cell, S100 proteins, in the form of heterodimers or homodimers, control the localization and activity of a variety of target proteins; however, the S100 proteins S100A8 and A9 are also secreted from cells as calprotectin, a heterodimeric proinflammatory cytokine [5]. Calprotectin exerts its effects by binding to a variety of receptors on the surface of target cells, including Toll-like receptor 4 (TLR4), the receptor for advanced glycation end-products (RAGE), and extracellular matrix metalloproteinase inducer (EMM-PRIN) [5–7]. S100A8 and A9 are expressed at extremely low levels in unperturbed keratinocytes, but their expression is readily stimulated by a variety of insults, including UVR exposure [8]. Calprotectin is chemotactic for leukocytes and keratinocytes; thus, it stimulates keratinocyte motility and recruits inflammatory cells to the skin [9]. Melanocytes and melanoma cells themselves do not appear to express significant levels of S100A8 and A9 [10], although they do express the calprotectin receptors RAGE, TLR4, and EMMPRIN [7, 11, 12]. Based on these observations, we investigated a possible role for calprotectin in the paracrine activation of melanocytes and melanoma cells.

2. Materials and Methods

2.1. Cells. Normal human melanocytes (NHM) and normal human keratinocytes of neonatal origin were obtained from the American Type Culture Collection (Manassas, VA) and were maintained in dermal basal medium supplemented with a melanocyte or keratinocyte growth kit (ATCC) as

140

Diagnosis and Management of Skin Cancer

appropriate. The WC62 melanoma cell line (Coriell Institute, Camden, NJ), derived from the primary melanoma of a patient with metastatic disease, was grown in Eagle's modified essential medium (ATCC) supplemented with 10% normal calf serum (Thermo Scientific, Hudson, NJ).

2.2. Immunofluorescence. Cells grown on coverslips were fixed briefly in paraformaldehyde and nonspecific binding was blocked with 5% BSA in Tris-buffered saline containing 0.05% Tween. Coverslips were incubated with a rabbit polyclonal anti-RAGE primary antibody (Abcam, Cambridge, MA) diluted in blocking buffer for 2 hours at room temperature and then with Alexa 488-labeled goat anti-rabbit Fab secondary antibody (Life Technologies, Grand Island, NY) for 1 hour in the dark at room temperature. Control slides were incubated with normal goat IgG (R&D Systems, Minneapolis, MN) at a protein concentration equivalent to the primary antibody before addition of secondary antibody. Cells were examined by confocal microscopy.

2.3. qRT-PCR. To validate expression of RAGE, mRNA was isolated from normal human keratinocytes, NHM, and WC62 cells using the Qiagen RNeasy kit followed by QIAshredder treatment (Qiagen, Valencia, CA). After reverse transcription and DNAse treatment, RAGE and GAPDH mRNA levels were determined using TaqMan gene expression assays (Hs00542584_g1 and Hs02758991_g1, Life Technologies, Grand Island, NY) as directed together with TaqMan Universal Master Mix (4304437, Applied Biosystems). Amplifications were performed on a 7900HT real-time PCR analyzer (Applied Biosystems). Relative gene expression was calculated using the comparative C(T) method [13], using GAPDH expression to calculate delta CT and determining fold change compared to expression in normal human keratinocytes.

2.4. Cell Proliferation Assay. To assay the effect of calprotectin on melanocyte and melanoma cell proliferation, we treated the cells with calprotectin, using recombinant S100A8 and S100A9 (Abnova, Taiwan) allowed to dimerize *in vitro* [14]. Cells were seeded at $1–5 \times 10^4$ cells per well in 96-well dishes in standard medium or medium containing calprotectin at a final concentration of 100 pg/mL S100A8 and 1 ng/mL S100A9. On the succeeding 5 days, 3-[4,5-dimethylthiazol-2-yl]-2,5-diphenyl tetrazolium bromide (MTT) (Sigma, St. Louis, MO) dissolved in freshly prepared 0.1 N HCl in anhydrous isopropanol at a concentration of 5 mg/mL was added and cells were incubated for 3 hours. Absorbance was measured at 570 nm.

2.5. Cell Migration Assay. To evaluate the effect of calprotectin on migration, cells were plated into uncoated or Matrigel-coated transwell chambers (Becton, Dickinson and Company Biosystems, Bedford, MA). Lower chambers were filled with medium alone or with medium containing recombinant S100A8 and S100A9 [14]. After 24 hours, upper chambers were cleaned of remaining cells and membranes were fixed and stained to visualize migrating cells (DiffQuick kit, Sigma, St. Louis, MO). Dye was extracted from transwell membranes using methanol and absorbance measured with a spectrophotometer at 550 nm. All migration assays were conducted in the presence of 10 µg/mL mitomycin c (Sigma, St. Louis, MO) to block proliferation.

3. Results and Discussion

As shown in Figure 1(a), both cell types expressed detectable levels of surface RAGE, the canonical calprotectin receptor, in agreement with previous reports [11]. Expression of RAGE mRNA was confirmed by qRT-PCR (Figure 1(b)). Compared to normal human keratinocytes, NHM expressed more than twice the level and WC62 cells expressed a comparable level of RAGE mRNA. Previous studies have demonstrated RAGE expression in cultured normal human keratinocytes [15]. Both immunofluorescence and qRT-PCR results suggest higher expression of RAGE in NHM than in WC62 cells.

As shown in Figure 2(a), a significant difference in cell number between control and calprotectin-treated cells appeared at 4 days of treatment in NHM and at 2 days of treatment in WC62 cells. Calprotectin stimulated a maximum increase in cell number of 1.8-fold in NHM and 2.5-fold in WC62 cells compared to control cells. Movement through untreated membranes (migration) and through Matrigel-coated membranes (invasion) was significantly enhanced by 2- to 3-fold in both melanocytes and melanoma cells treated with calprotectin compared to control cells (Figure 2(b)).

It is important to note that these studies do not indicate that RAGE is the calprotectin receptor responsible for the effect of calprotectin on NHM and WC62 melanoma cell proliferation and migration, only that these cells express at least one calprotectin receptor. Another study has shown that overexpression of RAGE in a human melanoma cell line is associated with not only increased migration but also reduced proliferation in contrast with our study, [16]. Other calprotectin receptors, including TLR4 and EMMPRIN, may play important roles in mediating calprotectin effects on cells of melanocytic origin. Indeed, a recent study demonstrates that S100A9, probably also calprotectin, is a ligand for EMMPRIN and that EMMPRIN overexpression enhances and EMMPRIN blockade suppresses the migration of melanoma cell lines in response to S100A9 treatment [7]. Moreover, downregulation of EMMPRIN expression in melanoma cells reduces both proliferation and migration [17]. However, it does not appear that EMMPRIN is expressed at appreciable levels on normal human melanocytes [18].

It is clear from these studies that exogenous calprotectin can activate melanocytes and melanoma cells to proliferate and to migrate. Thus, calprotectin appears to be one of the numerous paracrine factors released by UVR-exposed keratinocytes that may promote melanomagenesis. Blocking the induction, release, or activity of calprotectin may thus represent a potential preventative or therapeutic strategy for melanoma. TLRs and RAGEs, receptors for calprotectin and for a variety of other ligands, are being considered as therapeutic targets for a wide array of diseases, including sepsis, asthma, and diabetes [19, 20]. A number of approaches to blocking signaling through these receptors are under investigation and may prove valuable in preventing

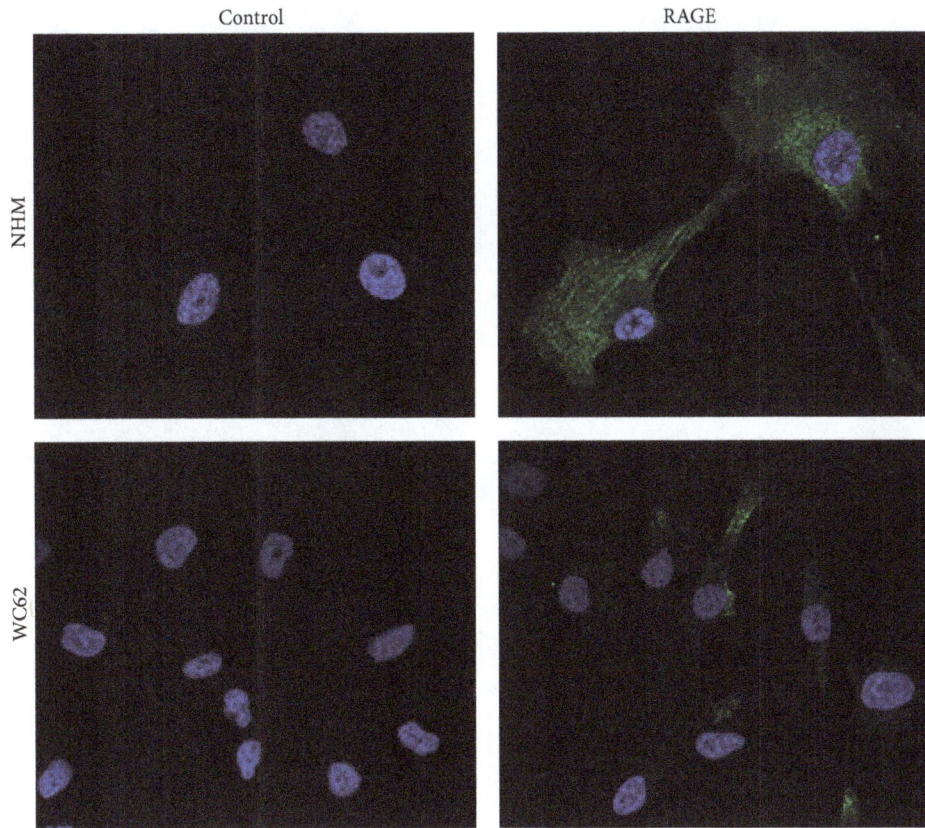

(a)

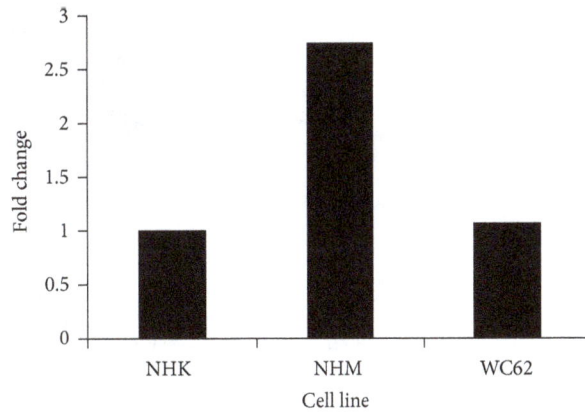

(b)

FIGURE 1: Expression of the calprotectin receptor RAGE on melanocytes and melanoma cells. NHM or WC62 cells were labeled with anti-RAGE primary antibodies followed by fluorescently labeled secondary antibody, as described in Materials and Methods, and examined by confocal microscopy. Control samples were treated with a protein concentration of normal goat IgG equivalent to that of the primary antibody.

or treating melanoma. However, further studies are clearly needed to determine the importance of calprotectin in melanoma development and progression and the therapeutic benefit of blocking its activity.

4. Conclusion

Calprotectin is one of many proinflammatory mediators released from UVR-exposed keratinocytes. We have shown that melanocytes and melanoma cells express RAGE,

the canonical calprotectin receptor, and that calprotectin stimulates these cells to proliferate and to migrate. Because calprotectin activates melanocytes and melanoma cells, it is a potential target for intervention in melanomagenesis.

Abbreviations

EMMPRIN: Extracellular matrix metalloproteinase inducer
MTT: 3-[4,5-Dimethylthiazol-2-yl]-2,5-diphenyl tetrazolium bromide

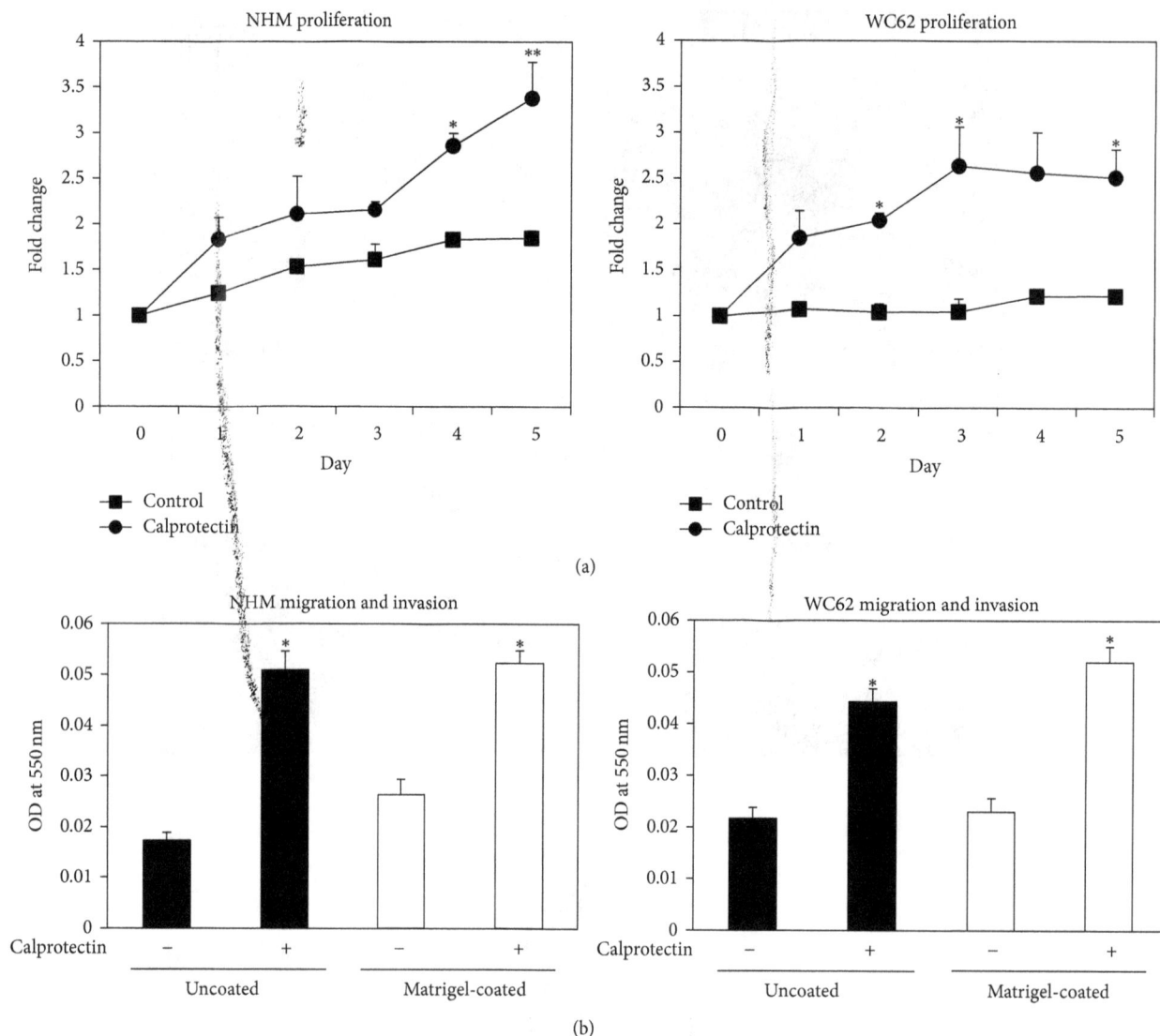

FIGURE 2: Melanocyte and melanoma cell proliferation and migration in response to calprotectin. (a) NHM or WC62 cells were plated in 96-well plates, treated with a mixture of recombinant S100A8 (100 pg/mL) and S100A9 (1 ng/mL), and allowed to dimerize *in vitro*. Cell number was determined using the MTT assay. Triplicate samples were run for each treatment in each experiment and the experiments were repeated 5 times. Bars indicate SEM. Asterisks indicate a significant difference ($P < 0.05$) between control and calprotectin-treated cells as determined by 2-tailed Student t-test assuming unequal variance. (b) NHM or WC62 cells were plated in uncoated or Matrigel-coated transwell chambers containing the appropriate growth medium. Lower chambers were filled with medium alone or with medium containing recombinant S100A8 (100 pg/mL) and S100A9 (1 ng/mL) (Abnova, Taiwan) and were allowed to dimerize *in vitro*. Twenty-four hours later, the number of cells that had migrated through the membrane was determined as described in the text. Three replicate experiments were performed. Bars indicate SD. Asterisks indicate a significant difference ($P < 0.05$) between control and calprotectin-treated cells as determined by 2-tailed Student t-test assuming unequal variance.

NHM: Normal human melanocytes
RAGE: Receptor for advanced glycation end-products
TLR: Toll-like receptor
UVR: Ultraviolet radiation.

Acknowledgment

This research was supported by the National Institutes of Health (USA) Grants R21AR061641 and P30 CA16672.

References

[1] J. T. Lee and M. Herlyn, "Microenvironmental influences in melanoma progression," *Journal of Cellular Biochemistry*, vol. 101, no. 4, pp. 862–872, 2007.

[2] M. Brenner, K. Degitz, R. Besch, and C. Berking, "Differential expression of melanoma-associated growth factors in keratinocytes and fibroblasts by ultraviolet A and ultraviolet B radiation," *British Journal of Dermatology*, vol. 153, no. 4, pp. 733–739, 2005.

[3] G. Imokawa, "Autocrine and paracrine regulation of melanocytes in human skin and in pigmentary disorders," *Pigment Cell Research*, vol. 17, no. 2, pp. 96–110, 2004.

[4] A. Richmond, J. Yang, and Y. Su, "The good and the bad of chemokines/chemokine receptors in melanoma," *Pigment Cell and Melanoma Research*, vol. 22, no. 2, pp. 175–186, 2009.

[5] J. M. Ehrchen, C. Sunderkötter, D. Foell, T. Vogl, and J. Roth, "The endogenous Toll-like receptor 4 agonist S100A8/S100A9 (calprotectin) as innate amplifier of infection, autoimmunity, and cancer," *Journal of Leukocyte Biology*, vol. 86, no. 3, pp. 557–566, 2009.

[6] R. Donato, "S100: a multigenic family of calcium-modulated proteins of the EF-hand type with intracellular and extracellular functional roles," *International Journal of Biochemistry and Cell Biology*, vol. 33, no. 7, pp. 637–668, 2001.

[7] T. Hibino, M. Sakaguchi, S. Miyamoto et al., "S100A9 is a novel ligand of EMMPRIN that promotes melanoma metastasis," *Cancer Research*, vol. 73, no. 1, pp. 172–183, 2013.

[8] C. Marionnet, F. Bernerd, A. Dumas et al., "Modulation of gene expression induced in human epidermis by environmental stress in vivo," *Journal of Investigative Dermatology*, vol. 121, no. 6, pp. 1447–1458, 2003.

[9] R. L. Eckert, A. Broome, M. Ruse, N. Robinson, D. Ryan, and K. Lee, "S100 proteins in the epidermis," *Journal of Investigative Dermatology*, vol. 123, no. 1, pp. 23–33, 2004.

[10] S. Petersson, E. Shubbar, L. Enerbäck, and C. Enerbäck, "Expression patterns of S100 proteins in melanocytes and melanocytic lesions," *Melanoma Research*, vol. 19, no. 4, pp. 215–225, 2009.

[11] E. Leclerc, C. W. Heizmann, and S. W. Vetter, "RAGE and S100 protein transcription levels are highly variable in human melanoma tumors and cells," *General Physiology and Biophysics*, vol. 28, pp. F65–F75, 2009.

[12] J. H. Ahn, T. J. Park, S. H. Jin, and H. Y. Kang, "Human melanocytes express functional toll-like receptor 4," *Experimental Dermatology*, vol. 17, no. 5, pp. 412–417, 2008.

[13] T. D. Schmittgen and K. J. Livak, "Analyzing real-time PCR data by the comparative CT method," *Nature Protocols*, vol. 3, no. 6, pp. 1101–1108, 2008.

[14] A. Saha, Y. Lee, Z. Zhang, G. Chandra, S. Su, and A. B. Mukherjee, "Lack of an endogenous anti-inflammatory protein in mice enhances colonization of B16F10 melanoma cells in the lungs," *The Journal of Biological Chemistry*, vol. 285, no. 14, pp. 10822–10831, 2010.

[15] N. Djerbi, P. J. Dziunycz, D. Reinhardt et al., "Influence of cyclosporin and prednisolone on RAGE, S100A8/A9, and NFκB expression in human keratinocytes," *JAMA Dermatology*, vol. 149, no. 2, pp. 236–237, 2013.

[16] V. Meghnani, S. W. Vetter, and E. Leclerc, " RAGE overexpression confers a metastatic phenotype to the WM115 human primary melanoma cell line," *Biochimica Biophysica Acta*, vol. 1842, no. 7, pp. 1017–1027, 2014.

[17] X. Chen, J. Lin, T. Kanekura et al., "A small interfering CD147-targeting RNA inhibited the proliferation, invasiveness, and metastatic activity of malignant melanoma," *Cancer Research*, vol. 66, no. 23, pp. 11323–11330, 2006.

[18] J. Su, X. Chen, and T. Kanekura, "A CD147-targeting siRNA inhibits the proliferation, invasiveness, and VEGF production of human malignant melanoma cells by down-regulating glycolysis," *Cancer Letters*, vol. 273, no. 1, pp. 140–147, 2009.

[19] S. Yamagishi, K. Nakamura, T. Matsui, S. Ueda, K. Fukami, and S. Okuda, "Agent that block advanced glycation end product (AGE)-RAGE (receptor for AGEs)-oxidative stress system: a novel therapeutic strategy for diabetic vascular complications," *Expert Opinion on Investigational Drugs*, vol. 17, no. 7, pp. 983–996, 2008.

[20] C. Zuany-Amorim, J. Hastewell, and C. Walker, "Toll-like receptors as potential therapeutic targets for multiple diseases," *Nature Reviews Drug Discovery*, vol. 1, no. 10, pp. 797–807, 2002.

19

Six Years of Experience in Photodynamic Therapy for Basal Cell Carcinoma: Results and Fluorescence Diagnosis from 191 Lesions

M. Fernández-Guarino,[1] A. Harto,[1] B. Pérez-García,[1] A. Royuela,[2] and P. Jaén[1]

[1] Dermatology Department, Ramon y Cajal University Hospital, Carretera de Colmenar Km 9,100, 28034 Madrid, Spain
[2] Statistics Department, Ramon y Cajal University Hospital, Carretera de Colmenar Km 9,100, 28034 Madrid, Spain

Correspondence should be addressed to M. Fernández-Guarino; montsefdez@msn.com

Academic Editor: Arash Kimyai-Asadi

Background. Photodynamic therapy (PDT) has become a therapeutic option for basal cell carcinoma (BCC) in the last decade. *Objectives.* To study the results and predictors of BCC response to treatment with PDT and to evaluate fluorescence diagnosis of BCC. *Methods.* A descriptive, retrospective, and observational study was carried out. Patients with biopsy-confirmed BCC who were treated with methyl aminolevulinate and red light according to standard treatment protocols (2 sessions separated by 2 weeks, 630 nm, 37 J/cm², 8 minutes, Aktilite) were selected. Response was scored as clinically complete and incomplete and the patients were followed up every three months. *Results.* Data from 191 BCC in 181 patients with a mean age of 69.55 years and a mean follow-up period of 34.4 months were collected. The overall response was 74% of the BCC treated, with the best response in superficial BCC with a 95% of complete response. The regression analysis revealed that the superficial histological type was the primary factor predictive of a complete response. *Conclusions.* In the treatment of BCC with PDT, the most significant factor for predicting response is the histological type.

1. Introduction

PDT with MAL was approved in Europe in 2005 for the treatment of superficial (sBCC) and nodular (nBCC) basal cell carcinoma (BCC) [1]. The results of PDT on BCC have been evaluated in several studies, most of them clinical trials. The cure rates achieved in these studies were 80–90% for sBCC [2–5] and 52–73% for nBCC [2, 3, 6, 7]. The level of recommendation in sBCC treatment guidelines is A with a level of evidence of I and B for nBCC with a level of evidence of I (surgery continues to be the gold standard for nBCC) [8]. However, since its approval, few large retrospective studies that study the results of its daily use and on fluorescence diagnosis have been published [9–11]. These studies, though having less statistical power than the clinical trials, reveal new aspects of PDT on BCC by describing what happens in routine clinical practice. This study summarizes the findings of six years of experience in the treatment and fluorescence diagnosis using PDT on BCC in a series of 181 patients and also provides a long follow-up period.

2. Materials and Methods

A descriptive, retrospective observational study was carried out between May of 2005 and May of 2011. Data from patients with BCC treated with PDT were collected from three dermatologists at the same center. All of the office visits from the three dermatologists' schedules were collected using an Excel spreadsheet and patients diagnosed with BCC by skin biopsy, cross-checked with the pathology database from the same hospital ("Cajal" program), were selected. Cases that lacked sufficient clinical and photographic follow-up were excluded. Patients who were treated for more than two BCCs were also excluded in order to avoid inclusion of extraneous variables or a hypothetical case of undiagnosed Gorlin syndrome.

TABLE 1: Clinical caracteristics of the 191 lesions and their P values in the trunk-head distribution.

Location	Body 73 (38%) Head 118 (62%)	Body ($n = 73$)	Head ($n = 118$)	$P = 0.043$
Histological type	Superficial 87 (46%)	50 (57%)	37 (43%)	
	Nodular 49 (26%)	7 (14%)	42 (86%)	
	Not specified 31 (16%)	10 (32%)	21 (68%)	$P < 0.001$
	Infiltrating 22 (11%)	6 (27%)	16 (73%)	
	Sclerosing 2 (1%)	0 (0%)	2 (100%)	
Size	Less than or equal to 1 cm: 60 (31%)	5 (8%)	55 (92%)	
	Between 1 and 2 cm: 99 (52%)	45 (45%)	54 (55%)	$P < 0.001$
	Greater than or equal to 2 cm: 32 (17%)	23 (72%)	9 (28%)	
Fluorescence	Exact 99 (52%)	65 (65%)	34 (34%)	
	Excessive 79 (41%)	4 (5%)	75 (95%)	$P < 0.000$
	Defective 13 (7%)	4 (31%)	9 (69%)	

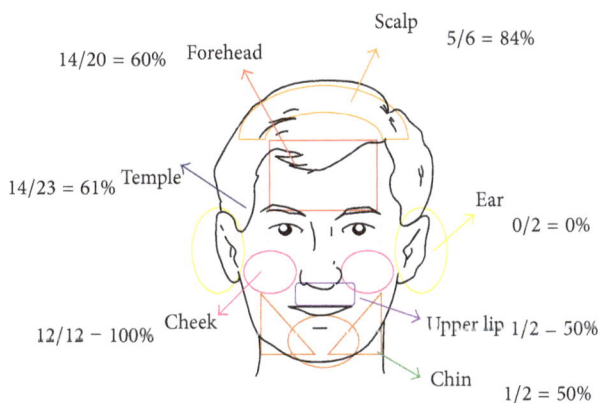

Scalp 5/6 = 84%
14/20 = 60% Forehead
14/23 = 61% Temple
Ear 0/2 = 0%
12/12 = 100% Cheek
Upper lip 1/2 − 50%
Chin 1/2 = 50%

FIGURE 1: Number of BCC, location, and response in the head.

Only patients who received conventional two-session treatment were selected [1]. Methyl aminolevulinic acid (MAL) was occluded for 3 hours followed by illumination with red 630 nm light at 37 J/cm^2 for 7 minutes (Aktilite). The BCC lesions were only subjected to cleaning with gauze and saline solution prior to application of MAL and nBCC lesions also underwent light and superficial curettage as defined in treatment guidelines [1].

Data on the patient's age and gender, BCC histological type, response, location and size of the lesion, fluorescence, and follow-up period were collected. The histological type was determined by the pathologist and divided into superficial, nodular, infiltrating, sclerodermiform, and not specified. The locations were divided into head (face and neck) and body. Locations on the face were specified in different zones: scalp, forehead, temple, nose, cheeks, earlobes, upper lip, and chin-mandible. The nose was also subdivided into the base of the nose, nostril, and tip of the nose. The response was classified as complete or incomplete and in the case of the latter, it was specified whether subsequent simple surgery or Mohs surgery was required. The size of the lesions was measured using the Photoshop "ruler" tool, which allows for the maximum diameter to be calculated using clinical

photographs, and they were classified into three categories: 1: ≤1 cm; 2: 1-2 cm; 3: ≥2 cm. The fluorescence photographs were taken using an Olympus C5060 camera with ultraviolet flashes (Clearstone). The fluorescence of the lesions was classified as negative or positive. When the lesion was positive, it was classified in relation to the clinical margin appreciated by the dermatologist. The positive fluorescence was divided into excessive, exact, or defective, based on whether it extended beyond the clinical edge of the lesion, it perfectly delineated the lesion, or it did not reach the clinical edge of the lesion.

Statistical analysis of the data was carried out using SPSS. The chi-squared test was used for contingency analysis of the variables for histological type, location, size, fluorescence, and response. The interaction between all of the variables was quantified using logistical regression analysis.

3. Results

A total of 191 BCCs were collected (see Table 1), 110 in men and 81 in women, from 181 patients with a mean age of 69.55 years (range 34–98). Of the 191 BCCs, 73 (38%) were located on the body and 118 (62%) on the head with the following distribution: 44 on the nose (25 on the tip of the nose, 12 at the base of the nose, and 7 on the nostril), 20 on the forehead, 2 on the chin, 7 on the neck, 2 on the ears, 2 on the lip, 12 on the cheek, 23 on the temple, and 6 on the scalp (see Figure 1). Regarding the histological type, as shown in Table 1, 87 (46%) were superficial, 49 (26%) were nodular, 31 (16%) were not specified, 22 (11%) were infiltrating, and 2 (1%) were sclerosing. Regarding the distribution, the majority of the sBCCs (57%) were located on the trunk and the majority of nBCCs were located on the head ($P < 0.001$). The size of the BCCs collected was less than 1 cm in 60 (31%) and 1 to 2 cm in 99 (52%), and 32 (17%) were greater than 2 cm. Once again, the distribution is not random but rather statistically significant ($P < 0.001$). The BCCs smaller than 1 cm that were treated were more frequent on the head (92%), while the larger treated lesions were more frequent on the trunk. Fluorescence was exact in 98 (52%) of lesions, excessive in 80 (41%), and defective in 13 (7%). Negative fluorescence was

TABLE 2: Response according to the measured variables: location, histological type, size, and fluorescence.

Variable	Response		P
	Complete ($n = 141$)	Incomplete ($n = 50$)	
Location			
Trunk ($n = 73$)	63 (86%)	10 (14%)	$P < 0.001$
Head ($n = 118$)	78 (66%)	40 (34%)	
Histological type			
Superficial ($n = 87$)	83/87 (95%)	4/87 (5%)	
Not specified ($n = 31$)	22/31 (71%)	9 (19%)	
Nodular ($n = 49$)	24/49 (49%)	24/49 (51%)	$P < 0.001$
Infiltrating ($n = 22$)	11/22 (50%)	11/22 (50%)	
Morpheaform ($n = 2$)	0/2 (0%)	2/2 (100%)	
Size			
Size 1 ($n = 60$)	41 (68%)	19 (32%)	
Size 2 ($n = 99$)	72 (73%)	27 (27%)	$P < 0.063$
Size 3 ($n = 32$)	28 (87%)	4 (13%)	
Fluorescence			
Exact ($n = 99$)	87 (88%)	12 (12%)	$P < 0.029$
Inexact ($n = 82$)	54 (63%)	38 (47%)	

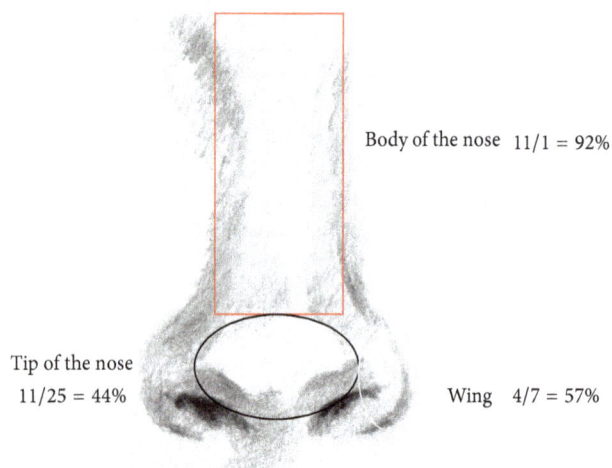

FIGURE 2: Location and response of the BCC in the nose.

The responses based on location, histological type, size, and fluorescence are described in Table 2. It is noted that the BCCs treated on the trunk responded better than those on the head, 86% versus 66%, respectively ($P < 0.001$). Superficial BCC responds best to PDT with a 95% complete response rate and this response is statistically significant ($P < 0.001$) versus the other histological types. Nodular BCC had a complete response in 49% of cases, not specified types in 71%, infiltrating in 50%, and neither of the two morpheaform BCCs treated responded to treatment. The same table (see Table 2) reveals that no association was found between the size of the BCC and the response to treatment ($P < 0.063$). BCCs that showed exact fluorescence achieved better response rates ($P < 0.029$).

Figure 1 shows the results obtained in the face. In this case, the small sample size did not allow for inferential statistical analysis to be carried out, but we can see the tendencies. There are areas that have a very good response, such as the check and the scalp with 100% and 84% of complete responses, respectively. Areas with an intermediate response such as the temple, forehead, upper lip, and chin had complete response rates of 61%, 60%, 50%, and 50%, respectively. The ear was an area of poor response to treatment with no complete responses, though only two BCCs were treated in this area. Figures 3, 4 and 5 shows the results of some patients treated.

Figure 2 shows the results obtained on the nose. The response on the body of the nose is greater, 92%, than on the tip of the nose or the nostril with 44 and 57%, respectively.

Table 3 shows the fluorescence pattern of the lesions studied. Fluorescence was statistically more precise on the trunk ($P < 0.000$), more precise in sBCC ($P < 0.000$), and more precise in large BCCs, sizes 2 and 3 ($P < 0.000$).

A logistical regression analysis was carried out in order to evaluate the interaction between the response variable

not observed in any cases. Exact fluorescence is much more frequent on the trunk ($P < 0.000$, 65%) than the head, where excessive fluorescence was more frequent (95%).

The response was complete in 141 lesions and incomplete in 50, which translates to an overall response rate of 74% (141/191). The mean follow-up period for the BCCs in complete response (CR) was 34.4 months (range 6–72 months). Of the 50 BCCs that did not respond to PDT, 48 were surgically extirpated (28 of these 48 using Mohs surgery) and the other two were considered inoperable. Curiously, all of the incomplete responses (IR) or recurrences after treatment that required subsequent extirpation occurred in the first 6 months after PDT sessions.

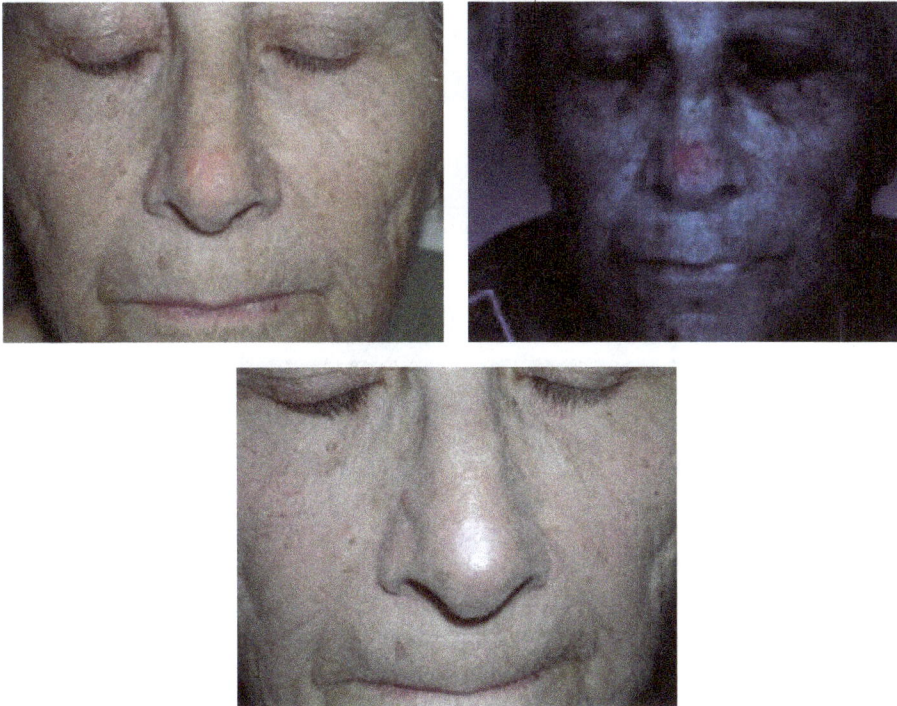

FIGURE 3: Superficial BCC in the nose. Inexact fluorescence and complete response (24 months).

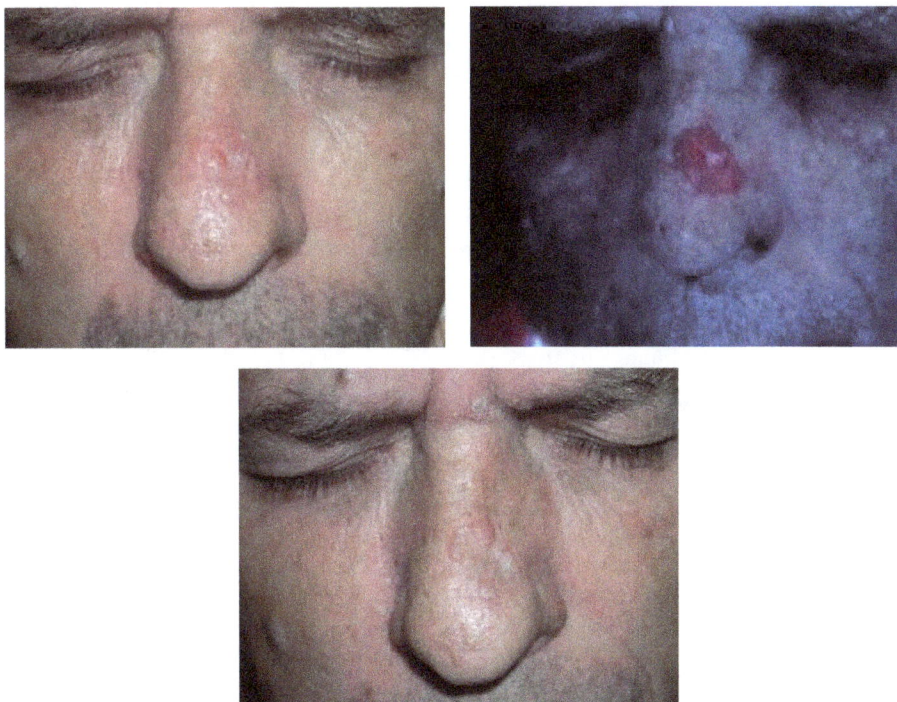

FIGURE 4: Nodular BCC in the nose. Exact fluorescence and incomplete response.

and fluorescence and the rest of the variables measured (see Table 4). Evaluation of the response revealed the same contingency table for all variables. In other words, there was no interaction or confounding factors between the response variable and the rest of the variables. The possibility of a complete response from nBCC to sBCC was reduced by 0.034 times (96.6%) and for the nonspecified type versus sBCC it was reduced by 0.087 times (91.3%). This means only the histological type influenced response. Conversely, on evaluation of the fluorescence result, three different contingency tables

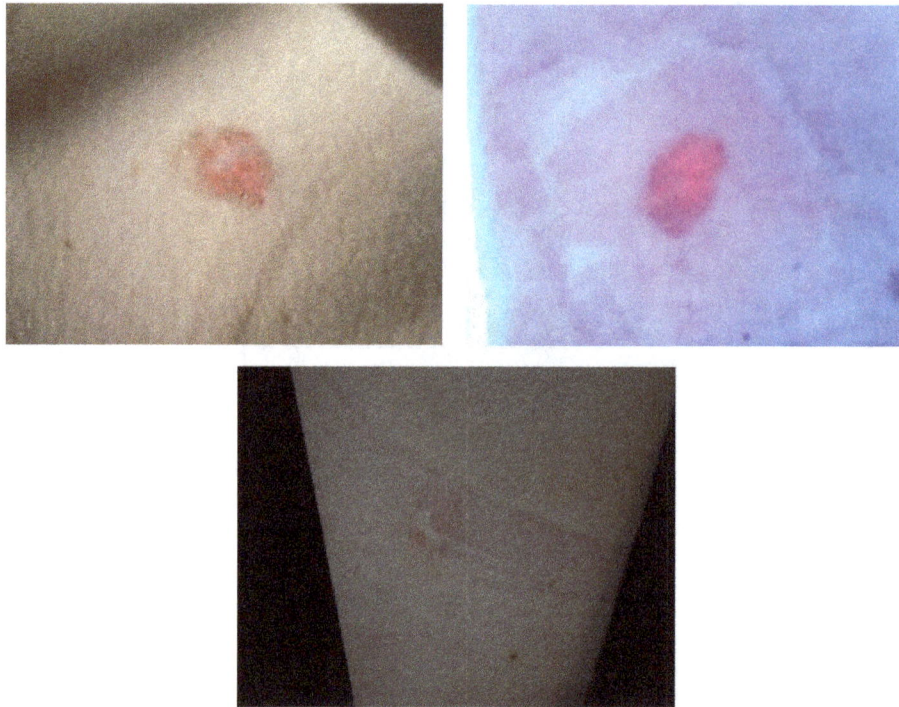

FIGURE 5: Superficial BCC in the lower limb, exact fluorescence, and complete response (72 months).

TABLE 3: Fluorescence pattern based on the variables studied.

Variable	Fluorescence			P
	Exact ($n = 99$)	Excessive ($n = 79$)	Defective ($n = 13$)	
Location				
Head ($n = 118$)	34 (29%)	75 (64%)	9 (7%)	$P < 0.000$
Trunk ($n = 73$)	65 (90%)	4 (5%)	4 (5%)	
Histological type				
Superficial ($n = 87$)	63 (72%)	21 (24%)	3 (4%)	
Not specified ($n = 31$)	10 (32%)	18 (58%)	3 (10%)	$P < 0.000$
Nodular ($n = 49$)	19 (39%)	25 (51%)	5 (10%)	
Infiltrating ($n = 22$)	6 (27%)	16 (73%)	0 (0%)	
Size				
Size 1 ($n = 60$)	11 (18%)	45 (75%)	4 (7%)	
Size 2 ($n = 99$)	62 (63%)	31 (31%)	6 (93%)	$P < 0.000$
Size 3 ($n = 32$)	26 (82%)	3 (9%)	3 (9%)	

were obtained. This means that the size, histological type, and location are confounding factors on BCC fluorescence.

4. Discussion

The objective of this study was to describe our center's experience after six years of treating BCC with PDT. We tried to find and describe parameters that would be predictive of response in order to improve selection of BCCs to be treated with PDT and to optimize the technique.

This is a descriptive, retrospective, observations study with less statistical power than clinical trials. However, it reproduces routine clinical practice. The primary limitations

of our study were those derived from its retrospective design, compiling patients treated by three different dermatologists and biopsies of the BCCs. Despite its histological diagnosis being simple, they were evaluated by different pathologists. Patients who had more than two BCCs and those who did not complete the standard two-session protocol were excluded. This was done to avoid selecting patients who possibly had undiagnosed Gorlin syndrome, to practically evaluate one lesion per patient and to be able to compare our results with other studies. Nevertheless, there is the possibility of selection bias given that many patients were excluded and BCCs that had a very good response in one session and those that required several sessions but also achieved a complete

TABLE 4: Interaction between response and fluorescence and the remaining variables measured.

(a) Response (type, size, and location)

Response	OR (95% CI)	P
Type		
Superficial	REF	REF
Nodular	0.034 (0.010; 0.123)	<0.001
NS	0.087 (0.022; 0.350)	0.001

(b) Fluorescence (type, size, and location)

Fluorescence	OR (95% CI)	P
	Type location	
Type		
Superficial	REF	REF
Nodular	0.551 (0.233; 1.305)	0.176
NS	0.191 (0.063; 0.576)	0.003
Size		
Size 3	REF	REF
Size 1	5.963 (2.394; 14.849)	<0.001
Size 2	19.521 (108.963);	0.001
	Size type	
Size		
Size 3	REF	REF
Size 1	10.536 (4.524; 24.534)	<0.001
Size 2	60.000 (11.990; 300.251)	<0.001

response were also excluded. The variables for histological type, size, and location were chosen because they are variables that the dermatologist can manage in routine practice. The reason for dividing the location into head (face and neck) and trunk, and the sizes into three groups, was to obtain sufficient statistical power. The precise locations of the BCCs on the face were specified because our group has observed a worse response in some locations. However, we did not have sufficient power to perform an inferential statistical analysis.

The patients treated were older and the majority had moderately sized BCCs on the truck. It is notable that, despite the long follow-up period (34.4 months), the majority of recurrences in our sample occurred in the first six months after treatment, practically making them incomplete responses that end up requiring surgical removal. This may suggest that patients with a complete clinical response do not require a longer follow-up period. However, the guidelines recommend follow-up for one year after treatment [12] and other studies have found more delayed recurrences [4, 7, 13]. One recent retrospective study on 157 BCCs revealed the majority of recurrences in the two years after treatment in 19% of BCCs (26% had incomplete responses or recurrences in our series) [11]. This study also revealed independently that the nodular histological type had the highest rates of recurrences [11].

In our sample, sBCC responded better to PDT overall than nBCC, 95% versus 49%, and this difference was statistically significant ($P < 0.001$). This fact was already noted in another large retrospective study [9] where a complete response rate of 82% was found for sBCC and 33% for nBCC ($P < 0.000$). Together these findings suggest that nBCC is not a good indication for PDT and, as recommended in their treatment guidelines, and surgery continues to be the gold standard for treatment [8]. This finding also calls into question the use of curettage prior to submitting the nBCC to occlusion with the photosensitizer. In our patient group and according to the published recommendations [1], nBCCs are subjected to superficial scraping prior to treatment. Perhaps if this scraping was more intense, we would achieve a better response, though perhaps this procedure would not be PDT but rather curettage plus PDT.

When the lesions are analyzed by location, BCC on the trunk responds better than on the head (86% versus 66%; $P < 0.001$). No association was found between size and the response ($P < 0.063$), but BCCs with exact fluorescence had better complete responses ($P < 0.029$). However, we have a sample in which the sBCCs, which are those that responded best to treatment, were statistically significantly located more in the trunk, their fluorescence is more exact and they were of intermediate size. In other words, it is possible that what was being measured was the same and therefore demonstrated a covariate analysis that revealed that, out of all the variables measured, the only variable that influences response is the histological type. In a 2012 study, Fantini et al. [9] found very similar findings measuring the same variables on 194 BCCs. Nevertheless, when a regression analysis is performed, it is noted that the histological type and the location are independent predictors of response. The study also was of a sample which significantly ($P < 0.000$) consisted of sBCCs located on the trunk.

Regarding BCCs on the face, they are more frequently nodular and small ($P < 0.05$), which accounts for the inferior response to treatment. Regarding the locations, it is noted that some areas have a tendency to have a good or intermediate response such as the scalp, cheeks, temple, forehead, lip, and chin. There are also areas that tend to have a poorer response such as the ears, tip of the nose, and nostril. Clearly one cannot draw conclusions from such a small sample size; however, it is notable that these areas coincide with locations defined as high-risk BCC [8]. High-risk BC is defined as those located in the H zone of the face (eyes, nose, lips, and ears), which coincides with those in our patient group who had a poorer response to PDT.

Fluorescence of the lesions prior to illumination has been a parameter described in many PDT studies as a possible predictive factor for response to treatment. Exact fluorescence in our BCC group is more frequent in lesions that subsequently achieved a complete response ($P < 0.05$). Exact fluorescence is more common in the trunk, sBCCs, and sizes 2 and 3 ($P < 0.05$). These findings appear logical if we think that in the face, where there is more endogenous fluorescence from porphyrins, excessive fluorescence is more frequent and there are more nBCCs which have poorer fluorescence. However, when a covariate analysis of all these variables is performed, it is noted that fluorescence acts as a confounding factor. That is to say, there is no association between fluorescence, histological type, and location and, therefore, there is no association between fluorescence and response. Our study is the only study in the literature that has evaluated the interaction between these factors. There is a previous study that also revealed that there is no association between BCC fluorescence and its response to treatment [10].

5. Conclusions

In the treatment of BCC with PDT, the most significant factor for predicting response is the histological type. Superficial BCC responds significantly better than other histological types. BCC fluorescence is influenced by the histological type, the size of the BCC, and the location and cannot predict treatment response. Larger studies are needed in order to evaluate the interaction between all the variables studies and the BCC's response to PDT.

References

[1] C. A. Morton, K. E. McKenna, and L. E. Rhodes, "Guidelines for topical photodynamic therapy: update," *British Journal of Dermatology*, vol. 159, no. 6, pp. 1245–1266, 2008.

[2] W. M. Star, A. J. Van't Veen, D. J. Robinson, K. Munte, E. R. M. de Haas, and H. J. C. M. Sterenborg, "Topical 5-aminolaevulinic acid mediated photodynamic therapy of superficial basal cell carcinoma using two light fractions with a two-hour interval: long-term follow-up," *Acta Dermato-Venereologica*, vol. 86, no. 5, pp. 412–417, 2006.

[3] T. Surrenti, L. De Angelis, A. Di Cesare, M. C. Fargnoli, and K. Peris, "Efficacy of photodynamic therapy with methyl aminolevulinate in the treatment of superficial and nodular basal cell carcinoma: an open-label trial," *European Journal of Dermatology*, vol. 17, no. 5, pp. 412–415, 2007.

[4] N. Basset-Seguin, S. H. Ibbotson, L. Emtestam et al., "Topical methyl aminolaevulinate photodynamic therapy versus cryotherapy for superficial basal cell carcinoma: a 5 year randomized trial," *European Journal of Dermatology*, vol. 18, no. 5, pp. 547–553, 2008.

[5] K. Caekelbergh, A. F. Nikkels, B. Leroy, E. Verhaeghe, M. Lamotte, and V. Rives, "Photodynamic therapy using methyl aminolevulinate in the management of primary superficial basal cell carcinoma: clinical and health economic outcomes," *Journal of Drugs in Dermatology*, vol. 8, no. 11, pp. 992–996, 2009.

[6] L. E. Rhodes, M. de Rie, Y. Enström et al., "Photodynamic therapy using topical methylaminolevulinate vs surgery for nodular basal cell carcinoma: results of a multicenter randomized prospective trial," *Archives of Dermatology*, vol. 140, no. 1, pp. 17–23, 2004.

[7] P. Foley, M. Freeman, A. Menter et al., "Photodynamic therapy with methyl aminolevulinate for primary nodular basal cell carcinoma: results of two randomized studies," *International Journal of Dermatology*, vol. 48, no. 11, pp. 1236–1245, 2009.

[8] N. R. Telfer, G. B. Colver, and C. A. Morton, "Guidelines for the management of basal cell carcinoma," *British Journal of Dermatology*, vol. 159, no. 1, pp. 35–48, 2008.

[9] F. Fantini, A. Greco, C. Del Giovane et al., "Photodynamic therapy for basal cell carcinoma: clinical and pathological determinants of response," *Journal of the European Academy of Dermatology and Venereology*, vol. 25, no. 8, pp. 896–901, 2011.

[10] C. Sadberg, J. Paoli, M. Gillstedt et al., "Fluorescende diagnosis of basal cell carcinomas comparing mehtylaminolevulinate and aminoaevulinic acid and correlation with visual tumour size," *Acta Dermato-Venereologica*, vol. 91, pp. 398–403, 2011.

[11] R. Lindberg-Larsen, H. Solvsten, and K. Kragballe, "Evaluation of recurrence after photodynamic therapy with topical methylaminolevulinate for 157 basal cell carcinomas in 90 patients," *Acta Dermato-Venereologica*, vol. 92, no. 2, pp. 144–147, 2011.

[12] L. R. Braathen, R. Szeimies, N. Basset-Seguin et al., "Guidelines on the use of photodynamic therapy for nonmelanoma skin cancer: an international consensus," *Journal of the American Academy of Dermatology*, vol. 56, no. 1, pp. 125–143, 2007.

[13] C. Vinciullo, T. Elliott, D. Francis et al., "Photodynamic therapy with topical methyl aminolaevulinate for "difficult-to-treat" basal cell carcinoma," *British Journal of Dermatology*, vol. 152, no. 4, pp. 765–772, 2005.

20

Prediction of Sentinel Node Status and Clinical Outcome in a Melanoma Centre

Vera Teixeira,[1] Ricardo Vieira,[1,2] Inês Coutinho,[1] Rita Cabral,[1]
David Serra,[1] Maria José Julião,[3] Maria Manuel Brites,[1]
Anabela Albuquerque,[4] João Pedroso de Lima,[2,4] and Américo Figueiredo[1,2]

[1] Dermatology Department, Coimbra University Hospital, Praceta Mota Pinto, 3000-075 Coimbra, Portugal
[2] Faculty of Medicine, University of Coimbra, 3000-075 Coimbra, Portugal
[3] Pathology Department, Coimbra University Hospital, 3000-075 Coimbra, Portugal
[4] Nuclear Medicine Department, Coimbra University Hospital, 3000-075 Coimbra, Portugal

Correspondence should be addressed to Vera Teixeira; vera.teixeira.derm@gmail.com

Academic Editor: Giuseppe Argenziano

Background. Sentinel lymph node biopsy (SLNB) is a standard procedure for patients with localized cutaneous melanoma. The National Comprehensive Cancer Network (NCCN) Melanoma Panel has reinforced the status of the sentinel lymph node (SLN) as an important prognostic factor for melanoma survival. We sought to identify predictive factors associated with a positive SLNB and overall survival in our population. *Methods.* We performed a retrospective chart review of 221 patients who have done a successful SLNB for melanoma between 2004 and 2010 at our department. Univariate and multivariate analyses were done. *Results.* The SLNB was positive in 48 patients (21.7%). Univariate analysis showed that male gender, increasing Breslow thickness, tumor type, and absence of tumor-infiltrating lymphocytes were significantly associated with a positive SLNB. Multivariate analysis confirmed that Breslow thickness and the absence of tumor-infiltrating lymphocytes are independently predictive of SLN metastasis. The 5-year survival rates were 53.1% for SLN positive patients and 88.2% for SLN negative patients. Breslow thickness and the SLN status independently predict overall survival. *Conclusions.* The risk factors for a positive SLNB are consistent with those found in the previous literature. In addition, the SLN status is a major determinant of survival, which highlights its importance in melanoma management.

1. Introduction

Sentinel lymph node biopsy (SLNB) is the standard practice for pathological staging in patients with localized melanoma in most melanoma centers worldwide [1, 2]. With a 20% likelihood of yielding positive results, it spares most patients to a complete lymph node dissection (CLND), a more invasive procedure [1–6].

Although several factors have been identified as predictors of a positive SLNB, only few have been proved to be independent predictors after adjusting for confounding variables. Breslow thickness is the most consistently reported and well-established predictor of sentinel lymph node (SLN) metastasis. Other reported predictive factors are age, gender, primary site, ulceration, tumor mitotic rate, Clark level, lymphovascular invasion, and absence of tumor-infiltrating lymphocytes [5–9]. SLN status is an important prognostic factor in melanoma patients [1]. According to this, management guidelines issued by the National Comprehensive Cancer Network (NCCN) emphasize the role of SLN biopsy as staging and prognostic procedure [10].

We investigated the association of several clinical and pathological variables with an increased likelihood of positive SLNB and factors that have an impact in melanoma-related death in our population.

2. Material and Methods

The study was approved by the Research Ethics Board of Coimbra University Hospital. We did a retrospective chart review of 221 cases of cutaneous melanoma which had a successful SLNB. The cases were all from our department and refer to the period from January 2004 to December 2010. The followup was extended to June 2012. The procedure was performed in the presence of melanoma >1.0 mm, or even thinner if adverse prognostic features were present, as recommended by NCCN guidelines. Most of the patients were staged up to T1b, but nine patients were in T1a, seven of them with exactly 1 mm Breslow thickness. Only patients without clinical or radiological evidence of nodal or distant metastases were selected to be submitted to SLNB.

3. SLN Biopsy Technique

Lymphoscintigraphy was performed the day before surgery by intradermal injection of technetium 99 m sulfur colloid around the primary lesion or biopsy site to identify lymphatic basins by gamma imaging. Single-photon emission computed tomography (SPECT) drainage was used in patient's complex lymphatic drainage. The site of the sentinel lymph node (hot spot) was marked on the skin. On the day of surgery, with the aid of a hand-held gamma probe, a 10–15 mm incision was made over the marked lymph node basin and after careful exploration of the tissue, the SLB was localized and excised. All nodes with radioactive counts exceeding 10% of the node with the highest radioactive count were removed and sent for histopathological analysis [11].

4. Data Collection

Our data contains patient characteristics like age, gender, and location of the primary lesion (categorized into four anatomic locations: head and neck, trunk, upper limb, and lower limb) and histological features of the primary melanoma such as Breslow thickness, tumor type, mitotic rate, ulceration, neurotropism, angioinvasion, and presence/absence of tumor-infiltrating lymphocytes.

A pathologist (Maria José Julião) reviewed the histological sections of all positive SLN in our data to exclude misinterpretations in the original pathology reports. The slides were stained with hematoxylin-eosin and immunohistochemistry examination involved S100 and HMB45. The following micromorphometric features were registered: SLN basin site, number of positive SLN, size of largest metastatic deposit in SLN (stratified into 2 groups: ≤1 mm and >1 mm), intranodal location of tumor deposits (subcapsular, parenchymal, both, or extensive), number of metastatic foci, and presence of extranodal invasion and perinodal lymphatic invasion. CLND positivity (when performed), melanoma recurrence (peritumoral skin), and survival outcomes were assessed.

5. Statistical Analysis

Statistical analysis was performed using Software Package for Statistical Science (SPSS for Windows, version 18.0, Chicago, IL, USA). Categorical data are presented as frequency (percentage) and continuous data are presented as mean ±

standard deviation. For the comparison of categorical data, a Chi-square test was done.

We used univariate and multivariate logistic regressions to test the correlation of each variable with SLNB positivity. Odds ratios of the significant predictors are provided along with 95% confidence intervals (CI). Some histological variables were reported inconsistently and were not included in the data.

Overall survival (OS) was calculated from the SLNB to the date of death or last follow-up visit for all patients. Only deaths due to melanoma were considered "events." Kaplan-Meier survival curves were compared with the logrank test; multivariate analysis was performed using a Cox regression model to estimate significant independent prognostic factors on survival. A test statistic with a P value < 0.05 was considered significant.

6. Results

6.1. Clinical and Pathological Features. Forty-eight (21.7%) out of 221 patients with localized primary melanoma were tested positive upon SLN biopsy (Table 1). CLND was performed in 44 patients (4 patients refused the procedure), showing additional metastases in 13 patients (29.5%) (Table 2). The mean age of the cohort was 59.3 years (range 18–88), and 61.5% (N = 136) were females. Forty-three percent of melanomas were located on the lower limbs and 21.3% of all melanomas were located in the feet. The average Breslow thickness was 3.08 mm (±2.88 mm), and ulceration was present in 46.7% of cases. Local recurrence was observed in 11% of patients, on average after 15.6 months of SLN biopsy (Table 3). Melanoma-related death occurred in 14.9% (N = 33). The median follow-up duration was 44 months (range 3–110).

6.2. Predictors of Positive SLN. Table 1 shows the descriptive statistics of the clinical and pathological differences between patients according to SLN status. The univariate logistic regression showed that patient's gender (male), tumor type, Breslow thickness, and the absence of tumor-infiltrating lymphocytes are associated with a higher likelihood of a positive SLNB (Table 1). Mean Breslow thickness in negative SLNB group was 2.60 mm compared to 4.74 mm in positive SLN group (P < 0.001). Only 13.8% of the patients with lymphocytic infiltrate in the primary lesion had SLN positive compared to 30.2% of the patients without lymphocytic infiltrate (P = 0.021). No significant correlation was found between SLN status, patient's age (even after stratification by age groups, data not shown), tumor location, and SLN basin.

The multivariate analysis showed that Breslow thickness and absence of tumor-infiltrating lymphocytes were independent predictors of positive SLNB (Table 4). Others variables were no longer statistically significant.

The frequency of SLN metastasis is positively correlated with an increase in Breslow thickness: only one patient in T1 stage (4.8%) showed SLN involvement compared to almost half of the patients in T4 category (46.5%) (P < 0.001, Figure 1). For each additional mm in Breslow thickness, the likelihood of positive SLN increased by 12%.

TABLE 1: Clinical and pathological features of patients who underwent sentinel lymph node biopsy (SLNB) between 2004 and 2010 by SLN status and univariable association with positive SLN.

	Total N (%)/mean ($\pm$SD)	SLN negative N (%)/mean ($\pm$SD)	SLN positive N (%)/mean ($\pm$SD)	P value	OR (95% CI)
Number of patients	221	173 (78.3)	48 (21.7)		
Age, yr	59.3 ($\pm$15.9)	58.8 ($\pm$16.4)	60.0 ($\pm$14.0)	NS	
Gender					
Female	136 (61.5)	116 (85.3)	20 (14.7)	<0.001	2.85 (1.48–5.49)
Male	85 (38.5)	57 (67.1)	28 (32.9)		
Tumor location					
Head and neck	23 (10.5)	20 (87)	3 (13)		
Upper limb	33 (15)	30 (90.9)	3 (9.1)	NS	
Lower limb	95 (43)	70 (73.7)	25 (26.3)		
Trunk	69 (31.4)	52 (75.4)	17 (24.6)		
Histologic type					
Superficial spreading	38 (17.2)	35 (92.1)	3 (7.9)		
Nodular	45 (20.4)	30 (66.7)	15 (33.3)	0.001	
Acral lentiginous	47 (21.3)	30 (63.8)	17 (36.2)		
Unknown/others (spitzoid, desmoplastic, nevoid, amelanotic)	91 (41.2)	78 (85.7)	13 (14.3)		
Breslow (mean, mm)	3.08 ($\pm$2.88)	2.60 ($\pm$3.88)	4.74 ($\pm$2.32)		<0.001
Breslow category					
T1 ($\leq$1 mm)	21 (10)	20 (95.2)	1 (4.8)		
T2 (1.01–2 mm)	89 (42.4)	79 (88.8)	10 (11.2)	<0.001	
T3 (2.01–4 mm)	57 (27.1)	41 (71.9)	16 (28.1)		
T4 ($\geq$4 mm)	43 (20.5)	23 (53.5)	20 (46.5)		
Ulceration					
Absent	97 (53.3)	79 (81.4)	18 (18.6)	NS	
Present	85 (46.7)	60 (70.6)	25 (29.4)		
Tumor-infiltrating lymphocytes					
Present	80 (60.2)	69 (86.3)	11 (13.8)	0.021	2.71 (1.42–6.44)
Absent	53 (39.8)	37 (69.8)	16 (30.2)		
SLN site					
Axilla	92 (41.8)	72 (78.3)	20 (21.7)		
Inguinal	100 (45.5)	75 (75)	25 (25)	NS	
Cervical	28 (12.7)	25 (89.3)	3 (10.7)		

NS: not statistically significant; CI: confidence interval.

6.3. *Clinical Outcome.* A Kaplan-Meier analysis identified a significant negative effect on overall survival of male gender ($P < 0.05$), age > 60 years ($P < 0.05$), ulceration ($P < 0.001$), increasing Breslow thickness ($P < 0.001$), positive SLNB ($P < 0.001$), maximum size of the largest tumor deposit >1 mm ($P < 0.05$), and local recurrence ($P < 0.001$) (Figure 2). We found no significant correlation between overall survival and extracapsular invasion, perinodal lymphatic involvement, intranodal location of tumor, number of metastatic foci, or CLND.

On multivariate Cox proportional hazard analyses, independent significant prognostic factors for melanoma-specific survival were Breslow thickness and SLN status, whilst the other variables lose their association (Table 5). The 5-year overall survival was significantly shorter in SLN positive patients than in SLN negative patients (53.1% versus 88.2%, $P < 0.001$), and about 35.4% of SLN positive patients ($N = 17$) had melanoma-related death compared with 9.2% SLN negative patients ($N = 16$) ($P < 0.001$, OR 5.38, 95% CI 2.46–11.78) (Table 2).

TABLE 2: Micromorphometric features of SLN positive patients.

Micromorphometric features	N (%)
Size of metastasis	
≤1 mm	15 (31.3)
>1 mm	24 (50.0)
Unknown	9 (18.7)
Intranodal location	
Subcapsular	16 (33.3)
Parenchymal	9 (18.7)
Both	15 (31.3)
Extensive	6 (12.5)
Unknown	2 (4.2)
Number of metastatic foci	
1	15 (35.7)
2–5	16 (38.1)
>5	11 (26.2)
Unknown	6 (12.5)
Extranodal invasion	
Presence	9 (19.1)
Lymphatic invasion	
Presence	10 (21.3)
CLND	
Positive	13 (29.5)

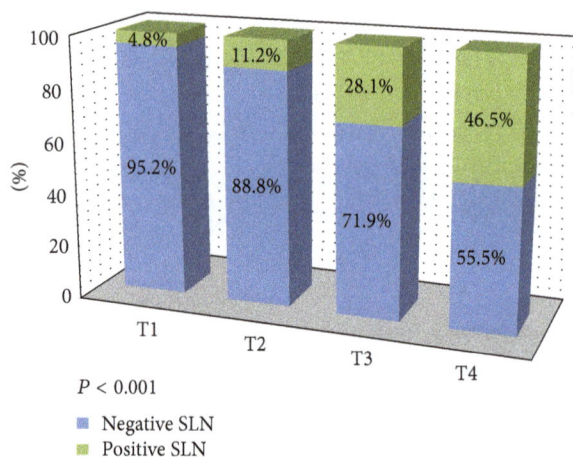

FIGURE 1: Association between Breslow category and SLN status.

Of the 21 patients in T1 stage none died of melanoma (Table 6). Instead, the cases of melanoma-related death (MRD) increased with Breslow thickness (34.9% in T4 category, $P < 0.001$).

7. Discussion

Despite the small number of patients in our study, our major findings are consistent with previous large trials. In particular, the SLNB positivity rate and the percentage of additional lymph node metastasis reported in the previous literature are both about 20%, in line with our results [3, 5].

Some authors have questioned the role of SLN biopsy in melanoma management. Multicentre selective lymphadenectomy trial I (MSLT-I) showed that patients with positive SLNB who underwent immediate CLND had higher survival rates than those who only had lymph node dissection if clinical disease appeared (72% versus 52%) [1]. This result highlights the staging and prognostic value of SLN biopsy, with an attempted intervention when the nodal tumor burden in SLN positive patients is lower compared with clinically detected nodal metastases. Our results confirm the predictive significance of Breslow thickness and support the efficacy of SLN biopsy as a staging and prognostic procedure.

The previous literature shows conflicting results among predictors of positive SLNB. This reflects in part the heterogeneity in the measurement of the variables used in different studies, especially in the histological variables for which there is no standardized reporting [12].

Despite these findings, the practical indications for an SLNB have not substantially changed in the last years. Nowadays, an SLNB is formally recommended for patients over the stage IB in the AJCC melanoma staging system [10]. Stage IB includes cutaneous melanomas greater than 1 mm in thickness, or thinner melanomas that also have ulceration or at least 1 mitosis per millimeter squared [13]. An SLNB biopsy should also be discussed and considered for patients with stage IA (≤1 mm in Breslow thickness and no ulceration or mitoses) if adverse prognostic features are present [10]. Although there is no consensus about what defines "adverse prognostic features," such features could include thickness over 0.75 mm, positive deep margins, lymphovascular invasion, or young age [10]. Although only 5% of positive SLNB results are found in T1 melanomas, a small group of patients will benefit from a therapeutic procedure such as CLND, or inclusion in control trials [14–16]. This explains our low threshold for an SLNB, and our results are consistent with other studies. As expected, we find that this subset of patients has a better prognosis, with no melanoma-related death among the 21 patients staged in T1.

The interaction between different factors is complex. Cadili and Dabbs (2010) found a higher rate of SLN metastasis in nodular melanoma, and they hypothesized an inherent biological characteristic of nodular melanomas as an explanation for this finding [12]. In addition, the presence of lymphocytic infiltrate was associated with a lower likelihood of a positive SLNB, which highlights its protector value against SLN metastasis [4, 17]. In contrast to other studies, we did not find any association of SLN positivity with age, even after stratification by age groups.

The SLN status was shown to be a highly significant prognostic factor of overall survival, with a 5-year survival of about 88% in patients with negative SLNB and 53% in those with positive SLNB. It is worth noting that factors predictive of SLN metastasis are similar to the prognostic factors for survival in melanoma patients [17]. The impact of SLN tumor features on survival is controversial. Some authors have demonstrated that the prognosis of SLN positive patients correlates with sentinel node tumor features, such as the maximum size of metastatic foci, intranodal location of tumor, extranodal spread, and perinodal lymphatic invasion [18–21].

TABLE 3: Local recurrence and melanoma-related death.

	Total N (%)/mean (±SD)	Negative SLN N (%)/mean (±SD)	Positive SLN N (%)/mean (±SD)	OR (95% CI)	P value*
Local recurrence	24 (11)	8 (4.7)	16 (34.8)	10.93 (4.30–27.81)	<0.001¥
Time to local recurrence (median, months)	15.6 (±13.7)	17.8 (±19.0)	14.7 (±9.9)	—	NS†
Melanoma-related death	33 (14.9)	16 (9.2)	17 (35.4)	5.38 (2.46–11.78)	<0.001¥

NS: not statistically significant; CI: confidence interval; *P value of the Chi-square test (¥) or t-Student's test (†) as appropriate.

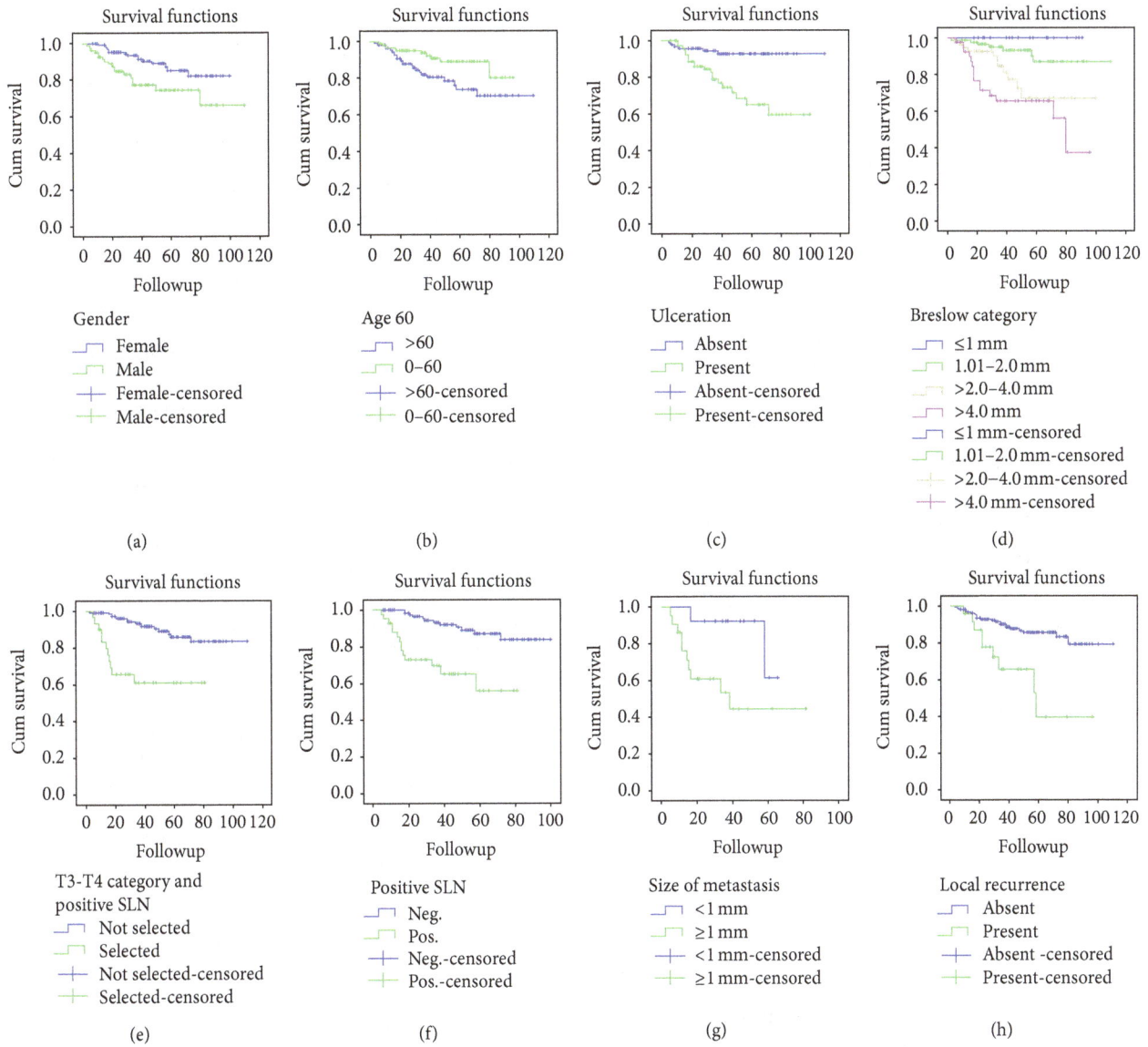

FIGURE 2: Association of melanoma-specific survival with clinical and pathological parameters. Survival estimates using Kaplan-Meier method; significance levels (P values) calculated using logrank tests. Not selected: all patients who are not positive SLN and T3 or T4 Breslow's category.

Positivity of CLND was not significantly associated with a worse prognosis, perhaps due to the small sample in our study. To point out that the prognostic impact of local recurrence (peritumoral skin) was lost after adjustment for the others factors.

We share our clinical experience in 7 years of SLNB practice for cutaneous melanoma. This study has some limitations, as it is based on a relatively small sample and the variables were assessed retrospectively. Moreover, information about the mitotic rate, a recently T1b criterion [22], was

TABLE 4: Multivariate analysis of factors predicting a positive SLN.

Factor	Adjusted odds ratio (95% CI)	P value
Male gender	2.01 (0.77–5.22)	0.154
Breslow thickness (per mm)	1.12 (1.03–1.34)	0.020
Histologic type		
Superficial spreading	1.00*	
Nodular	3.35 (1.21–1.70)	0.193
Acral lentiginous	5.41 (1.69–3.44)	0.640
Unknown/others (spitzoid, desmoplastic, nevoid, amelanotic)	0.57 (0.57–0.27)	0.602
Tumor-infiltrating lymphocytes (absence)	2.77 (1.06–7.24)	0.038

CI: confidence interval; *this group served as the reference group.

TABLE 5: Cox multivariate analysis of the factors that were significant predictors of melanoma-related death.

Factor	Melanoma-related death	
	Hazard ratio (95% CI)	P value
Age (per yr of age)	1.011 (0.018–0.361)	NS
Gender (male versus female)	1.486 (0.450–0.774)	NS
Ulceration (present versus absent)	2.124 (0.541–1.937)	NS
Breslow thickness (per mm)	1.216 (1.118–1.323)	<0.001
SLN status (positive versus negative)	2.901 (1.254–6.713)	<0.001
Local recurrence	0.365 (0.591–2.914)	NS

CI: confidence interval; NS: not statistically significant.

TABLE 6: Melanoma-related death (MRD) and Breslow thickness.

Breslow category	Total (N)	MRD (N, %)
T1 (≤1 mm)	21	0
T2 (1.01–2.0 mm)	89	7 (7.9%)
T3 (2.01–4.0 mm)	57	11 (19.3%)
T4 (>4.0 mm)	43	15 (34.9%)
Total	210	33

not always present, and some incomplete histological reports did not allow to incorporate more variables for statistical treatment.

An interesting particularity in our melanoma patient's population is a remarkable high number of melanomas on the lower limbs, mainly on the feet (21.3% of all cases). The biological behavior of melanoma is influenced by numerous factors (genetic, environment) which can vary from one region to another. It is thus worth knowing more about our particular population, combining clinical and histological features, and identifying subgroups of patients to allow for an individual clinical decision supported by evidence-based guidelines.

Acknowledgment

The authors are indebted to Dr. Margarida Marques, Department of Informatics, Coimbra University Hospital, for her assistance with the statistical analysis.

References

[1] D. L. Morton, J. F. Thompson, A. J. Cochran et al., "Sentinel-node biopsy or nodal observation in melanoma," *The New England Journal of Medicine*, vol. 355, no. 13, pp. 1307–1317, 2006.

[2] J. F. Thompson and H. M. Shaw, "Sentinel node mapping for melanoma: results of trials and current applications," *Surgical Oncology Clinics of North America*, vol. 16, no. 1, pp. 35–54, 2007.

[3] J. H. Lee, R. Essner, H. Torisu-Itakura, L. Wanek, H. Wang, and D. L. Morton, "Factors predictive of tumor-positive nonsentinel lymph nodes after tumor-positive sentinel lymph node dissection for melanoma," *Journal of Clinical Oncology*, vol. 22, no. 18, pp. 3677–3684, 2004.

[4] J. E. Gershenwald, W. Thompson, P. F. Mansfield et al., "Multi-institutional melanoma lymphatic mapping experience: the prognostic value of sentinel lymph node status in 612 stage I or II melanoma patients," *Journal of Clinical Oncology*, vol. 17, no. 3, pp. 976–983, 1999.

[5] L. L. Kruper, F. R. Spitz, B. J. Czerniecki et al., "Predicting sentinel node status in AJCC stage I/II primary cutaneous melanoma," *Cancer*, vol. 107, no. 10, pp. 2436–2445, 2006.

[6] L. Kretschmer, H. Starz, K.-M. Thoms et al., "Age as a key factor influencing metastasizing patterns and disease-specific survival after sentinel lymph node biopsy for cutaneous melanoma," *International Journal of Cancer*, vol. 129, no. 6, pp. 1435–1442, 2011.

[7] R. L. White Jr, G. D. Ayers, V. H. Stell et al., "Factors predictive of the status of sentinel lymph nodes in melanoma patients from a large multicenterdatabase," *Annals of Surgical Oncology*, vol. 8, no. 13, pp. 3593–3600, 2011.

[8] S. C. Paek, K. A. Griffith, T. M. Johnson et al., "The impact of factors beyond breslow depth on predicting sentinel lymph node positivity in melanoma," *Cancer*, vol. 109, no. 1, pp. 100–108, 2007.

[9] Z. I. Nowecki, P. Rutkowski, A. Nasierowska-Guttmejer, and W. Ruka, "Sentinel lymph node biopsy in melanoma patients with clinically negative regional lymph nodes—one institution's experience," *Melanoma Research*, vol. 13, no. 1, pp. 35–43, 2003.

[10] "NCCN Clinical Practice Guidelines in Oncology (NCCN Guidelines): melanoma," Version v1.2013, 2012.

[11] R. E. Emery, J. S. Stevens, R. W. Nance, C. L. Corless, and J. T. Vetto, "Sentinel node staging of primary melanoma by the "10% rule": pathology and clinical outcomes," *American Journal of Surgery*, vol. 193, no. 5, pp. 618–622, 2007.

[12] A. Cadili and K. Dabbs, "Predictors of sentinel lymph node metastasis in melanoma," *Canadian Journal of Surgery*, vol. 53, no. 1, pp. 32–36, 2010.

[13] American Joint Committee on Cancer, *Cancer Staging Handbook*, Springer, New York, NY, USA, 7th edition, 2010.

[14] J. M. Ranieri, J. D. Wagner, S. Wenck, C. S. Johnson, and J. J. Coleman III, "The prognostic importance of sentinel lymph node biopsy in thin melanoma," *Annals of Surgical Oncology*, vol. 13, no. 7, pp. 927–932, 2006.

[15] S. S. Venna, S. Thummala, M. Nosrati et al., "Analysis of sentinel lymph node positivity in patients with thin primary melanoma," *Journal of the American Academy of Dermatology*, vol. 68, no. 4, pp. 560–567, 2013.

[16] R. H. I. Andtbacka and J. E. Gershenwald, "Role of sentinel lymph node biopsy in patients with thin melanoma," *Journal of the National Comprehensive Cancer Network*, vol. 7, no. 3, pp. 308–317, 2009.

[17] R. C. Taylor, A. Patel, K. S. Panageas, K. J. Busam, and M. S. Brady, "Tumor-infiltrating lymphocytes predict sentinel lymph node positivity in patients with cutaneous melanoma," *Journal of Clinical Oncology*, vol. 25, no. 7, pp. 869–875, 2007.

[18] M. Wiener, K. M. Acland, H. M. Shaw et al., "Sentinel node positive melanoma patients: prediction and prognostic significance of nonsentinel node metastases and development of a survival tree model," *Annals of Surgical Oncology*, vol. 17, no. 8, pp. 1995–2005, 2010.

[19] A. A. Ghaferi, S. L. Wong, T. M. Johnson et al., "Prognostic significance of a positive nonsentinel lymph node in cutaneous melanoma," *Annals of Surgical Oncology*, vol. 16, no. 11, pp. 2978–2984, 2009.

[20] E. H. Wright, P. R. W. Stanley, and A. Roy, "Evaluation of sentinel lymph nodes positive for melanoma for features predictive of non-sentinel nodal disease and patient prognosis: a 49 patient series," *Journal of Plastic, Reconstructive and Aesthetic Surgery*, vol. 63, no. 5, pp. e500–e502, 2010.

[21] R. Murali, C. Desilva, J. F. Thompson, and R. A. Scolyer, "Factors predicting recurrence and survival in sentinel lymph node-positive melanoma patients," *Annals of Surgery*, vol. 253, no. 6, pp. 1155–1164, 2011.

[22] C. M. Balch, J. E. Gershenwald, S.-J. Soong et al., "Final version of 2009 AJCC melanoma staging and classification," *Journal of Clinical Oncology*, vol. 27, no. 36, pp. 6199–6206, 2009.

21

Diet and Skin Cancer: The Potential Role of Dietary Antioxidants in Nonmelanoma Skin Cancer Prevention

Rajani Katta[1] and Danielle Nicole Brown[2]

[1]Department of Dermatology, Baylor College of Medicine, 1977 Butler Boulevard, Suite E6.200, Houston, TX 77030, USA
[2]Department of Dermatology, Baylor College of Medicine, Houston, TX 77030, USA

Correspondence should be addressed to Rajani Katta; rkatta@bcm.edu

Academic Editor: Silvia Moretti

Nonmelanoma skin cancer (NMSC) is the most common cancer among Americans. Ultraviolet (UV) radiation exposure is the major risk factor for the development of NMSC. Dietary AOs may prevent free radical-mediated DNA damage and tumorigenesis secondary to UV radiation. Numerous laboratory studies have found that certain dietary AOs show significant promise in skin cancer prevention. These results have been substantiated by animal studies. In human studies, researchers have evaluated both oral AO supplements and dietary intake of AOs via whole foods. In this review, we provide an overview of the role of AOs in preventing tumorigenesis and outline four targeted dietary AOs. We review the results of research evaluating oral AOs supplements as compared to dietary AOs intake via whole foods. While these specific supplements have not shown efficacy, intake of AOs via consumption of whole foods has shown some promise. Lessons learned from the field of hypertension research may provide important guidance in future study design. Further research on the role of dietary AOs in the prevention of NMSC is warranted and should focus on intake via whole food consumption.

1. Introduction

Nonmelanoma skin cancer (NMSC) is the most common cancer among Americans. The number of cases of NMSC, which includes basal cell carcinoma (BCC) and squamous cell carcinoma (SCC), exceeds that of breast, lung, prostate, and colon cancer combined. Ultraviolet (UV) exposure is the major risk factor for the development of skin cancer, and while public health campaigns have been somewhat successful in modifying the behaviors that increase UV exposure, there is still significant exposure that occurs through intentional tanning, use of tanning beds, and incidental exposure. Researchers have therefore studied other avenues of skin cancer prevention, including dietary modification through the intake of antioxidants (AOs).

In this review, we provide an overview of the role of dietary AOs in preventing tumorigenesis. Laboratory and animal studies have outlined potential mechanisms of action and have shown promise. There have been a limited number of large, longer-term human studies, and these have evaluated four AOs in depth. Researchers have also begun to evaluate the dietary intake of AOs via whole foods. While these specific supplements have not shown efficacy, intake of AOs via consumption of whole foods has shown some promise. Lessons learned from the field of hypertension research may provide important guidance in future study design. Further research on the role of dietary AOs in the prevention of NMSC is warranted. While such research may include evaluation of other supplements, or combinations of supplements, it must include further evaluation of intake of dietary AOs via whole food consumption.

2. Antioxidants and Their Role in Photocarcinogenesis

NMSC tumorigenesis is an extended, multistage process, consisting of initiation, promotion, and progression. Damage from free radicals is known to play a role in the initiation of this process [1]. UV radiation and exposure to environmental pollution generate free radicals. Both UVA and UVB radiation induce DNA damage; however, UVA radiation is more associated with free radical-mediated damage [1].

Free radicals are molecules that contain unpaired electrons and induce direct oxidative damage to proteins, lipids, and DNA. Most free radicals in the body exist in the form of reactive oxygen species (ROS) [1]. ROS are known to damage the bases and deoxyribosyl backbone of DNA [2]. More specifically, free radicals (mainly as singlet oxygen or hydroxyl radicals) damage DNA through the formation of oxidized pyrimidine bases and single strand DNA breaks [3]. This DNA damage may lead to tumorigenesis.

Free radicals damage not only DNA, but also cellular proteins and lipids. Direct oxidation of enzymatic proteins leads to activation of pathways that produce new proteins. These processes can increase cell proliferation and inflammation [4]. Free radical-mediated peroxidation of lipids promotes destruction of the cell phospholipid bilayer. Through these mechanisms, the accumulation of oxidative stress has been found to promote apoptosis [5].

Furthermore, UV radiation can lead to immunosuppression, hampering the ability of immune cells to recognize and combat cancer cells. As tumorigenesis progresses, other biochemical changes can result in increased angiogenesis and capacity for tumor invasion [6].

AOs combat these processes. They work through a number of mechanisms that prevent these oxidative reactions and subsequent DNA and cellular damage. Some have also been shown to act through upregulation of genes encoding for enzymes, which are capable of neutralizing ROS [7]. There are many naturally present AOs in the skin, and there exists a decreasing concentration gradient of these substances from the epidermis to the dermis [8]. These innate skin AOs include enzymes such as superoxide dismutase and glutathione peroxidase, as well as nonenzymatic substances such as vitamin C and vitamin E [1, 9].

While the body has mechanisms in place to neutralize ROS, accumulative oxidative stress from UV exposure can inundate these mechanisms. Therefore, researchers have turned to exogenous AOs. Preliminary studies in humans have shown that individuals with BCC have higher serum markers of oxidative stress and lower serum levels of dietary AOs [10]. Therefore, dietary AOs have been evaluated for their potential efficacy at reducing UVA-induced photocarcinogenesis.

Multiple animal studies, some ranging back decades, have found that AOs provide protection against skin cancer. Some have focused on supplementation with single AOs, while others have focused on varying combinations. In hairless mice exposed to UV light, a significant reduction in incidence of malignant and precancerous lesions was seen in mice that had received supplemental vitamin C in the diet [11]. In another study of mice exposed to a topical carcinogen, supplementation with beta-carotene reduced the number of tumors by 32%, while vitamin E supplementation reduced number of tumors by 25% [12]. In another study, selenium supplementation in the diet prior and during UV irradiation of mice was shown to provide significant dose-dependent protection against skin cancer [13].

In another study of hairless mice exposed to UV radiation, 30% of the mice fed a regular diet developed frank SCC, while only 7% of those fed a special diet developed SCCs [14]. This diet included a mixture of vitamins C and E with glutathione and butylated hydroxytoluene. In a later study of mice treated with a potent carcinogen, a nutrient mixture added to their diet significantly inhibited the incidence and multiplicity of skin tumors. This mixture included vitamin C, selenium, green tea extract, and other naturally occurring AOs [15].

Laboratory studies and further animal studies have identified potential mechanisms of action for these effects. It is important to note that the beneficial effects noted in these studies may be dependent on other factors. In fact, researchers write that "under certain conditions both water soluble antioxidants (e.g. vitamin C and urate) and the lipid soluble antioxidant tocopherol (vitamin E), promote or even induce peroxidation [16]." For example, in vitro studies have found that in mild oxidative states and in the absence of other co-AOs such as vitamin C, vitamin E may act as a prooxidant [17]. This mechanism, and the associated potential for adverse effects of AOs, is further described in the later section detailing the biochemical process of oxidation.

While there is clear benefit in multiple laboratory and animal studies, studies performed in human subjects have provided conflicting results. While there are a large number of identified AOs, this review focuses on four specific AOs for which longer-term human studies have been performed: vitamins C and E, beta-carotene, and selenium [18].

2.1. Vitamin C. Vitamin C, or ascorbic acid, is a water-soluble vitamin present most abundantly in fruits and vegetables. It serves as a cofactor of multiple different enzymes in the human body including prolyl and lysyl hydroxylase [7]. These enzymes are essential for the synthesis, cross-linkage, and stability of collagen. Vitamin C also serves as an intracellular antioxidant, and in studies it has been shown to provide protection against UV radiation and carcinogenesis.

In a study of cultured keratinocytes, researchers found that vitamins C and E counteracted the increase in ROS induced by acute UVB irradiation, and in combination protected against UVB-induced apoptosis [19]. In normal human oral keratinocytes, researchers compared the protective roles of vitamins C and E in oxidative stress imposed by smokeless tobacco. Vitamins C and E, alone and in combination, offered significant protection [20]. Vitamin C also impacts DNA repair. In a study of human dermal fibroblasts treated with vitamin C, researchers found an increased expression of genes associated with DNA replication and repair, and the fibroblasts demonstrated faster repair of oxidatively damaged DNA bases [21].

2.2. Vitamin E. Vitamin E differs from the other AOs reviewed here in that it actually represents a group of closely related molecules. These 8 different molecules include 4 tocotrienols and 4 tocopherols [22]. These fat-soluble substances are found in foods such as soybeans and wheat germ, and the naturally occurring form D-alpha tocopherol has the greatest biological activity. When synthesized, however, it forms together with l-alpha tocopherol, and this l-isomer has less biological activity. Therefore, when referring to vitamin E, the international unit (IU) designation is utilized and refers to the same level of biological activity, regardless of the form of vitamin E utilized.

Vitamin E is lipid soluble and has been shown to prevent membrane lipid peroxidation by ROS. In a study of mouse keratinocytes, vitamin E treatment prior to UVB radiation was able to reduce the UVB-associated epidermal damage [23]. In human fibroblasts exposed to UVA light, vitamins C and E showed photoprotective potential [24].

2.3. Carotenoids. Carotenoids are a group of plant compounds which impart a bright color to the different fruits and vegetables in which they are found, such as carrots, squash, and sweet potatoes. There are hundreds of carotenoids, with about 40 said to be present in the typical human diet [25]. Beta-carotene stands as the most studied, since in the majority of countries it is the most common carotenoid consumed.

In laboratory and animal studies, carotenoids have been shown to impact carcinogenesis, with several postulated mechanisms. Carotenoids can be converted by the body to retinoids, which have suppressed carcinogenesis in multiple animal tumor models [26].

Another mechanism focuses on the AO capabilities of carotenoids, which have the ability to quench singlet oxygen and scavenge free radicals. In a study of cells from a human liver cell line, carotenoids provided protection against oxidant-induced lipid peroxidation [27]. Of note, this protection was found to be independent of any proretinoid activity [28]. In animal studies, beta-carotene has suppressed lipid peroxidation [29, 30].

2.4. Selenium. Selenium is a trace mineral and is found in different food sources, including plants grown in soil with high selenium concentrations, as well as some meats, fish, and other sources. Selenoproteins are proteins that contain selenium in the form of an amino acid. In knockout mice studies, mice lacking selenoproteins in keratinocytes developed skin abnormalities, and it was found that selenoproteins are essential AOs which play an important role in keratinocyte growth and viability [31].

In laboratory studies, selenium has demonstrated effects against carcinogenesis. Selenium derivatives have induced apoptosis in different human tumour-derived cell lines, including skin cancer [32]. In a mouse carcinogenesis model, a selenium compound significantly reduced preneoplastic skin lesions, with significant decrease in cell proliferation and significant enhancement of apoptosis [33]. In the same carcinogenesis model, treatment with selenium also resulted in inhibition of lipid peroxidation in skin, as well as elevation of AO enzymes, including catalase and superoxide dismutase [34].

3. Human Subject Studies: Antioxidant Supplements

There are four AO supplements for which large, longer-term human research studies are available. Studies of these four supplements in humans have not supported their role in skin cancer prevention. Randomized controlled trials (RCT) of beta-carotene, selenium, and combination supplements (including various combinations of vitamin C, vitamin E, beta-carotene, selenium, and other substances) have not been shown to reduce the incidence of NMSC in men or women [35–41]. Details of these studies are provided in Table 1.

4. Human Subject Studies: Estimated Dietary Intake via Supplements Combined with Food

Studies estimating dietary intake of AOs via the combination of supplements and whole foods have not shown promise in reducing the incidence of NMSC (Table 2). However, these studies have considered the intake of AOs to be simply additive. Research supports the idea that AOs provided in the form of isolated supplements function in a different manner than that provided in the form of whole foods. Therefore, it would be ideal to differentiate between these forms of AO intake.

5. Human Subject Studies: Serum Levels

At this time, there are limited studies evaluating serum levels of these specific AOs in NMSC prevention (Table 3). The largest of these studies is a cohort study of 485 adults.

Conflicting results have been seen in these small studies. In addition, the issue of timing when performing serum studies is an important one. While in one study lower than mean selenium levels were associated with skin cancer, it was noted that neoplastic tissue sequesters selenium [42]. This may then lower serum levels, thus magnifying the importance of timing when performing serum studies.

In addition, it is not known how well serum AO levels reflect dietary intake. In the case of serum cholesterol, for example, it is well known that genetic differences can result in markedly different serum cholesterol levels despite the same level of dietary intake.

6. Human Subject Studies: Antioxidant Intake via Whole Foods

Designing a study to evaluate the effects of AO intake via whole foods is very challenging. One small, well-designed dietary intervention trial showed promise [43]. While the intervention did result in increased intake of vitamin C, beta-carotene, and fiber, the study was focused on the effects of a low-fat diet. A larger experimental study also looked at the effects of a low-fat diet. The subjects were given a dietary plan which entailed decreasing fat intake to less than 20% of caloric intake and consuming at least 5 servings of fruits and vegetables daily [44]. This study did not demonstrate efficacy, but the study design must be considered in evaluating the

TABLE 1: Experimental studies of AO supplements and NMSC incidence in human subjects.

Study	Study design	Antioxidant and other supplements studied	Effect on NMSC risk	Statistically significant results	Study location
Frieling et al., 2000 [35]	RCT of 22,071 male physicians over 12 years	50 mg beta-carotene, QOD	None	NA	USA
Duffield-Lillico et al., 2003 [36]	RCT of 1312 patients with previous NMSC over 10 years	200 mcg selenium, QD	BCC: none SCC: increased risk	BCC: NA SCC: RR: 1.14; 95% CI, 0.93–1.39	USA
Reid et al., 2008 [37]	RCT of 424 adults followed for 6 years, and a subset of 315 adults in the NPC study [37]	200 mcg selenium [NPC subset], QD	NMSC: increased risk	200 mcg cohort: RR: 1.49; 95% CI: 1.10–2.03; P: 0.008	USA
		400 mcg selenium, QD	None	NA	
Greenberg et al., 1990 [38]	RCT of 1805 patients with history of NMSC over 5 years	50 mg beta-carotene, QD	None	RR: 1.05; 95% CI, 0.91–1.22	USA
Hercberg et al., 2007 [39]	RCT of 13,017 adults followed over median of 7.5 years	Daily combination of: 120 mg vitamin C 30 mg vitamin E 6 mg beta-carotene 100 mcg selenium 20 mg zinc	BCC: none SCC: increased risk in women	BCC: NA SCC: Women: aHR: 1.68; P: 0.03	France
Vinceti et al., 2014 [40]	Meta-analysis which included 3 RCTs of NMSC	Selenium+	NMSC: increased risk	RR: 1.44; 95% CI: 0.95–1.17	Asia, Europe, US, and Australia
Chang et al., 2011 [41]	Meta-analysis of 10 RCTs	Vitamin A+ Vitamin C+ Vitamin E+ B-carotene+	None	NA	USA, Netherlands, Australia, UK, and Canada

+Dosages varied. aHR: adjusted hazard ratio; BCC: basal cell carcinoma; CI: confidence interval; NA: not applicable; NMSC: nonmelanoma skin cancer; mg: milligrams; mcg: micrograms; QD: daily dosing; QOD: every other day dosing; P: P value; RCT: randomized control trial. RR: relative rate; SCC: squamous cell carcinoma.

results. A separate prospective observational study did not focus on macronutrients (i.e., fat), but rather focused on the "combined consumption of foods," and it did find that a "vegetable and fruit" pattern decreased NMSC as opposed to a "meat and fat" pattern [45]. Details of these studies are shown in Table 4.

7. The Biochemical Process of Antioxidation: A Proposed Explanation for the Lack of Efficacy of Supplements

Given the results of large-scale, randomized, placebo-controlled trials, we conclude that these 4 AO supplements, in the reported doses and for the studied duration of intake, are not effective tools for skin cancer prevention. On the other

hand, while analysis of dietary intake of AOs via whole foods has not provided clear conclusions, some promising trends have emerged.

One reason for this reported difference in efficacy may be due to the biochemistry of AOs and their downstream effects. The process of oxidation, and correspondingly antioxidation, is not a straightforward, single-step process, nor is it a straightforward chain of events. It represents instead a finely balanced system, as has been shown in studies of beta-carotene and lung cancer.

In an interventional study, male smokers treated with beta-carotene supplements over 5–8 years had a higher incidence of lung cancer [46]. A later study of smokers also showed an increase in lung cancer among subjects taking beta-carotene supplements with vitamin A supplements [47]. Animal studies helped to identify a possible explanation. In a

TABLE 2: Observational studies of dietary intake via supplements combined with food and NMSC incidence.

Study	Study design	Method of assessing dietary intake	Antioxidant and other supplements studied	Effect on NMSC risk	Statistically significant results	Study location
van Dam et al., 2000, Health Professionals Follow-Up Study (HPFS) [64]	Prospective cohort study of 3,217 males followed for 8 years	FFQs	Retinol Vitamin C Vitamin E	BCC: no reduction	NA	USA
Fung et al., 2002, Nurses Health Study (NHS) [65]	Prospective cohort study of 85,836 women followed for 12 years	FFQs	Vitamin A Vitamin C Vitamin E B-carotene	BCC: no reduction; weakly positive trends seen	NA	USA
Fung et al., 2003 [66]	Prospective cohort study of HPFS and NHS followed women for 14 years and men for 10 years	FFQs	Retinol Vitamin A Vitamin C Vitamin E Carotenoids	SCC: no reduction	NA	USA

BCC: basal cell carcinoma; FFQs: food frequency questionnaires; NA: not applicable; NMSC: nonmelanoma skin cancer; SCC: squamous cell carcinoma.

study of ferrets exposed to smoke, markedly different effects were seen with low dose of beta-carotene supplementation (corresponding to dietary intake) versus high dose intake (corresponding to pharmacologic doses). With high doses of beta-carotene, increased cell proliferation was seen [48].

The biochemistry of this process provides an explanation. Free radicals can cause damage due to the presence of an unpaired electron. AOs such as beta-carotene may neutralize free radicals by providing an electron of their own. In the process, though, the AO itself now contains an unpaired electron. Vitamin C can act to neutralize this newly created prooxidant. Smokers, who are known to have a lower intake of vitamin C, would therefore be at higher risk from isolated beta-carotene supplements.

Further animal studies have shown that the explanation is likely to be even more complex. In cases of a limited (as opposed to a well-balanced) diet, beta-carotene supplements have resulted in significant exacerbation of UV carcinogenesis. The researchers explained that, when beta-carotene exerts its AO effects, the newly created beta-carotene radical cation contains an unpaired electron and is therefore strongly oxidizing. The researchers concluded that "the photoprotective effect of beta-carotene reported earlier by others...might depend on interaction with other dietary factors that are either absent, or present in ineffectual concentrations, in the semi-defined diet in which exacerbation of UV carcinogenesis occurs. Those factors could be other carotenoids, their isomers, or some yet unidentified phytochemical(s) [43]."

A related conclusion was drawn by Chang et al. While their meta-analysis of 10 large RCTs with vitamins and supplements known to have AO properties showed no reduction of NMSC incidence, the researchers did draw a distinction between supplements and whole foods [41]. They stated that when consumed in a fruit or vegetable, these AOs are consumed in relative quantities with one another that may be vital to their AO qualities.

8. Directions for Future Study: The Need to Study Whole Foods

Large RCTs of 4 specific AO supplements have not shown efficacy. While research is underway on the potential of other AO supplements, and combinations of AO supplements, it is imperative that future studies also target interventions that integrate dietary AOs in the form of whole foods. In this respect, much can be learned from accomplishments made in the area of diet and hypertension control. Hypertension researchers have had limited results with isolated dietary supplementation but have had success through interventions of whole foods, specifically the Dietary Approaches to Stop Hypertension (DASH) diet.

Prior to whole food investigations, one study showed that nutritional supplementation with calcium, magnesium, potassium, or fish oil had no effect on reducing blood pressure [49]. Another study found the effects from calcium supplementation alone to be too small to be clinically significant [50]. Furthermore, magnesium supplementation had equivocal results [51].

After concluding that dietary supplements lacked promise, a RCT of the DASH diet, a diet rich in fruits and vegetables and low in fat, was conducted. This diet significantly reduced both systolic and diastolic blood pressure in US adults when compared to a typical American diet [52]. Further studies have shown that the DASH diet in combination with a diet low in sodium is the most effective dietary intervention for reducing blood pressure [53].

A major reason to study whole foods is that the nutrients present in supplements are by necessity limited to those that researchers have thus far isolated, identified, and determined to be most worthy of study. As further research in the area of phytonutrients has progressed, researchers have discovered many other potential protective plant compounds.

TABLE 3: Serum AO levels and NMSC incidence.

Study	Study design	Antioxidant supplements studied	Effect on NMSC risk	Statistically significant results	Study location
Clark et al., 1984 [42]	Case-control study of 240 subjects with NMSC	Selenium	Significantly lower levels in patients with NMSC	BCC: OR: 3.91; 95% CI: 1.2–13.1	USA
Breslow et al., 1995 [67]	Nested case-control study of 30 BCC and 37 SCC patients using serum obtained prior to diagnosis of NMSC	Retinol Beta-carotene α-Tocopherol Selenium	None	NA	USA
Dorgan et al., 2004 [68]	Prospective cohort study of 302 subjects with history of BCC followed for 5 years	Carotenoids Vitamin E	None	NA	USA
van der Pols et al., 2009 [69]	Prospective cohort study of 485 Australian adults followed for 8 years	Carotenoids	None	NA	Australia
		Selenium	60% decreased incidence high serum levels	BCC: RR: 0.43; 95% CI: 0.21–0.86; P: 0.02 SCC: RR: 0.36; 85% CI: 0.15–0.82; P: 0.02	
		Vitamin E	None	NA	

BCC: basal cell carcinoma; CI: confidence interval; NA: not applicable; NMSC: nonmelanoma skin cancer; OR: odds ratio; P: P value; RR: relative rate; SCC: squamous cell carcinoma.

In vitro studies have shown that a number of other phytochemicals may have significant AO effects. Studies have found that compounds such as grape seed extract, resveratrol [from grapes], and ellagic acid [found in foods such as raspberries] are potent scavengers of superoxide radicals and that these compounds are able to protect cells from hydrogen peroxide-induced DNA damage [54]. Other laboratory and animal studies have supported the effects of multiple other phytonutrients, including curcumin (found in the spice turmeric), lycopene (found in tomatoes), and genistein (found in soy) [55, 56].

Animal studies have found that some polyphenols have the ability to protect the skin from the damaging effects of UV radiation, including a reduction in skin inflammation, oxidative stress, and DNA damage [57]. The compounds studied cover a wide range, including green tea polyphenols, grape seed proanthocyanidins, resveratrol, and genistein.

While some of these phytonutrients may be isolated and serve as the subjects of further study in the future, it is important to take into account the role of synergy. Multiple phytochemicals have demonstrated synergistic effects, as has been documented in both laboratory and animal studies. In a study of reconstituted human serum, beta-carotene, vitamin C, and vitamin E provided synergistic protection against oxidation [58]. In a study of murine skin, researchers administered various combinations of phytochemicals including topical resveratrol and oral ellagic acid, calcium D-glucarate, and grape seed extract [59]. Different combinations acted as potent inhibitors of skin tumorigenesis, and all combinations showed either additive or synergistic effects.

It is well recognized that there is a complex interplay of nutrients present in naturally occurring foods. In consuming a diet based on whole foods, the finely balanced proportion of nutrients, the large number of potentially protective compounds, and the other plant constituents (such as fiber) may all be necessary. Some compounds may potentiate the effects of others, and the role of synergy may make the whole more powerful than the sum of its parts. While there has historically been a focus on the effects of isolated nutrients in human subjects, it is just as vital, if not more so, to continue to study the effects of the entire package of interacting nutrients and substances found in whole foods.

9. Future Study Design

Studies performed to date on diet and nonmelanoma skin cancer have had notable limitations, including small sample sizes in some as well as the research methodology challenges that arise in any study of diet and cancer. To begin with, almost all studies that examine the link between diet and cancer are based on data provided by the patients. Researchers determine nutrient intake based on food frequency questionnaires (FFQ). Participants are asked to estimate their food intake over a specified time period. For example, participants may be given a FFQ which requires estimating their intake of 129 food groups over timespans of 6 months [60]. It is well-recognized that there are issues with the reliability and validity of FFQs. As one research group has stated, "Researchers now recognize that data from FFQs and other dietary assessment methods can have substantial

TABLE 4: AO intake via whole foods and NMSC incidence.

Study	Study design	Method of assessing dietary intake	Diet(s) studied	Effect on NMSC risk	Reported statistical results	Study location
Observational studies						
Ibiebele et al., 2007[a] [45]	Prospective observational study of 1360 adults followed over the course of 11 years	FFQs every 6 months	Meat & fat pattern	SCC: increased risk	RR: 3.77; 95% CI: 1.65–8.63; P: 0.002[b]	Australia
			Vegetable & fruit pattern	SCC: decreased risk by 54%[c]	RR: 0.46; 95% CI: 0.23–0.91; P: 0.02[b,c]	
van der Pols et al., 2011[a] [60]	Prospective observational study of 1056 Australian adults over the course of 11 years	FFQs every 6 months	129 different food groups	None	No significant findings among food groups	Australia
Experimental studies						
Black et al., 1995 [70]	Randomized control trial of 101 skin cancer patients followed over the course of 2 years	Complete daily food records	Low fat, high in beta-carotene, vitamin C, and fiber	Significant reduction	$P < 0.05$	USA
Gamba et al., 2013 [44]	Randomized control trial of over 48,000 postmenopausal women followed over the course of 8 years	FFQs at baseline, year one, and then every 3 years	Low fat, high in fruits, vegetables, and grains	None	NA	USA

[a]Used data from the ongoing Nambour Skin Cancer Study [71]. [b]Reported between lowest and highest tertiles of antioxidant intake. [c]In individuals with a history of skin cancer. BCC: basal cell carcinoma; CI: confidence interval; FFQs: food frequency questionnaires; NA: not applicable; NMSC: nonmelanoma skin cancer; OR: odds ratio; P: P value; RR: relative rate; SCC: squamous cell carcinoma.

measurement errors, both systematic and random, which may lead to biased disease risk estimates [61]."

Another important issue regarding dietary interventions is that of timing. Given that sunburns in childhood can influence the development of skin cancer decades later, at what point in this process are we able to successfully intervene? The duration of dietary changes necessary to impact change is not known either. Is a 1-year dietary change sufficient, or would a decade of change be necessary?

While larger studies are certainly warranted, they entail other challenges. In one RCT described earlier, over 48,000 women were randomly assigned to a control diet or a study diet [44]. Participants in the intervention arm were given a dietary plan which entailed decreasing fat intake to less than 20% of caloric intake and consuming at least 5 servings of fruits and vegetables daily. While mandatory nutritional counseling sessions were provided, only 57% of individuals in the study arm were compliant with attendance at 3 years, and only 31% were compliant at 6 years (in contrast, the control group had compliance rates of 87% and 75%). To assess dietary intake, the FFQ was used at baseline, year one, and then every three years. These limitations must be considered when evaluating these results.

Further research is warranted, and lessons learned from the DASH trial may help in future dietary intervention trials. In designing the study, researchers blindly and randomly assigned participants to one of three diets. During an initial three-week phase, participants were studied to see if they

would be fully compliant with the study design. Compliant participants then advanced to the intervention portion of the study, in which they ate one meal daily at the study center. Other meals were prepared for them to eat at home.

Adherence, reported as greater than 95% for all groups, was assessed through attendance at daily meals, daily diet diaries, and 24-hour urinary studies to verify dietary compliance. While this hypertension study was only 8 weeks in duration, it does serve as an example of a well-controlled dietary intervention in humans [52, 53, 62].

10. Conclusion

Dietary AOs may prevent free radical-mediated DNA damage and tumorigenesis secondary to UV radiation. Numerous laboratory studies have found that certain dietary AOs show significant promise in skin cancer prevention. These results have been substantiated by animal studies.

In human studies, researchers have evaluated both oral AO supplements and dietary intake of AOs via whole foods. Large RCTs of 4 specific AO supplements have been performed and have not shown efficacy. At this point in time these supplements are not recommended for NMSC prevention. Evaluation of other AO supplements, or AO combination supplements, may be warranted in the future based on laboratory and animal studies. Even this approach must be taken with caution, as research has already shown that some combinations of AOs may be linked to increased cancer risk. For example, the SU.VI.MAX trial found an increased risk of certain cancers in some subpopulations taking an AO combination supplement, specifically an increased risk of melanoma in supplemented women and an increased incidence of prostate cancer in men with an elevated prostate specific antigen at baseline [63].

In contrast, the results of human studies have indicated some promising trends when dietary AOs are provided via whole food intake. Regardless of the scientific interest in supplements, it is imperative that future studies evaluate the effects of dietary AOs provided via intake of whole foods. This is a vital area of research, especially given what we know of the mechanisms of oxidation, the evidence of benefit from many other phytonutrients in food, and the evidence of food synergy. Further research is warranted, despite the well-known challenges of studying whole food dietary interventions. In the meantime, there are many other reasons to recommend a diet strong in AOs, primarily the lack of side effects and known utility in the prevention of other cancers.

References

[1] L. Chen, J. Y. Hu, and S. Q. Wang, "The role of antioxidants in photoprotection: a critical review," *Journal of the American Academy of Dermatology*, vol. 67, no. 5, pp. 1013–1024, 2012.

[2] M. Valko, M. Izakovic, M. Mazur, C. J. Rhodes, and J. Telser, "Role of oxygen radicals in DNA damage and cancer incidence," *Molecular and Cellular Biochemistry*, vol. 266, no. 1-2, pp. 37–56, 2004.

[3] J. Cadet and T. Douki, "Oxidatively generated damage to DNA by UVA radiation in cells and human skin," *Journal of Investigative Dermatology*, vol. 131, no. 5, pp. 1005–1007, 2011.

[4] D. R. Bickers and M. Athar, "Oxidative stress in the pathogenesis of skin disease," *Journal of Investigative Dermatology*, vol. 126, no. 12, pp. 2565–2575, 2006.

[5] D. E. Godar, "UVA1 radiation triggers two different final apoptotic pathways," *Journal of Investigative Dermatology*, vol. 112, no. 1, pp. 3–12, 1999.

[6] W. L. Camp, J. W. Turnham, M. Athar, and C. A. Elmets, "New agents for prevention of ultraviolet-induced nonmelanoma skin cancer," *Seminars in Cutaneous Medicine and Surgery*, vol. 30, no. 1, pp. 6–13, 2011.

[7] E. Cadenas and L. Packer, *Handbook of Antioxidants*, Marcel Dekker, New York, NY, USA, 2nd edition, 2002.

[8] Y. Shindo, E. Witt, D. Han, W. Epstein, and L. Packer, "Enzymic and non-enzymic antioxidants in epidermis and dermis of human skin," *Journal of Investigative Dermatology*, vol. 102, no. 1, pp. 122–124, 1994.

[9] A. Godic, B. Poljšak, M. Adamic, and R. Dahmane, "The role of antioxidants in skin cancer prevention and treatment," *Oxidative Medicine and Cellular Longevity*, vol. 2014, Article ID 860479, 6 pages, 2014.

[10] B. E. De Almendra Freitas, L. L. De Castro, J. R. S. Aguiar et al., "Antioxidant capacity total in non-melanoma skin cancer and its relationship with food consumption of antioxidant nutrients," *Nutrición Hospitalaria*, vol. 31, no. 4, pp. 1682–1688, 2015.

[11] L. Pauling, R. Willoughby, R. Reynolds, B. E. Blaisdell, and S. Lawson, "Incidence of squamous cell carcinoma in hairless mice irradiated with ultraviolet light in relation to intake of ascorbic acid (vitamin C) and of D, L-alpha-tocopheryl acetate (vitamin E)," *International Journal for Vitamin and Nutrition Research Supplement*, vol. 23, pp. 53–82, 1982.

[12] L. A. Lambert, W. G. Wamer, R. R. Wei, S. Lavu, S. J. Chirtel, and A. Kornhauser, "The protective but nonsynergistic effect of dietary β-carotene and vitamin E on skin tumorigenesis in Skh mice," *Nutrition and Cancer*, vol. 21, no. 1, pp. 1–12, 1994.

[13] K. Overvad, E. B. Thorling, P. Bjerring, and P. Ebbesen, "Selenium inhibits UV-light-induced skin carcinogenesis in hairless mice," *Cancer Letters*, vol. 27, no. 2, pp. 163–170, 1985.

[14] H. S. Black and J. T. Chan, "Suppression of ultraviolet light induced tumor formation by dietary antioxidants," *Journal of Investigative Dermatology*, vol. 65, no. 4, pp. 412–414, 1975.

[15] M. W. Roomi, N. W. Roomi, T. Kalinovsky, V. Ivanov, M. Rath, and A. Niedzwiecki, "Inhibition of 7,12-dimethyl-benzanthracene-induced skin tumors by a nutrient mixture," *Medical Oncology*, vol. 25, no. 3, pp. 333–340, 2008.

[16] I. Pinchuk, H. Shoval, Y. Dotan, and D. Lichtenberg, "Evaluation of antioxidants: scope, limitations and relevance of assays," *Chemistry and Physics of Lipids*, vol. 165, no. 6, pp. 638–647, 2012.

[17] A. Kontush, B. Finckh, B. Karten, A. Kohlschütter, and U. Beisiegel, "Antioxidant and prooxidant activity of α-tocopherol in human plasma and low density lipoprotein," *Journal of Lipid Research*, vol. 37, no. 7, pp. 1436–1448, 1996.

[18] L. J. Johnson, S. L. Meacham, and L. J. Kruskall, "The antioxidants—vitamin C, vitamin E, selenium, and carotenoids," *Journal of Agromedicine*, vol. 9, no. 1, pp. 65–82, 2003.

[19] G.-H. Jin, Y. Liu, S.-Z. Jin, X.-D. Liu, and S.-Z. Liu, "UVB induced oxidative stress in human keratinocytes and protective effect of antioxidant agents," *Radiation and Environmental Biophysics*, vol. 46, no. 1, pp. 61–68, 2007.

[20] M. Bagchi, C. A. Kuszynski, J. Balmoori, S. S. Joshi, S. J. Stohs, and D. Bagchi, "Protective effects of antioxidants against smokeless tobacco-induced oxidative stress and modulation of Bcl-2 and p53 genes in human oral keratinocytes," *Free Radical Research*, vol. 35, no. 2, pp. 181–194, 2001.

[21] T. L. Duarte, M. S. Cooke, and G. D. D. Jones, "Gene expression profiling reveals new protective roles for vitamin C in human skin cells," *Free Radical Biology and Medicine*, vol. 46, no. 1, pp. 78–87, 2009.

[22] V. Treloar, "Chemoprevention and vitamin E," *Journal of the American Academy of Dermatology*, vol. 57, no. 5, p. 903, 2007.

[23] S. Maalouf, M. El-Sabban, N. Darwiche, and H. Gali-Muhtasib, "Protective effect of vitamin E on ultraviolet B light-induced damage in keratinocytes," *Molecular Carcinogenesis*, vol. 34, no. 3, pp. 121–130, 2002.

[24] E. A. Offord, J.-C. Gautier, O. Avanti et al., "Photoprotective potential of lycopene, β-carotene, vitamin E, vitamin C and carnosic acid in UVA-irradiated human skin fibroblasts," *Free Radical Biology and Medicine*, vol. 32, no. 12, pp. 1293–1303, 2002.

[25] S. A. R. Paiva, R. M. Russell, and S. K. Dutta, "β-Carotene and other carotenoids as antioxidants," *Journal of the American College of Nutrition*, vol. 18, no. 5, pp. 426–433, 1999.

[26] F. Alizadeh, A. Bolhassani, A. Khavari, S. Z. Bathaie, T. Naji, and S. A. Bidgoli, "Retinoids and their biological effects against cancer," *International Immunopharmacology*, vol. 18, no. 1, pp. 43–49, 2014.

[27] K. R. Martin, M. L. Failla, and J. C. Smith Jr., "Beta-carotene and lutein protect HepG2 human liver cells against oxidant-induced damage," *Journal of Nutrition*, vol. 126, no. 9, pp. 2098–2106, 1996.

[28] L. Lomnitski, S. Grossman, M. Bergman, Y. Sofer, and D. Sklan, "In vitro and in vivo effects of β-carotene on rat epidermal lipoxygenases," *International Journal for Vitamin and Nutrition Research*, vol. 67, no. 6, pp. 407–414, 1997.

[29] T. Iyama, A. Takasuga, and M. Azuma, "β-Carotene accumulation in mouse tissues and a protective role against lipid peroxidation," *International Journal for Vitamin and Nutrition Research*, vol. 66, no. 4, pp. 301–305, 1996.

[30] F. O. Zwald and M. Brown, "Skin cancer in solid organ transplant recipients: advances in therapy and management: part II. Management of skin cancer in solid organ transplant recipients," *Journal of the American Academy of Dermatology*, vol. 65, no. 2, pp. 263–279, 2011.

[31] A. Sengupta, U. F. Lichti, B. A. Carlson et al., "Selenoproteins are essential for proper keratinocyte function and skin development," *PLoS ONE*, vol. 5, no. 8, Article ID e12249, 2010.

[32] R. J. Jariwalla, B. Gangapurkar, and D. Nakamura, "Differential sensitivity of various human tumour-derived cell types to apoptosis by organic derivatives of selenium," *British Journal of Nutrition*, vol. 101, no. 2, pp. 182–189, 2009.

[33] R. K. Das, S. K. U. Hossain, and S. Bhattacharya, "Diphenylmethyl selenocyanate inhibits DMBA-croton oil induced two-stage mouse skin carcinogenesis by inducing apoptosis and inhibiting cutaneous cell proliferation," *Cancer Letters*, vol. 230, no. 1, pp. 90–101, 2005.

[34] R. K. Das and S. Bhattacharya, "Anti-tumour promoting activity of diphenylmethyl selenocyanate against two-stage mouse skin carcinogenesis," *Asian Pacific Journal of Cancer Prevention*, vol. 6, no. 2, pp. 181–188, 2005.

[35] U. M. Frieling, D. A. Schaumberg, T. S. Kupper, J. Muntwyler, and C. H. Hennekens, "A randomized, 12-year primary-prevention trial of beta carotene supplementation for nonmelanoma skin cancer in the physicians' health study," *Archives of Dermatology*, vol. 136, no. 2, pp. 179–184, 2000.

[36] A. J. Duffield-Lillico, E. H. Slate, M. E. Reid et al., "Selenium supplementation and secondary prevention of nonmelanoma skin cancer in a randomized trial," *Journal of the National Cancer Institute*, vol. 95, no. 19, pp. 1477–1481, 2003.

[37] M. E. Reid, A. J. Duffield-Lillico, E. Slate et al., "The nutritional prevention of cancer: 400 Mcg per day selenium treatment," *Nutrition and Cancer*, vol. 60, no. 2, pp. 155–163, 2008.

[38] E. R. Greenberg, J. A. Baron, T. A. Stukel et al., "A clinical trial of beta carotene to prevent basal-cell and squamous-cell cancers of the skin. The Skin Cancer Prevention Study Group," *The New England Journal of Medicine*, vol. 323, no. 12, pp. 789–795, 1990.

[39] S. Hercberg, K. Ezzedine, C. Guinot et al., "Antioxidant supplementation increases the risk of skin cancers in women but not in men," *Journal of Nutrition*, vol. 137, no. 9, pp. 2098–2105, 2007.

[40] M. Vinceti, G. Dennert, C. M. Crespi et al., "Selenium for preventing cancer," *The Cochrane Database of Systematic Reviews*, vol. 3, Article ID CD005195, 2014.

[41] Y. J. Chang, S.-K. Myung, S. T. Chung et al., "Effects of vitamin treatment or supplements with purported antioxidant properties on skin cancer prevention: a meta-analysis of randomized controlled trials," *Dermatology*, vol. 223, no. 1, pp. 36–44, 2011.

[42] L. C. Clark, G. F. Graham, R. G. Crounse, R. Grimson, B. Hulka, and C. M. Shy, "Plasma selenium and skin neoplasms: a case-control study," *Nutrition and Cancer*, vol. 6, no. 1, pp. 13–21, 1984.

[43] H. S. Black and J. Gerguis, "Modulation of dietary vitamins E and C fails to ameliorate β-carotene exacerbation of UV carcinogenesis in mice," *Nutrition and Cancer*, vol. 45, no. 1, pp. 36–45, 2003.

[44] C. S. Gamba, M. L. Stefanick, J. M. Shikany et al., "Low-fat diet and skin cancer risk: the women's health initiative randomized controlled dietary modification trial," *Cancer Epidemiology Biomarkers and Prevention*, vol. 22, no. 9, pp. 1509–1519, 2013.

[45] T. I. Ibiebele, J. C. van der Pols, M. C. Hughes, G. C. Marks, G. M. Williams, and A. C. Green, "Dietary pattern in association with squamous cell carcinoma of the skin: a prospective study," *American Journal of Clinical Nutrition*, vol. 85, no. 5, pp. 1401–1408, 2007.

[46] The Alpha-Tocopherol Beta Carotene Cancer Prevention Study Group, "The effect of vitamin E and beta carotene on the incidence of lung cancer and other cancers in male smokers," *The New England Journal of Medicine*, vol. 330, no. 15, pp. 1029–1035, 1994.

[47] G. S. Omenn, G. E. Goodman, M. D. Thornquist et al., "Effects of a combination of beta carotene and vitamin A on lung cancer and cardiovascular disease," *The New England Journal of Medicine*, vol. 334, no. 18, pp. 1150–1155, 1996.

[48] C. Liu, X.-D. Wang, R. T. Bronson, D. E. Smith, N. I. Krinsky, and R. M. Russell, "Effects of physiological versus pharmacological β-carotene supplementation on cell proliferation and histopathological changes in the lungs of cigarette smoke-exposed ferrets," *Carcinogenesis*, vol. 21, no. 12, pp. 2245–2253, 2000.

[49] The Trials of Hypertension Prevention Collaborative Research Group, "The effects of nonpharmacologic interventions on blood pressure of persons with high normal levels. Results of the Trials of Hypertension Prevention, phase I," *The Journal of the American Medical Association*, vol. 267, no. 9, pp. 1213–1220, 1992.

[50] P. S. Allender, J. A. Cutler, D. Follmann, F. P. Cappuccio, J. Pryer, and P. Elliott, "Dietary calcium and blood pressure: a meta-analysis of randomized clinical trials," *Annals of Internal Medicine*, vol. 124, no. 9, pp. 825–831, 1996.

[51] P. K. Whelton and M. J. Klag, "Magnesium and blood pressure: review of the epidemiologic and clinical trial experience," *The American Journal of Cardiology*, vol. 63, no. 14, pp. G26–G30, 1989.

[52] L. J. Appel, T. J. Moore, E. Obarzanek et al., "A clinical trial of the effects of dietary patterns on blood pressure," *The New England Journal of Medicine*, vol. 336, no. 16, pp. 1117–1124, 1997.

[53] F. M. Sacks, L. P. Svetkey, W. M. Vollmer et al., "Effects on blood pressure of reduced dietary sodium and the dietary approaches to stop hypertension (dash) diet," *The New England Journal of Medicine*, vol. 344, no. 1, pp. 3–10, 2001.

[54] M. C. Kowalczyk, Z. Walaszek, P. Kowalczyk, T. Kinjo, M. Hanausek, and T. J. Slaga, "Differential effects of several phytochemicals and their derivatives on murine keratinocytes *in vitro* and *in vivo*: implications for skin cancer prevention," *Carcinogenesis*, vol. 30, no. 6, pp. 1008–1015, 2009.

[55] T. I. Wright, J. M. Spencer, and F. P. Flowers, "Chemoprevention of nonmelanoma skin cancer," *Journal of the American Academy of Dermatology*, vol. 54, no. 6, pp. 933–946, 2006.

[56] M. J. Payette, J. Whalen, and J. M. Grant-Kels, "Nutrition and nonmelanoma skin cancers," *Clinics in Dermatology*, vol. 28, no. 6, pp. 650–662, 2010.

[57] J. A. Nichols and S. K. Katiyar, "Skin photoprotection by natural polyphenols: anti-inflammatory, antioxidant and DNA repair mechanisms," *Archives of Dermatological Research*, vol. 302, no. 2, pp. 71–83, 2010.

[58] K.-J. Yeum, G. Beretta, N. I. Krinsky, R. M. Russell, and G. Aldini, "Synergistic interactions of antioxidant nutrients in a biological model system," *Nutrition*, vol. 25, no. 7-8, pp. 839–846, 2009.

[59] M. C. Kowalczyk, P. Kowalczyk, O. Tolstykh, M. Hanausek, Z. Walaszek, and T. J. Slaga, "Synergistic effects of combined phytochemicals and skin cancer prevention in SENCAR mice," *Cancer Prevention Research*, vol. 3, no. 2, pp. 170–178, 2010.

[60] J. C. van der Pols, M. C. B. Hughes, T. I. Ibiebele, G. C. Marks, and A. C. Green, "Food intake and risk of basal cell carcinoma in an 11-year prospective study of Australian adults," *European Journal of Clinical Nutrition*, vol. 65, no. 1, pp. 39–46, 2011.

[61] C. L. Parr, M. B. Veierød, P. Laake, E. Lund, and A. Hjartåker, "Test-retest reproducibility of a food frequency questionnaire (FFQ) and estimated effects on disease risk in the Norwegian Women and Cancer Study (NOWAC)," *Nutrition Journal*, vol. 5, article 1, 2006.

[62] F. M. Sacks, E. Obarzanek, M. M. Windhauser et al., "Rationale and design of the Dietary Approaches to Stop Hypertension trial (DASH). A multicenter controlled-feeding study of dietary patterns to lower blood pressure," *Annals of Epidemiology*, vol. 5, no. 2, pp. 108–118, 1995.

[63] S. Hercberg, E. Kesse-Guyot, N. Druesne-Pecollo et al., "Incidence of cancers, ischemic cardiovascular diseases and mortality during 5-year follow-up after stopping antioxidant vitamins and minerals supplements: a postintervention follow-up in the SU.VI.MAX Study," *International Journal of Cancer*, vol. 127, no. 8, pp. 1875–1881, 2010.

[64] R. M. van Dam, Z. Huang, E. Giovannucci et al., "Diet and basal cell carcinoma of the skin in a prospective cohort of men," *The American Journal of Clinical Nutrition*, vol. 71, no. 1, pp. 135–141, 2000.

[65] T. T. Fung, D. J. Hunter, D. Spiegelman, G. A. Colditz, F. E. Speizer, and W. C. Willett, "Vitamins and carotenoids intake and the risk of basal cell carcinoma of the skin in women (United States)," *Cancer Causes and Control*, vol. 13, no. 3, pp. 221–230, 2002.

[66] T. T. Fung, D. Spiegelman, K. M. Egan, E. Giovannucci, D. J. Hunter, and W. C. Willett, "Vitamin and carotenoid intake and risk of squamous cell carcinoma of the skin," *International Journal of Cancer*, vol. 103, no. 1, pp. 110–115, 2003.

[67] R. A. Breslow, A. J. Alberg, K. J. Helzlsouer et al., "Serological precursors of cancer: malignant melanoma, basal and squamous cell skin cancer, and prediagnostic levels of retinol, β-carotene, lycopene, α-tocopherol, and selenium," *Cancer Epidemiology Biomarkers and Prevention*, vol. 4, no. 8, pp. 837–842, 1995.

[68] J. F. Dorgan, N. A. Boakye, T. R. Fears et al., "Serum carotenoids and alpha-tocopherol and risk of nonmelanoma skin cancer," *Cancer Epidemiology Biomarkers and Prevention*, vol. 13, no. 8, pp. 1276–1282, 2004.

[69] J. C. van der Pols, M. M. Heinen, M. C. Hughes, T. I. Ibiebele, G. C. Marks, and A. C. Green, "Serum antioxidants and skin cancer risk: an 8-year community-based follow-up study," *Cancer Epidemiology Biomarkers and Prevention*, vol. 18, no. 4, pp. 1167–1173, 2009.

[70] H. S. Black, J. I. Thornby, J. E. Wolf Jr. et al., "Evidence that a low-fat diet reduces the occurrence of non-melanoma skin cancer," *International Journal of Cancer*, vol. 62, no. 2, pp. 165–169, 1995.

[71] A. Green, G. Beardmore, V. Hart, D. Leslie, R. Marks, and D. Staines, "Skin cancer in a Queensland population," *Journal of the American Academy of Dermatology*, vol. 19, no. 6, pp. 1045–1053, 1988.

22

Comorbidity Assessment in Skin Cancer Patients: A Pilot Study Comparing Medical Interview with a Patient-Reported Questionnaire

Erica H. Lee,[1] Rajiv I. Nijhawan,[1,2] Kishwer S. Nehal,[1] Stephen W. Dusza,[1] Amanda Levine,[3] Amanda Hill,[3] and Christopher A. Barker[3]

[1]*Department of Medicine, Dermatology Service, Memorial Sloan Kettering Cancer Center, New York, NY 10022, USA*
[2]*Department of Dermatology, University of Texas Southwestern Medical Center, Dallas, TX 75390, USA*
[3]*Department of Radiation Oncology, Memorial Sloan Kettering Cancer Center, New York, NY 10065, USA*

Correspondence should be addressed to Erica H. Lee; leee@mskcc.org

Academic Editor: Lionel Larue

Background. Comorbidities are conditions that occur simultaneously but independently of another disorder. Among skin cancer patients, comorbidities are common and may influence management. *Objective.* We compared comorbidity assessment by traditional medical interview (MI) and by standardized patient-reported questionnaire based on the Adult Comorbidity Evaluation-27 (ACE-27). *Methods.* Between September 2011 and October 2013, skin cancer patients underwent prospective comorbidity assessment by a Mohs surgeon (MI) and a radiation oncologist (using a standardized patient-reported questionnaire based on the ACE-27, the PRACE-27). Comorbidities were identified and graded according to the ACE-27 and compared for agreement. *Results.* Forty-four patients were evaluated. MI and PRACE-27 identified comorbidities in 79.5% and 88.6% ($p = 0.12$) of patients, respectively. Among 27 comorbid ailments, the MI identified 9.9% as being present, while the PRACE-27 identified 12.5%. When there were discordant observations, PRACE-27 was more likely than MI to identify the comorbidity (OR = 5.4, 95% CI = 2.4–14.4, $p < 0.001$). Overall comorbidity scores were moderate or severe in 43.2% (MI) versus 59.1% (PRACE-27) ($p = 0.016$). *Limitations.* Small sample size from a single institution. *Conclusion.* Comorbidities are common in skin cancer patients, and a standardized questionnaire may better identify and grade them. More accurate comorbidity assessments may help guide skin cancer management.

1. Background

Skin cancer is the most common malignancy worldwide. Management recommendations rely primarily on characteristics of the cancer and patient. One important patient characteristic is comorbidity or the simultaneous presence of a medical condition independent of skin cancer. Comorbidities have been shown to predict outcomes such as infection rates, quality of life, life expectancy, and complications in cancer management, with a trend indicating inferior outcomes in individuals with additional comorbidities [1–5]. Comorbidity severity has been shown to guide treatment selection in a range of conditions from oral cancer to end-stage renal disease [6–9].

A method for assessing comorbidity in a standardized fashion could be valuable in the management of skin cancer patients; however, there are no specific tools for comorbidity evaluation for this population. The Charlson Comorbidity Index (CCI), a validated measure to predict survival, is frequently cited in publications [10]. A recent study evaluated comorbidities in patients ≥90 years old treated with Mohs micrographic surgery (MMS) and found no significant difference in survival among patients with and without comorbidities [11]. On the contrary, another study assessed patients ≥80 years old who underwent dermatologic surgery and found that comorbidities were associated with increased mortality [12]. Similarly, a study of those 90–99 years of age treated with Mohs surgery reported that patients with CCI scores of zero (no comorbidities) had longer survival compared to patients with CCI of three (advanced comorbidities) [13].

In addition to the CCI, there are several validated tools used to assess comorbidity such as the Kaplan-Feinstein Index, Adult Comorbidity Evaluation-27 (ACE-27), and the Elixhauser Comorbidity Measure [14–18]. In the general cancer population, the ACE-27 is a validated instrument used to identify and grade 27 comorbidities among nine organ systems plus substance abuse, obesity, and malignancy [14]. It was developed through modification of the Kaplan-Feinstein Comorbidity Index and validated in 19,268 cancer patients treated at Barnes-Jewish Hospital [5]. Studies have shown that the ACE-27 can detect comorbidities more often than the CCI [19–21] and also led to deviations from standard management in patients with comorbidities that were detected by the ACE-27 [9, 22].

In this pilot study, we sought to compare comorbidity assessments collected by the traditional medical interview (MI) in a dermatologic surgery practice and by a standardized patient-reported questionnaire based on the ACE-27 (referred to as PRACE-27 in this paper) ascertained by a radiation oncologist. We specifically used ACE-27 given its validation in a variety of cancer populations, its comprehensive approach, and its application using retrospective note review by cancer registrars [23, 24]. The objectives of this pilot study were to (1) assess the frequency, severity, and type of comorbidities among skin cancer patients presenting for outpatient management and (2) identify discrepancies in comorbidity assessment between MI and PRACE-27.

2. Methods

IRB exemption was obtained at Memorial Sloan Kettering Cancer Center. All patients with a biopsy proven skin cancer evaluated by both a radiation oncologist (CB) and one of two dermatologic surgeons (KN, EL) within a six month period between September 2011 and October 2013 were identified. Comorbidities were ascertained in a prospective manner using one of two techniques. The Mohs surgeons characterized comorbidities through a traditional medical interview (MI). The radiation oncologist performed comorbidity assessment by a patient-reported questionnaire based on the ACE-27 (referred to as PRACE-27).

Medical records were retrospectively reviewed and comorbidities were identified and graded according to the ACE-27. Individual organ systems and diseases were assessed based on specific criteria outlined by the grading guidelines on the following scale: 0 = no disease, grade 1 = mild decompensation, grade 2 = moderate decompensation, and grade 3 = severe decompensation. Based on the grading of the individual organ systems, an overall comorbidity score was calculated on a scale from 0 (no comorbidity) to 3 (severe comorbidity).

2.1. Statistical Analysis. The distributions of assessments for the twenty-seven comorbidities were evaluated for MI and PRACE-27. Cross-classifications between MI and PRACE-27 were completed to assess comorbidity prevalence, percent

agreement, kappa, and weighted kappa. The kappa (κ) value interpretations were graded as poor ($\kappa < 0.2$), fair ($\kappa = 0.2$–0.4), moderate ($\kappa = 0.41$–0.6), substantial ($\kappa = 0.61$–0.8), or excellent ($\kappa = 0.81$–1.0). McNemar's Chi-square and odds ratios with 95% confidence intervals were estimated for the paired observations. Trends in survival were also assessed. All statistical analyses were performed with Stata v.12.1, Stata Corporation, College Station, TX.

3. Results

Forty-four patients were studied. Patient demographic, cancer, and comorbidity data are listed in Table 1. Overall, 79.5% and 88.6% ($p = 0.12$) of patients were identified as having a comorbidity, according to the MI and PRACE-27, respectively. The most common comorbid ailments were hypertension, solid tumor, respiratory disease, and cardiac arrhythmia. Overall comorbidity scores were moderate or severe (scores of 2 or 3) in 43.2% (MI) versus 59.1% (PRACE-27) of patients, and this difference was statistically significant ($p = 0.016$; difference in paired proportions = 0.159 (95% CI: 0.028–0.29)).

As noted in Table 2, percent agreement and kappa scores for comorbidity identification in comorbid ailments between the MI and PRACE-27 were excellent (96%, range: 77.3–100%, kappa = 0.81). Among the comorbid ailments assessed by the ACE-27, 9.9% were identified using MI, while 12.5% were identified using the PRACE-27. When there were discordant observations, PRACE-27 was more likely than MI to identify the comorbidity (OR = 5.4, 95% CI = 2.4–14.4, $p < 0.001$). The respiratory system had the lowest percent agreement (94.7%), and, for this organ system, 10 patients were graded at a higher severity with the PRACE-27 compared to the MI. Table 3 presents the percent agreement and kappa between MI and PRACE-27 assessments for data grouped by organ system.

The PRACE-27 identified 4 patients (9%) with one or more comorbidities (related to respiratory disease, obesity, and gastrointestinal disease) that the MI identified as having no comorbidity, compared to 3 patients (6.8%) identified by the MI (related to solid organ malignancy) that was missed by the PRACE-27 ($p = 0.38$). PRACE-27 identified a greater severity of comorbidity when both assessments agreed to its presence. PRACE-27 rated 8 patients with a higher severity than the MI, whereas MI did not increase the severity score for any patients compared to PRACE-27. While there were discrepancies in the comorbidity grading severity of individual organ systems, the agreement in the overall comorbidity score for the patients was high (91.7%, $p < 0.001$) (Table 4).

The median follow-up for the 44 patients was 1.9 years from the first comorbidity assessment to the most recent follow-up. There were 7 deaths of which 5 (71.4%) were graded by the PRACE-7 as severe (i.e., 3) and 3 (42.8%) were graded by the MI as severe. Across comorbidity groups, there was a trend for lower survival for higher comorbidities that was significant for both the PRACE-7 and the MI groups ($p < 0.05$). Two-year survival rates were estimated as 100%,

TABLE 1: Patient demographic data, lesion information, and comorbidity data.

Demographic data							
Average age in years (median; range)				73.5 (76; 25–94)			
Female				22 (50.0%)			
Male				22 (50.0%)			

Diagnoses							
Basal cell carcinoma				22 (50.0%)			
Squamous cell carcinoma				12 (27.3%)			
Melanoma				7 (15.9%)			
Dermatofibrosarcoma protuberans				1 (2.3%)			
Merkel cell carcinoma				1 (2.3%)			
Microcystic adnexal carcinoma				1 (2.3%)			

Comorbidity data MI versus PRACE-27							
	MI				PRACE-27		
	0	1	2	3	0	1	2	3
Comorbid ailment								
Myocardial infarction	43	1	—	—	40	2	2	—
Angina/coronary artery disease	38	6	—	—	37	5	2	—
Congestive heart failure	44	—	—	—	42	—	2	—
Arrhythmias	36	—	8	—	35	1	8	—
Hypertension	22	22	—	—	19	20	5	—
Venous disease	40	2	1	1	40	1	2	1
Peripheral arterial disease	44	—	—	—	42	—	2	—
Respiratory system	42	1	1	—	34	6	2	2
Hepatic	44	—	—	—	43	—	—	1
Stomach/intestine	44	—	—	—	44	—	—	—
Pancreas	44	—	—	—	44	—	—	—
End-stage renal disease	44	—	—	—	44	—	—	—
Diabetes mellitus	39	3	2	—	39	2	1	2
Stroke	39	3	2	—	37	6	1	—
Dementia	41	2	—	1	41	1	1	1
Paralysis	43	1	—	—	41	2	—	1
Neuromuscular	41	2	—	1	40	2	—	2
Psychiatric	42	2	—	—	42	1	1	—
Rheumatologic	44	—	—	—	43	1	—	—
AIDS	44	—	—	—	44	—	—	—
Solid tumor including melanoma	28	9	6	1	31	7	4	2
Leukemia and myeloma	42	1	1	—	42	1	1	—
Lymphoma	41	3	—	—	41	2	—	1
Alcohol	44	—	—	—	44	—	—	—
Illicit drugs	44	—	—	—	44	—	—	—
Obesity	44	—	—	—	41	—	3	—
Overall comorbidity score	9	16	12	7	5	13	13	13

The comorbidity data section compares the number of patients identified as having a comorbid ailment between the MI and PRACE-27. Individual organ systems and diseases were assessed based on specific criteria outlined by the grading guidelines on the following scale: 0 = no disease, grade 1 = mild decompensation, grade 2 = moderate decompensation, and grade 3 = severe decompensation. Based on the grading of these individual organ systems, an overall comorbidity score was calculated on a scale from 0 (no comorbidity) to 3 (severe comorbidity).

92%, 91%, and 68% for grades 0, 1, 2, and 3 using the PRACE-27. Two-year survival rates were 100%, 86%, 91%, and 57% for grades 0, 1, 2, and 3 using the MI. These estimations are relatively similar to previously published estimations using the ACE-27: grade 0 (83%), grade 1 (80%), grade 2 (72%), and grade 3 (66%) [5].

4. Comment

The National Comprehensive Cancer Network (NCCN) emphasizes the importance of collecting and measuring comorbidities in cancer patients to guide medical care and for research. For skin cancer patients, comorbidities are

TABLE 2: Comorbid ailments captured and missed by medical interview (MI) and PRACE-27 in individual organ systems.

	Medical interview		Total
	Present	Absent	
PRACE-27			
Present	111	**38**	149
Absent	7	1032	1039
Total	118	1070	1188

There are a total of 1,188 possibilities for comorbid ailments to be identified among the forty-four patients in this study since each patient can potentially have twenty-seven comorbidities ($44 \times 27 = 1,188$). Both MI and PRACE-27 agreed upon 111 comorbidities being present and 1032 being absent. However, PRACE-27 identified 38 comorbidities that were deemed as being absent by MI while MI identified 7 comorbidities that were deemed absent by PRACE-27 [OR = 5.4, 95% CI: 2.4–14.4, $p < 0.001$].

TABLE 3: Percent agreement and kappa between medical interview (MI) and PRACE-27 assessments for data grouped by disease system and overall comorbidity scores.

Organ system	Percent agreement	Kappa	p value
Cardiovascular	98.7	0.80	<0.001
Respiratory	94.7	0.40	<0.001
Gastrointestinal	99.2	—	—
Renal	100	—	—
Endocrine	98.7	0.84	<0.001
Neurologic	98.8	0.77	<0.001
Psychiatric	96.0	−0.04	0.62
Rheumatologic	97.7	—	—
Immunological	100	—	—
Malignancy	98.7	0.84	<0.001
Substance abuse	100	—	—
Obesity	100	—	—

most commonly assessed using standard medical interview (MI) and rarely graded with a standardized approach. We sought to compare comorbidity collection between MI and a standardized patient-reported questionnaire based on the ACE-27 (PRACE-27).

Identification and agreement of comorbidities across 27 ailments as they relate to individual organ systems were high between the two data collection methods; however, PRACE-27 was more likely than MI to identify the existence of an ailment and determine that an ailment was of a greater severity. However, MI appeared to identify solid tumor malignancies more frequently, suggesting that additional attention to capture this ailment may be needed when using the PRACE-27. Nevertheless, the systematic collection of comorbidities with a questionnaire (e.g., PRACE-27) ensures that all organ systems are comprehensively queried. Severity grading may also provide a more accurate assessment of disease status, the overall picture of a patient's health, and potential survival status. Based on this pilot study, a standardized patient-reported questionnaire may better identify and grade individual comorbidities in skin cancer patients compared to standard MI. The concordance in the overall

comorbidity score, which is most commonly used to predict outcomes, was also high, suggesting that the PRACE-27 is an accurate assessment of comorbidities, compared to the gold-standard MI [25].

Comorbidity assessment using ACE-27 has been reported to be predictive of treatment modifications. In a study of cancer patients evaluated by a radiation oncologist, a change in treatment plan was noted for patients with moderate or severe indices more often than those with none or mild indices, while age had no contribution to predicting treatment change [22]. Comorbidity grading may similarly guide multidisciplinary management in the skin cancer population. Importantly, in skin cancer populations, patients with less comorbidity have also been shown to have better skin-related quality of life after treatment of both non-melanoma skin cancer (NMSC) and localized melanoma [26, 27]. However, the data is limited in the skin cancer population and additional research is needed to assess whether comorbidities affect outcomes and if systematic assessment should be included in skin cancer management algorithms.

There are a few limitations to this study. First, the number of patients studied was small and the follow-up period was limited to only 2 years. However, the power of the analysis is derived from the large number of binary endpoints used in the comparative analyses. Moreover, this pilot study required cotemporaneous evaluation by a small number of staff from two clinical services, thus limiting the number of potential patients eligible for study. Second, a single institution setting may not be representative of the general skin cancer population. Nevertheless, a study goal was to compare two methods of data collection, and identifying patients evaluated at a single center facilitated this objective. Third, comorbidity data extraction used information from an outpatient clinical assessment and did not utilize review of all of a patient's medical records. While this limited amount of clinical data may have led to underestimation of a patient's comorbid conditions, because most patients with skin cancer receive care by outpatient specialists, this is representative of general clinical practice. Moreover, retrospective chart review has previously been shown to provide sufficient information for comorbidity scoring using ACE-27 with minimal limitations [23, 24]. Finally, some might suggest that the results of the present study cannot be generalized because of the inability to implement a patient-reported comorbidity assessment in clinical practice. Although there are 27 comorbidities to identify and grade in the PRACE-27, there is a quick learning curve and computing severity scores takes less than three minutes [22].

Comorbidity assessment will likely become an important factor in individualizing treatment for all malignant diseases including skin cancer. It is well accepted that a single treatment approach should not be applied to all patients with skin cancer [28], and thus grading comorbidity severity in patients may help guide management. This pilot study shows that PRACE-27 was more likely to identify an ailment than the MI and better identified the higher grades. The ACE-27 is a validated tool that may be more applicable in the skin cancer population compared to other tools such as the Charlson Comorbidity Index (CCI), whose applicability to

TABLE 4: Percent agreement and kappa between medical interview (MI) and PRACE-27 assessments for overall comorbidity scores.

	PRACE-27							
	Medical interview					Percent agreement	Kappa	p value
Overall comorbidity score	0	1	2	3	Total # patients			
0	5*	0	0	0	5			
1	2**	11*	0	0	13	91.7	0.64	<0.001
2	1**	2**	9*	1***	13			
3	1**	3**	3**	6*	13			
Total # patients	9	16	12	7	44			

PRACE-27 and MI had identical overall comorbidity scores for 31/44 patients (marked with *). There were 12 patients for whom PRACE-27 had a higher overall comorbidity score (marked with **) compared to MI and 1 patient (marked with ***) for whom MI had a higher overall comorbidity score compared to PRACE-27.

skin cancer populations has been challenged [28]. Utilizing a patient-reported questionnaire like the PRACE-27 during the physician encounter may ensure that important components of the relevant medical history are not omitted. Further research is needed to better delineate the role of comorbidity assessment in the skin cancer population.

Ethical Approval

IRB exemption was obtained from MKSCC IRB.

Disclosure

Erica H. Lee and Rajiv I. Nijhawan are co-first authors. Dr. Christopher Barker serves as a paid consultant to Nucletron. MSKCC receives research funding from Nucletron for a study that Dr. Christopher Barker is leading. Nucletron was *not* involved in this study, in design or through financial support. No other authors have financial disclosure.

References

[1] P. C. Albertsen, P. C. Albertsen, D. G. Fryback et al., "The impact of co-morbidity on life expectancy among men with localized prostate cancer," *Journal of Urology*, vol. 156, no. 1, pp. 127–132, 1996.

[2] R. Yancik, M. N. Wesley, L. A. G. Ries, R. J. Havlik, B. K. Edwards, and J. W. Yates, "Effect of age and comorbidity in postmenopausal breast cancer patients aged 55 years and older," *The Journal of the American Medical Association*, vol. 285, no. 7, pp. 885–892, 2001.

[3] D. C. Miller, D. A. Taub, R. L. Dunn, J. E. Montie, and J. T. Wei, "The impact of co-morbid disease on cancer control and survival following radical cystectomy," *Journal of Urology*, vol. 169, no. 1, pp. 105–109, 2003.

[4] C. K. Wells, J. K. Stoller, A. R. Feinstein, and R. I. Horwitz, "Comorbid and clinical determinants of prognosis in endometrial cancer," *Archives of Internal Medicine*, vol. 144, no. 10, pp. 2004–2009, 1984.

[5] J. F. Piccirillo, R. M. Tierney, I. Costas, L. Grove, and E. L. Spitznagel Jr., "Prognostic importance of comorbidity in a hospital-based cancer registry," *Journal of the American Medical Association*, vol. 291, no. 20, pp. 2441–2447, 2004.

[6] C.-Y. Ma, T. Ji, A. Ow et al., "Surgical site infection in elderly oral cancer patients: is the evaluation of comorbid conditions helpful in the identification of high-risk ones?" *Journal of Oral and Maxillofacial Surgery*, vol. 70, no. 10, pp. 2445–2452, 2012.

[7] T. T. A. Peters, B. A. C. van Dijk, J. L. N. Roodenburg, B. F. A. M. van der Laan, and G. B. Halmos, "Relation between age, comorbidity, and complications in patients undergoing major surgery for head and neck cancer," *Annals of Surgical Oncology*, vol. 21, no. 3, pp. 963–970, 2014.

[8] I. K. Lægreid, K. Aasarod, A. Bye, T. Leivestad, and M. Jordhoy, "The impact of nutritional status, physical function, comorbidity and early versus late start in dialysis on quality of life in older dialysis patients," *Renal Failure*, vol. 36, no. 1, pp. 9–16, 2014.

[9] G. Baijal, T. Gupta, C. Hotwani et al., "Impact of comorbidity on therapeutic decision-making in head and neck cancer: audit from a comprehensive cancer center in India," *Head and Neck*, vol. 34, no. 9, pp. 1251–1254, 2012.

[10] M. E. Charlson, P. Pompei, K. A. Ales, and C. R. MacKenzie, "A new method of classifying prognostic comorbidity in longitudinal studies: development and validation," *Journal of Chronic Diseases*, vol. 40, no. 5, pp. 373–383, 1987.

[11] A. Delaney, I. Shimizu, L. H. Goldberg, and D. F. MacFarlane, "Life expectancy after Mohs micrographic surgery in patients aged 90 years and older," *Journal of the American Academy of Dermatology*, vol. 68, no. 2, pp. 296–300, 2013.

[12] J. C. Pascual, I. Belinchon, and J. M. Ramos, "Mortality after dermatologic surgery for nonmelanoma skin cancer in patients aged 80 years and older," *Journal of the American Academy of Dermatology*, vol. 69, no. 6, pp. 1051–1052, 2013.

[13] A. J. Charles Jr., C. C. Otley, and G. R. Pond, "Prognostic factors for life expectancy in nonagenarians with nonmelanoma skin cancer: implications for selecting surgical candidates," *Journal of the American Academy of Dermatology*, vol. 47, no. 3, pp. 419–422, 2002.

[14] V. Paleri and R. G. Wight, "A cross-comparison of retrospective notes extraction and combined notes extraction and patient interview in the completion of a comorbidity index (ACE-27) in a cohort of United Kingdom patients with head and neck cancer," *Journal of Laryngology and Otology*, vol. 116, no. 11, pp. 937–941, 2002.

[15] M. T. A. Sharabiani, P. Aylin, and A. Bottle, "Systematic review of comorbidity indices for administrative data," *Medical Care*, vol. 50, no. 12, pp. 1109–1118, 2012.

[16] B. S. Linn, M. W. Linn, and L. Gurel, "Cumulative illness rating scale," *Journal of the American Geriatrics Society*, vol. 16, no. 5, pp. 622–626, 1968.

[17] M. S. Litwin, S. Greenfield, E. P. Elkin, D. P. Lubeck, J. M. Broering, and S. H. Kaplan, "Assessment of prognosis with the total illness burden index for prostate cancer: aiding clinicians in treatment choice," *Cancer*, vol. 109, no. 9, pp. 1777–1783, 2007.

[18] M. H. Kaplan and A. R. Feinstein, "The importance of classifying initial comorbidity in evaluating the outcome of diabetes mellitus," *Journal of Chronic Diseases*, vol. 27, no. 7-8, pp. 387–404, 1974.

[19] R. Mayr, M. May, T. Martini et al., "Predictive capacity of four comorbidity indices estimating perioperative mortality after radical cystectomy for urothelial carcinoma of the bladder," *BJU International*, vol. 110, no. 6, pp. E222–E227, 2012.

[20] D. Kallogjeri, S. M. Gaynor, M. L. Piccirillo, R. A. Jean, E. L. Spitznagel Jr., and J. F. Piccirillo, "Comparison of comorbidity collection methods," *Journal of the American College of Surgeons*, vol. 219, no. 2, pp. 245–55, 2014.

[21] V. S. Nesic, Z. M. Petrovic, S. B. Sipetic, S. D. Jesic, I. A. Soldatovic, and D. A. Kastratovic, "Comparison of the Adult Comorbidity Evaluation 27 and the Charlson Comorbidity indices in patients with laryngeal squamous cell carcinoma," *Journal of Laryngology and Otology*, vol. 126, no. 5, pp. 516–524, 2012.

[22] J. B. Owen, N. Khalid, A. Ho et al., "Can patient comorbidities be included in clinical performance measures for radiation oncology?," *Journal of Oncology Practice*, vol. 10, no. 3, pp. e175–e181, 2014.

[23] V. Paleri and R. G. Wight, "Applicability of the adult comorbidity evaluation—27 and the Charlson indexes to assess comorbidity by notes extraction in a cohort of United Kingdom patients with head and neck cancer: a retrospective study," *Journal of Laryngology and Otology*, vol. 116, no. 3, pp. 200–205, 2002.

[24] J. F. Piccirillo, C. M. Creech, R. Zequeira, S. Anderson, and A. S. Johnston, "Inclusion of comorbidity into oncoogy data registries," *Journal of Registry Management*, vol. 26, pp. 66–70, 1999.

[25] N. Daver, K. Naqvi, E. Jabbour et al., "Impact of comorbidities by ACE-27 in the revised-IPSS for patients with myelodysplastic syndromes," *American Journal of Hematology*, vol. 89, no. 5, pp. 509–516, 2014.

[26] T. Chen, D. Bertenthal, A. Sahay, S. Sen, and M.-M. Chren, "Predictors of skin-related quality of life after treatment of cutaneous basal cell carcinoma and squamous cell carcinoma," *Archives of Dermatology*, vol. 143, no. 11, pp. 1386–1392, 2007.

[27] G. Schubert-Fritschle, A. Schlesinger-Raab, R. Hein et al., "Quality of life and comorbidity in localized malignant melanoma: results of a German population-based cohort study," *International Journal of Dermatology*, vol. 52, no. 6, pp. 693–704, 2013.

[28] J. F. Sobanko and S. T. Ross, "Mistaken conclusions in a nonmelanoma skin cancer article published in JAMA," *Dermatologic Surgery*, vol. 40, no. 5, pp. 489–496, 2014.

23

Cutaneous Human Papillomavirus Infection and Development of Subsequent Squamous Cell Carcinoma of the Skin

Shalaka S. Hampras,[1] **Rhianna A. Reed,**[1] **Spencer Bezalel,**[2]
Michael Cameron,[2] **Basil Cherpelis,**[3,4] **Neil Fenske,**[3,4] **Vernon K. Sondak,**[5] **Jane Messina,**[3,5,6]
Massimo Tommasino,[7] **Tarik Gheit,**[7] **and Dana E. Rollison**[1]

[1]*Department of Cancer Epidemiology, Moffitt Cancer Center, Tampa, Florida, USA*
[2]*University of South Florida, Morsani College of Medicine, Tampa, Florida, USA*
[3]*Department of Dermatology, University of South Florida, College of Medicine, Tampa, FL, USA*
[4]*Department of Cutaneous Surgery, University of South Florida, College of Medicine, Tampa, FL, USA*
[5]*Cutaneous Oncology Program, Moffitt Cancer Center, Tampa, Florida, USA*
[6]*Departments of Pathology and Cell Biology, University of South Florida, College of Medicine, Tampa, FL, USA*
[7]*Infections and Cancer Biology Group, International Agency for Research on Cancer-World Health Organization, Lyon 69372, France*

Correspondence should be addressed to Shalaka S. Hampras; shalaka.hampras@moffitt.org

Academic Editor: Günther Hofbauer

The role of cutaneous human papillomavirus (HPV) infection in the development of subsequent cutaneous squamous cell carcinoma (SCC) is unknown. Pathologically confirmed cases of SCC ($n = 150$) enrolled in a previously conducted case-control study were included in a retrospective cohort study to examine the association of cutaneous HPV at the time of SCC diagnosis with the risk of subsequent SCC development. Data on HPV seropositivity, HPV DNA in eyebrow hairs (EB) and SCC tumors were available from the parent study. Incidence of subsequent SCC was estimated using person-years of follow up. Cox Proportional Hazards ratios were estimated to evaluate the associations of both, HPV seropositivity and HPV DNA positivity with subsequent SCC. The five year cumulative incidence of subsequent SCC was 72%. Seropositivity to cutaneous HPV was not associated with the risk of subsequent SCC (HR = 0.83, 95% CI = 0.41–1.67). Any beta HPV infection in EB was associated with reduced risk (HR = 0.30, 95% CI = 0.11–0.78) of subsequent SCC among cases who were positive for beta HPV DNA in tumor tissue. Infection with beta HPV type 2 (HR = 0.32, 95% CI = 0.12–0.86) in EB was associated with reduced risk of subsequent SCC among HPV DNA positive SCCs. In conclusion, beta HPV infection was inversely associated with the risk of subsequent SCC.

1. Introduction

Keratinocyte cancer (KC), including squamous cell carcinoma (SCC) and basal cell carcinoma (BCC), is the most commonly diagnosed cancer in the United States [1]. While ultraviolet radiation is an established risk factor for KC [2], growing evidence suggests infection with cutaneous human papillomavirus (HPV) may increase the risk of cutaneous SCC [3–8]. We previously reported an increased risk of SCC associated with the presence of four or more types of cutaneous HPV DNA in eyebrow hairs [3]. Serological responses to genus beta HPV types were found to be associated with increased risk of SCC [4]. Further, poor tanning ability was associated with 6.9 times increased risk of SCC among those who were seropositive to beta HPV type [5]. Collectively, these findings suggest that cutaneous HPV may play a role in the pathogenesis of SCC. However, it should be noted that some previous case-control studies reporting an association between beta HPV and SCC included only primary cases of SCC [6, 9], while others [3, 4] did not differentiate between primary and subsequent SCCs. Therefore, the role of cutaneous HPV infection in the development of subsequent SCC is unknown.

As compared to BCCs, SCCs are more likely to be clinically aggressive with a propensity to recur and metastasize [1, 10]. As reviewed previously, patients with metastatic SCC have less than 20% survival rate over 10 years [1]. Varying recurrence rates for SCC have been reported based on the site of involvement, metastasis, and grade. In a retrospective study, 30% SCCs involving temporal bone were found to recur within an average of 5.8 months [11]. Others have reported lower SCC recurrence rates of 9–15% [12, 13]. As summarized by Alam and Ratner, risk factors for recurrence of SCCs include tumor size, site, tumor depth, perineural invasion, history of treatment for SCC, and tumor differentiation [1]. While these factors may aid in the identification of SCC cases at high risk of recurrence, they provide limited scope for intervention beyond treatment or close surveillance to prevent the recurrence of SCC.

SCC cases are also at a high risk of developing second primary SCCs. In a large population based study of over 25,000 Swedish SCC cases, a significantly increased risk of second primary SCC was observed (standardized incidence ratio = 15.6) [14]. Meta-analyses results have shown that the risk of developing SCC subsequent to an "index" SCC was 18% [15]. As cautioned by Marcil and Stern, some of the previous studies examining the risk of a subsequent SCC included index SCC cases with a history of >1 SCC or did not provide such information. Thus, the index SCCs may have comprised both first and recurrent SCCs [15]. The high morbidity associated with development of subsequent SCCs warrants further research.

Given the increased risk of SCC observed in association with cutaneous HPV infection as described above, it is reasonable to hypothesize that patients with SCCs associated with cutaneous HPV infection are more likely to develop subsequent SCCs compared to patients with SCCs that are not associated with HPV.

Using a subset of SCC cases ($n = 150$) from our previously conducted study [3, 4], we conducted a retrospective cohort study to examine the association between cutaneous HPV infection at the time of SCC diagnosis in the parent study with the risk of subsequent SCC. Infection with cutaneous HPV was assessed using three biomarkers: serum antibodies to HPV, presence of HPV DNA in eyebrow hairs, and presence of HPV DNA in SCC tumors.

2. Materials and Methods

2.1. Study Design and Population. The study population has been described previously [3, 4, 16]. Briefly, a clinic based case-control study was conducted at Moffitt Cancer Center in Tampa, Florida, in 2007–2009. Histologically confirmed cases of SCC ($n = 173$) were identified through the University of South Florida (USF) Dermatology Clinic. Both newly diagnosed primary SCCs and cases with a prior history of SCC were included in the case group. Controls included patients without history of any type of cancer and who were negative for skin cancer based on a full-body screening exam at the time of enrollment. Of the 173 SCC cases enrolled in

the parent case-control study, 150 SCC cases were followed through 2014. The remaining cases either did not return to the clinic or were only referred to USF Dermatology Clinic for Moh's surgery. Cases without complete follow-up were similar in age and gender distribution to the cases with complete follow-up. The 150 "index" SCC cases with complete follow-up through 2014 were included in the present analyses. Serology data on 33 cutaneous HPV types, including HPV types in the alpha, beta, and gamma genera ($n = 150$), as well as beta HPV DNA ($n = 25$ beta HPV types) status in eyebrow hairs ($n = 145$) and SCC tumor tissue ($n = 131$), at the time of enrollment of index SCC, were available from the parent study [3, 4]. Self-reported data on demographics, smoking, alcohol consumption, and skin cancer risk factors, including history of blistering sunburns, sun exposure, and tanning ability were also available from the parent study. For the current retrospective cohort, subsequent SCC was defined as the SCC, including recurrent and second primary SCC, detected after the index SCC was diagnosed at the enrollment biopsy in the parent case-control study [3, 4]. Medical charts of index SCCs were reviewed, and data on the date of past history of SCC prior to enrollment of an index SCC case in the parent case-control study, date of subsequent SCC diagnosed after the index SCC enrollment, site and tumor dimensions of subsequent SCC, other incident keratinocyte cancers and date of last contact or death were abstracted. All participants provided written informed consent, and the study protocol was approved by the Institutional Review Board at USF.

2.2. Serology. Serum samples obtained from the index SCC cases at the time of their enrollment in the parent study were examined for antibodies to major capsid protein L1 for 33 cutaneous HPV types including genera alpha (2, 3, 7, 10, 27, 57, and 77); beta [beta 1 (5, 8, 20, 24, 36), beta 2 (9, 15, 17, 23, 38, 107), beta 3 (49, 75, 76), beta 4 (92), and beta 5 (96)], gamma (4, 48, 50, 65, 88, 95, 101, 103), mu (1), and nu (41). As described previously [4], antibodies were detected using an enzyme linked immunosorbent assay [17, 18] and fluorescent bead-based multiplex serology [19].

2.3. HPV DNA in Eyebrow Hairs and SCC Tumor Tissue. Measurement of HPV DNA in eyebrow hairs and fresh-frozen SCC tumors has been described in detail previously [3, 4]. Briefly, HPV DNA was extracted from eyebrow hairs and SCC tumor tissue with the QIAGEN EZ1 DNA Tissue Kit, and HPV genotyping was performed using a type specific multiplex assay detecting DNA from 25 genus beta HPV types (5, 8, 9, 12, 14, 15, 17, 19, 20, 21, 22, 23, 24, 25, 36, 37, 38, 47, 49, 75, 76, 80, 92, 93, and 96) [20, 21].

2.4. Statistical Analyses. Follow-up time was defined as the time interval between the date of index SCC biopsy at enrollment in the parent study and date of diagnosis of subsequent SCC or date of last contact. Five-year cumulative incidence of subsequent SCC was estimated using person-years of follow-up. Demographic, lifestyle factors, and skin cancer risk factors were compared between those who developed a subsequent SCC and those who did not, using Chi Square and Fisher's exact tests, as appropriate. Cox Proportional Hazards ratios (HR) and corresponding 95% confidence intervals (CIs) were estimated for associations of seropositivity to cutaneous HPV, overall and by genera, with the risk of subsequent SCC, adjusting for age and gender. Seropositivity to "any" HPV was defined as proportions of SCC cases that were positive for an antibody to at least one HPV type across all genera (overall cutaneous HPV seropositivity), within the specific genera (genus specific seropositivity) or within specific species (species-specific seropositivity). Seropositivity to multiple HPV infections was defined as the presence of antibodies corresponding to ≥2 beta HPV types.

"Any" beta HPV infection in eyebrow hairs, overall and by species, was defined as the proportion of cases who had DNA corresponding to at least one HPV type in genus beta or in a given species within genus beta, respectively. Multiple HPV infections were defined as the presence of HPV DNA corresponding to ≥2 beta HPV types. Since SCC tumors have lower viral DNA load compared to eyebrow hairs [3], HPV DNA status in tumors was categorized as "negative for all of the 25 types of beta HPV DNA" or "positive for ≥1 type of beta HPV DNA" or "positive for ≥1 species-specific beta HPV DNA." Cox Proportional Hazards ratios and corresponding 95% CIs were estimated for associations of beta HPV DNA positivity, overall and by species, with the risk of subsequent SCC, adjusting for age and gender. Associations of both beta HPV seropositivity and beta HPV DNA positivity in eyebrow hairs with the risk of subsequent SCC were stratified by SCC tumor beta HPV DNA status.

3. Results and Discussion

As seen in Table 1, SCC cases included in this study were all White, with an average age at index SCC diagnosis of 64.5 years, with 92.8% cases reporting a prior history of SCC. Of the 150 index SCC cases, 105 (70%) were diagnosed with at least one KC during follow-up. Ninety-one out of the 150 SCC cases were found to have at least one subsequent SCC since their enrollment in the previous case-control study [3, 4]. Up to five SCC tumors per case, the majority in the head and neck region, were detected at the time of diagnosis of subsequent SCC. The median follow-up time was 1.15 years. The five-year cumulative incidence of subsequent SCC was 72%.

Subsequent SCCs were detected within an average of 1 year from the date of SCC biopsy at enrollment visit. SCC cases with a past history of SCC or BCC or both were significantly more likely to have a subsequent SCC (Table 2). None of the other demographic or lifestyle characteristics were associated with subsequent SCC (Table 2). Seropositivity to cutaneous HPV infections, overall, by genera and beta HPV species, was not associated with the risk of subsequent SCC (Table 3).

Presence of beta HPV DNA in eyebrow hairs was not associated with the risk of subsequent SCC, overall or by species (Table 4). However, after stratification by tumor beta HPV DNA, "any" beta HPV infection in eyebrow hairs was significantly associated with 70% reduced risk of subsequent SCC among cases who were positive for any beta HPV DNA in tumor tissue (Table 5). Further, species-specific analyses showed that "any" beta-2 HPV infection in eyebrow hairs was

associated with 68% significantly reduced risk of subsequent SCC among tumor DNA positive index SCC cases (Table 5). Beta HPV seropositivity was not associated with subsequent SCC after stratification by tumor beta HPV DNA status (Table 5).

Cutaneous SCCs contribute substantial morbidity due their tendency to recur [1] and associated high risk of development of second primary malignances of the skin and other organs [14]. With the rising incidence of SCC [22], the prevalence of recurrent and second primary SCCs will also increase contributing substantially to public health burden. It is important to identify factors predisposing to recurrent and second primary SCCs to guide development of better follow up protocols, characterize high risk SCCs, and inform preventive strategies aimed at reducing the morbidity associated with subsequent SCCs.

In this retrospective cohort study, while no association was observed between cutaneous HPV seropositivity and the risk of subsequent SCC, a significantly inverse association was observed between cutaneous beta HPV infection in eyebrow hairs detected at the time of index SCC diagnosis and subsequent SCC development, among SCC cases with HPV DNA positive index SCC tumors. These findings are in contrast to the positive association reported between cutaneous HPV infection, measured by HPV serology and presence of HPV in eyebrow hairs, and SCC [3, 4]. However, our findings are consistent with findings from previous studies on mucosal HPV infection associated cancers. Mucosal HPV infection has been previously associated with improved survival [23–25] or reduced rate of recurrence [26] in some cancers. For example, in a small study of 41 cases, recurrence rate of nasopharyngeal carcinoma was 75% in HPV tumor DNA negative patients compared to 11% in tumor DNA positive patients [26]. Ritchie et al. reported that HPV positive oropharyngeal cancers had 70% significantly improved survival compared to HPV negative cases, with significant survival benefits for men versus women [25]. As discussed previously [25], increased sensitivity to radiation treatment and reduced occurrence of P53 mutations in HPV tumor positive cases have been suggested as possible mechanisms of improved prognosis in association with mucosal HPV infection.

In the context of cutaneous SCC, which is mainly treated by excision, it is not clear whether the underlying mechanisms of improved prognosis of HPV positive SCCs are similar to those suggested for prognosis of mucosal HPV associated cancers. Cutaneous HPV infection is thought to be involved in the initiation, but not the maintenance of SCC [27, 28]. One explanation of the observed inverse association between beta HPV infection and subsequent SCC could be that beta HPV infection in index SCC tumors may be immunogenic and could potentially stimulate host immune response that prevents the development of subsequent SCCs.

Our findings may suggest different mechanisms driving tumor progression in HPV DNA positive versus HPV DNA negative SCC cases. Immunological and genetic factors that are associated with HPV DNA negative tumors should be explored further. Previously, we showed that, among a subset of SCC cases included in the present study, single nucleotide polymorphisms (SNPs) in epidermodysplasia verruciformis

TABLE 1: Demographic and baseline characteristics of 150 cutaneous squamous cell carcinoma (SCC) cases.

Variable	n (%)
Age in years [Mean (std)]	64.4 (10.20)
Gender	
Male	100 (66.7)
Female	50 (33.3)
Race	
White	134 (100.0)
Other	0 (0)
Education	
≤ 12th grade	23 (17.4)
>12th grade	109 (82.6)
Skin color	
Fair white	59 (44.4)
Medium white	69 (51.9)
Light brown	5 (3.8)
Skin's reaction to first time exposure in the sun	
A blistering sunburn	21 (16.0)
A sunburn without blisters	58 (44.3)
A mild sunburn that becomes a tan	35 (26.7)
A tan with no sunburn	164 (10.7)
No change in skin color	3 (2.3)
History of blistering sunburn prior to index SCC diagnosis	
No	29 (22.3)
Yes	101 (77.7)
Skin's reaction to repeated exposure in the sun	
Unable to tan	243 (17.6)
It can tan if you work at it	61 (46.6)
It tans easily	47 (35.9)
Job in sun for more than 3 months at any time in life prior to the index SCC diagnosis	
No	70 (53.0)
Yes	62 (47.0)
Number of moles on the entire body	
None	47 (35.3)
Less than 10 moles	62 (46.6)
10–25 moles	21 (15.8)
More than 25 moles	3 (2.3)
History of smoking	
Never	40 (30.8)
Ever	90 (69.2)
History of SCC	
No	8 (7.2)
Yes	103 (92.8)

genes, regulating immune response against HPV, were associated with reduced risk of beta HPV DNA positive SCC tumors [29]. These SNPs should be explored further in association with the risk of subsequent SCC.

The findings from our study should be interpreted with caution. A majority (92.8%) of index SCC cases had a history of SCC prior to their enrollment in the parent case-control study. Thus, external validity of our findings may be limited to those cases with a past history of SCC. Cutaneous HPV

infection status at the diagnosis of past SCCs was unknown. Therefore, association of change in HPV infection status over time with the risk of subsequent SCCs could not be evaluated. HPV DNA status in subsequent SCC tumors detected during follow-up was not measured. Due to limited sample size, robust statistical analyses for HPV type specific association with subsequent SCC development could not be conducted. The subsequent SCCs detected in this study could be recurrent SCCs, presenting at the same anatomic site as

TABLE 2: Associations between baseline skin cancer risk factors and subsequent cutaneous squamous cell carcinoma (SCC).

Variable	No subsequent SCC ($n = 59$) n (%)	Subsequent SCC ($n = 91$) n (%)	P value for Chi Square test
Age [mean (STD)]	62.9 (12.4)	65.4 (8.4)	0.16[1]
Gender			
Female	24 (40.7)	26 (28.6)	0.12
Male	35 (59.3)	65 (71.4)	
History of blistering sunburn prior to index SCC diagnosis			
No	15 (28.3)	14 (18.2)	
Yes	38 (71.7)	63 (81.8)	0.17
Tanning ability			
No	11 (21.6)	12 (15.0)	
Yes	40 (78.4)	68 (85.0)	0.33
Job in sun for more than 3 months at any time in life prior to the index SCC diagnosis			
No	31 (59.6)	39 (48.7)	0.22
Yes	21 (40.4)	41 (51.2)	
Smoking			
Never	17 (32.1)	23 (29.9)	
Ever	36 (67.9)	54 (70.1)	0.79
Alcohol			
Never drinker	12 (23.5)	15 (18.7)	0.51
1 or more drinks in past 1 year	39 (76.5)	65 (81.2)	
History of SCC prior to index SCC diagnosis			
No	7 (15.6)	1 (1.5)	
Yes	38 (84.4)	65 (98.5)	**0.007**[2]
History of BCC prior to index SCC diagnosis			
No	7 (21.2)	2 (3.6)	
Yes	26 (78.8)	53 (96.4)	**0.01**[2]
History of SCC and BCC prior to index SCC diagnosis			
No	7 (21.9)	1 (2.0)	**0.005**[2]
Yes	25 (78.1)	49 (98.0)	
Number of HPV types in index SCC tumors			
0	23 (42.6)	22 (28.6)	0.17
1	12 (22.2)	14 (18.2)	
2–5	17 (31.5)	33 (42.9)	
>5	2 (3.7)	8 (10.4)	

[1] Student's *t*-test. [2] Fisher's exact test.

primary SCC, or second primary SCCs and the analyses stratified by these two outcomes were not conducted due to small sample. Conversely, combining recurrent and second primary SCCs as one outcome may have attenuated the true effect of HPV infection in index SCC on the development of recurrent or second primary SCCs.

The study has several strengths. To our knowledge, this is the first prospective study reporting an association between cutaneous HPV infection in SCC cases and subsequent SCCs. Of the 173 SCC cases enrolled in the parent case-control study, 86.7% cases were included in the present analyses

highlighting complete follow-up on a large proportion of the cases. Since 92.8% SCC cases reported a prior history of SCC, the findings from our study may help further prognostic stratification of these SCCs using a biomarker of infection. These cases may represent ideal candidates to direct infection related prevention measures due to the high morbidity associated with risk of developing subsequent SCCs among SCCs. Based on the observed inverse association between HPV seropositivity and risk of subsequent SCC (Table 3), although not significant, immune response against HPV may protect against the development of subsequent

TABLE 3: Association of seropositivity to cutaneous human papillomavirus (HPV) types at the time of the diagnosis of index SCC and risk of subsequent squamous cell carcinoma (SCC) of the skin.

Viral infection at the time of the index SCC diagnosis	No subsequent SCC ($n = 59$) n (%)	Subsequent SCC ($n = 91$) n (%)	HR (95% CI)*
Any cutaneous HPV[1]			
Seronegative to 33 cutaneous HPV types	6 (10.2)	9 (9.9)	1.00
Seropositive to ≥1 cutaneous HPV	53 (89.8)	82 (90.1)	0.83 (0.41–1.67)
Alpha cutaneous HPV			
Seronegative to 33 cutaneous HPV types	6 (21.4)	9 (20.4)	1.00
Alpha HPV seropositive[2]	22 (78.6)	35 (79.6)	0.86 (0.40–1.82)
Alpha HPV seronegative	37 (62.7)	56 (61.5)	
Alpha HPV seropositive[3]	22 (37.3)	35 (38.5)	1.04 (0.68–1.59)
Beta HPV			
Seronegative to 33 cutaneous HPV types	6 (12.0)	9 (12.0)	1.00
Beta HPV seropositive[2]	44 (88.0)	66 (88.0)	0.80 (0.39–1.62)
Beta HPV seronegative	15 (25.4)	25 (27.5)	1.00
Beta HPV seropositive[3]	44 (74.6)	66 (72.5)	0.82 (0.51–1.30)
Any beta 1 HPV[4]			
Seronegative	6 (17.6)	9 (16.4)	1.00
Beta 1 HPV seropositive	28 (82.3)	46 (83.6)	0.77 (0.37–1.59)
Any beta 2 HPV[5]			
Seronegative	6 (17.6)	9 (15.0)	1.00
Beta 2 HPV seropositive	28 (82.3)	51 (85,0)	0.99 (0.48–2.04)
Multiple beta 1 HPV[6]			
Seronegative	18 (52.9)	24 (43.6)	1.00
Seropositive to ≥2 beta 1 HPV	16 (47.1)	31 (56.4)	1.06 (0.61–1.83)
Multiple beta 2 HPV[7]			
Seronegative	18 (52.9)	25 (41.7)	1.00
Seropositive to ≥2 beta 2 HPV	16 (47.1)	35 (58.3)	0.98 (0.58–1.67)
Gamma HPV			
Seronegative to 33 cutaneous HPV types	6 (15.0)	9 (13.2)	1.00
Seropositive[2]	34 (85.0)	59 (86.8)	0.93 (0.46–1.90)
Gamma HPV Seronegative	25 (42.4)	32 (35.2)	1.00
Seropositive[3]	34 (57.6)	59 (64.8)	1.21 (0.78–1.87)
Mu HPV			
Seronegative to 33 cutaneous HPV types	6 (22.2)	9 (20.5)	1.00
Seropositive[2]	21 (77.8)	35 (79.5)	0.78 (0.37–1.65)
Mu HPV seronegative	38 (64.4)	56 (61.5)	1.00
Seropositive[3]	21 (35.6)	35 (38.5)	1.05 (0.68–1.61)
Nu HPV			
Seronegative to 33 cutaneous HPV types	6 (66.7)	9 (39.1)	1.00
Seropositive[2]	3 (33.3)	14 (60.9)	0.96 (0.38–2.44)
Nu HPV seronegative	56 (94.9)	77 (84.6)	1.00
Seropositive[3]	3 (5.1)	14 (15.4)	1.31 (0.73–2.34)

[1]Seropositivity to any cutaneous HPV ($n = 33$ types) versus negative to all. [2]Seropositive to at least one genus specific type versus negative to all cutaneous ($n = 33$) types. [3]Seropositive to at least one genus specific HPV versus seronegative to all genus-specific HPV types. [4]Seropositive to at least one beta 1 type versus seronegative to 33 cutaneous HPV types. [5]Seropositive to at least one beta 2 type versus seronegative to 33 cutaneous HPV types. [6]Seropositive to ≥2 beta 1 HPV types versus seronegative to all cutaneous types or positive to at least one beta 1 HPV type. [7]Seropositive to ≥2 beta 2 HPV types versus seronegative to all cutaneous types or positive to at least one beta 2 HPV type. HR = hazards ratio, CI = confidence interval. *Adjusted for age and gender.

TABLE 4: Association between cutaneous human papillomavirus (HPV) infection in *eyebrow hair* and the risk of subsequent squamous cell carcinoma (SCC).

Eyebrow hair viral infection at the index SCC diagnosis	No subsequent SCC (*n* = 59)	Subsequent SCC (*n* = 91)	*HR (95% CI)
Any beta HPV[1]			
DNA negative	6 (10.5)	12 (13.6)	1.00
DNA positive	51 (89.5)	76 (86.4)	0.84 (0.45–1.56)
Any beta 1 HPV[2]			
DNA negative	6 (13.6)	12 (16.2)	1.00
DNA positive	38 (86.4)	62 (83.8)	0.84 (0.44–1.58)
Any beta 2 HPV[3]			
DNA negative	6 (12.0)	12 (16.2)	1.00
DNA positive	44 (88.0)	62 (83.8)	0.85 (0.45–1.59)
Multiple beta 1 HPV[4]			
DNA negative	25 (56.8)	37 (50.0)	1.00
DNA positive	19 (43.2)	37 (50.0)	1.18 (0.72–1.93)
Multiple beta 2 HPV[5]			
DNA negative	29 (58.0)	35 (47.3)	1.00
DNA positive	21 (42.0)	39 (52.7)	1.23 (0.75–2.01)

[1] Eyebrow hair DNA positive to any beta HPV type versus negative to all 25 beta HPV types. [2] Eyebrow hair DNA positive to at least one beta 1 HPV type versus DNA negative to 25 beta HPV types. [3] Eyebrow hair DNA positive to at least one beta 2 HPV type versus DNA negative to 25 beta HPV types. [4] Eyebrow hair DNA positive to 2 or more beta-1 HPV types versus DNA negative to 25 beta HPV types or positive to one beta 1 HPV type. [5] Eyebrow hair DNA positive to 2 or more beta 2 HPV types versus DNA negative to 25 beta HPV types or positive to one beta 2 HPV type. HR = hazards ratio, CI = confidence interval. *Adjusted for age and gender.

TABLE 5: Association of beta HPV infection in *eyebrow hair* and beta HPV *seropositivity* with the risk of subsequent SCC *by index tumor HPV DNA status*.

Viral infection at the time of index SCC diagnosis	HPV DNA negative index SCC			HPV DNA positive index SCC		
	No subsequent SCC (*n* = 23)	Subsequent SCC (*n* = 22)	HR (95% CI)	No subsequent SCC (*n* = 31)	Subsequent SCC (*n* = 55)	HR (95% CI)
HPV serology						
Any beta HPV[1,3]						
Beta HPV seronegative	7 (30.4)	10 (45.5)	1.00	7 (22.6)	12 (21.8)	1.00
Beta HPV seropositive	16 (69.6)	12 (54.5)	0.44 (0.18–1.03)	24 (77.4)	43 (78.9)	0.92 (0.48–1.75)
HPV infection in eyebrow hairs						
Any beta HPV[2,3]						
DNA negative to all beta HPV types	3 (13.6)	6 (27.3)	1.0	2 (6.7)	5 (9.4)	1.0
DNA positive to ≥1 beta HPV	19 (86.4)	16 (72.7)	0.97 (0.38–2.50)	28 (93.3)	48 (90.6)	**0.30 (0.11–0.78)**
Any beta 1 HPV[4]						
DNA negative	3 (25.00)	6 (33.3)	1.0	2 (11.1)	1 (2.8)	1.0
DNA positive	9 (75.0)	12 (66.7)	1.21 (0.45–3.24)	16 (88.9)	35 (97.2)	0.72 (0.09–5.45)
Any beta 2 HPV[4]						
DNA negative	3 (15.0)	6 (35.3)	1.0	1 (4.8)	5 (12.8)	1.0
DNA positive	17 (85.0)	11 (64.7)	0.85 (0.31–2.32)	20 (95.2)	34 (87.2)	**0.32 (0.12–0.86)**

[1] Any beta HPV seropositivity was defined as seropositive to ≥1 beta HPV types versus seronegative to all beta HPV types. [2] Any beta HPV infection in eyebrow hairs was defined as DNA positivity to ≥1 beta HPV types versus DNA negativity to all beta HPV types. [3] Tumor DNA status was defined as DNA positive to one or more beta HPV types versus DNA negative to all beta HPV types. [4] Tumor DNA status was defined as DNA positivity to species-specific beta HPV types versus DNA negative to all beta HPV types.

SCCs. Thus, acquired immunity through vaccination against cutaneous HPV could potentially be explored among SCC cases. Additional strengths of this study include, examination of biomarkers of both, present HPV infection (eyebrow hair DNA and HPV serology) and past HPV infection (HPV serology) and evaluation of HPV infection as a prognostic marker by HPV genera and species.

4. Conclusion

In conclusion, the results from our prospective cohort study suggest that cutaneous HPV infection in eyebrow hairs is inversely associated with the development of subsequent SCCs in a subset of SCC cases with HPV DNA positive tumors. The observed association supports previous reports of lack of a role for cutaneous HPV infection in progression of SCCs. While cutaneous HPV may not be directly involved in the prognosis of SCC, this line of research may eventually lead to discovery of underlying immunological factors involved in SCC development and progression. Cutaneous HPV infection status could potentially be used as a biomarker for prognostic stratification of SCCs.

Competing Interests

The authors declare that there is no conflict of interests regarding the publication of this paper.

Acknowledgments

The parent case-control study was supported by a Florida Biomedical grant awarded to Dana E. Rollison (06NIR-08). This research was also supported in part by the Miles for Moffitt Foundation Funds and by the Tissue Core and Survey Core at H. Lee Moffitt Cancer Center & Research Institute, an NCI-designated Comprehensive Cancer Center (P30-CA076292). The authors thank Kristen Jonathan, Jill Weber, Carolyn Gerow, and the USF/LCS staff for assistance with patient recruitment, and Monika Junk for technical assistance during the parent case-control study.

References

[1] M. Alam and D. Ratner, "Cutaneous squamous-cell carcinoma," *New England Journal of Medicine*, vol. 344, no. 13, pp. 975–983, 2001.

[2] R. M. Lucas, A. J. Mcmichael, B. K. Armstrong, and W. T. Smith, "Estimating the global disease burden due to ultraviolet radiation exposure," *International Journal of Epidemiology*, vol. 37, no. 3, pp. 654–667, 2008.

[3] M. R. Iannacone, T. Gheit, H. Pfister et al., "Case-control study of genus-beta human papillomaviruses in plucked eyebrow hairs and cutaneous squamous cell carcinoma," *International Journal of Cancer*, vol. 134, no. 9, pp. 2231–2244, 2014.

[4] M. R. Iannacone, T. Gheit, T. Waterboer et al., "Case-control study of cutaneous human papillomaviruses in squamous cell carcinoma of the skin," *Cancer Epidemiology Biomarkers and Prevention*, vol. 21, no. 8, pp. 1303–1313, 2012.

[5] M. R. Iannacone, W. Wang, H. G. Stockwell et al., "Sunlight exposure and cutaneous human papillomavirus seroreactivity in basal cell and squamous cell carcinomas of the skin," *Journal of Infectious Diseases*, vol. 206, no. 3, pp. 399–406, 2012.

[6] J. N. Bouwes Bavinck, R. E. Neale, D. Abeni et al., "Multicenter study of the association between betapapillomavirus infection and cutaneous squamous cell carcinoma," *Cancer Research*, vol. 70, no. 23, pp. 9777–9786, 2010.

[7] C. M. Proby, C. A. Harwood, R. E. Neale et al., "A case-control study of betapapillomavirus infection and cutaneous squamous cell carcinoma in organ transplant recipients," *American Journal of Transplantation*, vol. 11, no. 7, pp. 1498–1508, 2011.

[8] L. Struijk, J. N. B. Bavinck, P. Wanningen et al., "Presence of human papillomavirus DNA in plucked eyebrow hairs is associated with a history of cutaneous squamous cell carcinoma," *Journal of Investigative Dermatology*, vol. 121, no. 6, pp. 1531–1535, 2003.

[9] M. R. Karagas, H. H. Nelson, P. Sehr et al., "Human papillomavirus infection and incidence of squamous cell and basal cell carcinomas of the skin," *Journal of the National Cancer Institute*, vol. 98, no. 6, pp. 389–395, 2006.

[10] C. Prieto-Granada and P. Rodriguez-Waitkus, "Cutaneous squamous cell carcinoma and related entities: epidemiology, clinical and histological features, and basic science overview," *Current Problems in Cancer*, vol. 39, no. 4, pp. 206–215, 2015.

[11] T. R. Mcrackan, T.-Y. Fang, S. Pelosi et al., "Factors associated with recurrence of squamous cell carcinoma involving the temporal bone," *Annals of Otology, Rhinology and Laryngology*, vol. 123, no. 4, pp. 235–239, 2014.

[12] M. J. Veness, C. E. Palme, and G. J. Morgan, "High-risk cutaneous squamous cell carcinoma of the head and neck: results from 266 treated patients with metastatic lymph node disease," *Cancer*, vol. 106, no. 11, pp. 2389–2396, 2006.

[13] J. C. Melo, M. E. A. Marques, L. Vasconcelos, H. A. Miot, and L. P. F. Abbade, "Invasive head and neck cutaneous squamous cell carcinoma: clinical and histopathological characteristics, frequency of local recurrence and metastasis," *Anais Brasileiros de Dermatologia*, vol. 89, no. 4, pp. 562–568, 2014.

[14] C. Wassberg, M. Thörn, J. Yuen, U. Ringborg, and T. Hakulinen, "Second primary cancers in patients with squamous cell carcinoma of the skin: a population-based study in Sweden," *International Journal of Cancer*, vol. 80, no. 4, pp. 511–515, 1999.

[15] I. Marcil and R. S. Stern, "Risk of developing a subsequent nonmelanoma skin cancer in patients with a history of nonmelanoma skin cancer: a critical review of the literature and meta-analysis," *Archives of Dermatology*, vol. 136, no. 12, pp. 1524–1530, 2000.

[16] D. E. Rollison, A. R. Giuliano, J. L. Messina et al., "Case-control study of Merkel cell polyomavirus infection and cutaneous squamous cell carcinoma," *Cancer Epidemiology Biomarkers and Prevention*, vol. 21, no. 1, pp. 74–81, 2012.

[17] P. Sehr, M. Müller, R. Höpfl, A. Widschwendter, and M. Pawlita, "HPV antibody detection by ELISA with capsid protein L1 fused to glutathione S-transferase," *Journal of Virological Methods*, vol. 106, no. 1, pp. 61–70, 2002.

[18] P. Sehr, K. Zumbach, and M. Pawlita, "A generic capture ELISA for recombinant proteins fused to glutathione S-transferase: validation for HPV serology," *Journal of Immunological Methods*, vol. 253, no. 1-2, pp. 153–162, 2001.

[19] T. Waterboer, P. Sehr, K. M. Michael et al., "Multiplex human papillomavirus serology based on in situ-purified glutathione

S-transferase fusion proteins," *Clinical Chemistry*, vol. 51, no. 10, pp. 1845–1853, 2005.

[20] T. Gheit, G. Billoud, M. N. C. De Koning et al., "Development of a sensitive and specific multiplex PCR method combined with DNA microarray primer extension to detect betapapillomavirus types," *Journal of Clinical Microbiology*, vol. 45, no. 8, pp. 2537–2544, 2007.

[21] J. B. Ruer, L. Pépin, T. Gheit et al., "Detection of alpha- and beta-human papillomavirus (hpv) in cutaneous melanoma: a matched and controlled study using specific multiplex pcr combined with dna microarray primer extension," *Experimental Dermatology*, vol. 18, no. 10, pp. 857–862, 2009.

[22] M. R. Karagas, E. R. Greenberg, S. K. Spencer, T. A. Stukel, and L. A. Mott, "Increase in incidence rates of basal cell and squamous cell skin cancer in New Hampshire, USA," *International Journal of Cancer*, vol. 81, no. 4, pp. 555–559, 1999.

[23] M. Sugiyama, U. K. Bhawal, M. Kawamura et al., "Human papillomavirus-16 in oral squamous cell carcinoma: clinical correlates and 5-year survival," *British Journal of Oral and Maxillofacial Surgery*, vol. 45, no. 2, pp. 116–122, 2007.

[24] K. R. Dahlstrom, G. Li, C. S. Hussey et al., "Circulating human papillomavirus DNA as a marker for disease extent and recurrence among patients with oropharyngeal cancer," *Cancer*, vol. 122, no. 3, pp. 489–489, 2016.

[25] J. M. Ritchie, E. M. Smith, K. F. Summersgill et al., "Human papillomavirus infection as a prognostic factor in carcinomas of the oral cavity and oropharynx," *International Journal of Cancer*, vol. 104, no. 3, pp. 336–344, 2003.

[26] S. Atighechi, M. R. A. Baghdadabad, S. A. Mirvakili et al., "Human papilloma virus and nasopharyngeal carcinoma: pathology, prognosis, recurrence and mortality of the disease," *Experimental Oncology*, vol. 36, no. 3, pp. 215–216, 2014.

[27] J. T. Schiller and C. B. Buck, "Cutaneous squamous cell carcinoma: a smoking gun but still no suspects," *Journal of Investigative Dermatology*, vol. 131, no. 8, pp. 1595–1596, 2011.

[28] S. Jablonska, J. Dabrowski, and K. Jakubowicz, "Epidermodysplasia verruciformis as a model in studies on the role of papovaviruses in oncogenesis," *Cancer Research*, vol. 32, no. 3, pp. 583–589, 1972.

[29] S. S. Hampras, D. E. Rollison, M. Tommasino et al., "Genetic variations in the epidermodysplasia verruciformis (EVER/TMC) genes, cutaneous human papillomavirus infection and squamous cell carcinoma of the skin," *British Journal of Dermatology*, vol. 173, no. 6, pp. 1532–1535, 2016.

24

A Qualitative Study of Quality of Life Concerns following a Melanoma Diagnosis

Rachel I. Vogel,[1,2] **Lori G. Strayer,**[1] **Rehana L. Ahmed,**[1,3]
Anne Blaes,[1,4] **and DeAnn Lazovich**[1,5]

[1]*Masonic Cancer Center, University of Minnesota, Minneapolis, MN, USA*
[2]*Division of Gynecologic Oncology, University of Minnesota, Minneapolis, MN, USA*
[3]*Department of Dermatology, University of Minnesota, Minneapolis, MN, USA*
[4]*Department of Medicine, Division of Hematology and Oncology, University of Minnesota, Minneapolis, MN, USA*
[5]*Division of Epidemiology and Community Health, University of Minnesota, Minneapolis, MN, USA*

Correspondence should be addressed to Rachel I. Vogel; isak0023@umn.edu

Academic Editor: Nihal Ahmad

The goal of this study was to identify a relevant and inclusive list of quality of life issues among long-term survivors of melanoma. Individuals diagnosed with stage I-III cutaneous melanoma and had survived 1-5 years, ages 18-65 years at diagnosis, were recruited. Five focus groups were conducted with 33 participants in total. Discussions centered on participants' experiences at diagnosis, as well as ongoing physical, emotional, and social concerns, and behavioral changes since diagnosis. The majority of participants reported shock, fear, and feeling overwhelmed at the time of diagnosis. Some reported lingering physical concerns, including pain, numbness, and lymphedema, while a few reported no lasting issues. Emotional concerns were common, with most reporting anxiety. Several also noted feeling lonely and isolated. Social concerns included alteration of activities to avoid sun exposure, issues with family communication, and frustration with the lack of appreciation of the seriousness of melanoma by others. Finally, while many participants reported changes to their sun exposure and UV-protection behaviors, some reported little to no change. The shared experiences among participants in this study confirm the unique nature of melanoma and the need for interventions designed to improve the health and quality of life of melanoma survivors.

1. Background

Melanoma, one of the most serious types of skin cancer, is unlike most common cancer types in that the incidence has been increasing over the past 30 years [1–3]. With a 5-year survival rate of 91%, there are currently over one million melanoma survivors in the United States [4]. Melanoma can be aggressive and resistant to treatment and can have the ability to metastasize even at the earliest stages [5]. These factors, and the young age at diagnosis, lead to an estimated 15–20 years of potential life lost [6], ranking seventh in number of years lost among all cancers in the United States [7]. A better understanding of the long-term and late effects of a melanoma diagnosis is needed as clinicians and researchers develop appropriate follow-up care guidelines and create educational and other interventions aimed at improving the lifespan and quality of life (QOL) of melanoma survivors.

QOL is a multidimensional concept that incorporates physical, psychological, and social functioning; an individuals' overall life satisfaction, perceptions of their health status, and ability to take part in valued activities are important components. To date, a limited number of studies examining QOL issues have been carried out in long-term melanoma survivors. The majority of these studies relied on currently available generic and cancer-specific instruments to assess a narrow range of issues, primarily related to emotional distress, anxiety, depression and psychosocial adjustment, or overall QOL [8–12].

The objective of the research reported here was to conduct focus groups to identify a relevant and inclusive list of QOL

TABLE 1: Questions asked during focus groups.

(i) Think back to the time of your melanoma diagnosis.
(a) What ran through your mind?
(b) Was there anything particularly difficult or surprising about the surgery/treatment?
(ii) What changes have you noticed since diagnosis?
(a) Physical.
(b) Emotional.
(c) Social.
(iii) Have you changed any behaviors since your diagnosis?
(iv) Was there a silver lining to this experience for you?
(v) Do you consider yourself a cancer survivor?

issues among melanoma survivors. Instead of focusing solely on the period of time immediately surrounding melanoma diagnosis and treatment, as others have done, we were interested in studying the issues survivors face as they live beyond their treatment.

2. Methods

2.1. Study Participants and Recruitment. The study was approved by the University of Minnesota Institutional Review Board (1201M09423). A convenience sample of patients treated by dermatologists and oncologists at the University of Minnesota were identified for participation in this study. English speaking individuals diagnosed with cutaneous melanoma in Minnesota since 2008, ages of 18–65 years at diagnosis, were eligible for this study. The age limits were imposed to match the eligibility criteria of a previous study conducted by the Principal Investigator (PI, Lazovich) [13]. Eligible individuals were sent an invitation letter, cosigned by their dermatologist, oncologist, or surgeon, and the PI. Potential participants were called to see if they were willing to participate in a focus group. A reminder letter was sent including a consent form to review prior to arrival.

2.2. Focus Groups. Focus groups were conducted to identify survivorship issues faced by people diagnosed with stage I–III melanoma. Groups were conducted separately for those with early stage disease (I and II) and advanced stage disease (III). Due to previous reports of differences in psychological adjustment after a diagnosis of melanoma between genders [9], focus groups were also held separately for men and women when possible. Five groups were formed from 33 participants, consisting of two all-male early stage melanoma groups (n = 6 and 7), two all-female early stage melanoma groups (n = 8 and 7), and one mixed-gender advanced stage melanoma group (n = 5).

The 90-minute focus groups were held at the University of Minnesota, Minneapolis campus. Participants provided written informed consent immediately prior to the start of the discussion. Each session was digitally audio-recorded and participants received $75 for their participation. All groups had the same moderator and comoderator and followed established methods for conduct of focus groups [14].

The question guide for the focus groups was developed iteratively. First, an extensive review was conducted of the literature that included published reports of QOL in melanoma survivors. The data from these studies were used to generate a list of topics thought to be important among persons diagnosed with melanoma. These topics were reviewed by all investigators and then refined into broad questions to serve as the focus group moderator guide [15]. The final questions included are presented in Table 1 and related to experience at diagnosis, physical, emotional, and social concerns since diagnosis, and behavioral changes since diagnosis.

At the end of each session, the moderator summarized key points discussed during the focus group and requested feedback from the group regarding the accuracy of the summary. All recordings from the focus groups were transcribed.

2.3. Analysis. We used standard procedures of qualitative thematic text analysis to analyze the focus group transcripts [15]. Two researchers (DL and RIV) independently read the transcripts and agreed to broad themes from the focus group discussions. Each researcher then conducted an analysis using descriptive coding techniques [14]. Results were compared for consistency and thoroughness and overarching themes and subtopics were agreed upon. Notes taken during the focus group discussions were used to complement the conclusions. Exemplary quotes from participants are provided as appropriate and presented verbatim.

3. Results

We identified 105 eligible melanoma patients, of whom 72 (68.6%) indicated they were willing to participate; 33 ultimately participated (31.4%). Among those who expressed initial interest but did not participate, the most common reason given was a scheduling conflict. Those who participated were similar to those who did not participate in gender and age. Participants were evenly distributed by gender (54.5% female), and most had a history of stage I disease (63.6%) with 18.2% each with a history of either stage II or stage III disease; the mean age was 49 ± 13 years. Approximately 25% had a family history of melanoma. A summary of the overarching themes is presented in Figure 1; details and quotes from the focus groups follow.

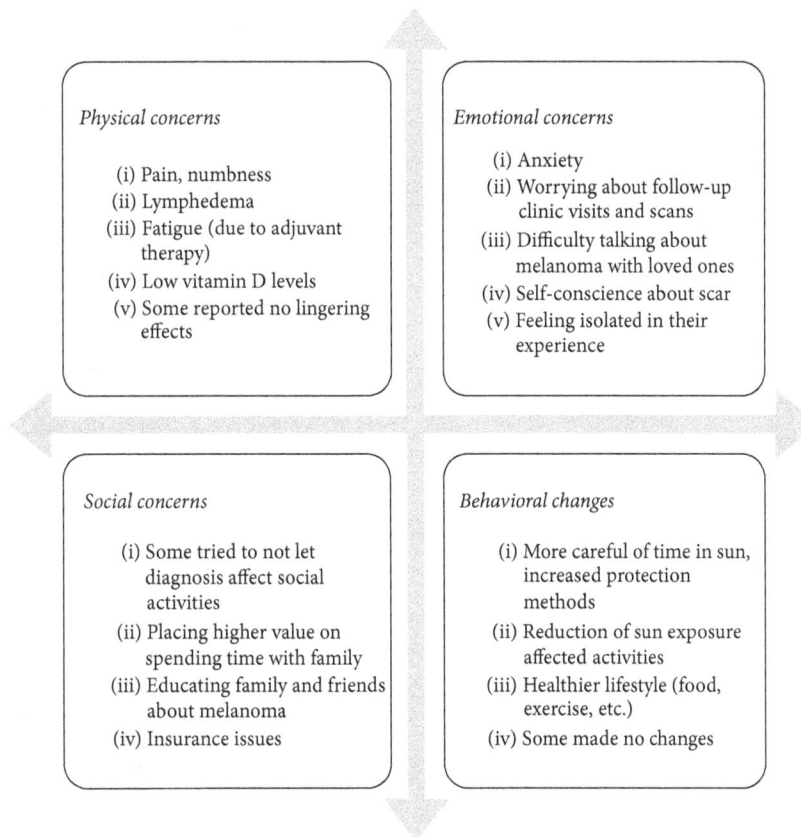

```
                        ↑
┌─────────────────────────┐  ┌─────────────────────────┐
│ Physical concerns       │  │ Emotional concerns      │
│                         │  │                         │
│  (i) Pain, numbness     │  │  (i) Anxiety            │
│  (ii) Lymphedema        │  │  (ii) Worrying about    │
│  (iii) Fatigue (due to  │  │       follow-up clinic  │
│        adjuvant therapy)│  │       visits and scans  │
│  (iv) Low vitamin D     │  │  (iii) Difficulty talking│
│       levels            │  │        about melanoma   │
│  (v) Some reported no   │  │        with loved ones  │
│      lingering effects  │  │  (iv) Self-conscience   │
│                         │  │       about scar        │
│                         │  │  (v) Feeling isolated in│
│                         │  │      their experience   │
└─────────────────────────┘  └─────────────────────────┘
←                                                        →
┌─────────────────────────┐  ┌─────────────────────────┐
│ Social concerns         │  │ Behavioral changes      │
│                         │  │                         │
│  (i) Some tried to not  │  │  (i) More careful of    │
│      let diagnosis      │  │      time in sun,       │
│      affect social      │  │      increased          │
│      activities         │  │      protection methods │
│  (ii) Placing higher    │  │  (ii) Reduction of sun  │
│       value on spending │  │       exposure affected │
│       time with family  │  │       activities        │
│  (iii) Educating family │  │  (iii) Healthier        │
│        and friends about│  │        lifestyle (food, │
│        melanoma         │  │        exercise, etc.)  │
│  (iv) Insurance issues  │  │  (iv) Some made no      │
│                         │  │       changes           │
└─────────────────────────┘  └─────────────────────────┘
                        ↓
```

FIGURE 1

3.1. *Experience at Diagnosis.* Each focus group started with a discussion of what participants experienced at the time of the melanoma diagnosis. The large majority of participants reported feeling shock, fear, and disbelief of the severity of the diagnosis.

> *Fear, screaming. It's a word [cancer] you don't ever want to hear. That was my initial reaction.*

A few said they had noticed changes in their skin but that their moles were assessed as normal by healthcare providers. They expressed anger when they finally received the diagnosis of melanoma.

> *I was angry [...] I had been questioning this spot for a year and had been told it was nothing and not to worry about it. So learning that it was melanoma, I was angry.*

Once diagnosed, most reported having surgery within a few days. Participants said the rapid pace of treatment was overwhelming as they tried to process the diagnosis, learn about melanoma, and undergo surgery. Many admitted they had little knowledge about melanoma before their diagnosis, which made the process more difficult. Those with early stage disease reported being thankful that their disease was caught early; however those with stage II and III disease described difficulty in making decisions regarding additional therapy.

Some described their melanoma diagnosis as a devastating and traumatic experience. In particular, those with younger children reported having concerns about their families and how family members would process the information.

> *I was sure that, at the time, this is it, I'm dying, this is it. I was absolutely petrified and absolutely scared to death.*

In contrast, while not the majority, a few reported their diagnosis was not particularly concerning, neither at the time of diagnosis nor in survivorship.

> *I feel like I'm in the wrong group because mine was no big deal.*

3.2. *Physical Concerns.* Next we asked about physical concerns, both at the time of diagnosis and in the survivorship period. Some participants reported lingering physical concerns, including pain, numbness, and lymphedema.

> *My melanoma was on the side of my face. So they went in to the neck resection and they went so deep that I was in a lot of pain ... I still have neck pain on that side of my neck.*

> *I wear compression garments on usually a daily basis to keep all that fluid from moving everywhere.*

A few noted some restrictions and limited motion during recovery that resolved with time and/or physical therapy.

The few participants who received adjuvant therapy reported additional side effects, with fatigue described as the most troublesome and pervasive.

A few with stage I disease and small tumors reported minor surgeries and no physical changes of note.

> *I didn't have any problem. I walked out of the doctor's office and went back to work. That's it.*

Lastly, some reported requiring extra vitamin D supplementation and a few noted still struggling with low levels and the resulting fatigue that they attributed to sun avoidance.

3.3. Emotional Concerns. The majority of participants reported longer-term concerns that were emotional in nature, with most experiencing some form of anxiety. A few reported general anxiety, whereas others were worried about follow-up checks and tests and their general health and were fearful of other cancers and melanoma for themselves and their children. Some reported that their anxiety improved with time, while for others the anxiety remained years after their diagnosis.

> *You listen to every one of us, the anxiety is the one thing that really got us. It's the anxiety, and the anxiety continues.*

> *… you get really uptight just before that scan. I don't even realize but my husband says, 'you're so bad the week before you scan'.*

A number of participants said they were surprised by the size of their scar and were self-conscious about it and the changes to their self-image.

> *It was just a teeny, tiny spot and they cut all the way down to the muscle and took all the tissue just for preventive.*

> *When they ended up taking that piece out of my cheek … I look in the mirror and I don't see my normal face.*

Many reported relying on their family for emotional support, whereas a few participants relied on faith and spirituality.

Some participants, however, reported difficulty discussing melanoma with their family.

> *I wish I could talk more about it because, I tell you, it's almost a taboo subject in my family. They just don't want to hear about it. It's fear or something.*

Several participants also noted feeling lonely and isolated despite family support. Interestingly, this issue came up not during the discussion of emotional health but at the end of the focus groups when we asked subjects about their motivation for participating in our study. We consistently heard how appreciative they were to participate in the discussion group as an opportunity to meet with others diagnosed with melanoma.

> *… it was kind of nice to be able to leave here today and not feel alone. Because that was my biggest thing, I constantly felt alone. Like I was the only person who had it ….*

3.4. Social Concerns. When asked about any social changes, participants noted a number of social concerns, including altering social activities to avoid sun exposure and wanting to educate others about melanoma. Most expressed a desire to not let their diagnosis affect their interactions; however some were careful to limit activities in the sun.

Some reported feeling the need to educate others about melanoma and prevention strategies. In particular, many reported being frustrated by the lack of appreciation by others of the seriousness of melanoma.

> *I was amazed by the number of people who hear melanoma, and they're like, oh that's skin cancer, not a big deal.*

A few reported not having insurance or having a high deductible plan and therefore faced difficulties with financial uncertainty and receiving optimal care. Quite a few also stated trouble obtaining life insurance after the diagnosis.

> *The reason I never got the mole taken off [earlier] was because I didn't have insurance initially.*

3.5. Behavioral Changes. When asked about any changes in health behaviors since diagnosis, many participants reported behavior changes. Some were limiting their time in the sun and increasing the use of protective clothing and sunscreen, particularly those with higher stage disease.

> *I don't see the sun.*

> *I have a lot of those long-sleeve shirts and it will be 86 degrees outside and I'll put on this long-sleeve shirt and I'm just sweating. But I wear them.*

Others, however, reported little to no change in their sun protection methods.

> *Probably not the right thing to do, but I very seldom use sunscreen.*

In addition, some reported adopting a healthier lifestyle, including losing weight, exercising more, and reducing work load. A few others also reported placing higher value on family and that their family became closer.

While most followed their physician's recommendations regarding surveillance, a few reported ignoring or postponing check-ups, particularly after the first year or two.

3.6. Identity as Cancer Survivor. As our goal was not only to summarize the experience of those diagnosed with melanoma but also to understand how future researchers might approach them, we asked participants whether they considered themselves to be cancer survivors. The responses were approximately evenly split between yes and no, but the explanations were diverse. All with stage III disease self-identified as cancer survivors, both indicating the literal stance that melanoma is cancer and also noting that it is a very serious cancer.

> I have a close friend that has breast cancer ... she was doing regular chemo and so I know all of that is just as grueling. But I don't think people realize sometimes that the stuff we do is just as grueling or it's the same thing. Cancer is cancer.

Some with early stage disease, when asked about being a cancer survivor, said yes as well, though a few participants noted they felt there was a spectrum of cancer survivorship.

> If you took a level of cancer survivor I would consider myself a one compared to a ten.

Participants who responded in the negative came from two different philosophies. Some did not consider melanoma serious enough or felt it was inappropriate because they did not have chemotherapy or radiation.

> I don't want to downplay melanoma, but when you say cancer survivor ... that's ... I don't want to upset anybody, but I really don't consider melanoma like pancreatic cancer or breast cancer.

> I feel like I didn't pay the full due with the chemo and the radiation and everything.

A few others, however, did not like the term because they felt they could develop another cancer.

> I've had cancer twice. I've gone through it twice, I've survived it twice. I don't consider myself a cancer survivor. I won't consider myself a cancer survivor until somebody looks me in the face and says, you know what honey, you're never going to get it again.

4. Discussion

The objective of the study was to document the experiences of persons diagnosed with melanoma further from their diagnosis using focus groups. The experiences shared by participants in this study highlight a number of QOL issues facing melanoma survivors. QOL among melanoma survivors has been an active area of research over the past few years and our study compliments the results of others, confirming many of the same themes.

As previously reported, most participants reported being shocked and overwhelmed at the time of diagnosis and having significant information needs [16–18]. Our data also support those of others who found melanoma survivors may experience treatment-specific symptoms such as fatigue and nausea, associated with adjuvant therapy [19–21], and lingering altered sensation and pain at the surgery site [22]. In addition, lymphedema was reported by a number of participants and resulted in notable complications, as reported by others with melanoma [16]. As important, some participants reported no physical concerns.

A systematic review found that most issues facing melanoma survivors are psychological in nature [12]. As noted by others, anxiety was the main concern of participants in this study, though it manifested in numerous ways: general anxiety, fear of recurrence or of a new cancer, and fear of family members getting cancer [23]. For most, the anxiety was worst around time of diagnosis and decreased over time. Similar to other reports, participants also reported concerns about their surgical scars, including feelings of disfigurement and discomfort with comments about the appearance of their scar by others [16, 17, 24]. We heard these concerns most notably among those with head or neck tumors and those with scars that were harder to disguise with clothing. The experiences shared by these survivors suggest that healthcare providers should inquire about emotional health when conducting surveillance exams and provide approaches for coping with anxiety.

As previously reported, for some participants their melanoma diagnosis had a positive impact on their life because it strengthened family relationships [10], whereas others felt socially isolated when they felt they could not join others in outdoor activities involving sun exposure [25]. We were, however, surprised by the level of isolation and loneliness reported despite having family support. This high level of isolation was also recently reported by Oliveria et al. [25]. Upon probing, it appeared to be caused by the lack of public awareness about the seriousness of melanoma. Compared to breast cancer survivors, for example, who have many opportunities to network with and meet other survivors, a need exists to increase both awareness of melanoma and chances for melanoma survivors to interact and support each other. Healthcare providers and advocates might consider promoting the creation of support groups and online forums for melanoma survivors, in addition to further educating the public about the serious nature of melanoma.

Studies to date on sun exposure and protection behaviors among melanoma survivors have been mixed; some have reported most survivors being conscious of sun exposure and protection [25–30], whereas others report risky sun behaviors despite their diagnosis [11, 30, 31]. The participants in this study suggest that both are true; while many alter their behaviors to avoid sun exposure, some report not changing their behavior. These data suggest at least some melanoma survivors need additional education and support regarding appropriate sun exposure and protection habits to reduce their risk of future melanomas.

Finally, participants were divided on whether they considered themselves a "cancer survivor." Similar responses have been reported in other cancers, including breast, prostate, colorectal, and hematologic cancers [32–37]. While most studies found the majority of survivors identify as being a cancer survivor, a significant proportion do not. Previous studies in other cancers have reported that those who do not endorse the term stated concerns about the cancer not being severe enough or the future being uncertain, particularly among those with a high risk of recurrence [33, 34, 38]. Due to the complexity of this issue, we encourage cautious use of the term "cancer survivor" when working directly with those who have been diagnosed with melanoma and instead recommend "person diagnosed with melanoma" until further research on the preferences of this population can be conducted.

Based on previous literature available at the time of the focus groups, we expected potential differences in experiences based on gender and wanted to ensure participant felt comfortable to share all concerns. In general, however, gender did not appear to drive differences in the experiences in our focus groups as much as disease stage and perceived seriousness of melanoma did. The numbers of groups were too limited to draw specific conclusions regarding gender differences.

The main strength of this study is the use of qualitative methods. Collecting data using focus groups allowed for a detailed and in-depth assessment of melanoma survivorship issues. These methods particularly permitted for capture of experiential personal information. We also focused on survivors of early stage disease, in contrast with most previous research. This study is not without limitations, however. The participants were one to four years from diagnosis and were from a single institution, an academic medical center. In addition few participants received adjuvant therapy. Therefore, the results here may not be generalizable to all melanoma survivors. Further, a portion of melanoma survivors had a family history of melanoma but this was not formally addressed during the focus groups and may have affected their concerns. In addition, qualitative research can be difficult to summarize in an objective way and despite efforts otherwise, our presence during data collection (i.e., conduct of focus groups) may have affected the subjects' responses.

5. Conclusions

With melanoma incidence on the rise and the unique nature of the disease in terms of both its potential early age of onset and severity, understanding the experiences of melanoma survivors is necessary from a public health perspective to promote optimal health and QOL in this growing population. Melanoma survivors participating in this study reported a diverse set of physical, emotional, and social concerns following diagnosis. The level of isolation and loneliness reported underscores the need to increase both awareness of melanoma and chances for melanoma survivors to interact and support each other. The shared experiences among participants in this study confirm the unique nature of melanoma and the need for interventions designed to improve the health and QOL of melanoma survivors.

Abbreviations

QOL: Quality of life
PI: Principal investigator.

Ethical Approval

The study was approved by the University of Minnesota Institutional Review Board (1201M09423).

Disclosure

The funders had no role in the design of the study, collection, analysis, and interpretation of data, or writing of the manuscript. These data were presented as a poster at the National Cancer Institute and American Cancer Society's Biennial Cancer Survivorship Research Conference, June 16–18, 2016.

Authors' Contributions

Rachel I. Vogel participated in study design and data collection, conducted data analysis, and wrote initial draft of the manuscript. Lori G. Strayer participated in study design and data collection. Rehana L. Ahmed participated in study design and interpretation of the results. Anne Blaes participated in interpretation of results. DeAnn Lazovich led study design and data collection and was a major contributor in writing the manuscript. All authors read and approved the final manuscript.

Acknowledgments

The study detailed here was funded by the Masonic Cancer Center of the University of Minnesota's Internal Grants Program and NIH grants from the National Cancer Institute (P30 CA77598) and National Center for Advancing Translational Sciences (UL1TR000114).

References

[1] A. C. Geller, R. W. Clapp, A. J. Sober et al., "Melanoma epidemic: an analysis of six decades of data from the connecticut tumor registry," *Journal of Clinical Oncology*, vol. 31, no. 33, pp. 4172–4178, 2013.

[2] E. P. Simard, E. M. Ward, R. Siegel, and A. Jemal, "Cancers with increasing incidence trends in the United States: 1999 through 2008," *CA Cancer Journal for Clinicians*, vol. 62, no. 2, pp. 118–128, 2012.

[3] G. P. Guy, C. C. thomas, T. Thompson, M. Watson, G. M. Massetti, and L. C. Richardson, "Vital signs: melanoma incidence and mortality trends and projectsion - united states, 1982–2030," Morbidity and Mortality Weekly Report 64, U.S. Department of Health and Human Services, 2015, Prevention CfDCa ed.

[4] American Cancer Society, *Cancer Treatment and Survivorship Facts & Figures 2014-2015*, American Cancer Society, Atlanta, GA, USA, 2014.

[5] M. F. Kalady, R. R. White, J. L. Johnson, D. S. Tyler, and H. F. Seigler, "Thin melanomas: predictive lethal characteristics from a 30-year clinical experience," *Ann Surg*, vol. 238, pp. 528–535, 2003.

[6] G. P. Guy Jr. and D. U. Ekwueme, "Years of potential life lost and indirect costs of melanoma and non-melanoma skin cancer," *PharmacoEconomics*, vol. 29, no. 10, pp. 863–874, 2011.

[7] N. Howlader, A. Noone, M. Krapcho et al., "SEER cancer statistics review, 1975–2008," Institute NC ed. Bethesda, MD, 2010.

[8] C. Holterhues, D. Cornish, L. V. Van De Poll-Franse et al., "Impact of melanoma on patients' lives among 562 survivors: a dutch population-based study," *Archives of Dermatology*, vol. 147, no. 2, pp. 177–185, 2011.

[9] Y. Hamama-Raz, "Does psychological adjustment of melanoma survivors differs between genders?" *Psycho-Oncology*, vol. 21, no. 3, pp. 255–263, 2012.

[10] C. Stava, M. Beck, L. T. Weiss, A. Lopez, and R. Vassilopoulou-Sellin, "Health profiles of 996 melanoma survivors: the M. D. Anderson experience," *BMC Cancer*, vol. 6, article 95, 2006.

[11] U. J. Mujumdar, J. L. Hay, Y. C. Monroe-Hinds et al., "Sun protection and skin self-examination in melanoma survivors," *Psycho-Oncology*, vol. 18, no. 10, pp. 1106–1115, 2009.

[12] N. A. Kasparian, J. K. McLoone, and P. N. Butow, "Psychological responses and coping strategies among patients with malignant melanoma: a systematic review of the literature," *Archives of Dermatology*, vol. 145, no. 12, pp. 1415–1427, 2009.

[13] D. Lazovich, R. I. Vogel, M. Berwick, M. A. Weinstock, K. E. Anderson, and E. M. Warshaw, "Indoor tanning and risk of melanoma: a case-control study in a highly exposed population," *Cancer Epidemiology Biomarkers and Prevention*, vol. 19, no. 6, pp. 1557–1568, 2010.

[14] R. Krueger and M. A. Casey, *Focus Groups: A Practical Guide for Applied Research*, Sage Publications, Thousand Oaks, Calif, USA, 4th edition, 2008.

[15] R. Krueger, *Focus Group Kit—Developing Questions for Focus Groups*, Sage Publications, Thousand Oaks, Calif, USA, 1998.

[16] J. D. Tan, P. N. Butow, F. M. Boyle, R. P. M. Saw, and A. J. O'Reilly, "A qualitative assessment of psychosocial impact, coping and adjustment in high-risk melanoma patients and caregivers," *Melanoma Research*, vol. 24, no. 3, pp. 252–260, 2014.

[17] J. B. Winstanley, E. G. White, F. M. Boyle, and J. F. Thompson, "What are the pertinent quality-of-life issues for melanoma cancer patients? Aiming for the development of a new module to accompany the EORTC core questionnaire," *Melanoma Research*, vol. 23, no. 2, pp. 167–174, 2013.

[18] O. Palesh, A. Aldridge-Gerry, K. Bugos et al., "Health behaviors and needs of melanoma survivors," *Supportive Care in Cancer*, vol. 22, no. 11, pp. 2973–2980, 2014.

[19] S. Ziefle, F. Egberts, S. Heinze et al., "Health-related quality of life before and during adjuvant interferon-α treatment for patients with malignant melanoma (DeCOG-trial)," *Journal of Immunotherapy*, vol. 34, no. 4, pp. 403–408, 2011.

[20] D. Rataj, E. Krajewska-Kułak, B. Jankowiak et al., "Quality-of-life evaluation in an interferon therapy after radical surgery in cutaneous melanoma patients," *Cancer Nursing*, vol. 28, no. 3, pp. 172–178, 2005.

[21] S. Dixon, S. J. Walters, L. Turner, and B. W. Hancock, "Quality of life and cost-effectiveness of interferon-alpha in malignant melanoma: results from randomised trial," *British Journal of Cancer*, vol. 94, no. 4, pp. 492–498, 2006.

[22] H. Høimyr, K. A. Rokkones, M. L. Von Sperling, K. Finnerup, T. S. Jensen, and N. B. Finnerup, "Persistent pain after lymph node excision in patients with malignant melanoma is neuropathic," *Pain*, vol. 152, no. 12, pp. 2721–2728, 2011.

[23] A. Molassiotis, L. Brunton, J. Hodgetts et al., "Prevalence and correlates of unmet supportive care needs in patients with resected invasive cutaneous melanoma," *Annals of Oncology: Official Journal of the European Society for Medical Oncology/ESMO*, vol. 25, no. 10, pp. 2052–2058, 2014.

[24] Z. Stamataki, L. Brunton, P. Lorigan, A. C. Green, J. Newton-Bishop, and A. Molassiotis, "Assessing the impact of diagnosis and the related supportive care needs in patients with cutaneous melanoma," *Supportive Care in Cancer*, vol. 23, no. 3, pp. 779–789, 2015.

[25] S. A. Oliveria, E. Shuk, J. L. Hay et al., "Melanoma survivors: health behaviors, surveillance, psychosocial factors, and family concerns," *Psycho-Oncology*, vol. 22, no. 1, pp. 106–116, 2013.

[26] E. Soto, H. Lee, R. N. Saladi et al., "Behavioral factors of patients before and after diagnosis with melanoma: a cohort study—are sun-protection measures being implemented?" *Melanoma Research*, vol. 20, no. 2, pp. 147–152, 2010.

[27] A. Freiman, J. Yu, A. Loutfi, and B. Wang, "Impact of melanoma diagnosis on sun-awareness and protection: efficacy of education campaigns in a high-risk population," *Journal of Cutaneous Medicine and Surgery*, vol. 8, no. 5, pp. 303–309, 2004.

[28] C. B. Novak and D. S. Young, "Evaluation of sun protection behaviour in patients following excision of a skin lesion," *Plastic Surgery*, vol. 15, no. 1, 2007.

[29] D. Mayer, A. Layman, and J. Carlson, "Sun-protection behaviors of melanoma survivors," *Journal of the American Academy of Dermatology*, vol. 66, no. 1, pp. e9-e10, 2012.

[30] R. Bränström, N. A. Kasparian, Y.-M. Chang et al., "Predictors of sun protection behaviors and severe sunburn in an international online study," *Cancer Epidemiology Biomarkers and Prevention*, vol. 19, no. 9, pp. 2199–2210, 2010.

[31] R. Bränström, Y.-M. Chang, N. Kasparian et al., "Melanoma risk factors, perceived threat and intentional tanning: an international online survey," *European Journal of Cancer Prevention*, vol. 19, no. 3, pp. 216–226, 2010.

[32] S. K. Chambers, P. Baade, X. Meng, P. Youl, J. Aitken, and J. Dunn, "Survivor identity after colorectal cancer: antecedents, prevalence and outcomes," *Psycho-Oncology*, vol. 21, no. 9, pp. 962–969, 2012.

[33] K. Kaiser, "The meaning of the survivor identity for women with breast cancer," *Social Science and Medicine*, vol. 67, no. 1, pp. 79–87, 2008.

[34] N. F. Khan, S. Harrison, P. W. Rose, A. Ward, and J. Evans, "Interpretation and acceptance of the term 'cancer survivor': a United Kingdom-based qualitative study," *European Journal of Cancer Care*, vol. 21, no. 2, pp. 177–186, 2012.

[35] D. Cho and C. L. Park, "Cancer-related identities in people diagnosed during late adolescence and young adulthood," *British Journal of Health Psychology*, vol. 20, no. 3, pp. 594–612, 2015.

[36] C. L. Park, I. Zlateva, and T. O. Blank, "Self-identity after cancer: 'survivor', 'victim', 'patient', and 'person with cancer'," *Journal of General Internal Medicine*, vol. 24, no. 2, pp. S430-S435, 2009.

[37] G. T. Deimling, K. F. Bowman, and L. J. Wagner, "Cancer survivorship and identity among long-term survivors," *Cancer Investigation*, vol. 25, no. 8, pp. 758–765, 2007.

[38] P. McGrath and H. Holewa, "What does the term 'survivor' mean to individuals diagnosed with a haematological malignancy? Findings from Australia," *Supportive Care in Cancer*, vol. 20, no. 12, pp. 3287–3295, 2012.

25

Current Data on Risk Factor Estimates Does Not Explain the Difference in Rates of Melanoma between Hispanics and Non-Hispanic Whites

Sonia Kamath,[1] **Kimberly A. Miller,**[2] **and Myles G. Cockburn**[1,2]

[1]*Department of Dermatology, Keck School of Medicine of the University of Southern California (USC), 1200 N State Street, Room 3250, Los Angeles, CA 90033, USA*
[2]*Department of Preventive Medicine, Keck School of Medicine of USC, 2001 N. Soto Street, Suite 318-A, Los Angeles, CA 90032, USA*

Correspondence should be addressed to Sonia Kamath; shkamath@med.usc.edu

Academic Editor: Günther Hofbauer

United States Hispanics have seven times lower melanoma incidence rates than non-Hispanic whites (NHW). It is unclear whether this difference can be explained solely by phenotypic risk factors, like darker skin, or whether modifiable risk factors, like sun exposure, also play a role. The purpose of this paper is to summarize what is currently known about melanoma risk factors among Hispanics and NHWs, and whether or not those differences could explain the difference in melanoma incidence. Through literature review, relative risks and prevalence of melanoma risk factors in Hispanics and NHWs were identified and used to calculate the expected rate in Hispanics and rate ratio compared to NHWs. We found that melanoma risk factors either have similar frequency in Hispanics and NHWs (e.g., many large nevi) or are less frequent in Hispanics but do not explain a high proportion of disease variation (e.g., red hair). Considering current knowledge of risk factor prevalence, we found that melanoma incidence rates in the two groups should actually be similar. Sun exposure behavior among Hispanics may contribute to the explanation for the 7-fold difference in melanoma rates. Currently, limited data exist on sun exposure behavior among Hispanics, but possibilities for improving primary prevention by further studying these practices are substantial.

1. Introduction

Hispanics are the largest ethnic group in the United States, and over the last few decades, rates of melanoma among Hispanics have steadily risen [1, 2]. In California, where Hispanics comprise almost 40% of the population, increases in melanoma have occurred for tumors with the worst prognosis [3–5]. Hispanics are diagnosed with melanoma at later stages than non-Hispanic whites (NHW), leading to increased likelihood of metastasis and higher mortality [3, 6, 7]. Still, the rates of melanoma in the Hispanic population remain approximately seven times lower than in the NHW population in California [3]. This difference in melanoma incidence between Hispanics and NHWs has traditionally been attributed to the protective effects of darker skin pigmentation [5]. However, Hispanics have significant heterogeneity of skin color and phenotype (including light skin color), and it is well known that ultraviolet (UV) exposure plays a role in the development of melanoma regardless of skin type [8, 9]. In fact, it is unclear whether key melanoma risk factors, including increased numbers of nevi, freckling, poor tanning ability, and fair complexion, differ substantially between Hispanics and NHWs [10, 11]. Few studies describe melanoma risk factors in Hispanics, or those risks relative to NHWs [12]. Most studies have focused on determining relative risks (RRs) for melanoma in NHWs, and few estimate melanoma burden attributable to each risk factor [13, 14].

In this review, we examined what is currently known about the risk factors for melanoma and their distribution among Hispanics and then calculated expected rate ratios (NHW compared to Hispanic) for each risk factor based on published estimates of relative risk and risk factor prevalence in the two groups. We found that, based on what is currently known about the risk factors, the rates of melanoma among

Hispanics and NHWs should be quite similar, and the fact that they are not similar may present an opportunity to investigate modifiable risk factors for melanoma—for which very little data exists in the Hispanic population—and to improve prevention efforts.

2. Materials and Methods

2.1. Defining the Risk Factors for Melanoma. For summary relative risk (RR) measures for melanoma risk factors, we used a comprehensive meta-analysis by Gandini et al. of 83 observational studies through September 2002 [20–22]. A PubMed search covering observational studies through April 2013 was conducted to provide a RR range for those risk factors not included in the meta-analysis.

Phenotypic risk factors for melanoma in the meta-analysis include blonde or red hair, many freckles, nevus counts, and Fitzpatrick phototype I or II. For freckles, the RR presented in the meta-analysis compared estimates for high versus low density of freckles. We focus on risk associated with increased numbers of common nevi, since dysplastic nevi have been noted to occur specifically in melanoma-prone families [22, 23]. Sunburn and sun exposure represent important risk factors for melanoma. Sun exposure was divided into total lifetime, intermittent, and chronic exposure. Intermittent sun exposure included estimates based on recreational activities, while chronic sun exposure was assessed as occupational exposure. Where multiple levels of exposure were reported, the highest level was included [20, 21].

For counts of large nevi, history of one or more childhood sunburns, and history of one or more lifetime sunburns, RRs were not summarized in the meta-analysis, so a literature search was conducted. Combinations of the following keywords and MeSH terms were used in PubMed: melanoma, etiology, epidemiology, prevention and control, risk factors, case-control studies, cohort studies, cross-sectional studies, nevus, skin pigmentation, skin color, hair color, sun exposure, sunlight, ultraviolet rays, sunburn, suntan, and sunbathing. Included studies were limited to those in English and those examining adult populations. Duplicates, reviews, and irrelevant articles were excluded. Other studies were excluded for ineligible study design (e.g., case series) (14 studies); using outcome of second primary melanoma (11 studies); not being independent of other included studies (3 studies); presenting data by gender, body site, or melanoma subtype (16 studies); or focusing on a restricted age group (1 study). An exception was made for Qureshi et al. and Han et al., as although they are based on the same cohort, the risk factors examined in each are different [24, 25].

We extracted study location, study design, number and source of cases and controls, age of study population, definitions and categories of risk factors, prevalence estimates, RR or odds ratio (OR) estimates, 95% confidence interval (CI), and variables for which statistical adjustment was done. For articles that presented multiple estimates, we recorded the one adjusted for the most confounders. For risk factors not included in the Gandini meta-analysis, the RR range represents estimates from all included studies, and the median of this range is reported in place of a summary statistic. For

other risk factors, the RR range is provided as an update of studies published after 2002.

2.2. Calculating the Expected Rate Ratio of Melanoma in Non-Hispanic Whites Compared to Hispanics. In order to compare the melanoma rates between Hispanics and NHWs in California, we obtained California population-based risk factor prevalence data wherever possible. The California Health Interview Survey (CHIS) provides information on sunburn prevalence in NHWs and Hispanics [18]. We obtained the prevalence of having more than three lifetime episodes of sunburn, as this was the highest exposure level reported in the majority of papers. The Los Angeles Multiethnic Cohort provided the prevalence of sunburn and red or blonde hair color in Hispanics and NHWs [15]. Prevalence of additional phenotypic characteristics and large nevi was obtained from the California Twin Program [16]. For phototype and chronic sun exposure, estimates were used from the National Health and Nutritional Examination Surveys (NHANES) and the National Health Interview Survey (NHIS) [17, 19]. Lastly, because of the lack of population-based prevalence information on sun exposure and counts of common nevi, we calculated a weighted average of the prevalence reported among controls of the included population-based studies.

We used the reported RR for each melanoma risk factor and the risk factor prevalence among Hispanics, to calculate the expected rate of melanoma incidence among Hispanics, and the ratio compared to that in NHWs. We present the rate ratio using an incidence rate of 29 per 100,000 in NHWs (observed in males in California), for which the comparable observed rate ratio is 7.25 (the comparable melanoma incidence rate in Hispanic males in California is approximately 4 per 100,000) [3].

Because so little data are available on the RR of melanoma risk factors specific to Hispanic populations, we have assumed that the RR in Hispanics is the same as in NHWs (discussed below). Where prevalence of risk factors was unknown in Hispanic populations, we could not calculate the expected rate ratio.

3. Results and Discussion

3.1. Does the Prevalence of Melanoma Risk Factor Phenotypes Explain the Lower Rate of Melanoma in Hispanics? Table 1 summarizes the risk factors, RR ranges, prevalence ranges, and calculated rate ratios [15–19, 24–95]. Of the risk factors for which an expected rate ratio could be calculated, skin phototype I or II was responsible for the highest expected rate ratio, but this was only 1.40. Blonde hair was associated with the second highest expected rate ratio (1.26) in NHWs compared to Hispanics. Having many large nevi, although carrying RR of 3.05, demonstrated an expected rate ratio of 1.04 (because the prevalence of large nevi is similar in NHW and Hispanics), and high chronic sun exposure accounted for no difference in expected melanoma rates between Hispanics and NHWs. In both cases the expected rate ratio was near null because of the similarity of prevalence of the risk factor in Hispanics and NHWs.

TABLE 1: Summary of relative risks (RR) and prevalence of risk factors.

Risk factor	Category	RR[a]	95% CI	RR range	Prevalence (%) NHW	Prevalence (%) Hispanic	Expected rate ratio[b] (Observed = 7.25)	Source
Hair color	Blonde	1.96	1.41–2.72	0.45–4.13	13.60–46.80	0.90–3.60	1.26	Park et al., 2012 [15] Cockburn et al., 2007 [16], CTP[c]
	Red	3.64	2.56–5.37	1.73–4.94	3.10–3.20	0.30–1.30	1.06	Park et al., 2012 [15] Cockburn et al., 2007 [16], CTP
Phototype	Fitzpatrick type I	2.09	1.67–2.58	2.36–2.64	5.00–7.60	1.00–3.30	1.04	Lin et al., 2012 [17] Galindo et al., 2007 [8]
	Fitzpatrick type II	1.84	1.43–2.36	1.82–4.13	26.70–39.00	10.70–12.00	1.16	Lin et al., 2012 [17] Galindo et al., 2007 [8]
	Fitzpatrick type I or II	2.99	1.75–5.12	1.31–2.90	34.30–44.00	13.00–14.00	1.40	Lin et al., 2012 [17] Galindo et al., 2007 [8]
Freckles	Many freckles	2.10	1.80–2.45	1.55–3.72	7.43 (controls)	Not available	~	
Nevi	Many nevi	4.82	3.05–7.62	1.50–6.50	11.66 (controls)	Not available	~	
	Many large nevi	3.05		1.19–5.70	5.70	3.60	1.04	CTP
Sunburn	Many sunburns (lifetime)	2.03	1.73–2.37	0.59–8.48	7.50–20.70	3.80–4.00	1.10	Park et al., 2012 [15] CHIS 2009 [18]
	Many sunburns (childhood)	2.24	1.73–2.89	1.00–6.22	13.70 (controls)	Not available	~	
	Ever had sunburn (lifetime)	1.21		1.10–5.70	61.8	21	1.08	Park et al., 2012 [15]
	Ever had sunburn (childhood)	1.47		0.90–3.56	28.19 (controls)	Not available	~	
Sun exposure	High total lifetime sun exposure	1.34	1.02–1.77	0.80–4.34	27.11 (controls)	Not available	~	
	High intermittent sun exposure	1.61	1.31–1.99	0.65–5.00	40.54 (controls)	Not available	~	
	High chronic sun exposure	0.95	0.87–1.04	0.33–2.57	5.44 (controls)	12.00	1.00	Coups et al., 2012 [19]

[a]RR represents summary statistic from meta-analysis by Gandini et al., 2005 [20–22] (I, II, and III) or median of RR range where summary statistic is not reported.

[b]Expected ratio of incidence rates (NHW/Hispanic) based on prevalence of risk factor in each population and RR provided. Median prevalence value is used when a range is provided.

[c]CTP: California Twin Program; prevalence data for NHWs is described by Cockburn et al., 2007 [16], and prevalence data for Hispanics comes from the same data set.

~Expected rate ratio cannot be calculated because prevalence in Hispanics is unknown.

Most studies comparing rates of melanoma in Hispanics and NHWs focus on delayed diagnosis and overall worse outcomes among Hispanics, while few specifically compare risk factors. Our review confirms that Hispanics do have lower prevalence of some of the major melanoma risk phenotypes, blonde or red hair color, Fitzpatrick skin type I or II, strong history of sunburn, and many large nevi. However, these risk factors are not sufficiently rare in Hispanics to explain their lower rate of melanoma compared to NHWs, largely because there is overlap in the prevalence of the risk factors between Hispanics and NHWs.

3.2. Could Sun Exposure Behavior Explain the Lower Rate of Melanoma in Hispanics? Hispanics may have a reduced melanoma risk if they practice better sun protection. Recent studies highlight differences in method of sun protection among subpopulations of Hispanics. Specifically, English-acculturated Hispanics display more sunscreen use but less use of sun protective clothing, while Spanish-acculturated Hispanics are more likely to wear sun protective clothing without sunscreen [19, 96]. Additionally, English-acculturated Hispanics are more likely to have had a sunburn in the past year compared to those less acculturated, consistent with data showing that sunscreen may not be as effective as sun protective clothing at preventing sunburn [19, 97]. Given the diversity of sun protective practices among Hispanics, studying the relationship between sun exposure behavior and melanoma stratified by level of acculturation would help clarify whether safer sun exposure behavior accounts for overall low rates of melanoma in this population.

Data from the Behavioral Risk Factor Surveillance System (BRFSS) shows that overall a smaller percentage of Hispanics reported having at least one sunburn in the preceding year compared to NHWs. Hispanics who reported having at least one sunburn in the past year were more likely to have had *only* one sunburn, compared to NHWs [98]. However, BRFSS data also show that sunburn among Hispanics is relatively common, which could contribute to their increasing incidence of melanoma. Compared to NHWs, Hispanics do have higher prevalence of chronic sun exposure, shown to be protective against melanoma compared to intermittent exposure [9, 10, 99].

3.3. Could Genetic Effects Explain the Lower Rate of Melanoma in Hispanics? A multitude of genetic factors, if substantially different in the two populations, could either protect Hispanics or make NHWs more susceptible to melanoma. Six loci have been implicated in melanoma susceptibility. While five of them represent genes involved in melanin production (*MC1R*, *TYR*, *TYRP1*, *SLC45A2*, and *ASIP*), the sixth locus is thought to represent two genes, both involved in nevus formation (*CDKN2A* and *MTAP*) [10, 100]. The *CDKN2A* gene is inherited in an autosomal dominant fashion and is associated with familial melanoma, which represents only 5 to 12% of melanoma cases [101]. The prevalence of these genotypes in Hispanics is unknown.

The *MC1R* gene codes for the melanocortin-1 receptor. Weak signaling of this receptor due to inactivating polymorphisms in the *MC1R* gene results in production of the red pigment pheomelanin ("red hair/fair skin" phenotype), instead of the brown/black eumelanin [102]. It has recently been shown that pheomelanin may be carcinogenic itself, independent of UV radiation, particularly in the context of an activating mutation in the kinase BRAF (the most common driver mutation in melanoma). Specifically, mice with an inactivating *MC1R* mutation and the BRAF mutation had red fur and developed melanoma, while mice who did not produce pheomelanin did not develop melanoma, despite having the BRAF mutation [103]. However, given the overlap in skin types between Hispanics and NHWs and the near-null expected rate ratio for skin type in our analysis, variations in the population prevalence of *MC1R* inactivating polymorphisms and pheomelanin are unlikely to fully explain the large difference in melanoma incidence.

BRAF mutations are more common in melanomas occurring in skin intermittently exposed to high amounts of sun compared with melanomas arising on unexposed or chronically exposed skin [104]. It is possible that fewer Hispanics have *BRAF* mutations, which could help to explain their lower incidence of melanoma. Since most clinical trials have been conducted in NHWs, there is a paucity of literature on genetic mutations in other populations [105]. Further studies

are necessary to elucidate the role of genotype in the risk for melanoma among Hispanics.

3.4. Limitations. The observation that Hispanics have more advanced melanomas at diagnosis than NHWs could be explained by lower awareness of melanoma in this population, resulting in lower likelihood of seeking care [106–109]. This presents the possibility that true rates of melanoma in the Hispanic population are higher than observed and that there is poorer detection of cases. However, 35.4 percent of tumors in Hispanic males in California are "thick" (>1.5 mm) at diagnosis, compared with 24.4 percent of tumors in NHWs, so the lack of detection of thin tumors through screening in Hispanics alone is unlikely to explain a 7-fold difference in the overall incidence rate [2].

We make a number of assumptions in our calculations, which are done for illustrative purposes. First, we assume that the RR for each risk factor is the same in Hispanics and NHWs. This is because there is little data assessing melanoma risk factors specifically in Hispanics. It is possible that RRs for melanoma risk factors differ for NHWs and Hispanics but that remains to be shown. For illustrative purposes, we have used incidence data only from NHW and Hispanic males in California, but the rate ratios for comparison among females in California provide similar results. Finally, we considered all invasive melanomas together, though the distributions of the various melanoma histologic subtypes are known to differ between NHW and Hispanics [5, 9]. However, risk factors for nodular and superficial spreading melanoma do not vary among NHWs, and there is limited data on other histology-specific risk factors [110].

4. Conclusions

To determine effective methods of primary prevention, it is useful to investigate characteristics associated with lower risk of melanoma. To that end, the melanoma experience of Hispanics, who have at least 7-fold lower risk of melanoma than NHWs, might provide clues to improved melanoma prevention. This review highlights the limited data on melanoma risk phenotypes in Hispanic populations; what is currently known about the differences in their prevalence between Hispanics and NHWs inadequately explains a 7-fold difference in melanoma rates.

While genotype may vary between Hispanics and NHWs, there is insufficient data about melanoma risk genes in Hispanic populations to attribute their lower melanoma rates to genetic factors alone. The association between genotype and melanoma risk phenotype might lead us to expect greater differences in skin type and nevi prevalence between Hispanics and NHWs if differentially expressed genetic factors explained the 7-fold difference in melanoma incidence.

While little data exist comparing sun exposure behaviors in Hispanics and NHWs, current data show that Hispanics sunburn less frequently. If sun exposure behaviors help protect Hispanics from melanoma, there could be great potential for improving prevention in all populations through behavioral change. Once the sun exposure behaviors of Hispanics are more clearly understood, prevention messages might be improved. The lower rate of melanoma in Hispanics should be formally investigated in future studies, providing direct comparison of measured risk factors in Hispanics versus NHWs and accounting for any differences in sun exposure behaviors, phenotypic and genotypic characteristics. Such an approach may better inform our methods of melanoma prevention in both Hispanics and NHWs.

Disclosure

The ideas and opinions expressed herein are those of the author(s) and endorsement by the State of California, Department of Public Health the National Cancer Institute, and the Centers for Disease Control and Prevention or their Contractors and Subcontractors is not intended nor should be inferred.

Competing Interests

The authors declare that there are no competing interests regarding the publication of this paper.

Acknowledgments

Dr. Myles G. Cockburn was supported in part by the National Cancer Institute's Surveillance, Epidemiology and End Results Program under Contract HHSN261201000140C awarded to the Cancer Prevention Institute of California, Contract HHSN261201000035C awarded to the University of Southern California, and Contract HHSN261201000034C awarded to the Public Health Institute and the Centers for Disease Control and Prevention's National Program of Cancer Registries, under Agreement U58DP003862-01 awarded to the California Department of Public Health.

References

[1] US Census Bureau, *Hispanics in the United States*, 2008, http://www.census.gov/population/hispanic/publications/hispanics_2006.html.

[2] M. G. Cockburn, J. Zadnick, and D. Deapen, "Developing epidemic of melanoma in the Hispanic population of California," *Cancer*, vol. 106, no. 5, pp. 1162–1168, 2006.

[3] R. A. Pollitt, C. A. Clarke, S. M. Swetter, D. H. Peng, J. Zadnick, and M. Cockburn, "The expanding melanoma burden in California Hispanics," *Cancer*, vol. 117, no. 1, pp. 152–161, 2011.

[4] US Census Bureau, *State & County Quick Facts—California*, 2012, http://quickfacts.census.gov/qfd/states/06000.html.

[5] R. D. Cress and E. A. Holly, "Incidence of cutaneous melanoma among non-Hispanic Whites, Hispanics, Asians, and blacks: an analysis of California Cancer Registry Data, 1988–93," *Cancer Causes and Control*, vol. 8, no. 2, pp. 246–252, 1997.

[6] X.-C. Wu, M. J. Eide, J. King et al., "Racial and ethnic variations in incidence and survival of cutaneous melanoma in the United States, 1999–2006," *Journal of the American Academy of Dermatology*, vol. 65, no. 5, supplement 1, pp. S26–S37, 2011.

[7] R. M. Merrill, N. D. Pace, and A. N. Elison, "Cutaneous malignant melanoma among white Hispanics and non-Hispanics in

the United States," *Ethnicity & Disease*, vol. 20, no. 4, pp. 353–358, 2010.

[8] G. R. Galindo, J. A. Mayer, D. Slymen et al., "Sun sensitivity in 5 US ethnoracial groups," *Cutis*, vol. 80, no. 1, pp. 25–30, 2007.

[9] S. Hu, F. Ma, F. Collado-Mesa, and R. S. Kirsner, "UV radiation, latitude, and melanoma in US Hispanics and blacks," *Archives of Dermatology*, vol. 140, no. 7, pp. 819–824, 2004.

[10] S. T. Chen, A. C. Geller, and H. Tsao, "Update on the epidemiology of melanoma," *Current Dermatology Reports*, vol. 2, no. 1, pp. 24–34, 2013.

[11] M. A. Tucker, "Melanoma epidemiology," *Hematology/Oncology Clinics of North America*, vol. 23, no. 3, pp. 383–395, 2009.

[12] N. Jaimes, S. Oliveria, and A. Halpern, "A cautionary note on melanoma screening in the Hispanic/Latino population," *JAMA Dermatology*, vol. 149, no. 4, pp. 396–397, 2013.

[13] C. M. Olsen, H. J. Carroll, and D. C. Whiteman, "Estimating the attributable fraction for cancer: a meta-analysis of nevi and melanoma," *Cancer Prevention Research*, vol. 3, no. 2, pp. 233–245, 2010.

[14] C. M. Olsen, H. J. Carroll, and D. C. Whiteman, "Estimating the attributable fraction for melanoma: a meta-analysis of pigmentary characteristics and freckling," *International Journal of Cancer*, vol. 127, no. 10, pp. 2430–2445, 2010.

[15] S. L. Park, L. Le Marchand, L. R. Wilkens et al., "Risk factors for malignant melanoma in white and non-white/non-African American populations: the multiethnic cohort," *Cancer Prevention Research*, vol. 5, no. 3, pp. 423–434, 2012.

[16] M. G. Cockburn, A. Hamilton, and T. Mack, "The simultaneous assessment of constitutional, behavioral, and environmental factors in the development of large nevi," *Cancer Epidemiology Biomarkers and Prevention*, vol. 16, no. 2, pp. 200–206, 2007.

[17] F. R. Lin, P. Maas, W. Chien, J. P. Carey, L. Ferrucci, and R. Thorpe, "Association of skin color, race/ethnicity, and hearing loss among adults in the USA," *Journal of the Association for Research in Otolaryngology*, vol. 13, no. 1, pp. 109–117, 2012.

[18] California Health Interview Survey, 2009, http://ask.chis.ucla.edu.

[19] E. J. Coups, J. L. Stapleton, S. V. Hudson, A. Medina-Forrester, A. Natale-Pereira, and J. S. Goydos, "Sun protection and exposure behaviors among Hispanic adults in the United States: differences according to acculturation and among Hispanic subgroups," *BMC Public Health*, vol. 12, pp. 985–993, 2012.

[20] S. Gandini, F. Sera, M. S. Cattaruzza et al., "Meta-analysis of risk factors for cutaneous melanoma: I. Common and atypical naevi," *European Journal of Cancer*, vol. 41, no. 1, pp. 28–44, 2005.

[21] S. Gandini, F. Sera, M. S. Cattaruzza et al., "Meta-analysis of risk factors for cutaneous melanoma: II. Sun exposure," *European Journal of Cancer*, vol. 41, no. 1, pp. 45–60, 2005.

[22] S. Gandini, F. Sera, M. S. Cattaruzza et al., "Meta-analysis of risk factors for cutaneous melanoma: III. Family history, actinic damage and phenotypic factors," *European Journal of Cancer*, vol. 41, no. 14, pp. 2040–2059, 2005.

[23] A. M. Goldstein and M. A. Tucker, "Dysplastic nevi and melanoma," *Cancer Epidemiology Biomarkers and Prevention*, vol. 22, no. 4, pp. 528–532, 2013.

[24] A. A. Qureshi, M. Zhang, and J. Han, "Heterogeneity in host risk factors for incident melanoma and non-melanoma skin cancer in a cohort of US women," *Journal of Epidemiology*, vol. 21, no. 3, pp. 197–203, 2011.

[25] J. Han, G. A. Colditz, and D. J. Hunter, "Risk factors for skin cancers: a nested case-control study within the Nurses' Health Study," *International Journal of Epidemiology*, vol. 35, no. 6, pp. 1514–1521, 2006.

[26] J. Wendt, O. Schanab, M. Binder, H. Pehamberger, and I. Okamoto, "Site-dependent actinic skin damage as risk factor for melanoma in a central European population," *Pigment Cell and Melanoma Research*, vol. 25, no. 2, pp. 234–242, 2012.

[27] E. De Vries, M. Trakatelli, D. Kalabalikis et al., "Known and potential new risk factors for skin cancer in European populations: a multicentre case-control study," *British Journal of Dermatology*, vol. 167, no. 2, pp. 1–13, 2012.

[28] O. C. Luiz, R. J. Gianini, F. T. Gonçalves et al., "Ethnicity and cutaneous melanoma in the city of Sao Paulo, Brazil: a case-control study," *PLoS ONE*, vol. 7, no. 4, Article ID e36348, 2012.

[29] C. Fortes, S. Mastroeni, P. Boffetta et al., "Polymorphisms of GSTM1 and GSTT1, sun exposure and the risk of melanoma: a case-control study," *Acta Dermato-Venereologica*, vol. 91, no. 3, pp. 284–289, 2011.

[30] A. E. Cust, M. A. Jenkins, C. Goumas et al., "Early-life sun exposure and risk of melanoma before age 40 years," *Cancer Causes and Control*, vol. 22, no. 6, pp. 885–897, 2011.

[31] J. A. Newton-Bishop, Y.-M. Chang, F. Elliott et al., "Relationship between sun exposure and melanoma risk for tumours in different body sites in a large case-control study in a temperate climate," *European Journal of Cancer*, vol. 47, no. 5, pp. 732–741, 2011.

[32] D. Lazovich, R. I. Vogel, M. Berwick, M. A. Weinstock, K. E. Anderson, and E. M. Warshaw, "Indoor tanning and risk of melanoma: a case-control study in a highly exposed population," *Cancer Epidemiology Biomarkers and Prevention*, vol. 19, no. 6, pp. 1557–1568, 2010.

[33] L. K. Dennis, C. F. Lynch, D. P. Sandler, and M. C. R. Alavanja, "Pesticide use and cutaneous melanoma in pesticide applicators in the agricultural heath study," *Environmental Health Perspectives*, vol. 118, no. 6, pp. 812–817, 2010.

[34] M. B. Veierød, H.-O. Adami, E. Lund, B. K. Armstrong, and E. Weiderpass, "Sun and solarium exposure and melanoma risk: effects of age, pigmentary characteristics, and nevi," *Cancer Epidemiology Biomarkers and Prevention*, vol. 19, no. 1, pp. 111–120, 2010.

[35] A. Chiarugi, M. Ceroti, D. Palli, G. Cevenini, M. Guarrera, and P. Carli, "Sensitivity to ultraviolet B is a risk factor for cutaneous melanoma in a Mediterranean population: results from an Italian case-control study," *Clinical and Experimental Dermatology*, vol. 34, no. 1, pp. 8–15, 2009.

[36] A. E. Cust, H. Schmid, J. A. Maskiell et al., "Population-based, case-control-family design to investigate genetic and environmental influences on melanoma risk," *American Journal of Epidemiology*, vol. 170, no. 12, pp. 1541–1554, 2009.

[37] C. Li, Z. Liu, L. E. Wang et al., "Haplotype and genotypes of the VDR gene and cutaneous melanoma risk in non-Hispanic whites in Texas: a case-control study," *International Journal of Cancer*, vol. 122, no. 9, pp. 2077–2084, 2008.

[38] V. A. Nikolaou, V. Sypsa, I. Stefanaki et al., "Risk associations of melanoma in a Southern European population: results of a case/control study," *Cancer Causes and Control*, vol. 19, no. 7, pp. 671–679, 2008.

[39] S. Rosso, R. Zanetti, M. J. Sánchez et al., "Is 2,3,5-pyrroletricarboxylic acid in hair a better risk indicator for melanoma than traditional epidemiologic measures for skin phenotype?" *American Journal of Epidemiology*, vol. 165, no. 10, pp. 1170–1177, 2007.

[40] C. S. Mantzoros, M. Trakatelli, H. Gogas et al., "Circulating adiponectin levels in relation to melanoma: a case-control study," *European Journal of Cancer*, vol. 43, no. 9, pp. 1430–1436, 2007.

[41] C. S. Lea, J. A. Scotto, P. A. Buffler, J. Fine, R. L. Barnhill, and M. Berwick, "Ambient UVB and melanoma risk in the United States: a case-control analysis," *Annals of Epidemiology*, vol. 17, no. 6, pp. 447–453, 2007.

[42] R. Zanetti, S. Rosso, C. Martinez et al., "Comparison of risk patterns in carcinoma and melanoma of the skin in men: a multi-centre case-case-control study," *British Journal of Cancer*, vol. 94, no. 5, pp. 743–751, 2006.

[43] Z. Tatalovich, J. P. Wilson, T. Mack, Y. Yan, and M. Cockburn, "The objective assessment of lifetime cumulative ultraviolet exposure for determining melanoma risk," *Journal of Photochemistry and Photobiology B*, vol. 85, no. 3, pp. 198–204, 2006.

[44] A. R. Shors, S. Kim, E. White et al., "Dysplastic naevi with moderate to severe histological dysplasia: a risk factor for melanoma," *British Journal of Dermatology*, vol. 155, no. 5, pp. 988–993, 2006.

[45] L. Naldi, G. Randi, A. Di Landro, and C. L. Vecchia, "Red hairs, number of nevi, and risk of cutaneous malignant melanoma: results from a case-control study in Italy," *Archives of Dermatology*, vol. 142, no. 7, pp. 935–936, 2006.

[46] T. Nijsten, C. Leys, K. Verbruggen et al., "Case-control study to identify melanoma risk factors in the Belgian population: the significance of clinical examination," *Journal of the European Academy of Dermatology and Venereology*, vol. 19, no. 3, pp. 332–339, 2005.

[47] E. De Vries, M. Boniol, G. Severi et al., "Public awareness about risk factors could pose problems for case-control studies: the example of sunbed use and cutaneous melanoma," *European Journal of Cancer*, vol. 41, no. 14, pp. 2150–2154, 2005.

[48] L.-E. Wang, P. Xiong, S. S. Strom et al., "In vitro sensitivity to ultraviolet B light and skin cancer risk: a case-control analysis," *Journal of the National Cancer Institute*, vol. 97, no. 24, pp. 1822–1831, 2005.

[49] L. Naldi, A. Altieri, G. L. Imberti, L. Giordano, S. Gallus, and C. La Vecchia, "Cutaneous malignant melanoma in women. Phenotypic characteristics, sun exposure, and hormonal factors: a case-control study from Italy," *Annals of Epidemiology*, vol. 15, no. 7, pp. 545–550, 2005.

[50] L. Titus-Ernstoff, A. E. Perry, S. K. Spencer, J. J. Gibson, B. F. Cole, and M. S. Ernstoff, "Pigmentary characteristics and moles in relation to melanoma risk," *International Journal of Cancer*, vol. 116, no. 1, pp. 144–149, 2005.

[51] V. Bataille, M. Boniol, E. De Vries et al., "A multicentre epidemiological study on sunbed use and cutaneous melanoma in Europe," *European Journal of Cancer*, vol. 41, no. 14, pp. 2141–2149, 2005.

[52] K. Lasithiotakis, S. Krüger-Krasagakis, D. Ioannidou, I. Pediaditis, and A. Tosca, "Epidemiological differences for cutaneous melanoma in a relatively dark-skinned caucasian population with chronic sun exposure," *European Journal of Cancer*, vol. 40, no. 16, pp. 2502–2507, 2004.

[53] M. C. Fargnoli, D. Piccolo, E. Altobelli, F. Formicone, S. Chimenti, and K. Peris, "Constitutional and environmental risk factors for cutaneous melanoma in an Italian population: a case-control study," *Melanoma Research*, vol. 14, no. 2, pp. 151–157, 2004.

[54] D. M. Freedman, A. Sigurdson, R. S. Rao et al., "Risk of melanoma among radiologic technologists in the United States," *International Journal of Cancer*, vol. 103, no. 4, pp. 556–562, 2003.

[55] Q. Wei, J. E. Lee, J. E. Gershenwald et al., "Repair of UV light-induced DNA damage and risk of cutaneous malignant melanoma," *Journal of the National Cancer Institute*, vol. 95, no. 4, pp. 308–315, 2003.

[56] A. C. Geller, A. J. Sober, Z. Zhang et al., "Strategies for improving melanoma education and screening for men age ≥ 50 years: gindings from the American Academy of Dermatology National Skin Cancer Screening Program," *Cancer*, vol. 95, no. 7, pp. 1554–1561, 2002.

[57] L. Bakos, M. Wagner, R. M. Bakos et al., "Sunburn, sunscreens, and phenotypes: some risk factors for cutaneous melanoma in southern Brazil," *International Journal of Dermatology*, vol. 41, no. 9, pp. 557–562, 2002.

[58] D. Loria and E. Matos, "Risk factors for cutaneous melanoma: a case-control study in Argentina," *International Journal of Dermatology*, vol. 40, no. 2, pp. 108–114, 2001.

[59] T. Dwyer, L. Blizzard, R. Ashbolt, J. Plumb, M. Berwick, and J. M. Stankovich, "Cutaneous melanin density of caucasians measured by spectrophotometry and risk of malignant melanoma, basal cell carcinoma, and squamous cell carcinoma of the skin," *American Journal of Epidemiology*, vol. 155, no. 7, pp. 614–621, 2002.

[60] A. R. Shors, C. Solomon, A. McTiernan, and E. White, "Melanoma risk in relation to height, weight, and exercise (United States)," *Cancer Causes and Control*, vol. 12, no. 7, pp. 599–606, 2001.

[61] M. T. Landi, A. Baccarelli, D. Calista et al., "Combined risk factors for melanoma in a Mediterranean population," *British Journal of Cancer*, vol. 85, no. 9, pp. 1304–1310, 2001.

[62] P. Kaskel, S. Sander, M. Kron, P. Kind, R. U. Peter, and G. Krähn, "Outdoor activities in childhood: a protective factor for cutaneous melanoma? Results of a case-control study in 271 matched pairs," *British Journal of Dermatology*, vol. 145, no. 4, pp. 602–609, 2001.

[63] A. Pfahlberg, K.-F. Kölmel, and O. Gefeller, "Timing of excessive ultraviolet radiation and melanoma: Epidemiology does not support the existence of a critical period of high susceptibility to solar ultraviolet radiation-induced melanoma," *British Journal of Dermatology*, vol. 144, no. 3, pp. 471–475, 2001.

[64] N. Håkansson, B. Floderus, P. Gustavsson, M. Feychting, and N. Hallin, "Occupational sunlight exposure and cancer incidence among Swedish construction workers," *Epidemiology*, vol. 12, no. 5, pp. 552–557, 2001.

[65] L. Naldi, G. L. Imberti, F. Parazzini et al., "Pigmentary traits, modalities of sun reaction, history of sunburns, and melanocytic nevi as risk factors for cutaneous malignant melanoma in the Italian population: results of a collaborative case-control study," *Cancer*, vol. 88, no. 12, pp. 2703–2710, 2000.

[66] G. Mastrangelo, C. R. Rossi, A. Pfahlberg et al., "Is there a relationship between influenza vaccinations and risk of melanoma? A population-based case-control study," *European Journal of Epidemiology*, vol. 16, no. 9, pp. 777–782, 2000.

[67] S. D. Walter, W. D. King, and L. D. Marrett, "Association of cutaneous malignant melanoma with intermittent exposure to ultraviolet radiation: results of a case-control study in Ontario, Canada," *International Journal of Epidemiology*, vol. 28, no. 3, pp. 418–427, 1999.

[68] S. Rosso, R. Zanetti, M. Pippione, and H. Sancho-Garnier, "Parallel risk assessment of melanoma and basal cell carcinoma: skin characteristics and sun exposure," *Melanoma Research*, vol. 8, no. 6, pp. 573–583, 1998.

[69] P. Wolf, F. Quehenberger, R. Müllegger, B. Stranz, and H. Kerl, "Phenotypic markers, sunlight-related factors and sunscreen use in patients with cutaneous melanoma: an Austrian case-control study," *Melanoma Research*, vol. 8, no. 4, pp. 370–378, 1998.

[70] M. A. Tucker, A. Halpern, E. A. Holly et al., "Clinically recognized dysplastic nevi: a central risk factor for cutaneous melanoma," *The Journal of the American Medical Association*, vol. 277, no. 18, pp. 1439–1444, 1997.

[71] J. M. Ródenas, M. Delgado-Rodríguez, C. Fariñas-Álvarez, M. T. Herranz, and S. Serrano, "Melanocytic nevi and risk of cutaneous malignant melanoma in southern Spain," *American Journal of Epidemiology*, vol. 145, no. 11, pp. 1020–1029, 1997.

[72] A. E. Grulich, V. Bataille, A. J. Swerdlow et al., "Naevi and pigmentary characteristics as risk factors for melanoma in a high-risk population: a case-control study in New South Wales, Australia," *International Journal of Cancer*, vol. 67, no. 4, pp. 485–491, 1996.

[73] V. Bataille, J. A. Newton Bishop, P. Sasieni et al., "Risk of cutaneous melanoma in relation to the numbers, types and sites of naevi: a case-control study," *British Journal of Cancer*, vol. 73, no. 12, pp. 1605–1611, 1996.

[74] K. J. Goodman, M. L. Bible, S. London, and T. M. Mack, "Proportional melanoma incidence and occupation among white males in Los Angeles County (California, United States)," *Cancer Causes and Control*, vol. 6, no. 5, pp. 451–459, 1995.

[75] J. Westerdahl, H. Olsson, A. Masback, C. Ingvar, and N. Jonsson, "Is the use of sunscreens a risk factor for malignant melanoma?" *Melanoma Research*, vol. 5, no. 1, pp. 59–65, 1995.

[76] P. Autier, J. F. Dore, F. Lejeune et al. et al., "Recreational exposure to sunlight and lack of information as risk factors for cutaneous malignant melanoma. Results of an European Organization for Research and Treatment of Cancer (EORTC) case-control study in Belgium, France and Germany. The EORTC Malignant Melanoma Cooperative Group," *Melanoma Research*, vol. 4, no. 2, pp. 79–85, 1994.

[77] P. J. Nelemans, H. Groenendal, L. A. L. M. Kiemeney, F. H. J. Rampen, D. J. Ruiter, and A. L. M. Verbeek, "Effect of intermittent exposure to sunlight on melanoma risk among indoor workers and sun-sensitive individuals," *Environmental Health Perspectives*, vol. 101, no. 3, pp. 252–255, 1993.

[78] L. D. Marrett, W. D. King, S. D. Walter, and L. From, "Use of host factors to identify people at high risk for cutaneous malignant melanoma," *Canadian Medical Association Journal*, vol. 147, no. 4, pp. 445–453, 1992.

[79] D. Zaridze, A. Mukeria, and S. W. Duffy, "Risk factors for skin melanoma in Moscow," *International Journal of Cancer*, vol. 52, no. 1, pp. 159–161, 1992.

[80] J. Weiss, J. Bertz, and E. G. Jung, "Malignant melanoma in southern Germany: different predictive value of risk factors for melanoma subtypes," *Dermatologica*, vol. 183, no. 2, pp. 109–113, 1991.

[81] J. M. Elwood, S. M. Whitehead, J. Davison, M. Stewart, and M. Galt, "Malignant melanoma in England: risks associated with naevi, freckles, social class, hair colour, and sunburn," *International Journal of Epidemiology*, vol. 19, no. 4, pp. 801–810, 1990.

[82] N. Dubin, B. S. Pasternack, and M. Moseson, "Simultaneous assessment of risk factors for malignant melanoma and non-melanoma skin lesions, with emphasis on sun exposure and related variables," *International Journal of Epidemiology*, vol. 19, no. 4, pp. 811–819, 1990.

[83] H. Beitner, S. E. Norell, U. Ringborg, G. Wennersten, and B. Mattson, "Malignant melanoma: aetiological importance of individual pigmentation and sun exposure," *British Journal of Dermatology*, vol. 122, no. 1, pp. 43–51, 1990.

[84] C. Garbe, S. Kruger, R. Stadler, I. Guggenmoos-Holzmann, and C. E. Orfanos, "Markers and relative risk in a German population for developing malignant melanoma," *International Journal of Dermatology*, vol. 28, no. 8, pp. 517–523, 1989.

[85] G. C. Roush, J. J. Nordlund, B. Forget, S. B. Gruber, and J. M. Kirkwood, "Independence of dysplastic nevi from total nevi in determining risk for nonfamilial melanoma," *Preventive Medicine*, vol. 17, no. 3, pp. 273–279, 1988.

[86] A. Osterlind, M. A. Tucker, K. Hou-Jensen, B. J. Stone, G. Engholm, and O. M. Jensen, "The Danish case-control study of cutaneous malignant melanoma. I. Importance of host factors," *International Journal of Cancer*, vol. 42, no. 2, pp. 200–206, 1988.

[87] E. A. Holly, J. W. Kelly, S. Shpall, and S.-H. Chiu, "Number of melanocytic nevi as a major risk factor for malignant melanoma," *Journal of the American Academy of Dermatology*, vol. 17, no. 3, pp. 459–468, 1987.

[88] C. M. J. Bell, C. M. Jenkinson, T. J. Murrells, R. G. Skeet, and J. D. Everall, "Aetiological factors in cutaneous malignant melanomas seen at a UK skin clinic," *Journal of Epidemiology and Community Health*, vol. 41, no. 4, pp. 306–311, 1987.

[89] M. Cristofolini, S. Franceschi, L. Tasin et al., "Risk factors for cutaneous malignant melanoma in a northern Italian population," *International Journal of Cancer*, vol. 39, no. 2, pp. 150–154, 1987.

[90] A. J. Swerdlow, J. English, R. M. MacKie et al., "Benign melanocytic naevi as a risk factor for malignant melanoma," *British Medical Journal*, vol. 292, no. 6535, pp. 1555–1559, 1986.

[91] A. Green, R. MacLennan, and V. Siskind, "Common acquired naevi and the risk of malignant melanoma," *International Journal of Cancer*, vol. 35, no. 5, pp. 297–300, 1985.

[92] C. D. J. Holman and B. K. Armstrong, "Pigmentary traits, ethnic origin, benign nevi, and family history as risk factors for cutaneous malignant melanoma," *Journal of the National Cancer Institute*, vol. 72, no. 2, pp. 257–266, 1984.

[93] J. M. Elwood, R. P. Gallagher, G. B. Hill, J. J. Spinelli, J. C. G. Pearson, and W. Threlfall, "Pigmentation and skin reaction to sun as risk factors for cutaneous melanoma: Western Canada Melanoma Study," *British Medical Journal*, vol. 288, no. 6411, pp. 99–102, 1984.

[94] V. Beral, S. Evans, H. Shaw, and G. Milton, "Cutaneous factors related to the risk of malignant melanoma," *British Journal of Dermatology*, vol. 109, no. 2, pp. 165–172, 1983.

[95] O. Klepp and K. Magnus, "Some environmental and bodily characteristics of melanoma patients. A case-control study," *International Journal of Cancer*, vol. 23, no. 4, pp. 482–486, 1979.

[96] V. A. Andreeva, J. B. Unger, A. L. Yaroch, M. G. Cockburn, L. Baezconde-Garbanati, and K. D. Reynolds, "Acculturation and sun-safe behaviors among US latinos: findings from the 2005 Health Information National Trends Survey," *American Journal of Public Health*, vol. 99, no. 4, pp. 734–741, 2009.

[97] E. Linos, E. Keiser, T. Fu, G. Colditz, S. Chen, and J. Y. Tang, "Hat, shade, long sleeves, or sunscreen? Rethinking US sun protection messages based on their relative effectiveness," *Cancer Causes and Control*, vol. 22, no. 7, pp. 1067–1071, 2011.

[98] Centers for Disease Control and Prevention, "Sunburn prevalence among adults—United States, 1999, 2003, and 2004," *Morbidity and Mortality Weekly Report*, vol. 56, no. 21, pp. 524–528, 2007.

[99] D. Carroll, R. M. Samardich, S. Bernard, S. Gabbard, and T. Hernandez, "Findings from the national agricultural workers survey (NAWS) 2001-2002: a demographic and employment profile of United States farm workers," Research Report 9, US Department of Labor, Washington, DC, USA, 2005.

[100] M. H. Law, S. MacGregor, and N. K. Hayward, "Melanoma genetics: recent findings take us beyond well-traveled pathways," *Journal of Investigative Dermatology*, vol. 132, no. 7, pp. 1763–1774, 2012.

[101] A. M. Goldstein and M. A. Tucker, "Genetic epidemiology of cutaneous melanoma: a global perspective," *Archives of Dermatology*, vol. 137, no. 11, pp. 1493–1496, 2001.

[102] N. Flanagan, E. Healy, A. Ray et al., "Pleiotropic effects of the melanocortin 1 receptor (MC1R) gene on human pigmentation," *Human Molecular Genetics*, vol. 9, no. 17, pp. 2531–2537, 2000.

[103] D. Mitra, X. Luo, A. Morgan et al., "A UV-independent pathway to melanoma carcinogenesis in the redhair-fairskin background," *Nature*, vol. 491, no. 7424, pp. 449–453, 2012.

[104] J. L. Maldonado, J. Fridlyand, H. Patel et al., "Determinants of BRAF mutations in primary melanomas," *Journal of the National Cancer Institute*, vol. 95, no. 24, pp. 1878–1880, 2003.

[105] S. Y. Morita and S. N. Markovic, "Molecular targets in melanoma: time for 'ethnic personalization'," *Expert Review of Anticancer Therapy*, vol. 12, no. 5, pp. 601–608, 2012.

[106] M. Pipitone, J. K. Robinson, C. Camara, B. Chittineni, and S. G. Fisher, "Skin cancer awareness in suburban employees: a hispanic perspective," *Journal of the American Academy of Dermatology*, vol. 47, no. 1, pp. 118–123, 2002.

[107] J. K. Robinson, K. M. Joshi, S. Ortiz, and R. V. Kundu, "Melanoma knowledge, perception, and awareness in ethnic minorities in Chicago: recommendations regarding education," *Psycho-Oncology*, vol. 20, no. 3, pp. 313–320, 2011.

[108] C. Roman, A. Lugo-Somolinos, and N. Thomas, "Skin cancer knowledge and skin self-examinations in the Hispanic population of North Carolina: the patient's perspective," *JAMA Dermatology*, vol. 149, no. 1, pp. 103–104, 2013.

[109] E. J. Coups, J. L. Stapleton, S. V. Hudson et al., "Skin cancer surveillance behaviors among US Hispanic adults," *Journal of the American Academy of Dermatology*, vol. 68, no. 4, pp. 576–584, 2013.

[110] B. Langholz, J. Richardson, E. Rappaport, J. Waisman, M. Cockburn, and T. Mack, "Skin characteristics and risk of superficial spreading and nodular melanoma (United States)," *Cancer Causes and Control*, vol. 11, no. 8, pp. 741–750, 2000.

26

Inflammatory Bowel Disease and Skin Cancer: An Assessment of Patient Risk Factors, Knowledge, and Skin Practices

Jessica N. Kimmel,[1] Tiffany H. Taft,[1] and Laurie Keefer[1,2]

[1]*Department of Medicine, Division of Gastroenterology and Hepatology, Northwestern University School of Medicine, Arkes Family Pavilion Suite 1400, 676 North Saint Clair Street, Chicago, IL 60611, USA*
[2]*Icahn School of Medicine, Mount Sinai Medical Center, Susan and Leonard Feinstein IBD Center, 17 East 102nd Street, 5th Floor, New York, NY 10029, USA*

Correspondence should be addressed to Jessica N. Kimmel; jessica.kimmel@northwestern.edu

Academic Editor: Günther Hofbauer

Objective. Patients with inflammatory bowel disease (IBD) are at increased risk from skin cancer. Aims include assessing IBD patients' risk factors and knowledge of skin cancer and current skin protection practices to identify gaps in patient education regarding skin cancer prevention in IBD. *Methods*. IBD patients ≥ 18 years were recruited to complete an online survey. *Results*. 164 patients (mean age 43.5 years, 63% female) with IBD (67% Crohn's disease, 31% ulcerative colitis, and 2% indeterminate colitis) were included. 12% ($n = 19$) of patients had a personal history and 34% ($n = 55$) had a family history of skin cancer. Females scored better on skin protection (16.94/32 versus 14.53/32, $P \leq 0.03$) and awareness (35.16/40 versus 32.98/40, $P \leq 0.03$). Patients over 40 years old scored better on prevention (17.45/28 versus 15.35/28, $P = 0.03$). Patients with skin cancer scored better on prevention (20.56/28 versus 15.75/28, $P \leq 0.001$) and skin protection (21.47/32 versus 15.33/32, $P \leq 0.001$). 61% of patients recognized the link between skin cancer and IBD. *Conclusions*. The majority of IBD patients are aware of the link between skin cancer and IBD; however, skin protection practices are suboptimal. This emphasizes the role of healthcare professionals in providing further education for skin cancer prevention in the IBD population.

1. Introduction

Skin cancer is the most common form of cancer in the United States and causes significant morbidity and mortality [1]. Inflammatory bowel disease (IBD) is a chronic autoimmune condition that is associated with increased risk of development of skin cancer. Proposed mechanisms predisposing IBD patients to skin cancer include chronic inflammation, cellular damage, and underlying immune dysfunction leading to altered tumor surveillance [2–4].

Use of immunosuppressants in IBD patients has been shown to lead to a 4–7-fold increased risk of skin cancer and approximately half of IBD patients are exposed to these medications within 5 years of diagnosis [3]. Specifically, the use of biologic and immunomodulating agents increases skin cancer risk [2–6]. Similarly, immunosuppression has been shown to accelerate the development of skin cancer in transplant patients; thus, routine skin exams are recommended [3, 4]. According to the United States Preventive Service Task Force, there is insufficient evidence to assess the risk versus benefit for general skin cancer screening [7]. In addition, there is a lack of data to support that early detection of skin cancer reduces morbidity and mortality [5]. However, patients with IBD have different risk factors for skin cancer development compared to the general population. Thus, these skin cancer screening recommendations may not be applicable to IBD patients. Despite the lack of specific standardized guidelines for screening, there is general consensus among gastroenterologists that IBD patients should protect themselves from the sun and that annual skin cancer surveillance should be considered, especially for patients on biologic and immunomodulating agents [5, 8, 9].

Thus, it is important for IBD patients to be aware of their risk of skin cancer and to adopt preventive strategies for modifiable risk factors. The aims of this study are to assess IBD patients' risk factors for and knowledge of skin cancer. In addition, we will assess patients' current skin protection practices. We anticipate that this survey will help to identify gaps in patient education regarding skin cancer prevention in the IBD population.

2. Methods

2.1. Patients. Patients 18 years of age or older with a diagnosis of inflammatory bowel disease were eligible for inclusion in the study. Due to the study design, a diagnosis of IBD was via self-report. Patients were recruited via email, by online sources, and by healthcare providers in gastroenterology offices at Northwestern Medicine. All subjects gave informed, signed consent prior to study registration. Eligible patients who agreed to participate were forwarded to an online, confidential, anonymous survey. Data was collected using Adobe FormsCentral. Study design was approved by the Northwestern University Institutional Review Board.

2.2. Survey Design. A cross-sectional research questionnaire queried patients about baseline demographics and IBD-related information, including medications, complications, and extent of their IBD. In addition, study participants were questioned about their individual skin cancer risk factors, sun exposure and skin protection practices, behaviors in the event that they identified a mole, and general skin cancer knowledge. Topics addressed in this study were compiled after critical review of published literature on skin cancer and its risk factors and included a compilation of questions in formats derived from other validated skin cancer assessments [6, 10–16]. Answers were formatted with Likert scales, true/false, and multiple-choice responses (Table 1). Questions were reviewed by dermatologists prior to administration.

2.3. Statistical Analyses. All responses were exported from the online system into SPSS v.22 for analysis. Data were tested for normal distribution. Descriptive statistics (percentages, mean (SD)) analyzed the demographic and clinical characteristics of the study sample. Scores for each skin cancer category were summed to produce total scores for skin cancer prevention (out of 28), awareness (out of 40), knowledge (out of 4), protection (out of 32), and exposure (out of 24). Each score was compared by demographic and clinical variables via a series of independent samples t-tests and one-way analysis of variance (ANOVA). Relationships between continuous variables were evaluated via Pearson's correlations while categorical variables were analyzed via Chi Square. Statistical significance was set to $P \leq 0.01$ for t-tests and ANOVA to control for type I error due to multiple comparisons.

3. Results

A total of 164 patients with inflammatory bowel disease completed the online survey. Patient demographics are reported in Table 2. The mean age of participants was 43.5 years

and 63% of patients were female. The majority of study participants were Caucasian (94%, $n = 153$) and non-Hispanic (98%, $n = 161$). Crohn's disease was reported in 67% of patients, ulcerative colitis in 31%, and indeterminate colitis in 2%. Ninety-five percent of patients were currently receiving IBD treatment at the time of survey response. Approximately two-thirds ($n = 105$) of patients reported either current or past treatment with immunomodulators (which include Imuran/Azathioprine and 6-mercaptopurine) and approximately two-thirds with biologics ($n = 103$).

Sunburn and skin cancer history were assessed and reported in Table 3. Twelve percent of patients ($n = 19$) reported a personal history of skin cancer, of which 7% were basal cell carcinoma, 2% squamous cell carcinoma, 1% melanoma, and 4% multiple types of skin cancer. Additionally, 34% ($n = 55$) reported having a first-degree relative with skin cancer. Sixty-two percent ($n = 102$) of patients had three or more episodes of bad sunburns. The majority of patients (70%) had seen a dermatologist, with 35% of patients receiving a full skin exam once per year, 30% less than once per year, and 24% having never received a skin exam. Half of patients (51%, $n = 84$) were self-referred to a dermatologist; gastroenterologists referred 13% of patients for dermatology consultation and primary care referred 17%.

Patient responses to standardized questions of skin cancer prevention, awareness, knowledge, protection, and sun exposure are reported in Table 1. Average scores for skin cancer prevention, awareness, knowledge, skin protection, and sun exposure were 16.24/28, 34.34/40, 2.93/4, 16.1/32, and 6.15/24, respectively. Patients over 40 years of age scored higher on prevention (17.45/28) compared to patients 40 years old or younger (15.35/28, $P = 0.03$). Females scored higher on skin protection (16.94/32 compared to 14.53/32 for males, $P = 0.02$) and awareness (35.16/40 compared to 32.98/40 for males, $P = 0.03$, Table 4). There were no statistically significant differences in scores between participants with or without exposure to immunomodulators. There was a difference in knowledge scores between those currently treated with biologic agents (3.01/4) compared to those with prior biologic exposure (2.91/4) or no exposure (2.85/4, $P \leq 0.01$). Additionally, those who had a personal history of skin cancer scored better on both skin protection (21.47/32) and prevention (20.56/28) questions compared to those without a personal history (15.33/32, 15.75/28, resp., $P \leq 0.001$). In addition, those with a family history scored higher on skin protection questions (18.46/32) compared to those without a first-degree relative with skin cancer (14.03/32, $P \leq 0.001$). When asked if IBD and its treatment increase the risk of skin cancer, 61% of patients agreed with the statement and 38% responded neutrally or disagreed (Table 5); patients currently or previously treated with immunomodulators scored higher than those who were not on these medications ($P = 0.000$).

4. Discussion and Conclusion

Patients with inflammatory bowel disease are at increased risk of development of skin cancer compared to the general population, independent of the use of immunosuppressants

TABLE 1: Categorized questions and answers for skin cancer variables (skin cancer prevention, awareness, knowledge, skin protection, and sun exposure).

(a) Skin cancer prevention

Questions addressed	Answers (%)				
	Very unlikely	Unlikely	Neutral	Likely	Very likely
How likely are you to visit a doctor if you noticed a new mole?	3.1	14.7	21.5	33.1	27.6
How likely are you to ignore a new mole?	1.9	16.0	22.2	29.0	30.9
How likely are you to check your own skin for moles?	7.5	14.4	23.8	36.3	18.1
If you found a new mole, how likely are you to see your primary care doctor right away?	32.7	37.7	19.1	5.6	4.9
If you found a new mole, how likely are you to see a dermatologist right away?	12.8	23.2	17.7	22.0	24.4
If you found a new mole, how likely are you to tell a family member or friend?	14.0	15.9	16.5	34.8	18.9
If you found a new mole, how likely are you to bring it up at your next doctor's appointment?	5.6	11.7	9.9	40.7	32.1

(b) Skin cancer awareness

Questions addressed	Answers (%)				
How worried would you be if a mole	Not at all worried (1) through very worried (5)				
	1	2	3	4	5
Had irregular borders	4.9	6.1	17.1	29.9	42.1
Was asymmetric	6.1	6.7	18.4	30.7	38.0
Had 2 or more colors	2.5	3.7	13.0	28.0	52.8
Is greater than 6 mm in diameter	1.2	2.5	16.0	25.8	54.6
Grew in size	1.8	0.6	8.0	23.3	66.3
Is painful	1.8	1.2	5.5	22.7	68.7
Itches	1.2	3.0	17.7	23.2	54.9
Bleeds	1.2	0.6	6.7	20.9	70.6

Which of the following factors increase melanoma risk?	Percent (N = # of responses)
None	0% (0)
Having lots of moles	46% (76)
Particular diets	10% (17)
Family history of skin cancer	77% (126)
Fair complexion	70% (114)
Alcohol use	9% (14)
Sunburns	80% (131)
Prolonged sun exposure	79% (130)
Smoking	30% (50)
Blue eyes	26% (42)
Green eyes	13% (22)
Red hair	26% (42)
Fair hair	29% (47)
Immunosuppression	58% (95)
All of the above	24% (40)

(c) Skin cancer knowledge

Questions addressed	Answers (%)	
	True	False
Skin cancer risk can be minimized by avoiding sun and using adequate sun protection	97.0	3.0
Skin cancer can be healed without treatment	1.8	98.2
Skin cancer can be cured if treated early	7.3	92.7
Skin cancer can lead to death if not treated	1.2	98.8

Inflammatory Bowel Disease and Skin Cancer: An Assessment of Patient Risk...

201

(d) Skin protection

Questions addressed	Answers (%)				
	Never	Rarely	Occasionally	Frequently	Always
I use sunscreen if I am going to be outside for more than 20 minutes	4.9	18.3	31.1	28.7	17.1
I use SPF 30 or higher	4.3	9.3	18.0	29.8	38.5
I use sunscreen if it is cloudy outside	28.4	28.4	24.1	14.8	4.3
I reapply sunscreen after swimming or heavily perspiring	13.5	16.0	25.8	27.6	17.2
I use sunscreen while on vacation or holiday	3.0	6.7	17.7	37.2	35.4
I wear protective clothing in the sun	9.9	19.3	40.4	25.5	5.0
I use an umbrella to protect me from the sun	57.7	22.1	11.7	5.5	3.1
I wear a hat outside	20.5	19.3	36.0	18.0	6.2

(e) Sun exposure

Questions addressed	Answers (%)				
	Never	Rarely	Occasionally	Frequently	Always
I spend more time outdoors than indoors	69.3	18.4	6.7	3.7	1.8
I try to get a suntan when outside	4.3	14.0	29.9	28.0	23.8
I spend a lot of time outdoors due to my occupation	1.3	10.0	42.5	35.0	11.3
	0		1–2	3–4	>5
How many sunny/beach/outdoor vacations have you been on in the last 5 years?	15.5		44.0	40.5	0.0
	Never			Current/prior use	
Have you ever used a tanning bed?	59.1			40.9	
	<10	10–25	25–50	50–100	>100
How many times have you used a tanning bed?	78.7	4.3	4.9	12.2	0.0

[2, 3]. Thus, this questionnaire aimed to assess IBD patients' actual and perceived risk factors for and knowledge of skin cancer as well as general skin protection strategies. Overall, we found that IBD patients are well informed about skin cancer and are cognizant of worrisome skin features. Despite this insight, they often practice suboptimal skin protection and prevention. According to the social-cognitive theory of health behavior, knowledge of risk alone is insufficient for behavior change; patients also require the perception of personal risk and skills training to change their habits [17]. This study highlights a potential opportunity for health professionals to teach and reinforce skin cancer prevention in IBD.

Other than treating the underlying inflammatory state of IBD, many of the factors that place these patients at additional risk of skin cancer development, including effective IBD treatments and early age at diagnosis, are not easily modifiable. However, similar to the general population, behavioral changes, such as avoidance of sun exposure and tanning beds and skin protection with use of sunscreen and protective clothing, can prevent or decrease the risk of skin cancer. One's perceived risk of skin cancer encourages these protective behaviors. On the contrary, a lack of awareness of skin cancer risk serves as a barrier to adoption of protective behaviors [14]. Overall, we found that IBD patients do have a modest understanding of skin cancer and are aware of worrisome signs and risk factors for skin cancer occurrence. In addition, our patient cohort does not report significant sun exposure. However, despite their knowledge and awareness, our patient population does not practice optimal sun protection or prevention strategies if they were to find a new mole.

Furthermore, when asked if IBD and its treatment increase one's skin cancer risk, 61% of patients agreed with this statement. Those with exposure to immunomodulators, which have been shown to increase the risk of skin cancer, did score higher for this variable. A proportion of our IBD population still does not recognize that their IBD increases their personal risk of skin cancer. Individuals adopt protective behavior (such as sun protection) if they perceive a health threat (such as skin cancer) [18, 19]. According to the health behavior model, if IBD patients do not perceive a personal risk of skin cancer development, they may not adopt effective skin protection behaviors [18]. Thus, it is our role as clinicians to discuss this topic with our patients. Furthermore, patients must understand that the proposed behavioral changes can mitigate this threat and that they can overcome barriers to achieving this [17, 18]. Accordingly, this highlights the importance of not only teaching patients about their own risk but also providing them with ways to minimize this risk with methods to protect oneself from the sun and its negative effects.

Moreover, we found that patients with a personal and family history of skin cancer tend to address worrying skin lesions with more vigilance and practice better sun protection than those without such histories. This further highlights that one's perceived risk of skin cancer development motivates one to adopt appropriate skin protection strategies. We found that females practice more appropriate sun protection and are

TABLE 2: Patient demographics.

Demographics	Percent of participants (N)
Gender	
Male	37% (61)
Female	63% (103)
Race	
White	94% (153)
Black	3% (5)
Multiple	2% (3)
Asian	1% (2)
Ethnicity	
Hispanic	2% (3)
Non-Hispanic	98% (161)
Married	57% (93)
College degree or higher	81% (132)
Employed full time	66% (108)
>$50,000 annual income	69% (111)
Private insurance	85% (139)
Smoking history	30% (48)
IBD diagnosis	
Crohn's disease	67% (109)
Ulcerative colitis	31% (51)
Indeterminate colitis	2% (4)
IBD surgery history	43% (71)
Current IBD treatment	95% (156)
Patient recruitment source	
Provider	75% (122)
Email	23% (37)
Other	3% (5)

TABLE 3: Patient skin cancer information.

	Percent of participants (N)
Skin biopsy history	43% (70)
Skin cancer history	12% (19)
Skin cancer type	
Basal cell	7% (12)
Squamous cell	2% (4)
Melanoma	1% (1)
Multiple types	4% (6)
First-degree relative skin cancer	34% (55)
Number of bad sunburns	
Never	6% (10)
1-2 times	31% (50)
3+ times	62% (102)
Unknown	1% (1)
Number of blistering sunburns	
Never	14% (23)
1-2 times	29% (48)
3+ times	14% (23)
Unknown	43% (70)
Skin exam frequency	
Less than once per year	30% (49)
Once per year	35% (57)
More than once per year	10% (17)
Never	24% (40)
Sees a dermatologist	70% (114)
Dermatologist referral source	
Gastroenterologist	13% (21)
Other specialists	2% (2)
Primary care	17% (27)
Self	51% (84)
Friend/family	2% (2)
Unknown	17% (28)

better informed about skin cancer risk factors and worrisome skin features, which is consistent with prior studies [11]. Previous reports have found that young age is associated with high-risk behavior for skin cancer development, less knowledge about skin cancer, and increased incidence of skin cancer, especially melanoma [3, 11–14]. We found that patients over 40 years of age are more cognizant of when to seek medical attention for worrisome skin features. IBD patients often present in early adulthood, thus increasing the cumulative risk of skin cancer development. Specifically, younger men with Crohn's disease have an increased risk of nonmelanoma skin cancer; therefore, this is a particularly important group to target [3].

Our study has a few limitations. There is inherent reporter bias associated with the study design. The questionnaire format may both over- and/or underestimate skin cancer risk factors and skin practices. The participatory nature inherent in a research questionnaire leads to selection bias. Furthermore, given the anonymous nature of the survey, a diagnosis of IBD was self-reported and not confirmed via chart review. In addition, this study is limited by a sample primarily recruited in GI clinics at one large academic medical center. Thus, the study population may not be representative of all patients with inflammatory bowel disease. In addition,

questionnaire items were compiled based on prior literature and skin cancer surveys; however, this specific survey has not been validated. Furthermore, some findings were statistically significant using a P value of <0.05 instead of 0.01; thus there is the possibility of a type I statistical error.

Our study shows that the majority of survey participants did recognize the connection between skin cancer and IBD. Comparatively, quality improvement studies have found even lower vaccination rates in the IBD population. Encouragingly, several studies have demonstrated remarkable improvements in vaccination rates with implementation of educational programs and increased access to vaccines [20–22]. As in vaccination studies, physician recommendations for skin cancer prevention may not be sufficient for behavioral change. Our study demonstrates that despite general knowledge about skin cancer and an overall understanding that they are at increased risk of skin cancer development, our IBD population continues to practice suboptimal skin protection. Educational modules may be necessary for IBD patients to further understand their personal risk of skin cancer

TABLE 4: Mean differences for skin cancer variables by various demographics and treatment.

	Scores				
	Protection (out of 32)	Exposure (out of 24)	Prevention (out of 28)	Awareness (out of 40)	Knowledge (out of 4)
Gender					
Male	14.53	6.49	15.52	32.98	2.95
Female	16.94*	5.96	16.64	35.16*	2.92
Immunomodulator treatment					
Currently treated	16.09	6.10	16.54	35.00	2.98
Previously treated	16.54	6.12	16.44	33.92	2.93
Never treated	15.58	6.23	15.82	34.14	2.90
Biologic treatment					
Currently treated	16.05	5.98	16.17	33.36	3.01**
Previously treated	16.19	6.40	16.55	34.34	2.91
Never treated	16.08	6.19	16.16	35.45	2.85
Personal history of skin cancer					
No	15.33	6.05	15.75	34.03	2.92
Yes	21.47***	6.91	20.56***	36.81	3.00
Family history of skin cancer					
No	14.03	6.13	15.30	33.59	2.92
Yes	18.46***	6.36	17.52	35.43	2.96

*$P \leq 0.03$, **$P \leq 0.01$, and ***$P \leq 0.001$ compared via t-tests.

TABLE 5: Patient responses to the following question: "Are you at increased risk of having skin cancer because of your IBD and the medications that you take for the treatment of IBD?"

Responses	Percent of participants (N)
Strongly agree	23.6% (39)
Agree	37.6% (62)
Neutral	33.9% (56)
Disagree	0.6% (1)
Strongly disagree	3.6% (6)

development and to provide more information regarding appropriate preventive and protective behaviors. According to the social-cognitive theory of health behavior, in addition to knowledge of risk, patients also require guidance in tools to minimize this risk. Given the young age at IBD diagnosis, there is ample opportunity to intervene, educate, and reduce the cumulative risk of skin cancer development in this population.

This study supports the hypothesis that primary prevention of skin cancer in the IBD population is suboptimal and emphasizes a potential opportunity for healthcare professionals to highlight this population's risk and reinforce skin cancer prevention strategies. Implementation for improvement includes clinical reminders at each visit and educational modules on proper skin protection techniques.

Authors' Contribution

All authors have made substantial contributions to the study design and concept, as well as data acquisition, analysis, and interpretation. Jessica N. Kimmel contributed to study concept and design, data acquisition, interpretation of data, and drafting and critical revision of the paper. Tiffany H. Taft contributed to data analysis and interpretation and revised the paper critically. Laurie Keefer contributed to study concept and design and revised the paper critically. All authors approve the final version.

Acknowledgments

The authors thank all of the patients who participated in this study. They also thank Amanda Nolan who contributed to patient recruitment.

References

[1] American Cancer Society, "Skin cancer," 2015, http://www.cancer.org/cancer/skincancer/index.

[2] S. Singh, S. J. S. Nagpal, M. H. Murad et al., "Inflammatory bowel disease is associated with an increased risk of melanoma: a systematic review and meta-analysis," *Clinical Gastroenterology and Hepatology*, vol. 12, no. 2, pp. 210–218, 2014.

[3] H. Singh, Z. Nugent, A. A. Demers, and C. N. Bernstein, "Increased risk of nonmelanoma skin cancers among individuals with inflammatory bowel disease," *Gastroenterology*, vol. 141, no. 5, pp. 1612–1620, 2011.

[4] M. D. Long, C. F. Martin, C. A. Pipkin, H. H. Herfarth, R. S. Sandler, and M. D. Kappelman, "Risk of melanoma and

nonmelanoma skin cancer among patients with inflammatory bowel disease," *Gastroenterology*, vol. 143, no. 2, pp. 390–399, 2012.

[5] M. D. Long, M. D. Kappelman, and C. A. Pipkin, "Non-melanoma skin cancer in inflammatory bowel disease: a review," *Inflammatory Bowel Diseases*, vol. 17, no. 6, pp. 1423–1427, 2011.

[6] G. W. Moran, A. W. K. Lim, J. L. Bailey et al., "Review article: dermatological complications of immunosuppressive and anti-TNF therapy in inflammatory bowel disease," *Alimentary Pharmacology and Therapeutics*, vol. 38, no. 9, pp. 1002–1024, 2013.

[7] *Screening for Skin Cancer, Clinical Summary of U.S. Preventive Services Task Force Recommendation*, US Preventive Services Task Force, Rockville, Md, USA, 2009, http://www.uspreventive-servicestaskforce.org/Page/Topic/recommendation-summary/skin-cancer-screening?ds=1&s=skin%20cancer.

[8] M. Moscandrew, U. Mahadevan, and S. Kane, "General health maintenance in IBD," *Inflammatory Bowel Diseases*, vol. 15, no. 9, pp. 1399–1409, 2009.

[9] C. S. Manolakis and B. D. Cash, "Health maintenance and inflammatory bowel disease," *Current Gastroenterology Reports*, vol. 16, article 402, 2014.

[10] H. S. Gillespie, T. Watson, J. D. Emery, A. J. Lee, and P. Murchie, "A questionnaire to measure melanoma risk, knowledge and protective behaviour: assessing content validity in a convenience sample of Scots and Australians," *BMC Medical Research Methodology*, vol. 11, pp. 123–131, 2011.

[11] A. Jackson, C. Wilkinson, and R. Pill, "Moles and melanomas—who's at risk, who knows, and who cares? A strategy to inform those at high risk," *British Journal of General Practice*, vol. 49, no. 440, pp. 199–203, 1999.

[12] S. N. Markovic, L. A. Erickson, R. D. Rao et al., "Malignant melanoma in the 21st century, part 1: epidemiology, risk factors, screening, prevention, and diagnosis," *Mayo Clinic Proceedings*, vol. 82, no. 3, pp. 364–380, 2007.

[13] E. J. Coups, S. L. Manne, and C. J. Heckman, "Multiple skin cancer risk behaviors in the U.S. population," *American Journal of Preventive Medicine*, vol. 34, no. 2, pp. 87–93, 2008.

[14] B. L. Diffey and Z. Norridge, "Reported sun exposure, attitudes to sun protection and perceptions of skin cancer risk: a survey of visitors to Cancer Research UK's SunSmart campaign website," *British Journal of Dermatology*, vol. 160, no. 6, pp. 1292–1298, 2009.

[15] V. Bataille and E. de Vries, "Melanoma—part 1: epidemiology, risk factors, and prevention," *British Medical Journal*, vol. 337, no. 7681, pp. 1287–1291, 2008.

[16] K. Glanz, E. Schoenfeld, M. A. Weinstock, G. Layi, J. Kidd, and D. M. Shigaki, "Development and reliability of a brief skin cancer risk assessment tool," *Cancer Detection and Prevention*, vol. 27, no. 4, pp. 311–315, 2003.

[17] A. Bandura, "Health promotion from the perspective of social cognitive theory," *Psychology and Health*, vol. 13, no. 4, pp. 623–649, 1998.

[18] K. M. Jackson and L. S. Aiken, "A psychosocial model of sun protection and sunbathing in young women: the impact of health beliefs, attitudes, norms, and self-efficacy for sun protection," *Health Psychology*, vol. 19, no. 5, pp. 469–478, 2000.

[19] M. A. Morales-Sánchez, M. L. Peralta-Pedrero, and M. A. Domínguez-Gómez, "Design and validation of a questionnaire for measuring perceived risk of skin cancer," *Actas Dermo-Sifiliográficas*, vol. 105, no. 3, pp. 276–285, 2014.

[20] S. Parker, L. C. White, C. Spangler et al., "A quality improvement project significantly increased the vaccination rate for immuno-suppressed patients with IBD," *Inflammatory Bowel Diseases*, vol. 19, no. 9, pp. 1809–1814, 2013.

[21] K. Huth, E. I. Benchimol, M. Aglipay, and D. R. Mack, "Strategies to improve influenza vaccination in pediatric inflammatory bowel disease through education and access," *Inflammatory Bowel Diseases*, vol. 21, no. 8, pp. 1761–1768, 2015.

[22] A. Fleurier, C. Pelatan, S. Willot et al., "Vaccination coverage of children with inflammatory bowel disease after an awareness campaign on the risk of infection," *Digestive and Liver Disease*, vol. 47, no. 6, pp. 460–464, 2015.

27

College Students' Perceptions of Worry and Parent Beliefs: Associations with Behaviors to Prevent Sun Exposure

Robert A. Yockey,[1] **Laura A. Nabors,**[2] **Oladunni Oluwoye,**[3] **Kristen Welker,**[2] **and Angelica M. Hardee**[2]

[1]*Department of Psychiatry and Behavioral Neuroscience and Department of Health Education and Promotion, University of Cincinnati, Cincinnati, OH 45221-0068, USA*
[2]*Health Promotion and Education Program, School of Human Services, University of Cincinnati, Cincinnati, OH 45221-0068, USA*
[3]*Initiative for Research and Education to Advance Community Health (IREACH), Washington State University, Spokane, WA 99210-1495, USA*

Correspondence should be addressed to Laura A. Nabors; naborsla@ucmail.uc.edu

Academic Editor: Robert Dellavalle

More research is needed to understand how attitudes impact behaviors that afford sun protection. The current study examined the impact of students' perceptions of parental beliefs about sun exposure and its influence on their practiced sun protection behaviors and worry about sun exposure. Participants were college students ($N = 462$) at a large Midwestern university. They completed a survey to examine their perceptions of risks and messages about sun exposure and sun exposure behaviors. Results indicated that gender and students' perceptions of parental beliefs about sun exposure were related to sun protection behaviors and their own worry over sun exposure. Specifically, males showed lower levels of sun protection behaviors, with the exception of wearing a hat with a brim, and lower levels of worry about sun exposure compared to females. Roughly a third of our sample had a family history of skin cancer, and this variable was related to worry about sun exposure and parental beliefs. Prevention messages and interventions to reduce sun risk for college students should address risks of sun exposure as well as educating young adults about the importance of wearing sunscreen, protective clothing, and hats to improve sun protection.

1. Introduction

Estimates from recent reports from the American Cancer Society indicated that 9,730 people die from melanoma each year, with the greatest casualties in men, and the reported numbers are continuing to rise [1, 2]. Parallel to the rising prevalence rates are the costs of treating dermatological cancers, thus creating economic hardships for some families. Guy et al. [3] reported a 126.2% increase in annual total costs in skin cancer treatment from 2002 to 2011, making the final total cost of skin cancer treatment, in 2011, $8.1 billion. Although skin cancer is a significant public health concern, sun protection behaviors often lag behind knowledge of this threat [4]. Young adults may not engage in use of sunscreen or other sun protection behaviors, such as wearing hats or avoiding sun exposure [5]. Estimates from 2015 indicated

that about 33% of adults reported wearing sunscreen with SPF 15+, 38% reported wearing protective clothing, and 39% sought shade to protect themselves from the sun [6]. Greater understanding of attitudinal factors that might motivate young adults to engage in sun protection behaviors will be important to inform prevention messages for this high risk group.

The Health Belief Model and the Protection Motivation Theory suggest that perceptions, such as people's views of social norms, influence their actions related to health prevention practices, such as wearing sunscreen and hats to protect one's skin from sun exposure [7, 8]. Research has found that adults' perceptions of social norms also may influence their health protection behaviors [9]. Reid et al. [10] proposed that perceptions about others' beliefs of the importance of a behavior may influence an individual's behavior. As such, students' perceptions toward parental beliefs about the importance of sun exposure may positively influence sun protection behaviors [11].

Researchers have reported that increased anticipatory emotion, such as worry, is related to increased health protection [9, 12]. Worrying over a potential health problem is an anticipatory emotion, which may influence protective behaviors [12, 13]. As such, worrying about sun exposure has been related to increased sun protection behaviors [10, 11, 14]. In addition to worry and parental influence, there may be differences in men's and women's sun protection behaviors. Specifically, women may engage in more sun protection behaviors and worry more about the harmful effects from sun exposure relative to men [9, 15, 16].

There were two main aims of this study. The first aim was to examine the influence of worry about sun exposure and young adults' perceptions of parent beliefs about the importance of sun exposure on their sun protection behaviors. It was hypothesized that greater worry about sun exposure would be related to reports of higher levels of sun protection behaviors. Additionally, it was anticipated that greater parents' perceived importance about sun exposure would be related to higher levels of sun protection behaviors. The second aim was to examine the influence of family history of skin cancer on worry about sun exposure and perceptions of parental beliefs about the importance of sun exposure. It was hypothesized that having a family history of skin cancer would be related to greater worry and higher levels of perceived parental beliefs about sun exposure.

2. Materials and Methods

2.1. Participants. Four hundred and sixty-two college students from a large Midwestern university participated in this study (see Table 1). Mean age was 19 years and 2 months (SD: 1 year, 5 months; age range: 16 to 33 years).

2.2. Measure. Questions used in the *Sun Exposure Survey* were developed after a literature review [17–21]. Health education professionals in the field provided expert review of questions in our survey. Questions about sun exposure behaviors were answered on a four-point scale ("Do not know = 0; 1 = never/rarely; 2 = sometimes; 3 = most of the time; and 4 = always"). The following questions were used to assess sun exposure behaviors: "I wear sunglasses"; "I wear sunscreen"; "I wear hats in the bright sun"; "I wear chap stick with sunscreen in it"; and "I wear a hat with a brim on it." One question was used to examine worry—"I worry about getting too much sun on my skin." Another question was "Has anyone in your family ever had skin cancer?" (response categories were "yes, no, and do not know"). Students then circled the members of their family who had skin cancer from the following list: "Mom, Dad, Brother, Sister, Grandpa, Grandma, Aunt, Uncle, Cousin or Other Relative." Student views of parent beliefs were assessed with the following question: "My parents think sun exposure is a big deal" (response categories were: "yes, no, and do not know").

TABLE 1: Demographic information and student responses for sun protection behaviors.

Variable	n	%
Sex		
Male	185	40%
Female	275	59.5%
Ethnic group		
White	359	77.7%
Black	36	7.8%
Asian	26	5.6%
Indian*	8	1.7%
Hispanic	6	1.3%
Biracial	21	4.5%
Other	5	.01%
College level		
Freshman and sophomores	404	87.4%
Juniors and seniors	58	12.6%

Notes. N = 462. Two students did not provide information about gender and one student did not provide information about ethnicity. *Indian does not refer to Native American Indians, but rather those students identifying with India.

2.3. Procedures. This study was approved by a university-based institutional review board (IRB). Participants reviewed an information form, which reviewed all informed consent procedures. The information form noted that college students who completed the *Sun Exposure Survey* for this study were providing their consent to participate. Participants independently completed the *Sun Exposure Survey* and when finished with the survey placed it in a sealed envelope or box in their college classroom.

A test-retest study was also completed to assess reliability of the survey. The sixteen students (a convenience sample of college students at the same university) participating in the test-retest study reviewed a second information form, explaining the test-retest study and procedures, which also was approved by the same university-based institutional review board. These participants completed the survey two times (retest 14 days later). They placed surveys in a sealed envelope when completing them.

2.4. Data Analyses. Descriptive analyses were conducted on student perceptions, sun protection behaviors, and reports about family history of skin cancer. SPSS Version 23 was used for analyses. A MANCOVA was used to examine the relationship between participant sex (male or female) and student perceptions of parent beliefs of sun exposure (yes, no, or do not know) and its effect on student report of sun protection behaviors (e.g., wearing sunscreen, chap stick with sunscreen, and wearing hats) and their worry about sun exposure. The different sun protection behaviors were considered dependent variables. Age was the covariate. Two chi-square analyses were used to examine whether having a history of skin cancer in the family influenced student worry about sun exposure and student perceptions of their parents' beliefs about sun exposure being important.

3. Results

Results for descriptive statistics assessing sun exposure protection behaviors and questions assessing level of worry about sun exposure are presented in Table 2.

Results indicated students were most likely to wear sunscreen sometimes, and 17% of students did not wear or rarely wore sunscreen. Twenty-eight percent never/rarely wore chap stick or lip balm with sunscreen, 37% did not wear/rarely wore hats in the bright sun, and 13% never/rarely wore sunglasses. Approximately 20% of participants were worried about sun exposure (see Table 2). Four hundred and fifty-seven students also reported their perceptions of their parents' beliefs about sun exposure being a big deal. Thirty-seven (8.1%) reported they did not know their parents' beliefs. Two hundred and ninety-five (64.6%) thought their parents believed sun exposure was a big deal, while 125 (27.4%) did not believe their parents thought sun exposure was a big deal. Mean scores and standard deviations for the questions were as follows: wearing sunglasses, M = 2.46 (SD = .90); wearing sunscreen, M = 2.25 (SD = .84); wearing hats in bright sun, 1.86, (SD = .83); wearing chap stick with sunscreen, M = 2.23 (SD = 1.08); wearing a hat with a brim, M = 1.83 (SD = .90); and worry about too much sun exposure on skin, M = 1.92 (SD = .95). In general, these scores indicated variable (e.g., "sometimes") engagement in sun protection behaviors among college students.

A 2 × 3 (sex × parent beliefs) MANCOVA with age in years as a covariate was used to examine the influence of sex and parent beliefs on college students' report of their sun protection behaviors and worry about getting too much sun exposure. Results were significant for sex, Wilks' lambda = .882, $p < .001$, and $\eta_p^2 = .118$, and for parental beliefs, Wilks' lambda = .903, $p < .001$, and $\eta_p^2 = .05$. The results for the interaction term were not significant, and age was not a significant covariate. Results of the univariate tests for the main effect of sex of the participants, with means and standard deviations, are presented in Table 3.

Results indicated females were more likely to wear sunglasses, sunscreen, and chap stick and worry about getting too much sun on their skin. Males were more likely to wear a hat in the sun or a hat with a brim in the sun (see Table 3).

Table 4 presents results of the univariate tests for the main effect of parent beliefs on student reports of sun protection behaviors and worry about sun exposure as well as means and standard deviations and results from Tukey's follow-up tests.

Results indicated a significant difference for all of the questions, with the exception of wearing sunglasses (see Table 4). Therefore, Tukey's follow-up tests were used to examine differences between "do not know," "yes," and "no" answers for student perceptions of parents' beliefs about sun exposure for wearing sunscreen, hats, chap stick, and a hat with a brim and worry about getting too much sun. College students were more likely to report engaging in wearing sunscreen, hats, and chap stick with sunscreen and to worry about getting too much sun if their parents viewed sun exposure as a big deal. Means for wearing sunscreen and chap stick with sunscreen were higher for students who reported, "yes"; their parents thought sun exposure was a big deal compared to those who reported they did not know their parents' beliefs about sun exposure (see Table 4).

One hundred and fifty students (32.5%) reported that a family member had experienced skin cancer. In terms of the family member who had skin cancer, 148 of the students reported who had experienced skin cancer. Specifically, 52 (35.1%) students reported the family member was a grandparent, 30 (20.3%) reported it was a parent, 40 (27%) reported multiple family members had skin cancer, and the remaining students ($n = 26$; 17.6%) reported that another family member had experienced skin cancer.

A chi-square analysis was used to examine the relationship between student perceptions of parent beliefs that sun exposure was a big deal and whether a family member had skin cancer. The family member having had skin cancer variable was recoded, combining "do not know" and "no" answers into "no" answers compared to "yes" answers. This coding occurred so that answers indicating a family history of skin cancer could be compared to other responses provided by participants. Students' reports about parent beliefs were recoded, and "do not know" and "no" answers were combined and compared to "yes" answers (using the logic of comparing "yes" responses to all other responses). The chi-square was significant, $\chi^2 = 13.53$, $p < .001$. When students viewed parents as thinking that sun exposure was a big deal, there was more likely to be skin cancer in the family (61.4%), compared to not having skin cancer in the family (38.6%). When students reported parents as not seeing sun exposure as a big deal, there was less likely to be skin cancer in the family. Specifically, for students reporting it was not viewed as a big deal by parents, 21.7% of the students reported skin cancer in the family, while 78.3% reported that there was no skin cancer in the family.

A chi-square analysis was performed to examine the relationship between personal worry and whether a family member had skin cancer. The variable for personal worry was recoded so that "never/rarely" and "sometimes" answers were combined to indicate low worry, and "most of the time" and "always" answers were combined to indicate high worry. This was compared to a family member having skin cancer (coded as "yes" or "no"). The chi-square was significant, $\chi^2 = 9.01$, $p = .002$. At the higher level of worry, 45.4% of the participants had a family member with skin cancer (54.6% did not have a family member with skin cancer). At the lower level of worry, 29.2% of the participants had a family member with skin cancer (while 70.8 did not have a family member with skin cancer).

As mentioned, a test-retest reliability study was conducted with 16 college students (female = 10; male = 6; 14 = white; 2 = black). These students completed the measure at a two-week interval. The mean age was 19 years and 7 months (SD = 1 year and 8 months; age range = 18–25 years). Correlations for the questions examining sun exposure behaviors at Time 1 and Time 2 were as follows: wearing sunglasses, $r = .912$, $p < .001$; wearing sunscreen, $r = .872$, $p < .001$; wearing hats in the bright sun, $r = .767$, $p < .001$; wearing

TABLE 2: Sun protection behaviors and worry reported by college students.

Area	Question	Do not know		Never/rarely		Sometimes		Most of the time		Always	
		n	%	n	%	n	%	n	%	n	%
Sun protection behaviors	I wear sunglasses	1	.2%	62	13.4%	187	40.6%	145	31.5%	66	14.3%
	I wear sunscreen	1	.2%	79	17.1%	221	47.8%	123	26.6%	37	8%
	I wear hats in the bright sun	1	.2%	174	37.7%	194	42.1%	74	16.1%	18	3.9%
	I wear chap stick with sunscreen in it	6	1.3%	130	28.2%	155	33.6%	92	20%	78	16.9%
	I wear a hat with a brim on it	2	.4%	195	42.4%	168	36.5%	67	14.6%	28	6.1%
Worry	I worry about getting too much sun on my skin	4	.9%	170	36.9%	190	41.1%	53	11.5%	44	9.5%

Note. Four hundred and sixty students answered the question about wearing a hat with a brim. Four hundred and sixty-one of the students answered the other sun protection questions.

TABLE 3: Univariate tests for gender and means and standard deviations for females and males.

Area	Question	F	p	η_p^2	Female		Male	
					M	SD	M	SD
Sun protection behaviors	I wear sunglasses	5.23	.023	.012	2.59	.88	2.26	.89
	I wear sunscreen	13.96	<.001	.030	2.43	.87	1.99	.72
	I wear hats in the bright sun	4.53	.034	.010	1.77	.82	1.97	.82
	I wear chap stick with sunscreen in it	26.82	<.001	.057	2.56	1.04	1.72	.92
	I wear a hat with a brim on it	9.99	.002	.022	1.71	.87	1.99	.89
Worry	I worry about getting too much sun on my skin	7.89	.005	.017	2.07	1.01	1.69	.81

Note. Including "Do not know" answers could have lowered mean scores.

chap stick, $r = .622$, $p = .01$; wearing a hat with a brim, $r = .629$, $p = .009$; and worry about getting too much sun on my skin, $r = .334$, $p = .205$. Kendall's tau-b for answers about parents believing sun exposure was a big deal at Time 1 and Time 2 were significant, $\tau = 2.75$, $p = .006$.

4. Discussion

Study results were consistent with other researches indicating that adults may neglect sun protection behaviors [4–6]. Over half of our sample reported low frequencies ("never/rarely", "sometimes") for participating in behaviors like wearing sunglasses, sunscreen, hats, and lip balm with SPF protection. Students who mentioned that sun exposure was a big deal to their parents were more likely to engage in sun protection behaviors and endorse worry about sun exposure. Almost a third of our sample reported having a family member who had experienced skin cancer. As expected, students with a higher level of worry reported that about 45% of their family members had experienced skin cancer, whereas those with lower worry reported that about 29% of their family members had experienced skin cancer. Of participants reporting greater perceptions of sun exposure being a big deal to parents, about 61% stated that a family member had experienced skin cancer, whereas participants with lower perceptions of parent beliefs about sun exposure being a big deal had fewer family members who had experienced skin cancer. This is consistent with research that has demonstrated that having skin cancer in the family may influence perceptions toward sun exposure [14].

In general, males engaged in lower sun protection behaviors, with the exception of wearing hats with a brim. College-age males in our sample may have been more likely to wear baseball caps, as a fashion accessory, compared to females. Our results support prior research, indicating that females are more likely to worry about sun exposure and engage in more sun protection behaviors compared to males [9, 15, 16]. Messages targeted at males should highlight information to increase their knowledge of greater risks for skin cancer and how sun protection behaviors, such as wearing sunscreen and lip balm with sunscreen, have the potential to substantially lower skin cancer risk. In addition, messages should include information about the benefits of sunscreen as well as staying out of the sun at peak hours, wearing protective clothing, and using hats and sunglasses [22]. Emphasizing risks of sunburns

for skin cancer and emphasizing the benefits of sunscreen and protective clothing and wearing hats may be critical components of health education messaging. Thus, there is a need for the development and use of educational materials about sun exposure dangers, especially for males who may engage in lower frequencies of sun protection behaviors.

Although our findings provide insight into college students' ideas about sun protection and potential areas for prevention and intervention campaigns, several limitations should be noted. For example, the survey used for this study was a self-report survey with a cross-sectional design, and, thus, social desirability bias may limit the generalizability of findings as does the fact that attitudes were assessed at only one point in time. Moreover, physical appearance attitudes (e.g., ideals about skin colors) were not examined, and differences in sun protection behaviors and worry about sun exposure may have been influenced by a desire to achieve an ideal skin color [22] Combining "do not know" and "no" answers for the family history questions is a limitation, because some of the participants who answered "do not know" may have had a positive family history for skin cancer. Combining the "do not know" and "no" answers for the perceptions of parental beliefs has similar limitations. Moreover, only one item was used to assess key variables. Some of the effect sizes for sun protection behaviors were fairly small; but, this was consistent with other literatures [9]. It is noteworthy that only one question had the wording "bright sun," whereas other questions were worded differently, which may have influenced participant responses. Moreover, the wording "parents think sun exposure is a big deal" could have been interpreted as encouraging sun exposure or as discouraging sun exposure. Finally, some test-retest correlations were low. It may be that responses do not remain consistent over time. It also was noteworthy that the sample size for the test-retest study was small, which may have influenced study findings. Thus, further research assessing study questions is needed.

5. Conclusion

Our results indicated that behaviors to prevent sun exposure in young adulthood are influenced by college students' perceptions of parental beliefs. Prevention and intervention programs such as sunscreen dispensers and messaging about sun protective behaviors in public places for this particular population decrease various risk factors associated with

TABLE 4: Univariate tests for parent values about sun exposure and means for student ratings of parent beliefs.

Area	Question	F	p	η_p^2	Ratings					
					Yes, important to parents		No, not important to parents		Do not know	
					M	SD	M	SD	M	SD
Sun protection behaviors	I wear sunglasses	2.57	.078	.011	2.41[ab]	.81	1.94[a]	.81	2.03[b]	.83
	I wear sunscreen	13.14	<.001	.056	1.91[a]	.84	1.69[a]	.75	1.86	.86
	I wear hats in the bright sun	3.59	.028	.016	2.35[ab]	1.06	2.00[a]	1.04	1.86[b]	1.11
	I wear chap stick with sunscreen in it	4.86	.008	.021	1.89[a]	.92	1.62[a]	.79	1.92	.86
	I wear a hat with a brim on it	4.90	.008	.021	2.10[a]	.97	1.54[a]	.75	1.78	1.00
Worry	I worry about getting too much sun on my skin	13.55	<.001	.057	2.41[ab]	.81	1.94[a]	.81	2.03[b]	.83

Notes. [a]Indicates a significant difference between yes and no answers using Tukey's follow-up tests; [b]indicates a significant difference between yes and do not know answers using Tukey's follow-up tests. Including "Do not know" answers could have lowered mean scores.

sun exposure. Early educational messages addressing youth perceptions may play an important role in shaping health behaviors. Parents should emphasize the use of sunscreen and products that include SPF as well as use of protective clothing and hats to reduce risk for sunburns and sun damage. Attitudes about beauty, ideal skin color, and knowledge and experience with sun burns were not assessed in this study and remain important areas for future research.

Ethical Approval

The current study was approved by a university-based institutional review board at a land grant university in the United States. All work was conducted in accordance with the Declaration of Helsinki (1964). Participants read an information form that explained the study and provided consent for participation.

References

[1] American Cancer Society, *Cancer Facts and Figures 2017*, American Cancer Society, Georgia, Ga, USA, 2017.

[2] ACS, "What are the key statistics about melanoma skin cancer?" http://www.cancer.org/cancer/skincancermelanoma/ detailedguide/melanoma-skin-cancer-key-statistics.

[3] G. P. Guy, S. R. Machlin, D. U. Ekwueme, and K. R. Yabroff, "Prevalence and costs of skin cancer treatment in the U.S., 2002-2006 and 2007-2011," *American Journal of Preventive Medicine*, vol. 48, no. 2, pp. 183-187, 2015.

[4] S. Prentice-Dunn, B. F. McMath, and R. J. Cramer, "Protection motivation theory and stages of change in sun protective behavior," *Journal of Health Psychology*, vol. 14, no. 2, pp. 297-305, 2009.

[5] P. H. Cohen, H. Tsai, and J. C. Puffer, "Sun-protective behavior among high-school and collegiate athletes in Los Angeles, CA," *Clinical Journal of Sport Medicine*, vol. 16, no. 3, pp. 253-260, 2006.

[6] "National Cancer Institute, Sun Protective Behavior: Cancer Trends Progress Report, 2017," https://progressreport.cancer .gov/prevention/sun_protection.

[7] I. M. Rosenstock, "The health belief model and preventive health behavior," *Health Education & Behavior*, vol. 2, no. 4, pp. 354-386, 1977.

[8] S. Prentice-Dunn and R. W. Rogers, "Protection motivation theory and preventive health: beyond the health belief model," *Health Education Research*, vol. 1, no. 3, pp. 153-161, 1986.

[9] P. Sheeran, P. R. Harris, and T. Epton, "Does heightening risk appraisals change people's intentions and behavior? A meta-analysis of experimental studies," *Psychological Bulletin*, vol. 140, no. 2, pp. 511-543, 2014.

[10] A. E. Reid, R. B. Cialdini, and L. S. Aiken, "Social norms and health behavior," in *Handbook of Behavioral Medicine*, pp. 263-274, Springer, New York, NY, USA, 2010.

[11] A. E. Reid and L. S. Aiken, "Correcting injunctive norm misperceptions motivates behavior change: a randomized controlled

[12] E. Janssen, L. Van Osch, H. De Vries, and L. Lechner, "Measuring risk perceptions of skin cancer: Reliability and validity of different operationalizations," *British Journal of Health Psychology*, vol. 16, no. 1, pp. 92-112, 2011.

[13] K. D. McCaul, A. B. Mullens, K. M. Romanek, S. C. Erickson, and B. J. Gatheridge, "The motivational effects of thinking and worrying about the effects of smoking cigarettes," *Cognition and Emotion*, vol. 21, no. 8, pp. 1780-1798, 2007.

[14] A. C. Geller, D. R. Brooks, G. A. Colditz, H. K. Koh, and A. L. Frazier, "Sun protection practices among offspring of women with personal or family history of skin cancer," *Pediatrics*, vol. 117, no. 4, pp. e688-e694, 2006.

[15] R. Branström, N. A. Kasparian, Y. Chang et al., "Predictors of sun protection behaviors and severe sunburn in an international online study," *Cancer Epidemiology, Biomarkers and Prevention*, vol. 19, no. 9, pp. 2199-2210, 2010.

[16] N. A. Kasparian, J. K. McLoone, and B. Meiser, "Skin cancer-related prevention and screening behaviors: a review of the literature," *Journal of Behavioral Medicine*, vol. 32, no. 5, pp. 406-428, 2009.

[17] V. E. Cokkinides, M. Weinstock, M. C. O'Connell et al., "Sun exposure and sun-protection behaviors and attitudes among U.S. Youth, 11 to 18 years of age," *Preventive Medicine*, vol. 33, no. 3, pp. 141-151, 2001.

[18] V. Cokkinides, M. Weinstock, K. Glanz, J. Albano, E. Ward, and M. Thun, "Trends in sunburns, sun protection practices, and attitudes toward sun exposure protection and tanning among US adolescents, 1998-2004," *Pediatrics*, vol. 118, no. 3, pp. 853-864, 2006.

[19] A. K. Day, C. Wilson, R. M. Roberts, and A. D. Hutchinson, "The skin cancer and sun knowledge (SCSK) scale: validity, reliability, and relationship to sun-related behaviors among young western adults," *Health Education and Behavior*, vol. 41, no. 4, pp. 440-448, 2014.

[20] K. Glanz, E. Schoenfeld, M. A. Weinstock, G. Layi, J. Kidd, and D. M. Shigaki, "Development and reliability of a brief skin cancer risk assessment tool," *Cancer Detection and Prevention*, vol. 27, no. 4, pp. 311-315, 2003.

[21] P. Rouhani, Y. Parmet, A. G. Bessell, T. Peay, A. Weiss, and R. S. Kirsner, "Knowledge, attitudes, and behaviors of elementary school students regarding sun exposure and skin cancer," *Pediatric Dermatology*, vol. 26, no. 5, pp. 529-535, 2009.

[22] M. Suppa, S. Cazzaniga, M. C. Fargnoli, L. Naldi, and K. Peris, "Knowledge, perceptions and behaviours about skin cancer and sun protection among secondary school students from Central Italy," *Journal of the European Academy of Dermatology and Venereology*, vol. 27, no. 5, pp. 571-579, 2013.

[11] sun protection intervention," *Health Psychology*, vol. 32, no. 5, pp. 551-560, 2013.

28

Is There a Relationship between the Stratum Corneum Thickness and That of the Viable Parts of Tumour Cells in Basal Cell Carcinoma?

Olav A. Foss,[1] **Patricia Mjønes,**[2,3] **Silje Fismen,**[4] **and Eidi Christensen**[2,5]

[1]*Orthopaedic Research Centre, Clinic of Orthopaedy, Rheumatology and Dermatology, St. Olavs Hospital,*
  Trondheim University Hospital, Trondheim 7030, Norway
[2]*Department of Cancer Research and Molecular Medicine, Faculty of Medicine, Norwegian University of Science and*
  Technology (NTNU), Trondheim 7030, Norway
[3]*Department of Pathology and Medical Genetics, St. Olavs Hospital, Trondheim University Hospital, Trondheim 7030, Norway*
[4]*Department of Pathology, University Hospital of North Norway, Tromsø 9019, Norway*
[5]*Department of Dermatology, Clinic of Orthopaedy, Rheumatology and Dermatology, St. Olavs Hospital,*
  Trondheim University Hospital, Trondheim 7030, Norway

Correspondence should be addressed to Eidi Christensen; eidi.christensen@ntnu.no

Academic Editor: Iris Zalaudek

Basal cell carcinoma (BCC) is an invasive epithelial skin tumour. The thickness of the outermost epidermal layer of the skin, the stratum corneum (SC), influences drug uptake and penetration into tumour and may thereby affect the response of BCC to topical treatment. The aim was to investigate a possible relationship between the thickness of the SC and that of the viable part of BCC. Histopathological evaluations of the corresponding SC and viable tumour thickness measurements of individual BCCs of different subtypes were explored. A total of 53 BCCs from 46 patients were studied. The median tumour thickness was 1.7 mm (0.8–3.0 mm), with a significant difference between subtypes ($p < 0.001$). The SC had a median thickness of 0.3 mm (0.2–0.4 mm), with no difference between tumour subtypes ($p = 0.415$). Additionally, no significant association between the thickness of the SC and that of the viable part of the tumour was demonstrated ($p = 0.381$). In conclusion our results indicate that SC thickness is relatively constant in BCC.

1. Introduction

The stratum corneum (SC) is the outermost epidermal layer of the skin. It consists of flattened, anucleated keratinized cells (corneocytes) enclosed in lipid bilayers including ceramides, free fatty acids, and cholesterol which together with enzymes, antimicrobial peptides, and structural proteins make a barrier function [1].

Basal cell carcinoma (BCC) is an epithelium tumour that primarily originates in the epidermis and its appendages. It is the most common type of invasive skin cancer in the fair skinned population of the world, causing significant patient morbidity, and should be managed properly [2]. Several types of treatment can be used of which minimally invasive methods such as topical photodynamic therapy

(PDT) have become an attractive option [3]. This method is recommended for treatment of superficial BCCs and for small nodular tumours. However, the treatment response of thick tumours is regarded as inferior, partly because of the limited penetration of topical drugs through the SC, and deep into the tumour [4]. The SC physiochemical properties provide the main barrier for drug penetration of the skin [1]. In addition, crusts may cover part or the whole of the BCC, thereby increasing the thickness of the outer barrier layer.

SC thickness has been closely investigated in normal skin and has been found to vary, depending on various factors such as body site [5, 6]. However, the knowledge of SC thickness in BCC as well as information as to whether its thickness varies with total tumour thickness and across tumour subtypes is lacking.

A clinical estimate of BCC thickness can readily be made before selecting an appropriate therapy. Nevertheless, it is the histopathological thickness that is considered the "gold standard" measurement for prediction of treatment response. Information about the agreement between clinical and histopathological evaluations of BCC thickness is, to our knowledge, limited to the results of a single study [7]. In that study, the estimation of tumour thickness by the two methods was poor between corresponding measurements for individual tumours. It should be noted that the clinical estimation of tumour thickness includes the SC and any overlying crusts, as opposed to histology. In accordance with standard practice, the histological thickness is measured from the upper part of the stratum granulosum (SG) and comprises the viable part of the tumour cells [8]. Hence, there is a systematic difference between clinical and histopathological evaluations of BCC thickness, which may bias comparisons of results between these two methods. For this reason, and because the SC is the main barrier to percutaneous penetration of topically applied drugs, we wanted to investigate SC thickness in BCC.

The main objective of the present study was to investigate a possible relationship between measurements of SC thickness and the thickness of the corresponding viable part of the BCC.

2. Materials and Methods

The study was performed at the outpatient clinic at the Department of Dermatology, St. Olavs Hospital, Trondheim University Hospital (Trondheim, Norway), and approved by the regional committee for medical research ethics (REK number 4.2007.558). Patients gave written informed consent before entry into the study.

Part of the study sample had been included in previous reports that compared measurements of BCC thickness from clinical investigations, punch biopsies, and excision specimens [7, 9]. Consecutive patients of both sexes, over 18 years of age, with primary histopathologically verified BCC suitable for excision surgery and over 9 mm in size to ensure sufficient material for investigation, were included. Pregnancy and lactation were exclusion criteria.

Three physicians (two dermatology consultants and an experienced dermatology registrar) performed the clinical examinations of, respectively, 12, 17, and 24 tumours. A single hospital pathologist performed the histopathological assessment of all the specimens.

Clinical evaluations and sampling of tumour tissue for histopathological investigations were performed on the same day. The tumour size (in mm) was clinically defined as the mean value of its measured maximum length and width. Details of study inclusions and exclusions, the particular tissue sampling procedures, and the tissue processing are given in an earlier report [9].

BCC thickness was measured on haematoxylin, eosin, and saffron- (HES-) stained slides using an ocular microm- eter (Vernier method) with a precision of 0.1 mm [10]. The BCC-free deep margin was defined as at least 0.1 mm of tumour-free tissue. The thicknesses were measured with the upper part of the SG as reference. The thickness of the viable part of the tumour was measured from this reference position to the bottom of the tumour nest and is referred to in this paper as the "tumour thickness." The thickness of the SC with any crust was measured from the reference position to the outermost surface and is referred to as the "SC thickness." The greatest thickness measurements for both the SC and the viable part of each tumour were used in the analysis as this was considered most relevant to the use of topical therapy. The tumours were histopathologically subclassified into three subtypes: superficial, nodular, and aggressive. The aggressive category included morpheaform, infiltrative, and basosquamous types [11]. They were classified according to the most aggressive component for those BCCs representing a mixed growth pattern.

All statistical calculations were performed using IBM SPSS Statistics (v.21, IBM Corp., Armonk, NY, USA). Visual inspection of Q-Q plots was used to examine whether data were normally distributed. The tumour size data were normally distributed and are presented as mean (SD). The tumour thickness measurements were normally distributed, whereas the SC thickness measurements were not. Therefore, all thickness data are presented as medians (quartiles). The Kruskal-Wallis test was used to compare SC thickness between subtypes. Regression analysis with tumour thickness and SC thickness was carried out to describe a possible relationship between these two parameters. A mixed linear model was used. All thickness measurement data had to be logarithmically transformed to achieve the assumption of normally distributed residuals in the models. Tumour size, location, and patient sex and age were initially included as covariates. For all tests, $p < 0.05$ was considered statistically significant.

3. Results

Measurements were taken of 53 BCCs from 46 patients. Of these tumours, 26 were located on the head/neck, 27 on the trunk, and six on the extremities. Histopathologically, 14 were superficial, 24 were nodular, and 15 were aggres- sive tumours. Twelve of the BCCs demonstrated crusts on histology.

The descriptive data are presented in Table 1. The median tumour thickness was 1.7 mm (0.8–3.0 mm) with a significant difference between subtypes ($p < 0.001$). Superficial tumours were significantly thinner than nodular and aggressive types (both $p < 0.001$), and there was no difference between the nodular and aggressive types ($p = 0.813$). The median SC thickness was 0.3 mm (0.2–0.4 mm) with no significant difference between subtypes ($p = 0.415$). Figure 1 presents a scatter plot of tumour thickness and SC thickness. The regression analyses showed no statistically significant asso- ciation between the tumour and SC thicknesses ($p = 0.381$). Three examples of BCCs of different subtype with different thicknesses for the viable cellular part but with similar SC thicknesses are shown in Figure 2. None of the following parameters were significant when included as covariates in the regression analyses: tumour size ($p = 0.432$), tumour location ($p = 0.992$), patient sex ($p = 0.497$), and patient age ($p = 0.776$).

TABLE 1: Descriptive data of patients and BCCs.

Tumour type	Age [years]	Sex [M/F]	Number	Location [H/T/E]	Tumour size [mm] Mean (SD)	Tumour thickness [mm] Median (quartiles)	Stratum corneum thickness [mm]
Superficial	69	7/7	14	2/9/3	17 ± 5	0.6 (0.4–0.7)	0.3 (0.2–0.4)
Nodular	76	17/7	24	12/10/2	18 ± 6	2.0 (1.6–3.7)	0.2 (0.2–0.3)
Aggressive	73	9/6	15	6/8/1	18 ± 4	2.2 (1.5–2.9)	0.3 (0.2–0.4)
All	73	33/20	53	20/27/6	18 ± 5	1.7 (0.8–3.0)	0.3 (0.2–0.4)

E: extremities; F: female; H: head/neck; M: male; SD: standard deviation; T: trunk.

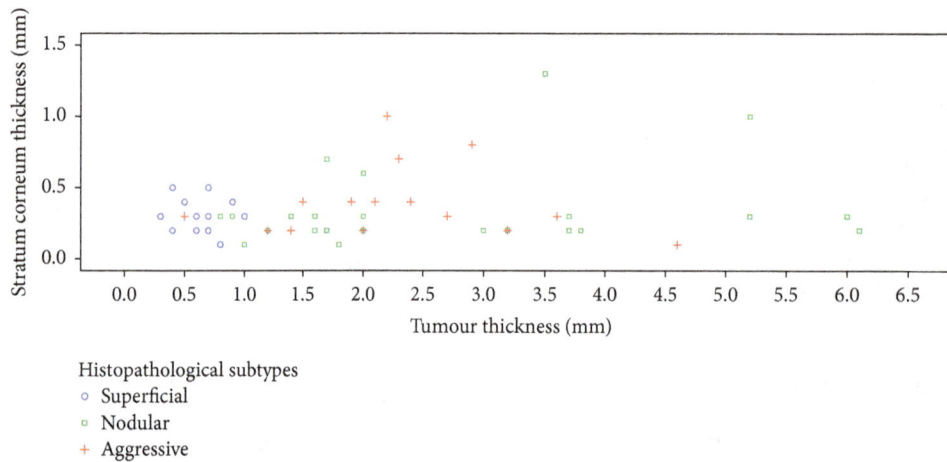

FIGURE 1: Plot of corresponding stratum corneum thickness versus tumour thickness of individual BCCs.

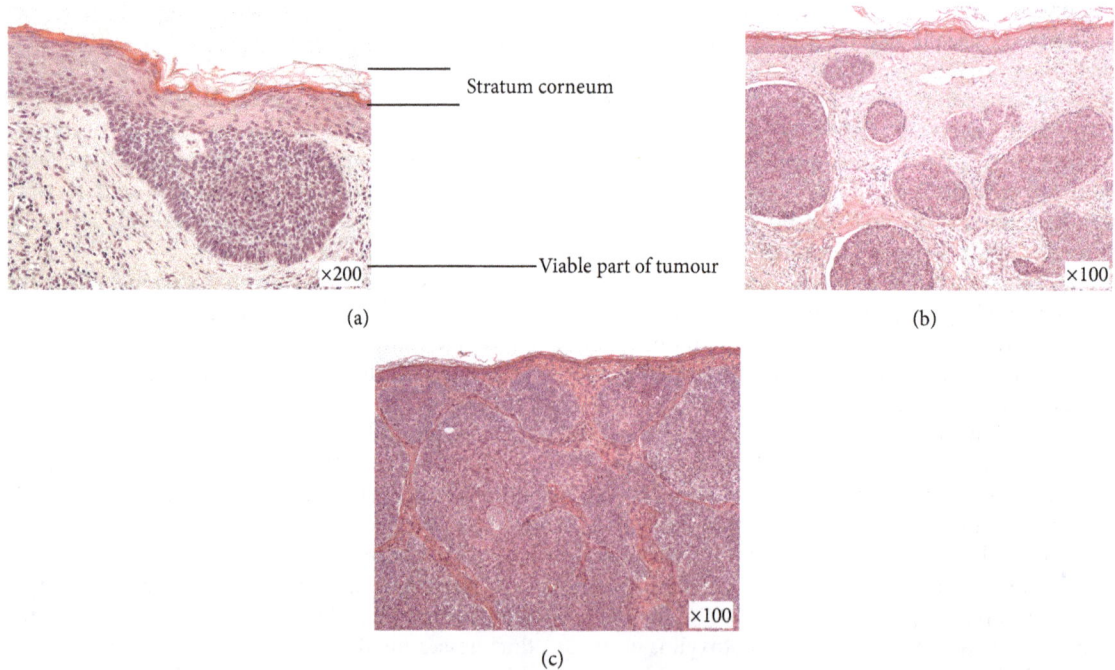

FIGURE 2: HES-stained histopathological images of sections of the stratum corneum and the viable parts of tumour cells from three basal cell carcinomas with different growth patterns: (a) superficial tumour from the back, (b) nodular tumour from the chest, and (c) aggressive tumour from the cheek.

4. Discussion

The main finding was the no significant relationship between the thickness of the SC and that of the viable part BCC, regardless of tumour size and subtype.

Knowledge of SC thickness in skin cancer is of interest in relation to PDT and may also be of interest to other topical therapies. PDT exerts its action by light activation of a photosensitizer, leading to destruction of targeted tumour cells. 5-Aminolaevulinic acid (ALA) and its ester derivate are the two most commonly used prodrugs for topical PDT of BCC [4]. After cellular uptake, ALA is metabolized to photosensitive porphyrins, and any factors limiting its penetration through skin may reduce the treatment effect. The thickness of SC has been shown to influence local uptake of ALA in viable cells [12, 13]. This was studied using fluorescence diagnosis with ALA-induced porphyrins in psoriatic plaque and actinic keratosis [14, 15]. When excited by blue light, porphyrin accumulating cells emit red fluorescence that is visualized. The SC proved thicker in lower fluorescent psoriatic plaques and a negative correlation between SC thickness and fluorescence intensity in actinic keratosis was observed. These findings indicate that SC thickness is a factor in differences of ALA uptake in viable cells and this may in turn be significant for treatment outcome. Thus, it was of interest to investigate whether the SC thickness varies in different subtypes of BCC when PDT efficacy is more superior in superficial than other subtypes of tumour. Although slight variation in SC thicknesses was observed between individual BCCs (lower quartile 0.2 mm, upper quartile 0.4 mm), the SC thickness does not appear to explain different treatment results on a group level between tumour subtypes.

In accordance with current PDT guidelines, SC and any crusts are commonly removed from the tumour surface and surrounding skin area before treatment in attempt to enhance drug permeation into tumour tissue [16, 17]. Various physical and/or chemical methods may be used [17, 18]. However, pre-PDT preparation can produce varying results because the procedures are, at present, not standardized and depend on both methods and physicians' assessments, aims, and skills.

We also wanted to examine whether SC thickness is a factor that may affect clinical assessment of tumour thickness. In an earlier aforementioned study, the results demonstrated that the clinicians overestimated the thickness of thin tumours and underestimated the thickness of thick tumours compared to histology [7]. The histopathological thickness was measured from the upper SG, whereas the clinical estimation of thickness included the SC and any crusts, as the clinician could not distinguish between microscopic tissue layers. The present results imply that the SC thickness probably could have contributed to the clinical overestimation of the thickness of thin BCCs.

The thickness of the SC in nonmelanoma skin cancers such as *in situ* and invasive squamous cell carcinomas has been studied previously, and no significant difference in SC thickness between the different histological diagnoses was shown [12]. Our results are in agreement, as we found no difference in SC thickness across BCC subtypes. However, in normal skin SC thickness may vary depending on body site,

and within-site variation has also been observed [19]. Results from investigations of relationship between the SC thickness and sex and age in humans have been contradictory [5, 6, 20]. In the present study, these factors were initially included as covariates in the regression analysis, and none of them was found to be significant. However, our findings apply only to the particular analyses described in this report and should not be considered as contradicting the findings presented in the earlier cited reports. The relatively small number of tumours included should be regarded as a study limitation, particularly with regard to subgroup analyses. Other factors can influence the results. It is important for accurate measurement of thickness that the cuts from the tissue blocks were taken perpendicular to the skin surface. Also, possible errors in thickness estimations may have occurred owing to alterations in the physical properties of tissue after excision and preparation and individual evaluation of specimens are subject to variation [6, 21, 22].

5. Conclusions

The study results indicate that the thickness of SC in BCC is fairly constant independent of the viable tumour thickness and across different tumour sizes and subtypes.

Ethical Approval

The study was approved by the regional committee for medical research ethics (4.2007.558).

Acknowledgment

The authors would like to thank Professor A. M. Bofin for the histological pictures.

References

[1] P. M. Elias, "Structure and function of the stratum corneum extracellular matrix," *Journal of Investigative Dermatology*, vol. 132, no. 9, pp. 2131–2133, 2012.

[2] A. N. Crowson, "Basal cell carcinoma: biology, morphology and clinical implications," *Modern Pathology*, vol. 19, supplement 2, pp. S127–S147, 2006.

[3] F. J. Bath-Hextall, W. Perkins, J. Bong, and H. C. Williams, "Interventions for basal cell carcinoma of the skin," *Cochrane Database of Systematic Reviews*, no. 1, Article ID CD003412, 2007.

[4] L. R. Braathen, R.-M. Szeimies, N. Basset-Seguin et al., "Guidelines on the use of photodynamic therapy for nonmelanoma skin cancer: an international consensus," *Journal of the American Academy of Dermatology*, vol. 56, no. 1, pp. 125–143, 2007.

[5] Z. Ya-Xian, T. Suetake, and H. Tagami, "Number of cell layers of the stratum corneum in normal skin—relationship to the anatomical location an the body, age, sex and physical parameters," *Archives of Dermatological Research*, vol. 291, no. 10, pp. 555–559, 1999.

[6] J. Sandby-Møller, T. Poulsen, and H. C. Wulf, "Epidermal thickness at different body sites: relationship to age, gender, pigmentation, blood content, skin type and smoking habits," *Acta Dermato-Venereologica*, vol. 83, no. 6, pp. 410–413, 2003.

[7] E. Christensen, P. Mjønes, Ø. Grimstad, O. M. Rørdam, and O. A. Foss, "Comparison of clinical and histopathological evaluations of basal cell carcinoma thickness," *British Journal of Dermatology*, vol. 173, no. 2, pp. 578–580, 2015.

[8] A. Breslow, "Thickness, cross-sectional areas and depth of invasion in the prognosis of cutaneous melanoma," *Annals of Surgery*, vol. 172, no. 5, pp. 902–908, 1970.

[9] E. Christensen, P. Mjønes, O. A. Foss, O. M. Rørdam, and E. Skogvoll, "Pre-treatment evaluation of basal cell carcinoma for photodynamic therapy: comparative measurement of tumour thickness in punch biopsy and excision specimens," *Acta Dermato-Venereologica*, vol. 91, no. 6, pp. 651–654, 2011.

[10] B. F. Warren and J. D. Davies, "Pierre Vernier's invention: a neglected tool of our trade," *Histopathology*, vol. 18, no. 4, pp. 361–362, 1991.

[11] J. J. Rippey, "Why classify basal cell carcinomas?" *Histopathology*, vol. 32, no. 5, pp. 393–398, 1998.

[12] M. M. Kleinpenning, E. W. Wolberink, T. Smits et al., "Fluorescence diagnosis in actinic keratosis and squamous cell carcinoma," *Photodermatology Photoimmunology and Photomedicine*, vol. 26, no. 6, pp. 297–302, 2010.

[13] R. F. Donnelly, P. A. McCarron, and A. D. Woolfson, "Drug delivery of aminolevulinic acid from topical formulations intended for photodynamic therapy," *Photochemistry and Photobiology*, vol. 81, no. 4, pp. 750–767, 2005.

[14] M. M. Kleinpenning, T. Smits, E. Ewalds, P. E. J. van Erp, P. C. M. van de Kerkhof, and M. J. P. Gerritsen, "Heterogeneity of fluorescence in psoriasis after application of 5-aminolaevulinic acid: an immunohistochemical study," *British Journal of Dermatology*, vol. 155, no. 3, pp. 539–545, 2006.

[15] T. Smits, M. M. Kleinpenning, W. A. M. Blokx, P. C. M. van de Kerkhof, P. E. J. van Erp, and M.-J. P. Gerritsen, "Fluorescence diagnosis in keratinocytic intraepidermal neoplasias," *Journal of the American Academy of Dermatology*, vol. 57, no. 5, pp. 824–831, 2007.

[16] C. A. Morton, R.-M. Szeimies, A. Sidoroff, and L. R. Braathen, "European guidelines for topical photodynamic therapy part 1: treatment delivery and current indications—actinic keratoses, Bowen's disease, basal cell carcinoma," *Journal of the European Academy of Dermatology and Venereology*, vol. 27, no. 5, pp. 536–544, 2013.

[17] E. Christensen, T. Warloe, S. Kroon et al., "Guidelines for practical use of MAL-PDT in non-melanoma skin cancer," *Journal of the European Academy of Dermatology and Venereology*, vol. 24, no. 5, pp. 505–512, 2010.

[18] E. Touitou, "Drug delivery across the skin," *Expert Opinion on Biological Therapy*, vol. 2, no. 7, pp. 723–733, 2002.

[19] K. Robertson and J. L. Rees, "Variation in epidermal morphology in human skin at different body sites as measured by reflectance confocal microscopy," *Acta Dermato-Venereologica*, vol. 90, no. 4, pp. 368–373, 2010.

[20] E. Boireau-Adamezyk, A. Baillet-Guffroy, and G. N. Stamatas, "Age-dependent changes in stratum corneum barrier function," *Skin Research and Technology*, vol. 20, no. 4, pp. 409–415, 2014.

[21] J. N. Dauendorffer, S. Bastuji-Garin, S. Guéro, N. Brousse, and S. Fraitag, "Shrinkage of skin excision specimens: formalin fixation is not the culprit," *British Journal of Dermatology*, vol. 160, no. 4, pp. 810–814, 2009.

[22] M. J. J. Kerns, M. A. Darst, T. G. Olsen, M. Fenster, P. Hall, and S. Grevey, "Shrinkage of cutaneous specimens: formalin or other factors involved?" *Journal of Cutaneous Pathology*, vol. 35, no. 12, pp. 1093–1096, 2008.

29

Responsiveness of the Spanish Version of the "Skin Cancer Index"

M. de Troya-Martín,[1,2] F. Rivas-Ruiz,[2,3] N. Blázquez-Sánchez,[1,2]
I. Fernández-Canedo,[1] M. Aguilar-Bernier,[1] J. B. Repiso-Jiménez,[1] J. C. Toribio-Montero,[1]
M. Jones-Caballero,[4] and J. Rhee[5]

[1]Department of Dermatology, Agencia Sanitaria Costa del Sol, Marbella, Spain
[2]Red de Investigación en Servicios de Salud en Enfermedades Crónicas (REDISSEC), Spain
[3]Unit of Investigation, Agencia Sanitaria Costa del Sol, Marbella, Spain
[4]Department of Dermatology, University of Sydney, Sydney, NSW, Australia
[5]Department of Otolaryngology and Communication, Sciences Medical College of Wisconsin, Milwaukee, WI, USA

Correspondence should be addressed to M. de Troya-Martín; magdalenatroya@gmail.com

Academic Editor: Günther Hofbauer

Background. Skin Cancer Index (SCI) is a specific questionnaire measuring health related quality of life (HRQL) in patients with cervicofacial non-melanoma skin cancer (CFNMSC). The original scale has recently been adapted and validated into Spanish. *Objectives.* Evaluate the responsiveness of the Spanish version of SCI. *Methods.* Patients with CFNMSC candidate for surgical treatment were administered the questionnaire at time of diagnostic (t_0), 7 days after surgery (t_1), and 5 months after surgery (t_2). The scale and subscales scores (C1: social/appearance, C2: emotional) were then evaluated. Differences between t_0-t_1, t_1-t_2, and t_0-t_2 were determined and a gender-and-age segmented analysis was performed. *Results.* 88 patients, 54.8% male, mean age 62.5 years, completed the study. Differences between t_0-t_1 and t_1-t_2 scores were statistically significant ($p < 0.05$). The lowest values were found at time of diagnosis and postsurgery. Women and patients under 65 years showed the lowest values at the three times. *Limitations.* Concrete geographic and cultural area. Clinical and histological variables are not analysed. *Conclusions.* Our results confirm responsiveness of the Spanish version of the SCI. Further development of the instrument in Spanish-speaking countries and populations will make it possible to extend worldwide research and knowledge horizons on skin cancer.

1. Introduction

Non-melanoma skin cancer (NMSC), basal cell carcinoma (BCC), and squamous cell carcinoma (SCC) are the most common malignant tumours among humans [1, 2]. Their incidence has increased dramatically over the past 20 years, especially among women and people aged 30–39 years [3, 4], as a result of excessive exposure to ultraviolet radiation [5]. Although NMSC has a low mortality rate (0.1–0.3%), its morbidity is high; in over 80% of cases it is located in the face, where the tumour itself or surgical treatment often causes functional and aesthetic problems of diverse types [6, 7]. In addition, there is an accumulated risk of around 40% of developing a second NMSC within three years [8], making this

tumour a chronic and mutilating disease [9]. Health related quality of life (HRQL) is a measure of particular interest with respect to cervicofacial NMSC (CFNMSC). However, the lack of specific instruments and the low sensitivity of the questionnaires previously used have hampered understanding of this essential aspect of the disease, producing results that are sometimes confusing [10–21].

In 2005, Rhee et al. created the first specific HRQL questionnaire for patients with CFNMSC, termed the Skin Cancer Index (SCI), consisting of 15 items exploring three dimensions about HRQL in this patients (emotional, social, and appearance) [22]. In further studies the instrument demonstrated excellent psychometric properties (validity, reliability, and responsiveness) [23, 24]. The Spanish version of SCI has recently been developed, showing also an excellent level of internal consistency and an adequate level of reliability [25]. The aim of the present study is to assess responsiveness of the Spanish scale.

2. Material and Methods

A prospectively longitudinal study was designed and approved by the Bioethics Committee of our hospital.

Patients were selected consecutively among subjects diagnosed with CFNMSC candidate for surgical treatment at the Dermatology Service of the Costa del Sol Hospital during the period April 2009 to November 2011. All patients included in the study were new-onset patients with CFCCNM confirmed by biopsy (BCC or SCC), aged over 18 years, that correctly understand spoken and written Spanish, and who gave their informed consent to participate. Those who presented intellectual impairment or suffered a severe physical or mental illness were excluded.

The participants were invited to complete the quality-of-life questionnaire at three different time points during the surgical process: t_0 (time of diagnostic confirmation), t_1 (7 days after surgery), and t_2 (5 months after surgery). The Spanish version of the SCI [25] is linguistically and semantically equivalent to the original scale but differs in the number of items, because during the validation process three items were dismissed by not meeting criteria of validity. The final version is composed of 12 items, with two underlying dimensions which we termed (following the original model) "social/appearance" (7 items) and "emotional" (5 items). Both components presented an excellent level of internal consistency, with Cronbach's alpha values above 0.85. In addition, the Spanish scale provided an adequate level of reliability, with weighted kappa values greater than 0.4 and percentages of absolute agreement exceeding 60% in most items. As the original version, the answers are given on a Likert 5-point scale. The standardised final score ranges from 0 (lowest quality of life) to 100 (highest quality of life).

Responsiveness was assessed as the difference in the mean score in the scale at stages t_0, t_1, and t_2. Second outcome measure might be described as differences in the mean score in age (> or <65 y-o) and sex (male, female) groups.

2.1. Statistical Analysis. The global scores on the scale and its components were obtained at each of the three time points. To assess the sensitivity to change of the instrument, the paired Student's t-test was used (or the Mann-Whitney test if the criteria for parametric testing were not met). We recorded the differences of the means (DM) of the scores for the scale and its components and the corresponding 95% confidence intervals (95% CI). In addition, an age-and-gender segmented analysis was performed. The level of significance was set at $p < 0.05$. The statistical analysis was carried out using SPSS v15.

3. Results

88 of the 100 patients included in the study completed the survey at all three time points. Of these respondents, 54.8%

TABLE 1: Scale results for all patients assessed ($n = 88$).

	t_0		t_1		t_2	
	Mean	SD	Mean	SD	Mean	SD
Total	59.2	21.2	63.9	20.2	75.3	20.2
C1	79.4	24.8	84.4	23.4	90.5	19.5
C2	31.0	27.0	35.1	28.0	54.1	31.5

TABLE 2: Sensitivity to change.

	Mean	95% confidence interval		p
		Lower	Upper	
Total for the Scale				
Difference t_0-t_1	4.66	1.32	8.01	*0.007*
Difference t_0-t_2	16.10	12.08	20.12	*<0.001*
Difference t_1-t_2	11.43	8.05	14.81	*<0.001*
Component 1				
Difference t_0-t_1	3.98	0.78	7.18	*0.015*
Difference t_0-t_2	8.86	5.47	12.26	*<0.001*
Difference t_1-t_2	4.84	2.41	7.26	*<0.001*
Component 2				
Difference t_0-t_1	3.42	−0.73	7.56	*0.105*
Difference t_0-t_2	18.50	13.29	23.71	*<0.001*
Difference t_1-t_2	15.18	10.11	20.25	*<0.001*

were men, with a mean age of 62.5 years (SD: 14.1). On a standardized scale 0–100, the mean total scores were 59.2 (t_0), 63.9 (t_1), and 75.3 (t_2). The mean scores for the CI scale component were 79.4 (t_0), 84.4 (t_1), and 90.5 (t_2), and those for the C2 component were 31.0 (t_0), 35.1 (t_1), and 54.1 (t_2) (Table 1).

The differences in the total score for the scale, in all the pairwise comparisons, were statistically significant: t_0 versus t_1 (DM: 2.24; 95% CI 0.63–3.84), t_0 versus t_2 (DM: 7.73; 95% CI 5.80–9.66), and t_1 versus t_2 (DM: 5.49; 95% CI 3.86–7.11), except for t_0-t_1 in C2 (Table 2).

In the gender-and age segmented analysis, women and subjects younger than 65 years had lower scores at all three time points, and the changes over time were statistically significant in all tests for t_0-t_2 and t_1-t_2, except for t_1-t_2 in Cl in the subjects aged over 65 years (Tables 3 and 4).

4. Discussion

Responsiveness, defined as "the ability of an instrument to detect change over time in the construct to be measured," is the third main psychometric property, together with validity and reliability, to consider in health related questionnaires [26, 27].

Our results confirm responsiveness of the Spanish version of the SCI. We have used the same methodology the authors did to test responsiveness of the original questionnaire [16], following the recommendations of the international guidelines for validating health questionnaires [26–28]. Our study has been carried out in patients with CFNMSC undergoing surgery at three different time points of the medical care process. For the overall scale and the subscales, the capacity

TABLE 3: Scale results, segmented by sex ($n = 88$).

	t_0		t_1		t_2		$p\ t_0\text{-}t_1$	$p\ t_0\text{-}t_2$	$p\ t_1\text{-}t_2$
	Mean	SD	Mean	SD	Mean	SD			
Total									
Male	61.6	22.5	65.2	20.8	78.9	20.5	0.073	<0.001	<0.001
Female	57.4	19.1	62.9	19.3	70.6	20.0	0.081	<0.001	0.005
C1									
Male	82.8	24.0	86.8	22.2	92.3	18.2	0.021	<0.001	0.007
Female	76.3	25.1	82.5	24.9	88.3	21.8	0.15	0.005	0.029
C2									
Male	32.1	30.2	35.0	30.5	60.1	32.4	0.425	<0.001	<0.001
Female	30.9	23.7	35.5	25.2	45.8	29.7	0.278	0.002	0.014

TABLE 4: Scale results, segmented by age ($n = 88$).

	t_0		t_1		t_2		$p\ t_0\text{-}t_1$	$p\ t_0\text{-}t_2$	$p\ t_1\text{-}t_2$
	Mean	SD	Mean	SD	Mean	SD			
Total									
<65	55.0	20.0	58.7	19.5	70.7	20.0	0.166	<0.001	<0.001
≥65	62.6	21.6	68.3	19.8	79.3	19.7	0.014	<0.001	<0.001
C1									
<65	75.8	26.2	79.2	24.7	88.0	20.8	0.293	0.001	0.001
≥65	82.4	23.3	89.2	21.3	92.6	18.3	0.015	<0.001	0.08
C2									
<65	25.9	21.5	30.1	25.5	46.5	30.8	0.241	<0.001	0.001
≥65	35.0	30.7	39.1	29.5	60.7	30.7	0.316	<0.001	<0.001

of the instrument to identify changes in the subjects' HRQL has been revealed.

Like similar studies in the USA, the UK, or Canada [16, 29–31], patients with CFNMSC experienced a significant impact on their HRQL at the moment of diagnosis, and surgical treatment produces a marked improvement, as indicated by the significant increase in the scale score. HRQL was found to be more severely affected among female patients and patients of both sexes aged under 65 years, as reported by Rhee et al. [16]. Unlike other studies conducted in Anglo-Saxon countries [16, 29, 30], the values for emotional subscale were considerably lower than those for the social-appearance component, for all time points and all groups of patients.

As this is the only version of the scale measuring HRQL in patients with NMSC developed in a language other than the original, its implementation in countries and populations belonging to a Spanish-language culture will make it possible to extend worldwide research horizons of the disease.

This is a single-center study conducted in a particular sociocultural context. Therefore, our data need to be confirmed, by extending this investigation to other areas of Spain and to Latin American countries.

In conclusion, our results confirm the ability of the Spanish version of the SCI to discriminate changes in the HRQL of patients with CFNMSC. In the future, its implementation in Spanish-speaking countries and populations will make it possible to extend worldwide research on skin cancer.

Abbreviations

NMSC: Non-melanoma skin cancer
BCC: Basal cell carcinoma
SCC: Squamous cell carcinoma
CFNMSC: Cervicofacial non-melanoma skin cancer
SCI: Skin Cancer Index
HRQL: Health related quality of life.

Disclosure

For this type of study, formal consent is not required.

Competing Interests

The authors declare that they have no conflict of interests.

Acknowledgments

This study was funded by Health Ministry of Andalucia (Grant no. PI-0093/2008).

References

[1] B. Ö. Cakir, P. Adamson, and C. Cingi, "Epidemiology and economic burden of nonmelanoma skin cancer," *Facial Plastic Surgery Clinics of North America*, vol. 20, no. 4, pp. 419–422, 2012.

[2] A. Lomas, J. Leonardi-Bee, and F. Bath-Hextall, "A systematic review of worldwide incidence of nonmelanoma skin cancer,"

British Journal of Dermatology, vol. 166, no. 5, pp. 1069–1080, 2012.

[3] P. Aceituno-Madera, A. Buendía-Eisman, S. Arias-Santiago, and S. Serrano-Ortega, "Evolución de la incidencia del cáncer de piel en el período 1978–2002," *Actas Dermo-Sifiliográficas*, vol. 101, no. 1, pp. 39–46, 2010.

[4] S. C. Flohil, I. Seubring, M. M. van Rossum, J.-W. W. Coebergh, E. de Vries, and T. Nijsten, "Trends in basal cell carcinoma incidence rates: a 37-year dutch observational study," *Journal of Investigative Dermatology*, vol. 133, no. 4, pp. 913–918, 2013.

[5] V. Molho-Pessach and M. Lotem, "Ultraviolet radiation and cutaneous carcinogenesis," *Current Problems in Dermatology*, vol. 35, pp. 14–27, 2007.

[6] T. H. Nguyen and D. Q.-D. Ho, "Nonmelanoma skin cancer," *Current Treatment Options in Oncology*, vol. 3, no. 3, pp. 193–203, 2002.

[7] V. Madan, J. T. Lear, and R.-M. Szeimies, "Non-melanoma skin cancer," *The Lancet*, vol. 375, no. 9715, pp. 673–685, 2010.

[8] N. Roberts, Z. Czajkowska, G. Radiotis, and A. Körner, "Distress and coping strategies among patients with skin cancer," *Journal of Clinical Psychology in Medical Settings*, vol. 20, no. 2, pp. 209–214, 2013.

[9] S. van der Geer, H. A. Reijers, H. F. J. M. van Tuijl, H. de Vries, and G. A. M. Krekels, "Need for a new skin cancer management strategy," *Archives of Dermatology*, vol. 146, no. 3, pp. 332–336, 2010.

[10] S. Blackford, D. Roberts, M. S. Salek, and A. Finlay, "Basal cell carcinomas cause little handicap," *Quality of Life Research*, vol. 5, no. 2, pp. 191–194, 1996.

[11] R. E. Davis and J. M. Spercer, "Basal and squamous cell cancer of the facial skin," *Current Opinion in Otolaryngology & Head and Neck Surgery*, vol. 5, pp. 86–92, 1997.

[12] J. S. Rhee, F. R. Loberiza, B. A. Matthews, M. Neuburg, T. L. Smith, and M. Burzynski, "Quality of life assessment in nonmelanoma cervicofacial skin cancer," *Laryngoscope*, vol. 113, no. 2, pp. 215–220, 2003.

[13] J. S. Rhee, B. A. Matthews, M. Neuburg, T. L. Smith, M. Burzynski, and A. B. Nattinger, "Skin cancer and quality of life: assessment with the dermatology life quality index," *Dermatologic Surgery*, vol. 30, no. 4, pp. 525–529, 2004.

[14] J. S. Rhee, B. A. Matthews, M. Neuburg, T. L. Smith, M. Burzynski, and A. B. Nattinger, "Quality of life and sun-protective behavior in patients with skin cancer," *Archives of Otolaryngology—Head and Neck Surgery*, vol. 130, no. 2, pp. 141–146, 2004.

[15] F. J. Moloney, S. Keane, P. O'Kelly, P. J. Conlon, and G. M. Murphy, "The impact of skin disease following renal transplantation on quality of life," *British Journal of Dermatology*, vol. 153, no. 3, pp. 574–578, 2005.

[16] J. S. Rhee, B. A. Matthews, M. Neuburg, B. R. Logan, M. Burzynski, and A. B. Nattinger, "The skin cancer index: clinical responsiveness and predictors of quality of life," *Laryngoscope*, vol. 117, no. 3, pp. 399–405, 2007.

[17] T. Chen, D. Bertenthal, A. Sahay, S. Sen, and M.-M. Chren, "Predictors of skin-related quality of life after treatment of cutaneous basal cell carcinoma and squamous cell carcinoma," *Archives of Dermatology*, vol. 143, no. 11, pp. 1386–1392, 2007.

[18] M.-M. Chren, A. P. Sahay, D. S. Bertenthal, S. Sen, and C. S. Landefeld, "Quality-of-life outcomes of treatments for cutaneous basal cell carcinoma and squamous cell carcinoma," *Journal of Investigative Dermatology*, vol. 127, no. 6, pp. 1351–1357, 2007.

[19] J. Steinbauer, M. Koller, E. Kohl, S. Karrer, M. Landthaler, and R.-M. Szeimies, "Quality of life in health care of non-melanoma skin cancer—results of a pilot study," *Journal of the German Society of Dermatology*, vol. 9, no. 2, pp. 129–135, 2011.

[20] M.-M. Chren, "The Skindex instruments to measure the effects of skin disease on quality of life," *Dermatologic Clinics*, vol. 30, no. 2, pp. 231–236, 2012.

[21] F. Sampogna, A. Spagnoli, C. Di Pietro et al., "Field performance of the skindex-17 quality of life questionnaire: a comparison with the skindex-29 in a large sample of dermatological outpatients," *Journal of Investigative Dermatology*, vol. 133, no. 1, pp. 104–109, 2013.

[22] J. S. Rhee, B. A. Matthews, M. Neuburg, M. Burzynski, and A. B. Nattinger, "Creation of a quality of life instrument for nonmelanoma skin cancer patients," *Laryngoscope*, vol. 115, no. 7, pp. 1178–1185, 2005.

[23] J. S. Rhee, B. A. Matthews, M. Neuburg, B. R. Logan, M. Burzynski, and A. B. Nattinger, "Validation of a quality-of-life instrument for patients with nonmelanoma skin cancer," *Archives of Facial Plastic Surgery*, vol. 8, no. 5, pp. 314–318, 2006.

[24] B. A. Matthews, J. S. Rhee, M. Neuburg, M. L. Burzynski, and A. B. Nattinger, "Development of the facial skin care index: a health-related outcomes index for skin cancer patients," *Dermatologic Surgery*, vol. 32, no. 7, pp. 924–934, 2006.

[25] M. de Troya-Martín, F. Rivas-Ruiz, N. Blázquez-Sánchez et al., "A Spanish version of the skin cancer index: a questionnaire for measuring quality of life in patients with cervicofacial nonmelanoma skin cancer," *British Journal of Dermatology*, vol. 172, no. 1, pp. 160–168, 2015.

[26] X. Badia, M. Salamero, and J. Alonso, *La Medida de la Salud. Guía de Escalas de Medición en Español*, Fundación Lilly, Barcelona, Spain, 3rd edition, 2002.

[27] A. Carvajal, C. Centeno, R. Watson et al., "How is an instrument for measuring health to be validated?" *Anales del Sistema Sanitario de Navarra*, vol. 34, pp. 63–72, 2011.

[28] J. M. Ramada-Rodilla, C. Serra-Pujadas, and G. L. Delclós-Clanchet, "Cross-cultural adaptation and health questionnaires validation: revision and methodological recommendations," *Salud Pública de México*, vol. 55, no. 1, pp. 57–66, 2013.

[29] J. Caddick, L. Green, J. Stephenson, and G. Spyrou, "The psycho-social impact of facial skin cancers," *Journal of Plastic, Reconstructive and Aesthetic Surgery*, vol. 65, no. 9, pp. e257–e259, 2012.

[30] G. Radiotis, N. Roberts, Z. Czajkowska, M. Khanna, and A. Körner, "Nonmelanoma skin cancer: disease-specific quality-of-life concerns and distress," *Oncology Nursing Forum*, vol. 41, no. 1, pp. 57–65, 2014.

[31] P. C. Maciel, F. E. M. Fonseca, J. Veiga-Filho, L. M. Ferreira, M. P. de Carvalho, and D. F. Veiga, "Quality of life and self-esteem in patients submitted to surgical treatment of skin carcinomas: long-term results," *Anais Brasileiros de Dermatologia*, vol. 89, no. 4, pp. 594–598, 2014.

30

Immune Toxicity with Checkpoint Inhibition for Metastatic Melanoma: Case Series and Clinical Management

Anna J. Lomax [iD],[1] Jennifer Lim,[1] Robert Cheng,[2,3] Arianne Sweeting,[4,5] Patricia Lowe,[4,5] Neil McGill,[4,5] Nicholas Shackel,[3,4,5] Elizabeth L. Chua [iD],[4,5] and Catriona McNeil[1,4,5]

[1]Chris O'Brien Lifehouse, Camperdown, NSW, Australia
[2]Concord Repatriation General Hospital, Sydney, NSW, Australia
[3]Centenary Institute, Sydney, NSW, Australia
[4]Sydney Medical School, University of Sydney, Camperdown, NSW, Australia
[5]Royal Prince Alfred Hospital, Camperdown, NSW, Australia

Correspondence should be addressed to Anna J. Lomax; anna.lomax@lh.org.au

Academic Editor: Arash Kimyai-Asadi

Immune checkpoint inhibitors (anti-PD-1 and anti-CTLA-4 antibodies) are a standard of care for advanced melanoma. Novel toxicities comprise immune-related adverse events (irAE). With increasing use, irAE require recognition, practical management strategies, and multidisciplinary care. We retrospectively evaluated the incidence, kinetics, and management of irAE in 41 patients receiving anti-PD-1 antibody therapy (pembrolizumab) for advanced melanoma. 63% received prior anti-CTLA-4 antibody therapy (ipilimumab). IrAE occurred in 54%, most commonly dermatological (24%), rheumatological (22%), and thyroid dysfunction (12%). Thyroiditis was characterised by a brief asymptomatic hyperthyroid phase followed by a symptomatic hypothyroid phase requiring thyroxine replacement. Transplant rejection doses of methylprednisolone were necessary to manage refractory hepatotoxicity. A bullous pemphigoid-like skin reaction with refractory pruritus responded to corticosteroids and neuropathic analgesia. Disabling grade 3-4 oligoarthritis required sulfasalazine therapy in combination with steroids. The median interval between the last dose of anti-CTLA-4 antibody and the first dose of anti-PD-1 therapy was 2.0 months (range: 0.4 to 22.4). Toxicities may occur late; this requires vigilance and multidisciplinary management which may allow effective anticancer therapy to continue. Management algorithms for thyroiditis, hypophysitis, arthralgia/arthritis, colitis, steroid-refractory hepatitis, and skin toxicity are discussed.

1. Introduction

Immune checkpoint inhibition is the established immunotherapy treatment for advanced melanoma. Induction of a tumour-directed immune response due to T-cell activation halts tumour evasion from immune surveillance [1, 2]. Blockade of cytotoxic T-lymphocyte antigen-4 (CTLA-4) with ipilimumab showed the first evidence of improved survival in advanced melanoma [3] and long-term survival can be achieved [3, 4]. Novel side-effects include autoimmune toxicities referred to as immune-related adverse events (irAE). With the increasing use of these agents (as monotherapy or in combination) irAE require recognition and practical management strategies.

Pembrolizumab and nivolumab are anti-programmed cell death 1 (PD-1) antibodies targeting the effector arm of the immune checkpoint pathway. Benefit has been demonstrated in ipilimumab pretreated and naïve patients [5]. Anti-PD-1 antibodies have superseded ipilimumab as a first-line immunotherapy treatment for advanced melanoma. Both anti-PD-1 agents have superior response rates (36–44%) [6, 7] compared to ipilimumab (13–19%) [6,7] and improved 3-year survival (40–52%) [7, 8] versus 20–34% [3, 7]. Estimates of anti-PD-1 efficacy outside of clinical trials have been reported with response rates of 14–39% [9–11]. Anti-PD-1 agents have activity in other solid cancers including non-small cell lung cancer, genitourinary cancers, and Hodgkin's lymphoma [12–15].

Combining anti-PD-1 and anti-CTLA-4 checkpoint inhibitors improves response rate (58–61%) but at the cost of increased toxicity [7, 16]. Grade 3-4 or 3–5 treatment-related adverse events for combination therapy and anti-PD-1 or anti-CTLA-4 monotherapies have been reported in randomised trials: 45–59%, 17–21%, and 20–28%, respectively [6, 7, 16]. 3-year overall survival with dual checkpoint inhibition (nivolumab plus ipilimumab) is also superior to ipilimumab alone (58% vs 20–34%) [7] but what is critical is whether this adds a survival benefit over anti-PD-1 therapy alone given the added toxicity with this regimen. IrAE due to CTLA-4 blockade have an earlier onset and are more commonly associated with diarrhoea, colitis, and hypophysitis. Fatigue, arthralgia, and thyroid irAE are more frequently seen with PD-1 blockade [17]. IrAE with combination checkpoint inhibition can have a rapid onset and be associated with a protracted duration [18].

In clinical practice, patients are older with poorer Eastern Cooperative Oncology Group (ECOG) performance status than those enrolled in clinical trials. An early study of pembrolizumab after prior ipilimumab therapy required patients to have received the final dose of ipilimumab ≥ 6 weeks before commencing pembrolizumab [5], a period not necessarily pragmatic in clinical practice. Reduced dosing intervals between therapeutic agents impact severity and pattern of toxicities as observed in patients receiving these checkpoint inhibitors, albeit in different sequence [19].

This is a retrospective review of patients with advanced melanoma that received pembrolizumab at Chris O'Brien Lifehouse through compassionate access. We evaluated patients who were ipilimumab naïve and pretreated with respect to irAE and describe the management of these irAE in real clinical practice.

2. Methods

Patients with advanced melanoma were included. In patients who had received prior ipilimumab, disease had to be documented as progressive, recurrent, or persistent. Patients were excluded if they were receiving or were eligible for treatment with a BRAF or MEK inhibitor. Patients were also excluded if they had significant autoimmune disease requiring chronic immunosuppression.

Pembrolizumab was administered intravenously at 2 mg/kg of body weight every three weeks. Drug supply was via a compassionate access program. At the time of patient enrolment into the program, pembrolizumab therapy was not yet approved for use in Australia on the Pharmaceutical Benefits Scheme. Therapy was continued until disease progression or unacceptable toxicity. Response to pembrolizumab was assessed at week 12 after commencement and 12 weekly thereafter or as clinically appropriate. Where available, imaging was assessed according to Response Evaluation Criteria in Solid Tumours (RECIST) version 1.1. IrAE were graded according to the National Cancer Institute Common Terminology Criteria for Adverse Events, version 4.0 (CTCAE). Ethics committee approval was obtained (X15-0193 LNR/15/RPAH/256).

3. Results

From November 2013 to August 2015, 41 patients were identified. Patient and disease characteristics are described (Table 1). Median age was 65, 81% had an ECOG performance status of 0 or 1 and 71% had an elevated LDH. BRAF V600 mutations were identified in 24% of patients and 76% had M1c disease. Twenty-six patients (63%) had received prior ipilimumab. The median interval between the last ipilimumab dose and the first pembrolizumab dose was 2.0 months (range: 0.4 to 22.4). The median duration of follow-up was 4.1 months (range: 0 to 14.9). The median and mean number of pembrolizumab cycles received were 4 and 6, respectively (range: 1 to 20). In 15 patients, treatment was ongoing.

In patients whose tumour harboured a BRAF V600 mutation, one patient received one dose of pembrolizumab on the compassionate program while awaiting results of BRAF molecular testing. Once it was known that his tumour harboured an actionable V600K mutation, he was transitioned to dabrafenib plus trametinib and achieved a partial response. A second patient received 2 doses of pembrolizumab before also confirming the presence of a V600K mutation. This patient was commenced on dabrafenib and trametinib but developed progressive disease. Initial testing had demonstrated a negative immunostain for BRAF VE1 for these 2 patients but due to symptomatic disease needing swift commencement of treatment, pembrolizumab was started while formal molecular testing was performed.

The remaining 8 patients with a BRAF V600 mutation had received prior BRAF/MEK inhibitor therapy. These numbers are small and make it difficult to draw conclusions regarding response in this subgroup.

Objective response rates (ORR) were 26% and disease control rates (DCR) were 49% ($n = 39$, excluding the $n = 2$ BRAF V600K patients that received pembrolizumab before formal molecular results were reported). This was determined by RECIST 1.1 assessment for $n = 20$; imaging assessment but not per RECIST 1.1 $n = 12$ (imaging modality was not uniform between serial scans or performed offsite, precluding formal RECIST 1.1 assessment); clinical progression in $n = 3$ and unknown $n = 4$ patients. The median time to response was 2.7 months (range: 0.9 to 4.9). Three (7%) patients achieved a complete response.

IrAE were documented in 22 (54%) patients while receiving anti-PD-1 therapy. Common irAE were dermatological (24%), rheumatological (22%), and thyroid dysfunction (12%) (Table 1). Grade 3-4 irAE were uncommon (15%) with individual event rates of 2–5%. Of the 26 patients that received prior ipilimumab, 13 patients (50%) developed irAE secondary to ipilimumab. Of these 13 patients, 10 (38%) experienced subsequent irAE while receiving pembrolizumab. Of these 10 patients, 8 had an event of grade 1-2 severity during treatment with pembrolizumab and 2 developed grade 3-4 hepatotoxicity in the context of a short interval between ceasing ipilimumab and commencing pembrolizumab. Of the 13 patients who did not have irAE on ipilimumab, 6 (23%) patients had subsequent irAE while receiving pembrolizumab.

TABLE 1: Patient characteristics and immune-related adverse events.

Characteristics	Compassionate pembrolizumab ($n = 41$)	
Median age (range), yr	65 (37–90)	
Male sex, number (%)	32 (78%)	
Primary type		
Cutaneous	31 (76%)	
Mucosal	2 (5%)	
Occult	7 (17%)	
Unknown	1 (2%)	
ECOG performance status, number (%)		
0-1	33 (81%)	
>1	7 (17%)	
Unknown	1 (2%)	
Lactate dehydrogenase, number (%)		
≤ULN (≤250 U/L)	7 (17%)	
>ULN (>250 U/L)	29 (71%)	
Unknown	5 (12%)	
Metastasis stage, number (%)		
In-transit disease	1 (2%)	
M1a	5 (12%)	
M1b	4 (10%)	
M1c	31 (76%)	
Number of organ sites of disease		
≤3	24 (58%)	
>3	15 (37%)	
Unknown	2 (5%)	
BRAF V600 mutation, number (%)	10 (24%)	
Prior lines of treatment, number (%)		
0	10 (24%)	
1	20 (49%)	
2-3	10 (24%)	
Unknown	1 (2%)	
Preexisting autoimmune condition	2 (5%)	
Ipilimumab pretreated, number (%)	26 (63%)	
Ipilimumab-related irAE, number (%)	13 (50%)	
Rates of irAE during anti-PD-1 therapy	Any grade	Grade 3 or 4
Any	22 (54%)	4 (15%)
Skin	10 (24%)	1 (2%)
Arthralgia/arthritis	9 (22%)	1 (2%)
Thyroid dysfunction	5 (12%)	0
Gastrointestinal*	3 (7%)	0
Hypophysitis	2 (5%)	2 (5%)
Hepatitis	2 (5%)	2 (5%)
Pneumonitis	2 (5%)	0
Uveitis	1 (2%)	0
Parotitis	1 (2%)	0

*Colitis and proctitis $n = 1$ and diarrhoea $n = 2$.

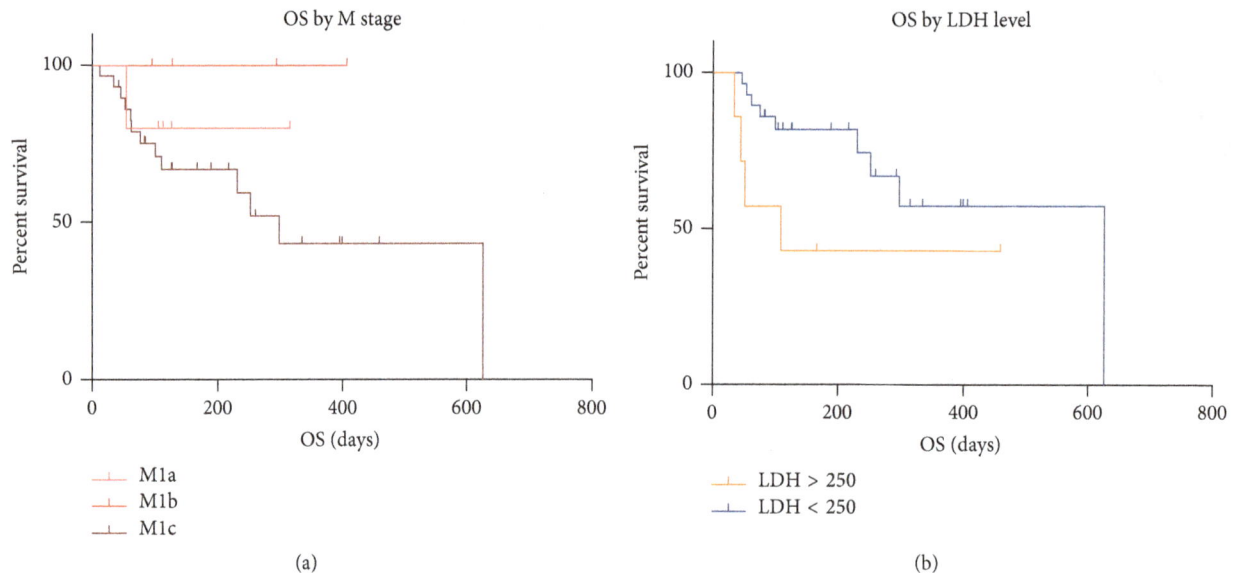

FIGURE 1: OS by M stage and LDH. Logrank statistic M stage ($p = 0.28$) and LDH level ($p = 0.06$).

Patients with M1c disease or an elevated LDH appeared to have worse survival outcomes (Figures 1(a) and 1(b)).

4. Organ Specific Toxicities and Treatment Algorithms

Owing to the mechanism of action of immunotherapy agents, manifestations of autoimmune toxicity can involve any organ. General principles of management revolve around managing mild (grade 1) toxicity with supportive measures and considering steroids in moderate (grade 2) toxicity. For severe (grades 3-4) toxicity, intervening with high-dose steroids or additional immunosuppressive therapy may be necessary. We outline management algorithms for the toxicities observed in our cohort of patients which overlap with established algorithms such as "eviQ Cancer Treatments Online" [20] but also include recommendations from our institutional experience. Specifically, we have documented general skincare supportive measures and the possible use of neuropathic analgesia for refractory pruritus. For endocrine toxicities, we have highlighted the expected clinical course of thyroiditis and have suggested a management algorithm for rheumatological irAE. Other guidelines, such as the ESMO Clinical Practice Guidelines [18], differ from the eviQ and our guidelines with respect to the grading of liver toxicity for autoimmune hepatitis. The ESMO statement refers to grade 3 ALT/AST elevation as 5–20x the upper limit of normal (ULN) and grade 4 elevation as >20x the ULN [18], whereas our algorithm and eviQ specify grade 3-4 AST/ALT elevation as >5x the ULN [20].

4.1. Dermatological Toxicity.

Cutaneous toxicity of any grade occurred in 10 (24%) patients (Table 1). Common presentations included pruritus, cutaneous eruptions, for example, maculopapular, eczematous, flare of Grover's disease (transient acantholytic dermatosis), and less commonly vitiligo.

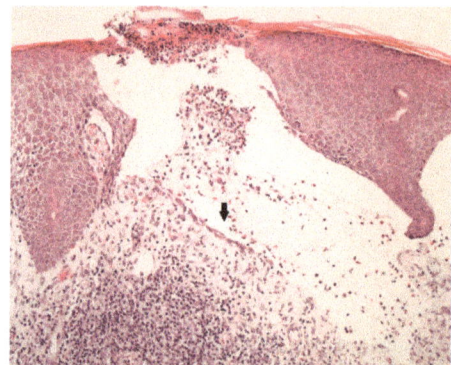

FIGURE 2: Pemphigoid-like reaction. Skin biopsies demonstrated a subepidermal blister (arrow) with inflammatory cells, predominantly eosinophils.

Nine patients had rash/pruritus (one case involved a bullous pemphigoid-like reaction described below) and 1 patient was documented to have developed vitiligo. No presentations had mucosal involvement.

An elderly female developed grade 3 skin toxicity on pembrolizumab [21] having displayed grade 1 toxicity (pruritic maculopapular eruption) during prior ipilimumab therapy. The latter improved with supportive therapy. Due to progressive metastatic disease, pembrolizumab was commenced 6 weeks after ipilimumab cessation. A bullous pemphigoid-like drug reaction developed after 8 months of pembrolizumab. Skin biopsies demonstrated a subepidermal blister with inflammatory cells, predominantly eosinophils. A perivascular and interstitial inflammatory cell infiltrate of lymphocytes, eosinophils, and neutrophils was within the dermis with adjacent spongiotic epidermis (Figure 2). Direct immunofluorescence was negative. Pembrolizumab was ceased. Although the rash was steroid responsive, the pruritus proved refractory until pregabalin was commenced (25 mg daily and titrated to 25 mg twice daily). Neuropathic analgesia [22, 23] has shown efficacy in the management of uraemic pruritus; however, oversedation was observed in 12–30% [23]. The patient had a complete disease response to pembrolizumab.

4.2. Dermatological irAE Management Algorithm. Rash due to anti-PD-1 antibodies may occur in 13–26% and 15–33% for anti-CTLA-4 therapy. Pruritus can occur in 14–19% and 25–35%, respectively [17, 24]. Skin toxicity due to anti-PD-1 therapy is potentially mediated by a shared antigen coexpressed by the dermoepidermal junction and tumour cells [25]. Most presentations are mild, usually a nonspecific maculopapular pruritic eruption, occasionally eczematous. As would be expected in immunotherapy of melanoma, hypopigmentation and depigmentation (vitiligo) have been reported [26, 27] with sites of predilection, including trunk and limbs, but can be limited to photoexposed sites. Rarely, life-threatening conditions such as Stevens-Johnson syndrome (SJS) or toxic epidermal necrolysis (TEN) occur [28–30].

Upon development of a nonspecific rash, flare of preexisting dermatosis and secondary cutaneous infections needs to be excluded. Perform skin swabs (bacterial MCS, viral PCR) and scrapings (fungal KOH) if indicated. Skin biopsy (with direct immunofluorescence if blisters present) and FBC may reveal eosinophilic infiltrate and eosinophilia, respectively, supporting the diagnosis of drug exanthem. Tissue reactions are most commonly spongiotic or lichenoid in nature.

The majority of skin irAE are managed supportively. Avoidance of common irritants (soap and excess water) should be reinforced. Liberal amounts of emollients and ointment-based preparations, if xerotic or pruritic, are advised. Specific therapies include moderate to very potent topical corticosteroid ointments (under wet dressing occlusion) and low to high doses of oral antihistamines. Severe skin toxicity requires hospital admission and high doses of corticosteroid administration [28–30] orally or intravenously. Consider commencement of IVIG and/or cyclosporine if SJS/TEN is suspected or confirmed on urgent skin biopsy. Transfer to a burns unit is essential if skin loss is >10%. The management of skin toxicity is outlined in Table 2.

4.3. Gastrointestinal and Hepatic Toxicity. Gastrointestinal irAE were infrequent, occurring in 3 (7%) patients, with none experiencing grade 3 or 4 toxicity (Table 1). One patient developed grade 2 colitis with proctitis and had never received prior ipilimumab. Two ipilimumab pretreated patients developed diarrhoea of grade 1-2 severity.

Two patients (5%) experienced grade 3-4 hepatotoxicity (Table 1). A 58-year-old male received 4 cycles of ipilimumab with the final dose administered 22 days before starting pembrolizumab. Liver function test derangement (LFT) of grade 4 severity with transaminases 15–30 times the ULN and elevated bilirubin occurred one month later. Biopsy confirmed lobular and portal hepatitis consistent with drug-induced injury. Methylprednisolone 0.5 mg/kg for 3 days was initiated and escalated to 1 g for 3 days with concurrent mycophenolate mofetil 500 mg twice daily due to lack of improvement. Prednisolone was weaned and mycophenolate

mofetil continued with resolution of biochemical abnormalities. Due to significant immunosuppression he developed presumed pneumocystis jiroveci pneumonia and died of respiratory failure and sepsis.

The second patient was a 67-year-old male who had a single dose of ipilimumab 27 days prior to commencing pembrolizumab. Following the second cycle of pembrolizumab he presented with fever and grade 3 ALT elevation at >5 times the ULN. Liver biopsy showed nonspecific mild portal and interface hepatitis. Methylprednisolone 1 mg/kg was commenced followed by weaning prednisolone and mycophenolate mofetil 1 g twice daily. The LFT derangement resolved. Due to this irAE and progressive disease, he did not receive subsequent therapy and died 6 months later.

4.4. Management of Refractory Hepatitis and Gastrointestinal Toxicity. Gastrointestinal toxicity is more commonly described with ipilimumab. Any grade of diarrhoea may occur in 23–33% with 3–6% of patients experiencing severe diarrhoea. Rates for significant colitis are 7–9% [17, 24]. Lower rates are documented with anti-PD-1 therapy with grade 3-4 or 3–5 diarrhoea described in 1–3% and similarly for severe colitis [17, 24]. Rates of severe diarrhoea or colitis for combined therapy are 9% and 8%, respectively [17, 24]. Management of colitis due to ipilimumab is well documented [31]. The management of single agent and combination checkpoint inhibitor induced colitis are outlined in Table 3.

In clinical trials, the rate of significant hepatitis or deranged liver function is identified at <1-2% for anti-CTLA-4 agents and 1-2% with anti-PD-1 therapies but increased to 6–8% with combined therapy [17, 24]. Grade 3-4 hepatotoxicity in our cohort was 5% and may reflect a short dosing interval between checkpoint inhibitors. The 2 patients in our cohort who developed hepatic toxicity required treatment with mycophenolic acid. Mycophenolate mofetil exerts its immunosuppressive effects through a cytostatic effect on lymphocytes [32]. Its use is outlined in clinical trial and ipilimumab irAE guidelines [31]. Doses of methylprednisolone required to treat transplant rejection have been used for ipilimumab-induced hepatotoxicity at our institution [33] and were necessary in 1 patient from our study cohort. From our experience, methylprednisolone 15 mg/kg (maximum 1 gm/day) is suggested for steroid-refractory hepatitis and is considered part of our management algorithm at our institution (Table 3).

4.5. Endocrine Toxicity, Thyroiditis-Kinetics, and Management. Thyroid dysfunction of grade 2 severity occurred in 5 (12%) patients (Table 1). Four patients had received prior ipilimumab. The onset of biochemical hyperthyroidism signalled the development of clinical thyroiditis in all patients. Thyroiditis was characterised by a brief asymptomatic hyperthyroid phase followed by a symptomatic hypothyroid phase (Figure 3(a)) requiring thyroxine replacement. This pattern is consistent with other case series [34, 35]. Hyperthyroidism occurred within 3–6 weeks of pembrolizumab initiation. The hypothyroid phase was generally evident within 3 weeks of the onset of thyroiditis. In most cases, the hypothyroid phase was evident by week 9 of pembrolizumab therapy and was

TABLE 2: Skin irAE: management algorithm.

Dermatology irAE	Investigations	Management
		Grade 1/mild
Rash < 10% body surface area (BSA), pruritus		Continue checkpoint inhibitor therapy *General skin care measures:* Avoid irritants: soap and excess water Emollients: creams and ointments Oral antihistamines: Nonsedating (daytime); sedating (nocte) Topical corticosteroids (moderate potency, ointment > cream vehicle) Phototherapy for pruritus: short course narrow band UVB, for example, 3x week for 4 weeks (relatively contraindicated with history of melanoma)
		Grade 2/moderate
Rash (10–30% BSA), pruritus	Skin swabs MCS, viral PCR, scrapings (fungal KOH) Prolonged symptoms (1-2 weeks): consider skin biopsy	Continue checkpoint inhibitor therapy Consider dermatology review General skin care measures and emollients as above Oral antihistamines (increased dosing may be required: 2–4x standard dose), depending on renal and liver function Topical corticosteroid (moderate to very potent, ointment > cream vehicle) Wet dressings (educate at outpatient dermatology treatment centre) *Prolonged symptoms:* Delay immunotherapy until resolving to ≤ Grade 1 Prednisolone 0.5–1 mg/kg/day with slow taper Consider hospital admission for wet dressings *Refractory pruritus:* Consider neuropathic analgesia, for example, pregabalin 25 mg daily and titrate to response
		Grade 3-4/severe/life-threatening
Rash (≥30% BSA), pruritus, blisters, ulceration	Skin biopsy (with direct immunofluorescence if blisters present)	Delay immunotherapy if Grade 3 until resolving to Grade ≤ 1 Cease immunotherapy if SJS/TEN (Grade 4) Urgent dermatology review and biopsy Prednisolone 1 mg/kg/day or pulse with methylprednisolone 1-2 mg/kg/day for 3 days*Consideration of IVIG and/or cyclosporin Transfer to burns unit if skin loss > 10%

*Switch to oral prednisolone 1 mg/kg/day with slow taper over 1 month or longer. PJP (e.g., bactrim DS 1/2 tablet daily) and GIT ulcer prophylaxis therapy when patients are on prolonged steroid taper. Monitor blood glucose.

TABLE 3: Gastrointestinal and hepatic irAE: management algorithm.

(a)

Gastrointestinal irAE	Investigations	Management
Diarrhoea (<4 stools/day over baseline)	Stool MCS	**Grade 1/mild** Continue checkpoint inhibitor monotherapy (If on dual checkpoint inhibitor therapy, patient will need careful consideration and monitoring closely) Antimotility agents, for example, loperamide Fluid replacement If prolonged symptoms, treat as Grade 2
Diarrhoea (4–6 stools/day over baseline) Colitis (pain, mucus, or blood)	Stool MCS Consider colonoscopy	**Grade 2/moderate** Delay immunotherapy until resolving to Grade ≤1 (If on dual checkpoint inhibitor therapy, consider ceasing anti-CTLA-4) Consider hospital admission Gastroenterology referral Oral prednisolone 1 mg/kg/day for colitis or persistent diarrhoea
Diarrhoea (≥7 stools/day over baseline, incontinence, life-threatening) Colitis (severe pain, blood, mucus, and peritonism)	Stools MCS Colonoscopy, if colitis suspected or persistent diarrhoea despite steroids AXR/CT if suspected perforation	**Grade 3-4/severe/life-threatening** Grade 3 toxicity: Delay anti-PD-1 until resolving to Grade ≤1 with careful consideration as to retreatment Cease anti-CTLA-4 Grade 4 toxicity (life-threatening, perforation): Discontinue immunotherapy permanently Hospital admission Gastroenterology referral Pulse with methylprednisolone 1-2 mg/kg/day* If no response to steroid therapy (3–5 days), consider infliximab 5 mg/kg (if no perforation/sepsis)

(b)

Hepatic irAE	Investigations	Management
		Grade 1/mild
Hepatic (AST/ALT < 3x ULN and/or total bilirubin < 1.5x ULN)	LFTs and viral serology; Monitor LFTs weekly; Exclude disease progression or medication-related causes	Continue checkpoint inhibitor therapy
		Grade 2/moderate
Hepatic (AST/ALT >3–≤5x ULN and/or total bilirubin >1.5–≤3x ULN)	LFTs and viral serology; Exclude disease progression or medication-related causes; LFTs every 3 days	Delay checkpoint inhibitor therapy until improving to baseline; Consider gastroenterology referral; Consider oral prednisolone 1 mg/kg/day with slow taper
		Grade 3–4/severe/life-threatening
Hepatic (AST/ALT >5x ULN and/or total bilirubin >3x ULN)	LFTs and viral serology; Exclude disease progression or medication-related causes; LFTs daily	Discontinue checkpoint inhibitor therapy; Hospital admission; Gastroenterology referral; Pulse with methylprednisolone 1–2 mg/kg/day for 3 days*; *Steroid refractory hepatitis:*; If no improvement after 3–5 days consider the following:; Mycophenolate mofetil 500 mg–1g bd and escalation of methylprednisolone to 15 mg/kg daily (maximum 1 gm/day) for 3 days

*Switch to oral prednisolone 1 mg/kg/day with slow taper over 1 month or longer. PJP (e.g., bactrim DS 1/2 tablet daily) and GIT ulcer prophylaxis therapy when patients are on prolonged steroid taper. Monitor blood glucose.

(a)

(b)

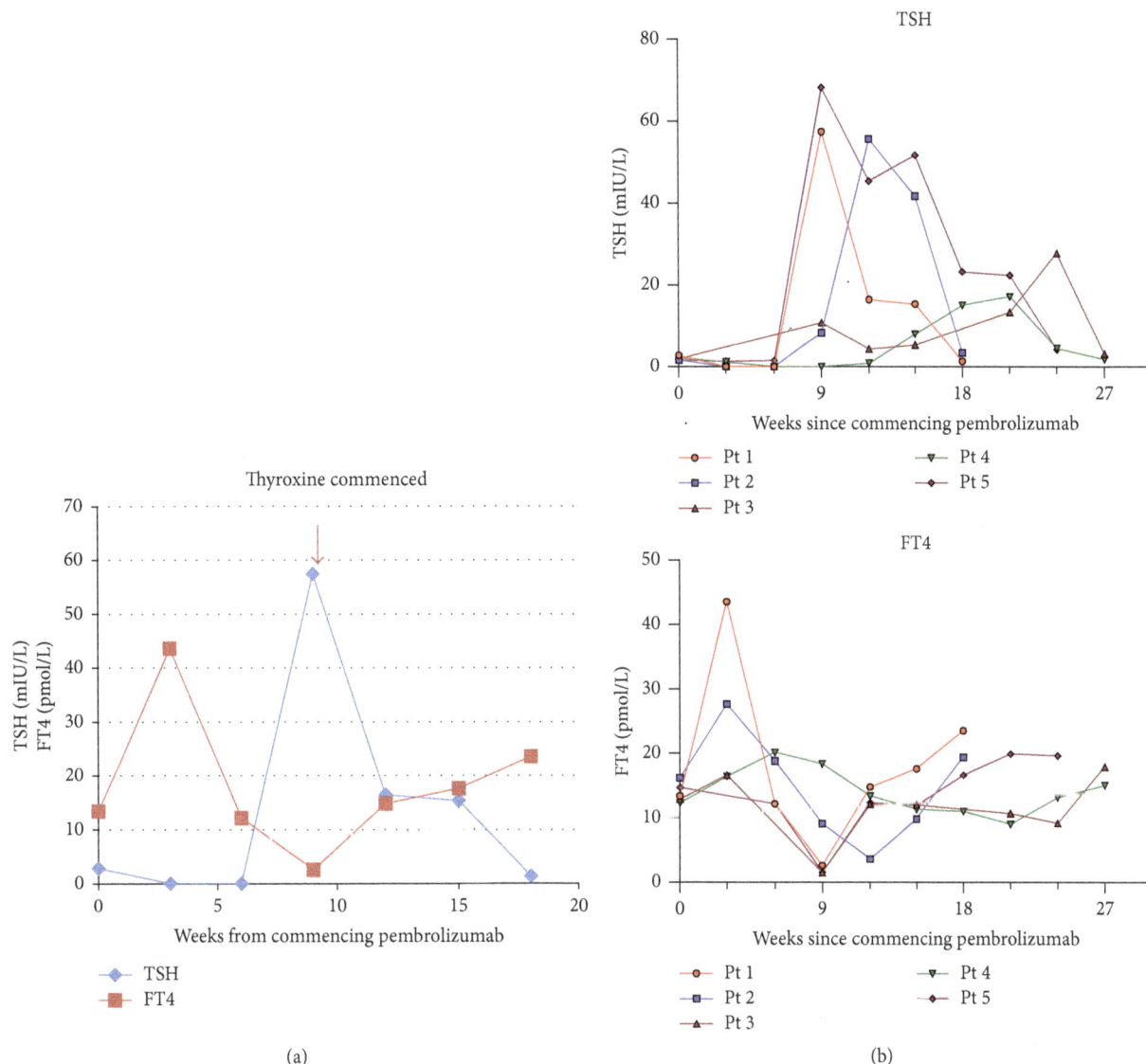

FIGURE 3: (a) Thyroiditis: hyperthyroid phase followed by hypothyroid phase in a patient treated with pembrolizumab. (b) Hyperthyroidism generally occurred within 3–6 weeks of initiation of pembrolizumab therapy (time = 0). Hypothyroid phase was evident by week 9 of pembrolizumab therapy and was characterised by markedly elevated TSH levels.

characterised by markedly elevated TSH levels (Figure 3(b)). Despite age and comorbidities of the patients, initiation of high-dose thyroxine (i.e., 100 mcg daily) at the onset of hypothyroidism was required. Thyroxine should be uptitrated to achieve normalisation of TSH. No evidence of thyroid function recovery occurred in our series, demonstrating the need for serial TSH monitoring.

From clinical trial data, hypophysitis is more commonly associated with ipilimumab and thyroid toxicity with anti-PD-1 agents [17]. In our cohort of 26 patients that had been pretreated with ipilimumab, 2 patients developed hypophysitis prior to receiving pembrolizumab and in 2 patients this occurred during anti-PD-1 therapy. Thyroiditis and hypophysitis management is described in Table 4.

4.6. Rheumatological Toxicity. Rheumatological toxicity occurred in 9 (22%) of patients (Table 1) and most events were

managed with low-dose prednisolone. One patient developed a grade 3-4 irAE. He received prior ipilimumab without complication. A disabling inflammatory arthropathy occurred 8 months after starting pembrolizumab. Synovial fluid aspirate showed an inflammatory infiltrate (white cell count 16.4 × 10^9/L) and no crystals were seen on microscopy, with CRP 60 and ESR 103 reflecting systemic inflammation. Rheumatoid factor, cyclic citrullinated peptide, and antinuclear antibodies and human leukocyte antigen B27 were negative. Anti-PD-1 therapy was ceased. The arthropathy was refractory to prednisolone doses up to 75 mg daily and required the addition of sulfasalazine, and the dose increased from 500 mg daily to 1 g twice daily over 10 days and continued with a good clinical response. Eight months after pembrolizumab cessation, prednisolone was weaned to 5 mg daily and sulfasalazine continued at 1 g twice daily. This patient achieved a complete disease response to pembrolizumab.

TABLE 4: Endocrine irAE management algorithm.

Endocrine irAE	Investigations	Management
		Grade 1/mild
Thyroid dysfunction (asymptomatic)	TFTs (TSH, FT4, FT3)	Continue checkpoint inhibitor therapy Mild biochemical abnormality: monitor TFTs prior to each infusion Consider endocrine referral
		Grade 2/moderate
Thyroiditis (initial hyperthyroid phase preceding prolonged hypothyroid phase)	TFTs prior to each infusion	Continue checkpoint inhibitor therapy Endocrine referral Hyperthyroidism may require medical management, if symptoms exist, but with close monitoring as this phase is usually short-lived *Onset of hypothyroid phase (generally by week 9 of treatment):* Commence thyroxine 50–100 mcg/daily Increase by 50 mcg in 3 weeks if TSH is still high until TSH is within normal range Continue thyroxine maintenance dose
Hypophysitis (symptomatic but clinically stable)	(AM) ACTH, cortisol, TFTs, LH, FSH, testosterone, oestrogen, prolactin, GH, IGF-1, blood glucose MRI pituitary	Consider delay of checkpoint inhibitor therapy Prednisolone 1 mg/kg/day Taper glucocorticoid to maintenance oral hydrocortisone (e.g., 10 mg hysone 0600/1500) It will generally require lifelong physiological replacement of steroid Adrenal sick day education Commence thyroxine/gonadal hormone replacement if required†
		Grade 3-4/severe/life-threatening
Hypophysitis (adrenal crisis: fatigue, headache, dizziness, hypotension, and hypoglycaemia shock)	(AM) ACTH, cortisol, TFTs, LH, FSH, testosterone, oestrogen, prolactin, GH, IGF-1, blood glucose MRI pituitary	Delay checkpoint inhibitor therapy Urgent endocrine review Pulse with methylprednisolone 1-2 mg/kg/day if indicated (e.g., headache); or high dose intravenous glucocorticoids (i.e., hydrocortisone 50 mg QID) Manage/exclude sepsis Fluid replacement Taper glucocorticoid to maintenance oral hydrocortisone (e.g., 10 mg hysone 0600/1500) It will generally require lifelong physiological replacement of steroid Adrenal sick day education Commence thyroxine/gonadal hormone replacement if required†

†Ensure steroid repletion prior to initiation of thyroxine to avoid precipitating adrenal crisis. Gonadal hormone replacement therapy can be initiated nonurgently when hypogonadotropic hypogonadism (secondary to hypophysitis) is confirmed to be persistent.

TABLE 5: Suggested algorithm arthralgia and arthritis.

Rheumatological irAE	Investigations	Management
Arthralgia and arthritis (minimal symptoms or signs)		*Grade 1/mild* Continue checkpoint inhibitor therapy Simple analgesia as required
Arthralgia and arthritis (moderate pain, inflammation, and impacting on daily function)	*Exclude:* Sepsis, crystal-induced arthritis, and coincidental inflammatory arthritis *Perform:* Synovial fluid cell count, polarised microscopy for crystals, gram stain and culture, blood culture RF, CCP, ANA, HLA-B27 (if positive, consider coincidental disease)	*Grade 2/moderate* Consider delay of checkpoint inhibitor therapy Consider rheumatology referral *Monoarthritis or oligoarthritis:* Consider intra-articular corticosteroid *Moderate inflammatory arthritis:* Consider low dose prednisolone 5–10 mg daily For more significant symptoms, higher doses may be required, for example, prednisolone 25 mg daily If response is not rapid, consider addition of sulphasalazine (immunomodulator without immunosuppressive effect)
Arthralgia and arthritis (severe pain or inflammation, disabling, and impacting on self-care)	*Exclude:* Sepsis, crystal-induced arthritis, and coincidental inflammatory arthritis *Perform:* Synovial fluid cell count, polarised microscopy for crystals, gram stain and culture, blood culture RF, CCP, ANA, HLA-B27 (if positive, consider coincidental disease)	*Grade 3–4/severe/life-threatening* Discontinue immunotherapy Rheumatology referral *Moderate-severe inflammatory arthritis:* Prednisolone 25 mg–40 mg daily If response is not rapid, consider addition of sulphasalazine *Severe:* Pulse with methylprednisolone 1-2 mg/kg/day for 3 days[*]

[*] Switch to oral prednisolone 1 mg/kg/day with slow taper over 1 month or longer. PJP (e.g., bactrim DS 1/2 tablet daily) and GIT ulcer prophylaxis therapy when patients are on prolonged steroid taper. Monitor blood glucose.

A 64-year-old male with a history of childhood glomerulonephritis developed significant sicca symptoms (xerophthalmia, xerostomia, and significant parotid swelling) after 3 cycles of pembrolizumab. Antinuclear antibody was elevated with high titres of 1 : 640 consistent with new onset immune-mediated Sjogren syndrome. He was treated with prednisolone 25 mg daily and the symptoms resolved, allowing steroids to be weaned. A postulated mechanism is an aberrant T-cell activation that is not dissimilar to that induced by graft versus host disease [36].

4.7. Arthralgia and Arthritis Management Algorithm. Rheumatological toxicity in clinical trials is higher for anti-PD-1 (8–12%) than anti-CTLA-4 therapy (5-6%) [17, 24]. Severe toxicity is rare but has also been reported in 2 patients that received prolonged pembrolizumab therapy [37]. Sulfasalazine was used with benefit and may be of use in conditions refractory to corticosteroids or to expedite steroid tapering. A suggested algorithm for the management of arthralgia and arthritis is outlined (Table 5).

4.8. Pneumonitis. Pneumonitis was observed in 2 (5%) patients of grade 2 severity. One patient had a short interval (47 days) between anti-CTLA-4 and anti-PD-1 dosing. Pneumonitis rates due to checkpoint inhibitors are low in the published literature (<1–4%) across several cancer types [12, 13, 17]. Pneumonitis is important to consider in the differential diagnosis of new cough or dyspnoea; however, other causes such as infection, exacerbation of airways disease, cancer progression, or sarcoidosis should be considered. Assessment requires imaging with CT, respiratory review, and in some circumstances, bronchoscopy. Grade 2 and Grade 3-4 pneumonitis require high-dose steroids with slow taper and prophylaxis against opportunistic infections [38].

No patients in our cohort experienced neurological toxicities. Fulminant myocarditis has been documented in patients receiving dual checkpoint inhibitor therapy [39] and in a patient that received prior combination therapy and later received single agent anti-PD-1 therapy [7].

5. Conclusion

Our cohort of patients receiving anti-PD-1 therapy for advanced melanoma included patients with poorer prognostic features with higher rates of elevated LDH, M1c disease, and poorer ECOG [5, 17], in comparison with patients enrolled on clinical trials. In the subset of patients that had a prior ipilimumab irAE, 62% and 23% developed mild irAE or no irAE on pembrolizumab, respectively, demonstrating that the development of irAE to anti-CTLA-4 therapy did not preclude subsequent treatment with another checkpoint inhibitor.

Recommencing anti-PD-1 therapy may be considered for selected significant irAE, dependent upon perceived benefits and risks of immunotherapy rechallenge. Toxicities may occur late and require vigilance and multidisciplinary management. This may allow effective anticancer therapy to continue. Limitations of the cohort are small patient numbers and retrospective nature of the data. Furthermore, a

significant number of patients received first-line anti-CTLA-4 therapy. The current evidence is for anti-PD-1 agents to be delivered first-line. However, the cases highlight a range of autoimmune toxicities and management in patients treated outside of a clinical trial. The use of overlapping anti-CTLA-4 and anti-PD-1 therapies demonstrates potentially added toxicity, having relevance in view of treatment approaches heading towards dual combinations of these and newer agents.

Acknowledgments

A. J. Lomax holds a position supported in 2015 and 2016 by the Simon Kerr Fellowship. The authors thank S. Anand at the Department of Tissue Pathology and Diagnostic Oncology, Royal Prince Alfred Hospital, Missenden Rd, Camperdown, NSW.

References

[1] A. Ribas, "Tumor immunotherapy directed at PD-1," *The New England Journal of Medicine*, vol. 366, no. 26, pp. 2517–2519, 2012.

[2] S. J. O'Day, O. Hamid, and W. J. Urba, "Targeting cytotoxic T-lymphocyte antigen-4 (CTLA-4): a novel strategy for the treatment of melanoma and other malignancies," *Cancer*, vol. 110, no. 12, pp. 2614–2627, 2007.

[3] F. S. Hodi, S. J. O'Day, D. F. McDermott et al., "Improved survival with ipilimumab in patients with metastatic melanoma," *The New England Journal of Medicine*, vol. 363, no. 8, pp. 711–723, 2010.

[4] D. Schadendorf, F. S. Hodi, C. Robert et al., "Pooled analysis of long-term survival data from phase II and phase III trials of ipilimumab in unresectable or metastatic melanoma," *Journal of Clinical Oncology*, vol. 33, no. 17, pp. 1889–1894, 2015.

[5] O. Hamid, C. Robert, A. Daud et al., "Safety and tumor responses with lambrolizumab (anti-PD-1) in melanoma," *The New England Journal of Medicine*, vol. 369, no. 2, pp. 134–144, 2013.

[6] J. Schachter, A. Ribas, G. V. Long, A. Arance, J-J. Grob, L. Mortier et al., *Pembrolizumab versus ipilimumab for advanced melanoma: final overall survival results of a multicentre, randomised, open-label phase 3 study (KEYNOTE-006)*, The Lancet.

[7] J. D. Wolchok, V. Chiarion-Sileni, R. Gonzalez et al., "Overall Survival with Combined Nivolumab and Ipilimumab in Advanced Melanoma," *The New England Journal of Medicine*, vol. 377, no. 14, pp. 1345–1356, 2017.

[8] C. Robert, A. Ribas, O. Hamid, A. Daud, J. D. Wolchok, A. M. Joshua et al., "Three-year overall survival for patients with advanced melanoma treated with pembrolizumab in KEYNOTE-001," *Journal of Clinical Oncology*, vol. 34, 2016.

[9] VG. Atkinson, V. Andelkovic, and B. Gunawan, "Poster Abstracts. Pembrolizumab for Metastatic Melanoma – One Year Results of Named Patient Access Program," *Asia-Pacific Journal of Clinical Oncology*, vol. 11, no. 117, 2015.

[10] T. C. Gangadhar, W. J. Hwu, M. A. Postow, O. Hamid, A. Daud, R. Dronca et al., "Society for Melanoma Research 2015 Congress. Safety and efficacy of pembrolizumab in US patients

enrolled in KEYNOTE-030, an Expanded Access Program (EAP)," *Pigment Cell and Melanoma Research*, vol. 28, no. 6, p. 774, 2015.

[11] AM. Grimaldi, E. Simeone, L. Festino, D. Giannarelli, M. Palla et al., "Society for Melanoma Research 2015 Congress. Correlation between immune-related adverse events and response to pembrolizumab in advanced melanoma patients," *Pigment Cell and Melanoma Research*, vol. 28, no. 6, p. 776, 2015.

[12] R. J. Motzer, B. Escudier, D. F. McDermott, S. George, H. J. Hammers, S. Srinivas et al., "Nivolumab versus Everolimus in Advanced Renal Cell Carcinoma," *The New England Journal of Medicine*, vol. 373, no. 19, 2015.

[13] H. Borghaei, L. Paz-Ares, L. Horn et al., "Nivolumab versus docetaxel in advanced nonsquamous non-small-cell lung cancer," *The New England Journal of Medicine*, vol. 373, no. 17, pp. 1627–1639, 2015.

[14] P. H. O'Donnell, E. R. Plimack, J. Bellmunt et al., "Pembrolizumab (MK-3475) for advanced urothelial cancer: Updated results and biomarker analysis from KEYNOTE-012," *Journal of Clinical Oncology*, vol. 33, pp. 296-296, 2015.

[15] S. M. Ansell, A. M. Lesokhin, I. Borrello et al., "PD-1 blockade with nivolumab in relapsed or refractory Hodgkin's lymphoma," *The New England Journal of Medicine*, vol. 372, no. 4, pp. 311–319, 2015.

[16] G. V. Long, V. Atkinson, J. S. Cebon et al., "Standard-dose pembrolizumab in combination with reduced-dose ipilimumab for patients with advanced melanoma (KEYNOTE-029): an open-label, phase 1b trial," *The Lancet Oncology*, vol. 18, no. 9, pp. 1202–1210, 2017.

[17] C. Robert, J. Schachter, G. V. Long et al., "Pembrolizumab versus ipilimumab in advanced melanoma," *The New England Journal of Medicine*, vol. 372, no. 26, pp. 2521–2532, 2015.

[18] J. B. Haanen, F. Carbonnel, C. Robert et al., "Management of Toxicities from Immunotherapy: ESMO Clinical Practice Guidelines," *Annals of Oncology*, vol. 28, 4, pp. iv119–iv142, 2017.

[19] S. Bowyer, P. Prithviraj, P. Lorigan et al., "Efficacy and toxicity of treatment with the anti-CTLA-4 antibody ipilimumab in patients with metastatic melanoma after prior anti-PD-1 therapy," *British Journal of Cancer*, vol. 114, no. 10, pp. 1084–1089, 2016.

[20] *Management of Immune-Related Adverse Events (irAEs)*, Cancer Treatment Online 2017, 1993, ID: 1993 v.2.

[21] A. J. Lomax, L. Ge, S. Anand, C. Mcneil, and P. Lowe, "Bullous pemphigoid-like reaction in a patient with metastatic melanoma receiving pembrolizumab and previously treated with ipilimumab," *Australasian Journal of Dermatology*, 2016.

[22] G. Aperis, C. Paliouras, A. Zervos, A. Arvanitis, and P. Alivanis, "The use of pregabalin in the treatment of uraemic pruritus in haemodialysis patients," *Journal of Renal Care*, vol. 36, no. 4, pp. 180–185, 2010.

[23] H. Rayner, J. Baharani, S. Smith, V. Suresh, and I. Dasgupta, "Uraemic pruritus: relief of itching by gabapentin and pregabalin," *Nephron Clinical Practice*, vol. 122, no. 3-4, pp. 75–79, 2012.

[24] J. Larkin, V. Chiarion-Sileni, R. Gonzalez et al., "Combined nivolumab and ipilimumab or monotherapy in untreated Melanoma," *The New England Journal of Medicine*, vol. 373, no. 1, pp. 23–34, 2015.

[25] J. Naidoo, D. B. Page, B. T. Li et al., "Toxicities of the Anti-PD-1 and Anti-PD-L1 Immune Checkpoint Antibodies," *Annals of Oncology*, vol. 26, no. 12, Article ID mdw141, 2016.

[26] C. Hua, L. Boussemart, C. Mateus et al., "Association of vitiligo with tumor response in patients with metastatic melanoma treated with pembrolizumab," *JAMA Dermatology*, vol. 152, no. 1, pp. 45–51, 2016.

[27] S. J. E. Hwang, G. Carlos, D. Wakade et al., "Cutaneous adverse events (AEs) of anti-programmed cell death (PD)-1 therapy in patients with metastatic melanoma: A single-institution cohort," *Journal of the American Academy of Dermatology*, vol. 74, no. 3, pp. 455–461, 2016.

[28] J. S. Weber, K. C. Kähler, and A. Hauschild, "Management of immune-related adverse events and kinetics of response with ipilimumab," *Journal of Clinical Oncology*, vol. 30, no. 21, pp. 2691–2697, 2012.

[29] M. A. Postow, "Managing immune checkpoint-blocking antibody side effects," *American Society of Clinical Oncology educational book / ASCO. American Society of Clinical Oncology. Meeting*, pp. 76–83, 2015.

[30] L. A. Fecher, S. S. Agarwala, F. Stephen Hodi, and J. S. Weber, "Ipilimumab and its toxicities: a multidisciplinary approach," *The Oncologist*, vol. 18, no. 6, pp. 733–743, 2013.

[31] "Yervoy (ipilimumab) immune-related adverse reaction (irAR) management guide," 2013.

[32] A. C. Allison and E. M. Eugui, "Mycophenolate mofetil and its mechanisms of action," *International Journal of immunopharmacology*, vol. 47, no. 2-3, pp. 85–118, 2000.

[33] R. Cheng, A. Cooper, J. Kench et al., "Ipilimumab-induced toxicities and the gastroenterologist," *Journal of Gastroenterology and Hepatology*, vol. 30, no. 4, pp. 657–666, 2015.

[34] R. Tanaka, Y. Fujisawa, H. Maruyama, Y. Nakamura, K. Yoshino, M. Ohtsuka et al., "Case series of thyroid dysfunction induced by nivolumab (anti-PD-1; ONO-4538)," *Annals of Oncology*, vol. 26, supplement 2, pp. ii34–ii35, 2015.

[35] C. Mace, S. Diem, M. Gore, J. Larkin, and D. Morganstein, "Thyroid abnormalities during anti-PD1 cancer immunotherapy," *Endocrine Abstracts*, vol. 38, p. 443, 2015.

[36] L. K. Jackson, D. B. Johnson, J. A. Sosman, B. A. Murphy, and J. B. Epstein, "Oral health in oncology: impact of immunotherapy," *Supportive Care in Cancer*, vol. 23, no. 1, pp. 1–3, 2015.

[37] M. M. K. Chan, R. F. Kefford, M. Carlino, A. Clements, and N. Manolios, "Arthritis and tenosynovitis associated with the anti-PD1 antibody pembrolizumab in metastatic melanoma," *Journal of Immunotherapy*, vol. 38, no. 1, pp. 37–39, 2015.

[38] M. A. Postow, *Managing immune checkpoint-blocking antibody side effects*, American Society of Clinical Oncology Educational Book, 2015, 76–83.

[39] D. B. Johnson, J. M. Balko, M. L. Compton et al., "Fulminant myocarditis with combination immune checkpoint blockade," *The New England Journal of Medicine*, vol. 375, no. 18, pp. 1749–1755, 2016.

31

Potential Role of Meiosis Proteins in Melanoma Chromosomal Instability

Scott F. Lindsey,[1] Diana M. Byrnes,[1] Mark S. Eller,[1] Ashley M. Rosa,[1] Nitika Dabas,[1] Julia Escandon,[1] and James M. Grichnik[1,2,3,4]

[1] Department of Dermatology and Cutaneous Surgery, University of Miami Miller School of Medicine, Miami, FL 33136, USA
[2] Anna Fund Melanoma Program Sylvester Comprehensive Cancer Center, University of Miami Miller School of Medicine, Miami, FL 33136, USA
[3] Frankel Family Division of Melanocytic Tumors, Department of Dermatology and Cutaneous Surgery, University of Miami Miller School of Medicine, Miami, FL 33136, USA
[4] Interdisciplinary Stem Cell Institute, University of Miami Miller School of Medicine, University of Miami, FL 33136, USA

Correspondence should be addressed to James M. Grichnik; grichnik@miami.edu

Academic Editor: Giuseppe Argenziano

Melanomas demonstrate chromosomal instability (CIN). In fact, CIN can be used to differentiate melanoma from benign nevi. The exact molecular mechanisms that drive CIN in melanoma have yet to be fully elucidated. Cancer/testis antigens are a unique group of germ cell proteins that are found to be primarily expressed in melanoma as compared to benign nevi. The abnormal expression of these germ cell proteins, normally expected only in the testis and ovaries, in somatic cells may lead to interference with normal cellular pathways. Germ cell proteins that may be particularly critical in CIN are meiosis proteins. Here, we review pathways unique to meiosis with a focus on how the aberrant expression of meiosis proteins in normal mitotic cells "meiomitosis" could impact chromosomal instability in melanoma and other cancers.

1. Introduction

Melanomas exhibit chromosomal instability (CIN). In fact, CIN is one of the most useful molecular markers to differentiate melanomas from benign nevi [1, 2]. Bastian et al. found that 96.2% of melanomas demonstrated chromosomal aberrations while only 13.0% of benign nevi showed these same abnormalities, of which all were Spitz nevi with stable 11p duplications [1]. Melanomas generally exhibit an increased number of overall chromosomes with frequent large translocations [1].

The fact that melanomas have such unstable genomes comes as no surprise, as genomic instability is widely regarded as the hallmark of cancer [3–7]. While genomic instability decreases the viability of most cells, it may also permit a subpopulation of cells to acquire genetic changes that lead them to escape normal growth control mechanisms. In addition, genomic instability allows established cancers to evolve and evade immunologic and pharmacologic destruction [8]. The extent to which different mechanisms play a role in genomic instability is controversial [4]; however three pathways are generally most accepted. These are defective DNA repair, telomere crisis, and mitotic spindle malfunction [3, 9–12]. An underappreciated but potentially important research area is the abnormal expression of germ cell proteins.

Expression of germ cell proteins has long been observed in cancer cells [13]. Cancer/testis antigens (CTAs) are a family of germ cell proteins expressed in a multitude of different histological tumor types [13, 14]. These proteins have been noted to have both diagnostic and prognostic value [2]. Studies have shown that expression of specific CTAs in melanoma can be used to predict tumor thickness, the presence of ulceration, and likelihood to undergo metastasis [15]. Melanomas have also been shown to express meiosis specific proteins including SCP1 (homologous chromosome pairing) [16], HORMAD1 (meiotic synapse regulation) [17], SPO11 (double stranded DNA breaks) [18], and REC8 (meiosis cohesion protein) [2]. We have also found three of these meiosis proteins, addition to a fourth not previously described, to be present in melanoma using western blot analysis (Figure 1) and immunofluorescence (Figure 2). Although the potential impact of the expression of meiotic proteins during mitosis in causing CIN has been suggested [17–21] and a role in reductional division in irradiated polyploid cells has been noted [22], thus far there has been no research directly evaluating the potential direct role of meiosis proteins in the creation of CIN. This review is focused on understanding meiosis pathways and explaining how the expression of these pathways during mitosis ("meiomitosis" [19, 20]) may result in chromosomal instability.

2. Meiosis General Overview: What Makes Meiosis Different from Mitosis?

Meiosis is a specialized type of cell division. In contrast to mitosis in which a diploid cell (2N) duplicates its DNA once and divides to produce two genetically identical diploid cells (2N), in meiosis a diploid cell (2N) duplicates its DNA once and undergoes two distinct rounds of cell division to produce four genetically unique haploid (1N) cells (Table 1). While mitosis occurs in all somatic cells of the human body, meiosis occurs naturally only in the male testis and female ovary.

The meiosis pathways are thought to have evolved from double-stranded DNA repair pathways [23]. In fact, meiosis still functions as a DNA repair process. This occurs through recombination events, where corresponding sections of DNA on the two homologous chromosomes are exchanged. This ensures that DNA damage is not passed on to progeny [24, 25], in addition to the obvious role of producing genetic diversity to facilitate species evolution [25–27].

Mitosis and meiosis have many similarities (Table 2). The second division of meiosis (meiosis II) has many aspects that are nearly identical to mitosis. The first division, on the other hand, exhibits three major modifications: (i) meiotic pairing to allow recombination, (ii) kinetochore coorientation to allow for homologous chromosome segregation during anaphase I, and (iii) stepwise loss of cohesion to ensure that sister chromatids segregate together in meiosis I [28]. These unique meiosis I pathways are the ones most likely to interfere with normal mitosis and will be the primary focus of this review.

3. Meiosis Gene Activation: The Regulatory Switch

The switch to meiosis from mitosis occurs in germ cells when the decision is made to produce gametes. Prior to this switch, germ cells use mitotic divisions as a way of self-renewal to increase their numbers and ensure the cell line does not become depleted [29]. The decision for cells to transition from a mitotic to meiotic cell cycle is complex and differs vastly among organisms. In most simple single-celled organisms that undergo asexual reproduction, this transition occurs as a result of environmental stressors. In yeast, nutrient deprivation triggers the dephosphorylation of the

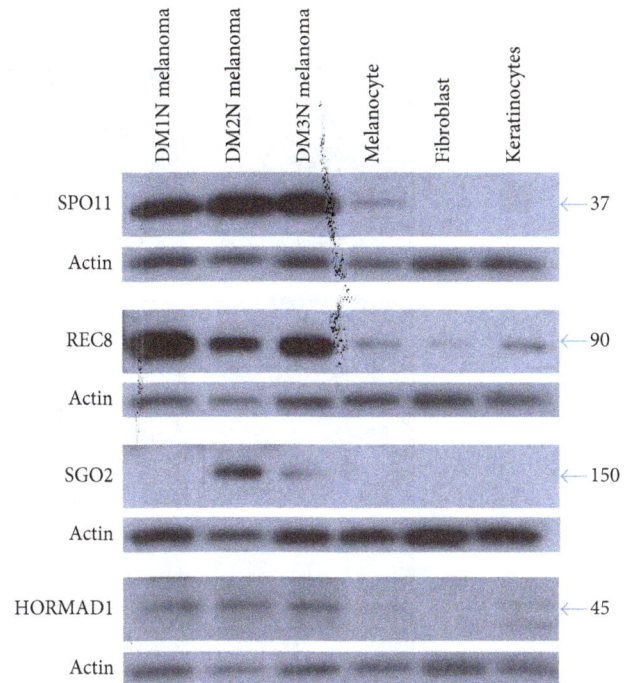

FIGURE 1: Analysis of meiosis proteins by western blot analysis. Western blot analysis was used to measure the expression of SPO11 (Abcam, ab81695), REC8 (Sigma, HPA031729), SGO2 (Sigma, HPA035163), and HORMAD1 (Abcam, ab57883) in melanoma lines compared to nontransformed melanocytes, fibroblasts, and keratinocytes. The cytoplasmic β-actin for each experiment is shown below its respective blot as a loading control.

RNA binding protein Mei2 by Pat1 Kinase which initiates the switch from mitosis to meiosis [30]. In Caenorhabditis elegans germline cells, GLD1 (quaking), GLD2 (Poly(A) polymerase), and GLD3 (Bicaudal C) have been shown to be critical for this switch [31, 32]. In mammals, the decision to transition from mitosis to meiosis is yet more complex and there are numerous regulatory molecules that govern this change. STRA8 is one of these proteins and is known to be imperative for the switch from mitosis to meiosis in both human male and female germ lines [33]. Data from Li et al. support this notion, showing that the spermatocytes in mice with depleted STRA8 failed to enter meiosis [34].

The crucial point in the cell cycle by which the cell must decide to make the mitotic-to-meiotic shift is at the G1/S checkpoint [35]. This is because the cell must undergo meiotic-specific events during S phase to ensure the proper progression of meiosis. The meiotic cohesin protein REC8 (discussed further below) must be incorporated into the newly replicated DNA during the premeiotic S phase so that the kinetochores can orient appropriately to allow for reduction division during meiosis I.

Although meiosis follows mitosis in the production of gametes, it is important to note that in the fertilized egg, mitosis is reestablished after meiosis. Thus the mitosis-meiosis pathways can be switched on and off and are reversible. Dysregulation of this switch causing the collision of the pathways could certainly cause CIN.

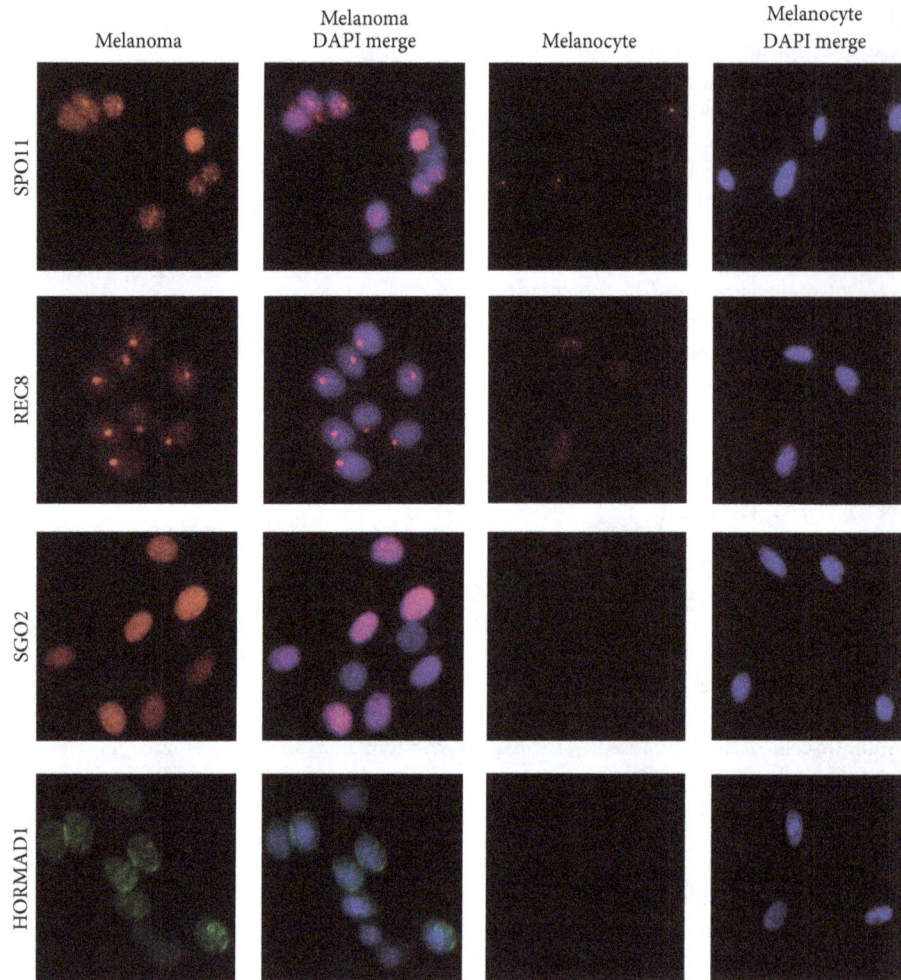

FIGURE 2: Analysis of meiosis proteins by immunofluorescence. Immunofluorescence was used to analyze the expression of SPO11, REC8, SGO2, and HORMAD1 in the DM2N melanoma line and nontransformed melanocytes using the same antibodies listed in Figure 1. Anti-rabbit secondary antibody was used for SPO11, REC8, and SGO2 and anti-mouse secondary was used for HORMAD1. The staining patterns varied between the different antibodies. SPO11, REC8, and SGO2 stained in a predominately nuclear manner with SPO11 demonstrating a fibular, dotted pattern, REC8 with discrete nuclear dots, and SGO2 with diffuse staining throughout the nucleus. HORMAD1 had a mostly cytoplasmic staining pattern although nuclear staining was also visualized. With all four antibodies, the staining in the melanoma was markedly stronger than the melanocytes.

4. DNA Double Strand Breaks: Rotating the Genes

The formation of crossover events lies at the heart of meiosis, as it allows for genetic recombination between homologous chromosomes and is necessary for the proper alignment of chromosomes during meiosis I. Crossovers are initiated by the creation of double-stranded breaks (DSBs) by the protein SPO11 [36].

SPO11 is a homolog of the archeal type II topoisomerase A subunit [37]. SPO11 creates DSBs using a catalytic tyrosine to attack the phosphodiester backbone of DNA, creating a covalent bond between itself and the $5'$ end of the break [37]. Each SPO11 protein associates with only one strand of DNA; thus two SPO11 molecules are needed for each DSB [37]. Once the DSB is formed, SPO11 is removed by polymerase β with the help of the MRE11 complex [36, 38] and the

$5'$ ends of the breaks are excised, leaving stretches of $3'$ ssDNA [36]. This single stranded DNA associates with DMC1 and RAD51, two proteins known to be involved in double-stranded DNA repair, to form a filament [37]. This filament then begins the search for a location of homology on the opposite chromosome.

Many of the factors which ensure that the single stranded DNA correctly associates with a corresponding DNA fragment on the homologous chromosome have yet to be elucidated. It is clear that the meiosis specific kinase MEK1 plays a role in ensuring interhomolog binding through its interaction with RAD54 and RAD51 [39, 40]. MEK1 also promotes recombination by suppressing DSB repairs [41]. Upon identification of the appropriate homologue, DMC1 begins the crossover recombination event using one of the $3'$ ends to mediate a stable invasion of the homologous chromosome [36]. DNA synthesis then extends the end of the

TABLE 1: Summary of the major events in each stage of the meiotic and mitotic cell cycle.

Stage of meiotic division	Outcome	Stage of mitotic division	Outcome
S Phase I	Duplication of genetic material, DNA double strand breaks induced by SPO11	S Phase	Duplication of genetic material
Prophase I	Chromosome condensation, homologous recombination	Prophase	Chromosome condensation
Metaphase I	Tetrad alignment at metaphase plate, cohesin degraded from chromosome arms but remains at centromere, monooriented sister kinetochores	Metaphase	Chromosome alignment at metaphase plate, cohesin degraded from centromere, bioriented sister kinetochores
Anaphase I	Homologous chromosomes separate to opposite sides of dividing cell, sister chromatids remain attached	Anaphase	Sister chromatids separate to opposite sides of dividing cell
Telophase I	Chromatid decondensation (sometimes just partial decondensation)	Telophase	Chromatid decondensation, two daughter cells are diploid
Prophase II	No chromosome duplication, chromosome recondensation		
Metaphase II	Sister chromatids align at metaphase plate, cohesin degraded from centromere, bi-oriented sister kinetochores		
Anaphase II	Sister chromatids separate to opposite sides of dividing cell		
Telophase II	Chromosome decondensation, four daughter cells are haploid		

TABLE 2: Summary of the differences between meiosis I, meiosis II, and mitosis.

	Meiosis I	Meiosis II	Mitosis
Reductional division	Yes	No	No
Equational division	No	Yes	Yes
Daughter Cells Genetically Identical	No	No	Yes
Double strand breaks introduced by SPO11	Yes	No	No
Pol β required for meiotic recombination and chromosome synapsis	Yes	No	No
Homologous chromosome recombination and segregation	Yes	No	No
Degradation of cohesion along chromosome arms	Yes	Not present	Not present
Degradation of cohesion at centromeres	No	Yes—during anaphase II	Yes—during anaphase
SGO2 protection of REC8 located at pericentromeric regions	Yes	No	No

invading strand. By recapture of this strand, a joint molecule is generated that contains a Holiday Junction, which can then be resolved into either a noncrossover or crossover event [36].

HORMAD1 also plays a critical role in synapsis formation through its role in DSB formation [42]. It ensures that adequate number DSBs are formed to allow for successful homology search [42]. Independently, HORMAD1 also promotes the proper formation of the synaptonemal complex, a proteinaceous structure which stabilizes the tetrad and ensures proper homolog pairing [42].

Together these factors cause DNA strand breaks and create a controlled number of crossover events. Deregulation, or simply the presence, of these pathways in otherwise mitotic cells would be expected to cause translocations as well as insertions and deletions. Although there is no data specifically implicating these pathways in cancer, it is important to note that SPO11 [18], DMC1 [22], and HORMAD1 [17] have all been shown to be increased in cancer. Both SPO11 and HORMAD1 have been specifically noted in melanoma [17, 18] and we found them to be overexpressed in melanoma compared to nontransformed cell types using western blot analysis (Figure 1) and immunofluorescence (Figure 2).

5. DNA Polymerase β: Potential Role Evolving the Genome

At least sixteen DNA polymerases exist in eukaryotes, each with its own unique role in maintaining the integrity of the genome [43]. Specific high fidelity DNA polymerases function in replicating the genome during the S phase of the cell cycle. More error-prone polymerases also exist and have specific functions including DNA repair and cell recombination [43]. While it is imperative that the cells employ methods to preserve the fidelity of DNA replication, error-prone polymerases may play a role in producing variability which could provide a selective advantage [43]. As such, in 1962 Magni and von Borstel observed that cells had a markedly higher rate of mutation during meiosis compared to mitosis [44].

DNA polymerase β (POL β) is one of the more error prone polymerases found in eukaryotes and is required for base excision repair during DNA replication and repair [45]. It has an error rate of one error per 10,000–100,000 nucleotides incorporated, up to 100x higher than the more accurate polymerases which the cell routinely uses for chromosomal replication [43]. Recently, POL β has also been found to have a critical role during meiotic synapsis [45]. POL β has been shown to localize to the synaptonemal complex during prophase I [46] where it facilitates the removal of the SPO11 complex from DNA breakage ends, facilitating the creation of ssDNA with which RAD51 and DMC1 associate [47]. Kidane et al. showed that POL β knockdown spermatocytes were unable to undergo chromosome synapsis and, instead, underwent apoptosis during prophase I [47].

Deregulated expression of POL β has been implicated in genomic instability in cancer [45]. Decreased POL β expression has been detected in one fifth of tumors [48] and this decrease has also been demonstrated to promote tumorigenesis [49] presumably due to decreased DNA repair. Conversely, increased levels of POL β have been noted in approximately one-third of tumors studied, with one sample showing a 286-fold increase [48]. Luo et al. used mouse embryonic fibroblasts to study the effect of varying levels of POL β on genomic instability by looking at three endpoints: DNA strand breaks, chromosomal breakage, and gene mutation [45]. POL β null cells showed a marked increase in genomic instability [45] due to their inability to repair DNA. POL β overexpressing cells showed a high frequency of mutations, but only after the introduction of DNA damaging agents [45], most likely because POL β was used to repair the DNA damage instead of one of its higher fidelity counterparts.

Servant et al. specifically studied the association between DNA POL β and melanoma and found that POL β was markedly overexpressed in melanoma tissue when compared to normal skin [50]. Mammalian cells which overexpressed POL β had a 1.5–2-fold higher resistance to UV radiation, though the surviving cells had a 2.6–50-fold increase in mutations [50]. POL β was able to repair both cyclobutane pyrimidine dimers (CPD) and pyrimidine-pyrimidone (6–4) photoproducts and had the ability to elongate the $3'$ strand after dATP addition [50]. This is significant because this period of elongation serves as a potential source of DNA point mutations due to POL β's markedly lower rate of fidelity than other polymerases.

Although POL β seems to be expressed at some level ubiquitously in all cells, it clearly plays an integral role in the meiotic pathways. It would be anticipated that cells activating meiosis pathways may exhibit increased POL β activity and increased mutations.

6. Cohesion: How Not to Let Go of Your Sister

The decision is made to enter the meiotic cycle prior to replicating the DNA. During the replication of DNA for meiosis, the newly duplicated strands are held together by a ring of proteins called cohesins. The mitotic cohesin complex normally includes the structural maintenance (SMC) proteins SMC1 and SMC2, the kleisin protein SCC1/RAD21, and an accessory subunit, SCC3 [51, 52]. In meiosis RAD21 is replaced by REC8 [53].

REC8 serves a number of functions including (1) acting within the synaptonemal complex to drive homologous recombination, (2) kinetochore orientation, and (3) sister chromatid adhesion.

6.1. Synaptonemal Complex/Homologous Recombination. The synaptonemal complex is a unique meiosis specific structure which is critical for chiasma (locations of crossover) formation, homologous chromosome binding, and chromosome segregation [54]. It bridges homologous chromosomes and is composed of three proteins: SCP1, 2, and 3. REC8 is critical in this structure for driving chiasma formation between homologous chromosomes [55, 56]. As the chromosomes condense, REC8 is cleaved on the chromosome arms and the cohesin complex is replaced by the condensin complex. The crossover point remains to ensure proper alignment, tension, and segregation of the homologous chromosomes.

6.2. Kinetochore Orientation. REC8 has also been shown to play a role in the monoorientation of sister kinetochores during meiosis I. When the mitotic cohesin protein RAD21 is expressed instead of REC8 in yeast, sister chromatids undergo equational rather than reductional chromosomal segregation during meiosis I [55, 57]. This suggests that the coorientation of kinetochores is lost, allowing sister chromatids to be pulled towards opposite poles of the dividing cell. Studies performed in maize support this theory, demonstrating that, in the absence of REC8, sister chromatids establish bioriented sister kinetochores in meiosis I [58]. While research suggests REC8 is required for monoorientation of sister kinetochores, its overexpression alone does not appear to always lead to chromosomal missegregation during mitosis [55, 57] but instead requires the cooperation of other factors such as monopolins, as reviewed below.

6.3. Kinetochore Adhesion. REC8 is retained around the centromere until the start of anaphase II [59] ensuring that sister chromatids do not become prematurely separated. Two of the factors that prevent the cleavage of REC8 at the centromere are SGO1 and SGO2. Although both of these proteins are ubiquitously expressed in mammals, SGO2 is found in higher concentrations in the testis, implying that it may play a more major role in meiosis [60]. Studies have supported this theory, showing that mice with a deleted *Sgo2* gene show no failure to thrive but are infertile, suggesting that this protein is not as critical in mitosis as meiosis [61].

The protease separase is required to remove cohesins from chromosomes [62]. REC8 can only be cleaved by separase when the former is hyperphosphorylated [60]. SGO2 protects REC8 from cleavage during meiosis I by ensuring its dephosphorylation at the centromeres. This is accomplished through the recruitment of protein phosphatase 2A (PP2A) to centromere proximal cohesins [28]. PP2A localization to centromeres results in dephosphorylation of centromere proximal REC8, inhibiting its cleavage by separase while allowing REC8 cleavage to occur along chromosome arms.

REC8/Synaptonemal complex proteins could play an important role in chromosomal missegregation and translocations. REC8 expression has been noted in melanoma [2] and we found it to be overexpressed in melanoma using western blot analysis (Figure 1) and immunofluorescence (Figure 2). REC8 has also been noted in irradiated lymphoma cells [22]. Forced expression of REC8 during mitosis leads to chromosome segregation defects [63]. Ishiguro et al. utilized yeast with overproduction of REC8 during mitosis to demonstrate this phenomenon [63]. Compared with the wild type yeast cells, the strains with upregulated REC8 showed bridged nuclei which were not able to divide appropriately [63]. Thus it is possible that high levels of REC8 may play a role in nuclear division abnormalities.

It has also been postulated that REC8 may play a role in reducing chromosome number in polyploid cancer cells by driving reductional divisions [22]. Interestingly, synaptonemal complex proteins SCP1 and SCP3 have been shown to be upregulated in cancer and are associated with tumor progression and survival [16, 22, 64]. SCP1 is a known cancer/testis antigen [64]. Türeci et al. found that in melanoma, four of the 28 samples tested showed positive synaptonemal complex protein expression [16]. Studies have demonstrated that when inserted into nongerm cells, these proteins are still able to produce a synaptonemal complex [54]. Thus it is possible that these proteins play a role in chromosomal missegregation and crossover events in cancer.

7. Kinetochore/Spindle Assembly: A Different Orientation

The kinetochore is a proteinaceous structure which forms on centromeres and serves as a spindle fiber attachment site used to pull chromosomes apart and to opposite poles of the nucleus during cell division. Every chromatid has its own kinetochore, thus after the duplication of genetic material each chromosome contains two kinetochores, one on each chromatid. During mitosis, the two kinetochores on each chromosome face in opposite directions so that spindle fibers from each pole attach to separate chromatids. This is known as amphitelic attachment. The kinetochore works as a sensing mechanism, ensuring that the chromosomes are appropriately amphitelically attached. It does this by detecting the tension produced from the counteracting pull from each spindle into the bidirectionally oriented sister kinetochores. Only when this tension is sensed does the cell proceed through the spindle assembly checkpoint (SAC) and begin anaphase.

This process is more complicated in meiosis, as the cell must undergo two subsequent rounds of chromosome segregation without intervening DNA duplication. This is accomplished by a different orientation of the kinetochores in meiosis I through the use of REC8, monopolin proteins, and Aurora B Kinase [58, 65]. In meiosis I, sister kinetochores are oriented on the same side of the chromosome (monooriented) and attach to spindle fibers in a syntelic fashion to ensure that sister chromatids are pulled towards the same pole of the dividing cell. The tension necessary to proceed through the checkpoint is created by the crossovers between homologous chromosomes, which are pulled in opposite directions. Resolution of the chiasma allows for separation of the joined homologous pairs in anaphase I. Meiosis II then proceeds similarly to mitosis.

Many of the details on kinetochore orientation and rotation in meiosis II have yet to be determined. REC8 is critical for mono-orientation [55, 58]. Condensins, proteins which play a major role in chromosome condensation and DSB repair during prophase I, are also known to play a role [66]. Brito et al. showed that in the absence of condensins, a portion of kinetochores biorient during meiosis I [66]. A third group of proteins called monopolins also play a key role [67–69]. Monopolins are meiosis specific proteins [69]. Through their interaction with Aurora B Kinase, monopolins help ensure that homologs are pulled towards opposite poles of the cell [67]. Although REC8 plays a clear role in maintaining monooriented sister kinetochores, monopolins alone are able to hold together sister kinetochores independently [67, 69].

Another critical part of this process is the spindle apparatus. In the female oocyte, the centrosome is destroyed before meiosis and the cell undergoes an acentrosomal spindle assembly [70, 71]. The spindle network is instead formed through the action of over 80 self-organized microtubule organized centers (MTOCs) that develop from the cytoplasmic microtubule complex and eventually aggregate into a bipolar network [70]. Very little is understood about acentrosomal spindle assembly and the differences between the mitotic and meiotic spindle, and further studies are needed.

During meiosis I, mechanisms exist to allow the unique process of homolog separation. Studies have shown that some SAC proteins specifically interact with REC8 and Shugoshin (SGO1 and 2) [56]. BUB1 is one of the SAC proteins shown to be specifically involved with this process. BUB1 is required for the localization of the meiosis cohesion regulators SGO1 and SGO2 to protect REC8 during meiosis I [72]. For this reason, BUB1 is thought to be essential for establishing proper kinetochore function [56, 73, 74]. BUB1 mutation results in chromosome fragmentation and missegregation in Drosophila [56, 73] and female specific germ cell aneuploidy in mice [56, 75].

BUB1 has been noted to be abnormally expressed in several cancers including gastric, colon, esophageal, breast, and melanoma [76–79]. The aberrant expression of BUB1 seems to have an especially strong correlation with melanoma [80]. Lewis et al. used qtPCR to identify molecular expression patterns in melanoma, benign nevi, and lymph nodes [80]. Of the 20 melanoma-related genes tested, BUB1 was one of the three genes found to have the highest discriminatory potential for distinguishing melanoma, benign nevi, and lymph nodes [80].

There is a delicate interplay between kinetochores, the spindle apparatus, and the SAC which, when not functioning properly, would be expected to result in chromosomal segregation abnormalities.

8. Conclusion and Future Directions

Melanomas are highly genomically unstable tumors and are known to express germ cell proteins. It is possible that these two phenomena are related due to the collision of

TABLE 3: The Potential ramifications of the aberrant expression of different meiotic proteins.

Meiotic Pathway	Potential ramification in mitosis	Potential Meiotic Proteins involved
DS DNA strand breaks	Insertions, deletions, translocations	SPO11
Error prone polymerase	Point mutations	POLB
Failure of cohesin ring digestion	Tetraplody, polyploidy	REC8/SGO2
Unresolved chismata	Anaphase bridging	REC8
Failure of kinetochore separation	Chromosomal missegregation	REC8/SGO2
Misalignment of kinetochores	Chromosomal missegregation	REC8/monopolins

meiotic germ cell pathways with the normal mitotic cell cycle pathways (meiomitosis). As discussed, these pathways could impact genomic instability at many levels including double stranded DNA breaks, crossover events, chromosomal cohesion, spindle defects, and direct introduction of point mutations (Table 3). Chromosomal instability is a hallmark of human cancer, and we hypothesize that the aberrant expression of meiosis proteins will prove to be a critical step in this process. Expression of these pathways may serve a diagnostic role in identifying tumor with particular aggressive behavior due to their capacity to continuously evolve. Further, these pathways may serve as therapeutic targets. Because meiosis proteins are largely limited to germ cells, targeted therapeutics could be designed to have very limited interactions with other cells in the body reducing potential adverse side effects. Meiomitosis is likely to play a critical role in cancer progression and we believe future research is needed to shed light on this promising field.

Disclosure

Scott F. Lindsey, Diana M. Byrnes, Ashley M. Rosa, Nitika Dabas, Mark S. Eller, and James M. Grichnik do not have any financial relationships relevant to this paper. Grichnik is a DigitalDerm, Inc., Major Shareholder. Scott F. Lindsey, Diana M. Byrnes, Ashley M. Rosa, Nitika Dabas, Mark S. Eller do not have any other financial relationships.

Funding

This study was supported by the Anna Fund Melanoma Program at Sylvester Comprehensive Cancer Center, the Melanoma Research Foundation, and the Frankel Family Division of Melanocytic Tumors, Department of Dermatology and Cutaneous Surgery, University of Miami.

Acknowledgments

The authors are indebted to the Anna Fund Melanoma Program at Sylvester Comprehensive Cancer Center, the Frankel Family Division of Melanocytic Tumors, the Department of Dermatology and Cutaneous Surgery, the Melanoma Research Foundation, and our many benefactors, especially William Rubin and his family and friends.

References

[1] B. C. Bastian, A. B. Olshen, P. E. LeBoit, and D. Pinkel, "Classifying melanocytic tumors based on DNA copy number changes," *American Journal of Pathology*, vol. 163, no. 5, pp. 1765–1770, 2003.

[2] A. M. Rosa, N. Dabas, D. M. Byrnes, M. S. Eller, and J. M. Grichnik, "Germ cell proteins in melanoma: prognosis, diagnosis, treatment, and theories on expression," *Journal of Skin Cancer*, vol. 2012, Article ID 621968, 8 pages, 2012.

[3] T. Davoli and T. de Lange, "The causes and consequences of polyploidy in normal development and cancer," *Annual Review of Cell and Developmental Biology*, vol. 27, pp. 585–610, 2011.

[4] S. Negrini, V. G. Gorgoulis, and T. D. Halazonetis, "Genomic instability—an evolving hallmark of cancer," *Nature Reviews Molecular Cell Biology*, vol. 11, no. 3, pp. 220–228, 2010.

[5] D. Hanahan and R. A. Weinberg, "Hallmarks of cancer: the next generation," *Cell*, vol. 144, no. 5, pp. 646–674, 2011.

[6] D. Hanahan and R. A. Weinberg, "The hallmarks of cancer," *Cell*, vol. 100, no. 1, pp. 57–70, 2000.

[7] M. Roh, O. E. Franco, S. W. Hayward, R. van der Meer, and S. A. Abdulkadir, "A role for polyploidy in the tumorigenicity of Pim-1-expressing human prostate and mammary epithelial cells," *PLoS ONE*, vol. 3, no. 7, Article ID e2572, 2008.

[8] G. Brkic, J. Gopas, N. Tanic et al., "Genomic instability in drug-resistant human melanoma cell lines detected by Alu-I-arbitrary-primed PCR," *Anticancer Research*, vol. 23, no. 3, pp. 2601–2608, 2003.

[9] V. M. Draviam, S. Xie, and P. K. Sorger, "Chromosome segregation and genomic stability," *Current Opinion in Genetics and Development*, vol. 14, no. 2, pp. 120–125, 2004.

[10] D. Gilley, H. Tanaka, and B. S. Herbert, "Telomere dysfunction in aging and cancer," *International Journal of Biochemistry and Cell Biology*, vol. 37, no. 5, pp. 1000–1013, 2005.

[11] W. T. Silkworth, I. K. Nardi, L. M. Scholl, and D. Cimini, "Multipolar spindle pole coalescence is a major source of kinetochore mis-attachment and chromosome mis-segregation in cancer cells," *PLoS ONE*, vol. 4, no. 8, Article ID e6564, 2009.

[12] A. G. Silva, H. A. Graves, A. Guffei et al., "Telomere-centromere-driven genomic instability contributes to karyotype evolution in a mouse model of melanoma," *Neoplasia*, vol. 12, no. 1, pp. 11–19, 2010.

[13] E. Fratta, S. Coral, A. Covre et al., "The biology of cancer testis antigens: putative function, regulation and therapeutic potential," *Molecular Oncology*, vol. 5, no. 2, pp. 164–182, 2011.

[14] P. Chomez, O. de Backer, M. Bertrand, E. de Plaen, T. Boon, and S. Lucas, "An overview of the MAGE gene family with the identification of all human members of the family," *Cancer Research*, vol. 61, no. 14, pp. 5544–5551, 2001.

[15] S. Svobodová, J. Browning, D. MacGregor et al., "Cancer-testis antigen expression in primary cutaneous melanoma has independent prognostic value comparable to that of Breslow thickness, ulceration and mitotic rate," *European Journal of Cancer*, vol. 47, no. 3, pp. 460–469, 2011.

[16] Ö. Türeci, U. Sahin, C. Zwick, M. Koslowski, G. Seitz, and M. Pfreundschuh, "Identification of a meiosis-specific protein as a member of the class of cancer/testis antigens," *Proceedings of the National Academy of Sciences of the United States of America*, vol. 95, no. 9, pp. 5211–5216, 1998.

[17] Y. T. Chen, C. A. Venditti, G. Theiler et al., "Identification of CT46/HORMAD1, an immunogenic cancer/testis antigen encoding a putative meiosis-related protein," *Cancer Immunity*, vol. 5, p. 9, 2005.

[18] A. J. G. Simpson, O. L. Caballero, A. Jungbluth, Y. T. Chen, and L. J. Old, "Cancer/testis antigens, gametogenesis and cancer," *Nature Reviews Cancer*, vol. 5, no. 8, pp. 615–625, 2005.

[19] J. M. Grichnik, "Genomic instability and tumor stem cells," *Journal of Investigative Dermatology*, vol. 126, no. 6, pp. 1214–1216, 2006.

[20] J. M. Grichnik, "Melanoma, nevogenesis, and stem cell biology," *Journal of Investigative Dermatology*, vol. 128, no. 10, pp. 2365–2380, 2008.

[21] M. Kalejs and J. Erenpreisa, "Cancer/testis antigens and gametogenesis: a review and "brain-storming" session," *Cancer Cell International*, vol. 5, no. 1, article 4, 2005.

[22] M. Kalejs, A. Ivanov, G. Plakhins et al., "Upregulation of meiosis-specific genes in lymphoma cell lines following genotoxic insult and induction of mitotic catastrophe," *BMC Cancer*, vol. 6, article 6, 2006.

[23] E. Marcon and P. B. Moens, "The evolution of meiosis: recruitment and modification of somatic DNA-repair proteins," *BioEssays*, vol. 27, no. 8, pp. 795–808, 2005.

[24] H. Bernstein, F. A. Hopf, and R. E. Michod, "The molecular basis of the evolution of sex," *Advances in Genetics*, vol. 24, pp. 323–370, 1987.

[25] H. Bernstein, H. C. Byerly, F. A. Hopf, and R. E. Michod, "Genetic damage, mutation, and the evolution of sex," *Science*, vol. 229, no. 4719, pp. 1277–1281, 1985.

[26] L. Hadany and J. M. Comeron, "Why are sex and recombination so common?" *Annals of the New York Academy of Sciences*, vol. 1133, pp. 26–43, 2008.

[27] S. P. Otto and A. C. Gerstein, "Why have sex? The population genetics of sex and recombination," *Biochemical Society Transactions*, vol. 34, no. part 4, pp. 519–522, 2006.

[28] G. A. Brar and A. Amon, "Emerging roles for centromeres in meiosis I chromosome segregation," *Nature Reviews Genetics*, vol. 9, no. 12, pp. 899–910, 2008.

[29] J. Kimble, "Molecular regulation of the mitosis/meiosis decision in multicellular organisms," *Cold Spring Harbor Perspectives in Biology*, vol. 3, no. 8, Article ID a002683, 2011.

[30] Y. Watanabe, S. Shinozaki-Yabana, Y. Chikashige, Y. Hiraoka, and M. Yamamoto, "Phosphorylation of RNA-binding protein controls cell cycle switch from mitotic to meiotic in fission yeast," *Nature*, vol. 386, no. 6621, pp. 187–190, 1997.

[31] J. Kimble and S. L. Crittenden, "Controls of germline stem cells, entry into meiosis, and the sperm/oocyte decision in *Caenorhabditis elegans*," *Annual Review of Cell and Developmental Biology*, vol. 23, pp. 405–433, 2007.

[32] C. R. Eckmann, S. L. Crittenden, N. Suh, and J. Kimble, "GLD-3 and control of the mitosis/meiosis decision in the germline of *Caenorhabditis elegans*," *Genetics*, vol. 168, no. 1, pp. 147–160, 2004.

[33] E. L. Anderson, A. E. Baltus, H. L. Roepers-Gajadien et al., "Stra8 and its inducer, retinoic acid, regulate meiotic initiation in both spermatogenesis and oogenesis in mice," *Proceedings of*

the *National Academy of Sciences of the United States of America*, vol. 105, no. 39, pp. 14976–14980, 2008.

[34] H. Li, K. Palczewski, W. Baehr, and M. Clagett-Dame, "Vitamin A deficiency results in meiotic failure and accumulation of undifferentiated spermatogonia in prepubertal mouse testis," *Biology of Reproduction*, vol. 84, no. 2, pp. 336–341, 2011.

[35] Y. Watanabe, S. Yokobayashi, M. Yamamoto, and P. Nurse, "Pre-meiotic S phase is linked to reductional chromosome segregation and recombination," *Nature*, vol. 409, no. 6818, pp. 359–363, 2001.

[36] J. L. Gerton and R. S. Hawley, "Homologous chromosome interactions in meiosis: diversity amidst conservation," *Nature Reviews Genetics*, vol. 6, no. 6, pp. 477–487, 2005.

[37] S. Keeney, "Spo11 and the formation of DNA double-strand breaks in meiosis," *Genome Dynamics and Stability*, vol. 2, pp. 81–123, 2008.

[38] V. Borde, "The multiple roles of the Mre11 complex for meiotic recombination," *Chromosome Research*, vol. 15, no. 5, pp. 551–563, 2007.

[39] H. Niu, L. Wan, B. Baumgartner, D. Schaefer, J. Loidl, and N. M. Hollingsworth, "Partner choice during meiosis is regulated by Hop1-promoted dimerization of Mek1," *Molecular Biology of the Cell*, vol. 16, no. 12, pp. 5804–5818, 2005.

[40] H. Niu, L. Wan, V. Busygina et al., "Regulation of meiotic recombination via Mek1-mediated Rad54 phosphorylation," *Molecular Cell*, vol. 36, no. 3, pp. 393–404, 2009.

[41] H. Niu, X. Li, E. Job et al., "Mek1 kinase is regulated to suppress double-strand break repair between sister chromatids during budding yeast meiosis," *Molecular and Cellular Biology*, vol. 27, no. 15, pp. 5456–5467, 2007.

[42] K. Daniel, J. Lange, K. Hached et al., "Meiotic homologue alignment and its quality surveillance are controlled by mouse HORMAD1," *Nature Cell Biology*, vol. 13, no. 5, pp. 599–610, 2011.

[43] A. J. Rattray and J. N. Strathern, "Error-prone DNA polymerases: when making a mistake is the only way to get ahead," *Annual Review of Genetics*, vol. 37, pp. 31–66, 2003.

[44] G. E. Magni and R. C. von Borstel, "Different rates of spontaneous mutation during mitosis and meiosis in yeast," *Genetics*, vol. 47, no. 8, pp. 1097–1108, 1962.

[45] Q. Luo, Y. Lai, S. Liu, M. Wu, Y. Liu, and Z. Zhang, "Deregulated expression of DNA polymerase beta is involved in the progression of genomic instability," *Environmental and Molecular Mutagenesis*, vol. 53, no. 5, pp. 325–333, 2012.

[46] A. W. Plug, C. A. Clairmont, E. Sapi, T. Ashley, and J. B. Sweasy, "Evidence for a role for DNA polymerase β in mammalian meiosis," *Proceedings of the National Academy of Sciences of the United States of America*, vol. 94, no. 4, pp. 1327–1331, 1997.

[47] D. Kidane, A. S. Jonason, T. S. Gorton et al., "DNA polymerase beta is critical for mouse meiotic synapsis," *The EMBO Journal*, vol. 29, no. 2, pp. 410–423, 2010.

[48] N. Bhattacharyya, H. C. Chen, L. Wang, and S. Banerjee, "Heterogeneity in expression of DNA polymerase β and DNA repair activity in human tumor cell lines," *Gene Expression*, vol. 10, no. 3, pp. 115–123, 2002.

[49] V. Poltoratsky, R. Prasad, J. K. Horton, and S. H. Wilson, "Down-regulation of DNA polymerase β accompanies somatic hypermutation in human BL2 cell lines," *DNA Repair*, vol. 6, no. 2, pp. 244–253, 2007.

[50] L. Servant, C. Cazaux, A. Bieth, S. Iwai, F. Hanaoka, and J.-S. Hoffmann, "A role for DNA polymerase β in mutagenic UV

lesion bypass," *The Journal of Biological Chemistry*, vol. 277, no. 51, pp. 50046–50053, 2002.

[51] K. I. Ishiguro and Y. Watanabe, "Chromosome cohesion in mitosis and meiosis," *Journal of Cell Science*, vol. 120, no. part 3, pp. 367–369, 2007.

[52] K. Nasmyth and C. H. Haering, "The structure and function of SMC and kleisin complexes," *Annual Review of Biochemistry*, vol. 74, pp. 595–648, 2005.

[53] S. L. Page and R. S. Hawley, "Chromosome choreography: the meiotic ballet," *Science*, vol. 301, no. 5634, pp. 785–789, 2003.

[54] R. Öllinger, M. Alsheimer, and R. Benavente, "Mammalian protein SCP1 forms synaptonemal complex-like structures in the absence of meiotic chromosomes," *Molecular Biology of the Cell*, vol. 16, no. 1, pp. 212–217, 2005.

[55] Y. Watanabe and P. Nurse, "Cohesin Rec8 is required for reductional chromosome segregation at meiosis," *Nature*, vol. 400, no. 6743, pp. 461–464, 1999.

[56] S. C. Sun and N. H. Kim, "Spindle assembly checkpoint and its regulators in meiosis," *Human Reproduction Update*, vol. 18, no. 1, pp. 60–72, 2012.

[57] S. Yokobayashi, M. Yamamoto, and Y. Watanabe, "Cohesins determine the attachment manner of kinetochores to spindle microtubules at meiosis I in fission yeast," *Molecular and Cellular Biology*, vol. 23, no. 11, pp. 3965–3973, 2003.

[58] S. Hauf and Y. Watanabe, "Kinetochore orientation in mitosis and meiosis," *Cell*, vol. 119, no. 3, pp. 317–327, 2004.

[59] M. Eijpe, H. Offenberg, R. Jessberger, E. Revenkova, and C. Heyting, "Meiotic cohesin REC8 marks the axial elements of rat synaptonemal complexes before cohesins SMC1β and SMC3," *Journal of Cell Biology*, vol. 160, no. 5, pp. 657–670, 2003.

[60] Y. Yao and W. Dai, "Shugoshins function as a guardian for chromosomal stability in nuclear division," *Cell Cycle*, vol. 11, no. 14, pp. 2631–2642, 2012.

[61] E. Llano, R. Gómez, C. Gutiéerrez-Caballero et al., "Shugoshin-2 is essential for the completion of meiosis but not for mitotic cell division in mice," *Genes and Development*, vol. 22, no. 17, pp. 2400–2413, 2008.

[62] N. R. Kudo, M. Anger, A. H. F. M. Peters et al., "Role of cleavage by separase of the Rec8 kleisin subunit of cohesin during mammalian meiosis I," *Journal of Cell Science*, vol. 122, no. part 15, pp. 2686–2698, 2009.

[63] T. Ishiguro, K. Tanaka, T. Sakuno, and Y. Watanabe, "Shugoshin-PP2A counteracts casein-kinase-1-dependent cleavage of Rec8 by separase," *Nature Cell Biology*, vol. 12, no. 5, pp. 500–506, 2010.

[64] J. Tammela, A. A. Jungbluth, F. Qian et al., "SCP-1 cancer/testis antigen is a prognostic indicator and a candidate target for immunotherapy in epithelial ovarian cancer," *Cancer Immunity*, vol. 4, p. 10, 2004.

[65] M. Petronczki, M. F. Siomos, and K. Nasmyth, "Un ménage à quatre: the molecular biology of chromosome segregation in meiosis," *Cell*, vol. 112, no. 4, pp. 423–440, 2003.

[66] I. L. Brito, H. G. Yu, and A. Amon, "Condensins promote coorientation of sister chromatids during meiosis I in budding yeast," *Genetics*, vol. 185, no. 1, pp. 55–64, 2010.

[67] F. Monje-Casas, V. R. Prabhu, B. H. Lee, M. Boselli, and A. Amon, "Kinetochore orientation during meiosis is controlled by Aurora B and the monopolin complex," *Cell*, vol. 128, no. 3, pp. 477–490, 2007.

[68] I. L. Brito, F. Monje-Casas, and A. Amon, "The Lrs4-Csm1 monopolin complex associates with kinetochores during

anaphase and is required for accurate chromosome segregation," *Cell Cycle*, vol. 9, no. 17, pp. 3611–3618, 2010.

[69] A. Tóth, K. P. Rabitsch, M. Gálová, A. Schleiffer, S. B. C. Buonomo, and K. Nasmyth, "Functional genomics identifies monopolin: a kinetochore protein required for segregation of homologs during meiosis I," *Cell*, vol. 103, no. 7, pp. 1155–1168, 2000.

[70] M. Schuh and J. Ellenberg, "Self-organization of MTOCs replaces centrosome function during acentrosomal spindle assembly in live mouse oocytes," *Cell*, vol. 130, no. 3, pp. 484–498, 2007.

[71] J. Dumont and A. Desai, "Acentrosomal spindle assembly and chromosome segregation during oocyte meiosis," *Trends in Cell Biology*, vol. 22, no. 5, pp. 241–249, 2012.

[72] T. S. Kitajima, S. A. Kawashima, and Y. Watanabe, "The conserved kinetochore protein shugoshin protects centromeric cohesion during meiosis," *Nature*, vol. 427, no. 6974, pp. 510–517, 2004.

[73] J. Basu, H. Bousbaa, E. Logarinho et al., "Mutations in the essential spindle checkpoint gene *Bub1* cause chromosome missegregation and fail to block apoptosis in *Drosophila*," *Journal of Cell Biology*, vol. 146, no. 1, pp. 13–28, 1999.

[74] S. Yamaguchi, A. Decottignies, and P. Nurse, "Function of Cdc2p-dependent Bub1p phosphorylation and Bub1p kinase activity in the mitotic and meiotic spindle checkpoint," *The EMBO Journal*, vol. 22, no. 5, pp. 1075–1087, 2003.

[75] S. Leland, P. Nagarajan, A. Polyzos et al., "Heterozygosity for a *Bub1* mutation causes female-specific germ cell aneuploidy in mice," *Proceedings of the National Academy of Sciences of the United States of America*, vol. 106, no. 31, pp. 12776–12781, 2009.

[76] C. Klebig, D. Korinth, and P. Meraldi, "*Bub1* regulates chromosome segregation in a kinetochore-independent manner," *Journal of Cell Biology*, vol. 185, no. 5, pp. 841–858, 2009.

[77] H. Shigeishi, N. Oue, H. Kuniyasu et al., "Expression of *Bub1* gene correlates with tumor proliferating activity in human gastric carcinomas," *Pathobiology*, vol. 69, no. 1, pp. 24–29, 2001.

[78] M. Shichiri, K. Yoshinaga, H. Hisatomi, K. Sugihara, and Y. Hirata, "Genetic and epigenetic inactivation of mitotic checkpoint genes hBUB1 and hBUBR1 and their relationship to survival," *Cancer Research*, vol. 62, no. 1, pp. 13–17, 2002.

[79] S. H. Doak, G. J. S. Jenkins, E. M. Parry, A. P. Griffiths, J. N. Baxter, and J. M. Parry, "Differential expression of the MAD2, BUB1 and HSP27 genes in Barrett's oesophagus—their association with aneuploidy and neoplastic progression," *Mutation Research*, vol. 547, no. 1-2, pp. 133–144, 2004.

[80] T. B. Lewis, J. E. Robison, R. Bastien et al., "Molecular classification of melanoma using real-time quantitative reverse transcriptase-polymerase chain reaction," *Cancer*, vol. 104, no. 8, pp. 1678–1686, 2005.

32

Oculocutaneous Albinism and Squamous Cell Carcinoma of the Skin of the Head and Neck in Sub-Saharan Africa

P. T. Lekalakala,[1] R. A. G. Khammissa,[2] B. Kramer,[3] O. A. Ayo-Yusuf,[4] J. Lemmer,[2] and L. Feller[2]

[1]Department of Maxillofacial and Oral Surgery, Sefako Makgatho Health Sciences University, Pretoria 0204, South Africa
[2]Department of Periodontology and Oral Medicine, Sefako Makgatho Health Sciences University, Pretoria 0204, South Africa
[3]School of Anatomical Sciences, Faculty of Health Sciences, University of the Witwatersrand, Johannesburg 2000, South Africa
[4]School of Oral Health Sciences, Sefako Makgatho Health Sciences University, Pretoria 0204, South Africa

Correspondence should be addressed to L. Feller; liviu.feller@smu.ac.za

Academic Editor: Iris Zalaudek

Oculocutaneous albinism which is characterised by impaired melanin biosynthesis is the most common inherited pigmentary disorder of the skin and it is common among Blacks in sub-Saharan Africa. All albinos are at great risk of developing squamous cell carcinoma of sun-exposed skin, and Black albinos in sub-Saharan Africa are at about a 1000-fold higher risk of developing squamous cell carcinoma of the skin than the general population. In Black albinos, skin carcinoma tends to run an aggressive course and is likely to recur after treatment, very probably because the aetiology and predisposing factors have not changed. Prevention or reduction of occurrence of squamous cell carcinoma of the skin in Black albinos might be achieved through educating the population to increase awareness of the harmful effects of exposure to sunlight and at the same time making available effective screening programs for early detection of premalignant and malignant skin lesions in schools and communities and for early treatment.

1. Introduction

Skin pigmentation varies between persons and is determined by multiple factors including the number and the metabolic activity of the melanocytes in the basal cell layer of the epidermis, the melanogenic activity of the melanosomes within these melanocytes, and differences in number, size, and distribution of the melanosomes. Differences in the type of melanins and differences in the degree of arborisation of the dendritic processes of the melanocytes and in the transfer of melanosomes from these processes to surrounding keratinocytes will also affect the pigmentation of the skin [1, 2].

Melanin biosynthesis is regulated by several factors, particularly by melanocortin-1 receptor (MC1R) on the melanocytes and its ligand, α-melanocyte stimulating hormone (αMSH). Cytokines and growth factors in the microenvironment and the degree of basal activity of tyrosinase, tyrosinase related protein 1 (TRP1), and membrane associated transport proteins are additional factors regulating this biosynthesis [2, 3]. One of the important functions of melanin is protecting the skin and eyes from the harmful effects of ultraviolet radiation (UVR).

Melanocytes of the skin and uveal tract of the eyes are derived from neural crest cells. A number of genes control the proliferation and differentiation of neural crest cells and also regulate the migration of precursor melanocytes to their ultimate positions in the skin and eye. Microphthalmia transcription factor (MITF) is the master regulator of melanocyte development, function, and survival [4] and is responsible for modulating expression of some melanocyte-specific proteins [5]. Following differentiation of melanocytes, MITF regulates expression of genes during exposure to UVR, thus assisting in tanning of the skin [6]. Transfer of the melanin to surrounding keratinocytes and the production of a nuclear cap protect the DNA from UVR damage [2, 7]. The degree of pigmentation of the skin is said to correlate inversely with the risk of sun-induced skin cancers [6].

Oculocutaneous albinism (OCA) is an autosomal recessive disorder of melanocyte differentiation brought about by defects in the pathway of melanin biosynthesis, by defects in melanosome biogenesis or function, or by dysregulation of intracellular transport and localization of proteins essential for melanin production [8]. The typical clinical manifestations of OCA can vary greatly and comprise partial or complete lack of melanin pigmentation of the skin, reduced visual acuity, and ocular nystagmus [8–10]. The number and distribution of melanocytes in OCA are normal. Albinos with total lack of melanin have white skin and hair and pink eyes, and they sunburn easily [11]. However, albinos with only partially reduced capacity for melanin biosynthesis will acquire some pigmentation during life [12].

OCA predisposes to squamous cell carcinoma of the skin (SCCS), particularly of the sun-exposed head and neck [13, 14]. SCCS is more frequent, runs a more aggressive course, and tends to have a higher rate of recurrence in Black albinos than in normally pigmented persons, whether Black or White [8, 15–17]. Surprisingly, in Black albinos, SCCS of the head and neck is more prevalent than basal cell carcinoma, and cutaneous melanoma of the head and neck is rare [18, 19]. In this short paper we will discuss some pathogenic mechanisms of SCCS in albinos and elaborate on public health measures to reduce its incidence.

2. Oculocutaneous Albinism

There are five types of OCA; of these OCA1 and OCA2 are by far the most frequent types. OCA type 1 (OCA1) occurs with a frequency of about 1/40 000 worldwide [20], affects different racial/ethnic groups equally, and is characterized by loss of function of the enzyme tyrosinase (TYR) as a result of a mutation in the TYR gene. Tyrosinase is the critical enzyme in the biosynthesis of both brown-black eumelanin and yellow-red pheomelanin. Persons with OCA1A have completely nonfunctional TYR, with no melanin production, while in persons with OCA1B there is some tyrosinase functional activity with limited melanin production [10, 12, 21].

OCA2 is the most common form of albinism worldwide [6], prevalent in southern Africa. It affects Blacks more commonly than Whites and is characterized by mutations in the OCA2 gene (formerly known as the P gene) that encodes the p protein [10, 21]. Its precise functions are not fully understood but p protein appears to be involved in transporting proteins to the melanosome, in stabilizing the melanosomal protein complex, and in regulating melanosomal pH and/or glutathione metabolism, all of which are important to melanin production [10, 21, 22]. Albinos with an OCA2 phenotype have no eumelanin but have some pheomelanin which may increase with age [9, 10, 23]. OCA2 is the most common phenotype affecting Black South African albinos, with an overall prevalence of OCA2 albinism of one in 3900 persons [23–25].

The OCA3 and the OCA4 phenotypes of albinism are caused by mutations in genes encoding tyrosinase related protein 1 (TRP1) and membrane associated transport protein (MATP), respectively [9]. TYPR1 is an enzyme which stabilizes tyrosinase. Mutations in TYPR1 are associated with early degradation of tyrosinase and with delayed maturation of melanosomes [16, 21]. MATP functions as a melanosomal

membrane transporter of proteins necessary for melanin biosynthesis, and mutations in the MATP gene consequently cause hypopigmentation and the OCA4 phenotype of albinism [16, 21]. OCA5 phenotype is linked to an as yet unidentified specific gene mapped to the 4q24 chromosomal region and was discovered in the members of a consanguineous Pakistani family [26, 27].

At birth, persons with the different phenotypic forms of OCA all have white hair and very pale and pink-white skin. Those with OCA1B, OCA2, OCA3, or OCA4 will acquire some pigmentation during life, but those with OCA1A will remain completely unpigmented [9, 21]. The degree of pigmentation associated with OCA5 phenotype is not clear [26, 27].

3. Melanin and SCCS

Cutaneous melanin, particularly brown/black eumelanin, provides protection both against sunlight and against oxidative stress-induced DNA damage so that dark-skinned persons have a lower frequency of SCCS than do light-skinned persons. However, the photoprotection afforded by melanin is not complete even in dark-skinned persons who can also sustain sunlight-induced DNA damage, but this damage is usually of a degree that can be repaired by cellular DNA repair mechanisms thus reducing the risk of malignant transformation. On the other hand, in light-skinned persons who lack sufficient melanin to provide effective protection against sunlight, the extent of the sunlight-induced DNA damage may exceed the capacity of these cellular DNA repair mechanisms, with increased risk of malignant transformation [12]. Albinos who have very little, if any, melanin in their skin are thus very susceptible to sunlight-induced SCCS.

In this connection it may be noted that xeroderma pigmentosum, in which there is inherently impaired functional activity of DNA repair mechanisms, can affect either dark-skinned or light-skinned persons, and both groups have equal frequency of SCCS [28]. This highlights the fact that effectively functioning cellular DNA repair mechanisms are more important in preventing SCCS than the quantum of melanin pigment in sun-exposed skin.

The melanin present in OCA is mainly pheomelanin, while the production of eumelanin is minimal [29]. Eumelanin has an important photoprotective role, but although pheomelanin does afford some sunlight photoprotection, during its biosynthesis, reactive oxygen species (ROS) which are carcinogenic are generated. Therefore, in albinos, both reduction in eumelanin photoprotection and elevation of pheomelanin-derived ROS are implicated in SCCS [9].

The biosynthesis of both types of melanin, brown/black eumelanin and yellow/red pheomelanin, is controlled to a large extent by the melanocortin-1 receptor (MC1R) on the melanocytes. Albinos with the OCA2 phenotype who possess polymorphic gene variants of MC1R, in contrast to most other albinos, may have reddish hair and a yellowish tinge to their skin [30]. In this regard, it has been reported that the OCA2 phenotype of albinism can be brought about solely by a mutated MC1R gene [31].

The activity of some MC1R variants can counteract apoptosis and reduce the capacity for the DNA repair of melanocytes. They can also indirectly reduce protection of keratinocytes from sunlight-induced DNA damage because of the reduced eumelanin production, thus increasing the risk of skin cancer. MC1R gene variants are associated not only with dysregulated melanin production and reduced tanning capacity, but also with modulation of host immunoinflammatory responses which are important in immune surveillance and in the killing of sunlight transformed keratinocytes [1, 29, 32]. In this regard, genetic polymorphisms of other genes encoding agents involved in melanin biosynthesis (TYR and TRP1), beside determining skin pigmentation, are in fact also factors contributing to the risk of developing skin cancer [1]; and it has been suggested that functionally active tyrosinase has the capacity to protect against oxidative DNA damage [33].

4. Sunlight-Induced Malignant Transformation

As most persons with severe forms of OCA are very prone to sunburn [21], the progenitor basal cell keratinocytes of sun-exposed skin of albinos are at great risk of undergoing sunlight-induced malignant transformation. SCCS in albinos can arise *de novo* or from premalignant actinic lesions such as sunlight keratosis, in which the keratinocytes have already undergone sunlight-induced initial transformation. The basal cell keratinocytes will sustain DNA damage of different degrees of severity according to the intensity and duration of exposure to sunlight. Normally, the p53 tumour-suppressor gene arrests the cell cycle, allowing for the repair of the damaged DNA, or promotes apoptosis if the DNA damage is irreparable. However, if sunlight induces mutations in p53 itself rendering it dysfunctional, there will be propagation of damaged DNA by cell division, resulting in a precancerized epithelial field composed of a clone of initially transformed keratinocytes with genomic instability. This genomic instability predisposes the initially transformed keratinocytes to additional genetic alterations and may drive the processes of clonal divergence with consequent clonal expansion of keratinocytes possessing a selective growth advantage, ultimately giving rise to a frank SCCS [12, 34, 35]. The risk of SCCS is proportional to the accumulated quantum of UVR absorbed by the keratinocytes [31], but ultimately the potential for malignant change is determined by the number of genetic insults. Thus, numerous smaller frequent exposures to sunlight are more likely to be carcinogenic than greater but infrequent exposures to sunlight [36], because each exposure event has the potential to cause a genetic change. The more the genetic alterations occur, the greater the chance of malignant transformation will be.

As albinos are photosensitive and tend to sunburn readily, sunlight-induced local inflammation in the skin can be an additional factor in bringing about an increase in proliferation and longevity of basal keratinocytes favouring initial malignant transformation. After sunburn, local inflammatory cell-derived ROS can directly cause DNA damage, dysregulating the mechanisms not only of DNA repair and of cell cycle checkpoint control but also of apoptosis, promoting evolution of SCCS [37].

At the molecular level, UVR-induced DNA damage is characterized by substitution of specific nucleotides, particularly C > T and CC > TT transitions found in the p53 gene that encodes the p53 protein, which normally regulates the cell cycle, apoptosis, and DNA repair. Sunlight regularly causes these genetic alterations that are referred to as UVR-associated "signature mutations," and these signature mutations drive the malignant transformation of sunlight-induced SCCS [36, 38].

Initially transformed keratinocytes are immunogenic and thus generate immune responses which can modulate or control tumourigenesis; but sunlight-induced immunosuppression may critically interfere with this protective mechanism [39].

The risk of SCCS in Black albinos is 1000 times greater than the risk in the general population, and the head and neck region is most frequently affected (Figure 1) [14, 40]. By the third decade of life, many Black albinos in Africa will have developed potentially fatal SCCS [16, 40], but if diagnosed at an early stage, SCCS is curable by surgical excision. Timely recognition of the disease is therefore crucial.

It is not clear what effect HIV-induced immune impairment or the virus itself may have on the aetiopathogenesis of SCCS [41, 42]. However, the frequency of squamous cell carcinoma of the lip (Figure 2) is reportedly increased in HIV-seropositive immunosuppressed subjects as compared to immunocompetent HIV-seronegative subjects [42, 43]. What the impact of HIV or HIV-induced immune impairment on SCCS in albinos is, is unknown and requires further research [42, 44].

5. Public Health Measures to Minimise SCCS in Albinos

The objectives of cancer management in the field of public health are reduction of the incidence, early detection, and prompt treatment of the disease when it occurs. Universal precautions against sunlight exposure should be introduced early in childhood, continue throughout life, and should include minimising of outdoor activities during peak sunlight hours, the wearing of protective clothing to cover as much of the skin as possible, and the use of sunscreen preparations for exposed skin [12, 34].

However in general, public health measures to minimise sunlight-induced damage to the skin of populations in Africa are often unsuccessful because of poverty, lack of understanding of the problem, and lack of compliance even when they have been informed about preventive measures [13, 40]. Moreover, in Africa, Black albinos are often subject to social discrimination because of superstitious beliefs and the stigma associated with albinism [12, 45, 46]. They are therefore often shunned by their communities with consequent delay in seeking and obtaining medical treatment until late in the course of any premalignant or malignant actinic lesions. Thus, by the time of diagnosis, SCCS in Black albinos is often advanced and has a poor prognosis [12, 47]. It has been

(a)

(b)

(c)

(d)

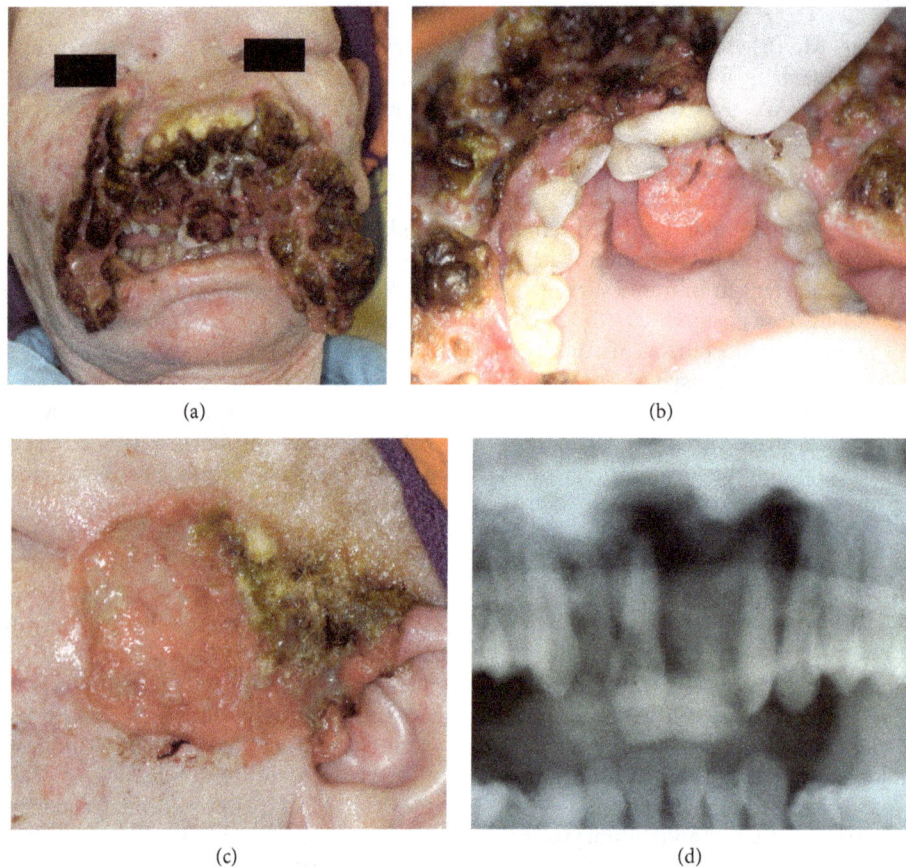

FIGURE 1: Squamous cell carcinomas (SCCs) in a 38-year-old HIV-seropositive Black albino woman. (a) SCC of the nose, cheeks and the lips, and (b) the labial mucosa and anterior part of the palate. The disease started as a small ulcer on the upper lip 18 months previously, progressing rapidly to involve the mouth and to destroy the lower face. (c) SCC of the left ear and temple started 8 months previously. (d) Panoramic radiograph showing destruction of the anterior maxilla. Histopathologically, the carcinoma was poorly differentiated. The patient died before investigation for metastases could be done. The extensive and striking sunlight-induced malignant facial damage is tragic evidence of the consequence of lack of sun-protection from an early age and of appropriate early medical care.

reported that on average Black albinos in Africa seek medical treatment 9–12 months after the onset of any actinic lesions [40, 47].

Sadly, about 40% of Black albinos in Africa with SCCS do not complete their treatment owing either to financial constraints [13] or to distance from medical facilities and are lost to follow-up. These may be the reasons why SCCS are more frequent and tend to have a higher rate of recurrence in Black albinos in Africa than in normally pigmented persons, whether Black or White [8, 15, 16].

It may be possible to reduce the prevalence of SCCS in Black albinos in Africa [47] if public health personnel were regularly to visit remote villages to screen for premalignant and malignant skin lesions in the albino population and to educate them on the harmful effects of exposure to solar radiation. This would need to be supplemented by accessible treatment centres, where treatment of early SCCS could be done [48], and by the establishment of educational support groups.

6. Conclusion

While there is still a need for further research on prevalence of albinism in Africa, measures directed at reducing the

incidence of SCCS in members of the albino community and at alerting those with premalignant actinic skin lesions to the benefits of early detection and treatment should include education about the risk factors associated with SCCS and about the hazards of delaying the seeking of professional advice. There is also a need to educate the population at large about albinism with the aim of promoting greater social integration of albinos into their communities.

Professional measures to prevent and control SCCS in albinos should include the institution of screening programmes with a view to identifying potentially malignant actinic skin lesions and detection of early SCCS and to make available immediate effective psychological and medical treatment.

Abbreviations

MC1R: Melanocortin-1 receptor
αMSH: α-melanocyte stimulating hormone
TRP1: Tyrosinase related protein
UVR: Ultraviolet radiation
MITF: Microphthalmia transcription factor
OCA: Oculocutaneous albinism

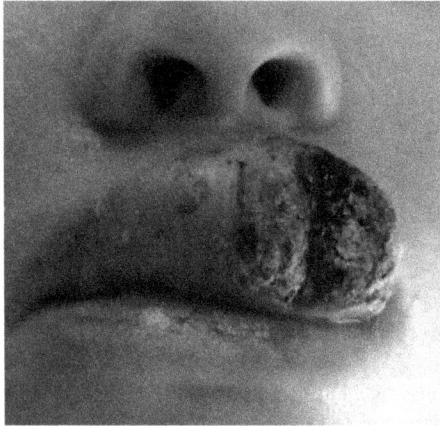

FIGURE 2: A 21-year-old HIV-seropositive Black albino woman with an exophytic crusted SCC of the upper lip, twelve months after she first noticed a small painless erosion. There was neither local lymph node involvement nor distant metastasis, and microscopically the carcinoma was moderately differentiated.

SCCS: Squamous cell carcinoma of the skin
TYR: Tyrosinase
MATP: Membrane associated transport protein
ROS: Reactive oxygen species.

Authors' Contribution

P. T. Lekalakala, R. A. G. Khammissa, B. Kramer, O. A. Ayo-Yusuf, J. Lemmer, and L. Feller provided the study concept and participated in its design and coordination. P. T. Lekalakala and R. A. G. Khammissa performed the clinical work and case management. B. Kramer, O. A. Ayo-Yusuf, J. Lemmer, and L. Feller were responsible for paper editing. B. Kramer, J. Lemmer, and L. Feller reviewed the paper. All authors read and approved the final paper.

References

[1] D. Scherer and R. Kumar, "Genetics of pigmentation in skin cancer—a review," *Mutation Research*, vol. 705, no. 2, pp. 141–153, 2010.

[2] L. Feller, A. Masilana, R. A. G. Khammissa, M. Altini, Y. Jadwat, and J. Lemmer, "Melanin: the biophysiology of oral melanocytes and physiological oral pigmentation," *Head and Face Medicine*, vol. 10, no. 1, article 8, 2014.

[3] G. Ficarra, S. Di Lollo, G. Asirelli, and I. Rubino, "Melanocytic activation in HIV disease: HMB-45 positivity in oral melanotic macules," *Oral Surgery, Oral Medicine, Oral Pathology, Oral Radiology, and Endodontology*, vol. 80, no. 4, p. 457, 1995.

[4] C. Levy, M. Khaled, and D. E. Fisher, "MITF: master regulator of melanocyte development and melanoma oncogene," *Trends in Molecular Medicine*, vol. 12, no. 9, pp. 406–414, 2006.

[5] A. Kawakami and D. E. Fisher, "Key discoveries in melanocyte development," *Journal of Investigative Dermatology*, vol. 131, no. 1, pp. E2–E4, 2011.

[6] P. Manga, R. Kerr, M. Ramsay, and J. G. R. Kromberg, "Biology and genetics of oculocutaneous albinism and vitiligo—common pigmentation disorders in southern Africa," *South African Medical Journal*, vol. 103, no. 12, pp. 984–988, 2013.

[7] M. Seiberg, "Keratinocyte—melanocyte interactions during melanosome transfer," *Pigment Cell Research*, vol. 14, no. 4, pp. 236–242, 2001.

[8] M. Castori, A. Morrone, J. Kanitakis, and P. Grammatico, "Genetic skin diseases predisposing to basal cell carcinoma," *European Journal of Dermatology*, vol. 22, no. 3, pp. 299–309, 2012.

[9] H. C. de Vijlder, J. J. M. de Vijlder, and H. A. M. Neumann, "Oculocutaneous albinism and skin cancer risk," *Journal of the European Academy of Dermatology and Venereology*, vol. 27, no. 3, pp. e433–e434, 2013.

[10] V. Nikolaou, A. J. Stratigos, and H. Tsao, "Hereditary non-melanoma skin cancer," *Seminars in Cutaneous Medicine and Surgery*, vol. 31, no. 4, pp. 204–210, 2012.

[11] N. H. Wood and A. Moodley, "Oral medicine case book 51: actinic cheilitis in a patient with oculocutaneous albinism," *Journal of the South African Dental Association*, vol. 68, no. 6, pp. 278–281, 2013.

[12] N. H. Wood, R. Khammissa, R. Meyerov, J. Lemmer, and L. Feller, "Actinic cheilitis: a case report and a review of the literature," *European Journal of Dentistry*, vol. 5, no. 1, pp. 101–106, 2011.

[13] J. B. Mabula, P. L. Chalya, M. D. Mchembe et al., "Skin cancers among Albinos at a University teaching hospital in Northwestern Tanzania: a retrospective review of 64 cases," *BMC Dermatology*, vol. 12, article 5, 2012.

[14] G. Mapurisa and L. Masamba, "Locally advanced skin cancer in an albino: a treatment dilemma," *Malawi Medical Journal*, vol. 22, no. 4, pp. 122–123, 2010.

[15] E. Berger, R. Hunt, J. Tzu, R. Patel, and M. Sanchez, "Squamous-cell carcinoma in situ in a patient with oculocutaneous albinism," *Dermatology Online Journal*, vol. 17, no. 10, p. 22, 2011.

[16] C. V. David, "Oculocutaneous albinism," *Cutis*, vol. 91, no. 5, pp. E1–E4, 2013.

[17] A. Yakubu and O. A. Mabogunje, "Skin cancer in African albinos," *Acta Oncologica*, vol. 32, no. 6, pp. 621–622, 1993.

[18] J. B. Mabula, P. L. Chalya, M. D. Mchembe et al., "Skin cancers among Albinos at a University teaching hospital in Northwestern Tanzania: a retrospective review of 64 cases," *BMC Dermatology*, vol. 12, article 5, pp. 5–13, 2012.

[19] M. E. Asuquo and G. Ebughe, "Major dermatological malignancies encountered in the University of Calabar Teaching Hospital, Calabar, southern Nigeria," *International Journal of Dermatology*, vol. 51, supplement 1, pp. 32–36, 2012.

[20] W. S. Oetting and R. A. King, "Molecular basis of Type I (tryrosinase-related) oculocutaneous albinism: mutations and polymorphisms of the human tyrosinase gene," *Human Mutation*, vol. 2, no. 1, pp. 1–6, 1993.

[21] K. Grønskov, J. Ek, and K. Brondum-Nielsen, "Oculocutaneous albinism," *Orphanet Journal of Rare Diseases*, vol. 2, no. 1, article 43, 2007.

[22] J. E. Hawkes, P. B. Cassidy, P. Manga et al., "Report of a novel *OCA2* gene mutation and an investigation of *OCA2* variants on melanoma risk in a familial melanoma pedigree," *Journal of Dermatological Science*, vol. 69, no. 1, pp. 30–37, 2013.

[23] G. Stevens, J. van Beukering, T. Jenkins, and M. Ramsay, "An intragenic deletion of the P gene is the common mutation causing tyrosinase-positive oculocutaneous albinism in southern African Negroids," *American Journal of Human Genetics*, vol. 56, no. 3, pp. 586–591, 1995.

[24] G. Stevens, M. Ramsay, and T. Jenkins, "Oculocutaneous albinism (OCA2) in sub-Saharan Africa: distribution of the common 2.7-kb P gene deletion mutation," *Human Genetics*, vol. 99, no. 4, pp. 523–527, 1997.

[25] R. Kerr, G. Stevens, P. Manga et al., "Identification of P gene mutations in individuals with oculocutaneous albinism in Sub-Saharan Africa," *Human Mutation*, vol. 15, no. 2, pp. 166–172, 2000.

[26] L. Montoliu, K. Grønskov, A.-H. Wei et al., "Increasing the complexity: new genes and new types of albinism," *Pigment Cell and Melanoma Research*, vol. 27, no. 1, pp. 11–18, 2014.

[27] T. Kausar, M. A. Bhatti, M. Ali, R. Shaikh, and Z. Ahmed, "OCA5, a novel locus for non-syndromic oculocutaneous albinism, maps to chromosome 4q24," *Clinical Genetics*, vol. 84, no. 1, pp. 91–93, 2013.

[28] L. Feller, M. Bouckaert, U. M. Chikte et al., "A short account of cancer–specifically in relation to squamous cell carcinoma.," *SADJ*, vol. 65, no. 7, pp. 322–324, 2010.

[29] M. Sengupta, D. Sarkar, M. Mondal, S. Samanta, A. Sil, and K. Ray, "Analysis of MC1R variants in Indian oculocutaneous albinism patients: highlighting the risk of skin cancer among albinos," *Journal of Genetics*, vol. 92, no. 2, pp. 305–308, 2013.

[30] R. A. King, R. K. Willaert, R. M. Schmidt et al., "MC1R mutations modify the classic phenotype of oculocutaneous albinism type 2 (OCA2)," *The American Journal of Human Genetics*, vol. 73, no. 3, pp. 638–645, 2003.

[31] S. B. Saleha, M. Ajaml, M. Jamil, M. Nasir, and A. Hameed, "MC1R gene mutation and its association with oculocutaneous albinism type (OCA) phenotype in a consanguineous Pakistani family," *Journal of Dermatological Science*, vol. 70, no. 1, pp. 68–70, 2013.

[32] D. Scherer, J. L. Bermejo, P. Rudnai et al., "MC1R variants associated susceptibility to basal cell carcinoma of skin: interaction with host factors and XRCC3 polymorphism," *International Journal of Cancer*, vol. 122, no. 8, pp. 1787–1793, 2008.

[33] A. Saran, M. Spinola, S. Pazzaglia et al., "Loss of tyrosinase activity confers increased skin tumor susceptibility in mice," *Oncogene*, vol. 23, no. 23, pp. 4130–4135, 2004.

[34] L. Feller, R. A. G. Khammissa, N. H. Wood, Y. Jadwat, R. Meyerov, and J. Lemmer, "Sunlight (actinic) keratosis: an update," *Journal of Preventive Medicine and Hygiene*, vol. 50, no. 4, pp. 217–220, 2009.

[35] L. L. Feller, R. R. A. G. Khammissa, B. B. Kramer, and J. J. Lemmer, "Oral squamous cell carcinoma in relation to field precancerisation: pathobiology," *Cancer Cell International*, vol. 13, no. 1, article 31, 2013.

[36] L. Andreassi, "UV exposure as a risk factor for skin cancer," *Expert Review of Dermatology*, vol. 6, no. 5, pp. 445–454, 2011.

[37] L. Feller, M. Altini, and J. Lemmer, "Inflammation in the context of oral cancer," *Oral Oncology*, vol. 49, no. 9, pp. 887–892, 2013.

[38] E. D. Pleasance, R. K. Cheetham, P. J. Stephens et al., "A comprehensive catalogue of somatic mutations from a human cancer genome," *Nature*, vol. 463, no. 7278, pp. 191–196, 2010.

[39] M. H. Motswaledi, R. A. Khammissa, N. H. Wood, R. Meyerov, J. Lemmer, and L. Feller, "Discoid lupus erythematosus as it relates to cutaneous squamous cell carcinoma and to photosensitivity," *Journal of the South African Dental Association*, vol. 66, no. 7, pp. 340–343, 2011.

[40] M. E. Asuquo, O. O. Otei, J. Omotoso, and E. E. Bassey, "Letter: skin cancer in albinos at the University of Calabar Teaching Hospital, Calabar, Nigeria," *Dermatology Online Journal*, vol. 16, no. 4, p. 14, 2010.

[41] L. Kinlen, "Infections and immune factors in cancer: the role of epidemiology," *Oncogene*, vol. 23, no. 38, pp. 6341–6348, 2004.

[42] A. E. Grulich, M. T. van Leeuwen, M. O. Falster, and C. M. Vajdic, "Incidence of cancers in people with HIV/AIDS compared with immunosuppressed transplant recipients: a meta-analysis," *The Lancet*, vol. 370, no. 9581, pp. 59–67, 2007.

[43] M. Frisch, R. J. Biggar, E. A. Engels, and J. J. Goedert, "Association of cancer with AIDS-related immunosuppression in adults," *Journal of the American Medical Association*, vol. 285, no. 13, pp. 1736–1745, 2001.

[44] E. A. Engels, "Non-AIDS-defining malignancies in HIV-infected persons: etiologic puzzles, epidemiologic perils, prevention opportunities," *AIDS*, vol. 23, no. 8, pp. 875–885, 2009.

[45] A. E. Cruz-Inigo, B. Ladizinski, and A. Sethi, "Albinism in Africa: stigma, slaughter and awareness campaigns," *Dermatologic Clinics*, vol. 29, no. 1, pp. 79–87, 2011.

[46] P. M. Lund and R. Gaigher, "A health intervention programme for children with albinism at a special school in South Africa," *Health Education Research*, vol. 17, no. 3, pp. 365–372, 2002.

[47] K. O. Opara and B. C. Jiburum, "Skin cancers in albinos in a teaching Hospital in eastern Nigeria—presentation and challenges of care," *World Journal of Surgical Oncology*, vol. 8, article 73, 2010.

[48] E. S. Hong, H. Zeeb, and M. H. Repacholi, "Albinism in Africa as a public health issue," *BMC Public Health*, vol. 6, article no. 212, 2006.

33

A Study of Basal Cell Carcinoma in South Asians for Risk Factor and Clinicopathological Characterization: A Hospital Based Study

Sumir Kumar,[1,2] **Bharat Bhushan Mahajan,**[1,2] **Sandeep Kaur,**[1,2] **Ashish Yadav,**[2,3] **Navtej Singh,**[2,3] **and Amarbir Singh**[1,2]

[1] *Department of Dermatology, Venereology & Leprology, Guru Gobind Singh Medical College & Hospital, Sadiq Road, Faridkot, Punjab 151203, India*
[2] *Department of Skin & V.D., OPD Block, Guru Gobind Singh Medical College & Hospital, Sadiq Road, Faridkot, Punjab 151203, India*
[3] *Department of Pathology, Guru Gobind Singh Medical College & Hospital, Sadiq Road, Faridkot, Punjab 151203, India*

Correspondence should be addressed to Sandeep Kaur; docsandeep_2005@yahoo.com

Academic Editor: Mark Lebwohl

Objectives. Although the incidence of skin cancers in India (part of South Asia) is low, the absolute number of cases may be significant due to large population. The existing literature on BCC in India is scant. So, this study was done focusing on its epidemiology, risk factors, and clinicopathological aspects. *Methods.* A hospital based cross-sectional study was conducted in Punjab, North India, from 2011 to 2013. History, examination and histopathological confirmation were done in all the patients visiting skin department with suspected lesions. *Results.* Out of 36 confirmed cases, 63.9% were females with mean ± SD age being 60.9 ± 14.2 years. Mean duration of disease was 4.7 years. Though there was statistically significant higher sun exposure in males compared to females (*P* value being 0.000), BCC was commoner in females, explainable by intermittent sun exposure (during household work in the open kitchens) in women. Majority of patients (88.9%) had a single lesion. Head and neck region was involved in 97.2% of cases, with nose being the commonest site (50%) with nodular/noduloulcerative morphology in 77.8% of cases. Pigmentation was evident in 22.2% of cases clinically. Nodular variety was the commonest histopathological variant (77.8%). *Conclusions.* This study highlights a paradoxically increasing trend of BCC with female preponderance, preferential involvement of nose, and higher percentage of pigmentation in Indians.

1. Introduction

Jacob Arthurin 1827 first coined the term "rodent ulcer" to describe what we now know as a basal cell carcinoma (BCC) [1]. It is the most common cutaneous malignancy worldwide, accounting for 65–75% of all skin cancers. Gross differences are noted in the percentage of skin cancer in the Asians (2–4%) and Blacks (1-2%) as compared to the Caucasians (35–40%) [2]. Although the incidence of skin cancers in India is lower as compared to the Western world, absolute number of cases may be significant due to large population. The existing literature on BCC in India is scant with lack of clinical studies with statistical analysis [3]. So, this study was undertaken to fill this deficit in literature of BCC with focus on epidemiology, risk factors, and clinical and pathological aspects of the disease.

BCC is a nonmelanocytic skin malignancy arising from basal cells of the epidermis or follicular structures and is seen mostly on sun exposed areas, especially head and neck, occasionally over the trunk and limbs, and rarely on the palms, soles, mucous membranes, and genitals [4, 5].

The anatomic distribution of BCC correlates with embryonic fusion planes. Recently, it has been indicated that BCC occurrence is higher along embryonic fusion planes as compared to other areas of the midface, evidence that supports this hypothesis for BCC pathogenesis [6].

Ninety-five percent of these neoplasms occur in patients aged more than 40 years, although cases in childhood and congenital basal cell epitheliomas have been reported [7–9]. In children, it is usually associated with a genetic defect, such as basal cell nevus syndrome, xeroderma pigmentosum, nevus sebaceous, epidermodysplasia verruciformis, Rombo syndrome, or Bazex syndrome.

Sunlight is the most frequent association with development of BCC; risk correlates with the amount and nature of accumulated exposure, especially during childhood. A latency period of 20–50 years is typical between the time of ultraviolet (UV) damage and BCC clinical onset. Both UVB radiation and UVA radiation contribute to the formation of BCC. UVB is believed to play a greater role in the development of BCC than UVA [10]. In a 2012 systematic review and meta-analysis of 12 studies with 9328 cases of nonmelanoma skin cancer, Wehner et al. found that indoor tanning was associated with a significantly increased risk of both basal and squamous cell skin cancers. The risk was highest among users of indoor tanning before age 25 [11]. Apart from UVR, X-ray and Grenz ray exposure is also linked with development of BCC.

Arsenic has been used as a medicinal agent, predominantly the Fowler solution of potassium arsenite, which was used to treat many disorders, including asthma and psoriasis, and is linked to the risk of development of multiple malignancies after a long latency period spanning many years.

The risk of developing new nonmelanoma skin cancer is reported to be 35% at 3 years and 50% at 5 years after an initial skin cancer diagnosis [12]. A study among adults in the United States reports a strong association between excessive alcohol drinking and higher incidence of sunburn, suggesting a linkage between alcohol consumption and skin cancer [13].

2. Methods

A hospital based study was conducted at a tertiary care hospital situated in Punjab, North India, from 2011 to 2013. Patients of all ages attending skin outpatient department with suspected lesions were screened for BCC after taking an informed written consent. Patients with histopathologically confirmed BCC were enrolled in the study.

Detailed history with recording of various patient variables like age, gender, duration of symptoms, Fitzpatrick skin phototype, skin color, average daily sun exposure (hours/day), occupation, residence place (rural or urban), exposure to chemicals including pesticides, radiation exposure history, treatment with psoralen UVA (PUVA) or narrow band UVB (NBUVB), smoking, alcohol intake, history of personal or family history of skin cancers, personal or family history of other cancers, history of genetic disorder like xeroderma pigmentosum, albinism, and history of previous treatment.

Clinical examination was done with data collection on various tumor variables which included the following: size, location, number, morphological subtype, and pigmentation. For descriptive purposes, the lesions were classified based on size into small (less than 1 cm in diameter), medium (1-2 cm in diameter), and large (>2 cm in diameter).

TABLE 1: Age-sex distribution of BCC.

Age (years)	Males	Females	Total	Fisher exact test P value
21–60	4	13	17	
61–100	9	10	19	0.177[NS]
Total	**13**	**23**	**36**	

For application of appropriate statistical tests, only two age groups were considered.
NS: not significant at 5% level of significance.

TABLE 2: Association between duration of disease and educational status.

Duration of disease (years)	Educational status Educated	Illiterate	Total	χ^2 value (d.f.)	P value
0–5	7	13	20		
More than 5	0	16	16	6.95 (1)	0.01[s]
Total	**7**	**29**	**36**		

S: significant at 5% level of significance.

Investigations included complete blood count with differentials, bleeding time, clotting time, renal function tests, liver function tests, and viral markers. Additional investigations were done depending upon the clinical scenario. Diagnosis was confirmed by histopathological examination of biopsy specimen with documentation of histopathological variant. To analyze the results, descriptive statistics such as mean, standard deviation (SD), and frequency tables were utilized. Various analytic tests such as χ^2 test, P value, and t-test were used. P value less than 5% was considered as significant.

3. Results

3.1. Demographic Data. A total of 36 histopathologically confirmed cases of BCC were enrolled in the study from 2011 to 2013. An increase was seen in absolute number of cases diagnosed per year with 9, 11, and 16 patients in 2011, 2012, and 2013, respectively (Figure 6).

Out of these patients, males were 36.1% (13/36) and females were 63.9% (23/36) with M : F being equal to 0.57 : 1 (Figure 7). Age of the affected cases ranged from 29 to 92 years of age. The mean ± SD age of the patients was 60.9 ± 14.2 years (65.92 ± 14.35 years for males and 57.96 ± 13.54 years in case of females). Although the difference in mean age between males and females was not statistically significant (data was analyzed using unpaired t-test), it carries a clinical relevance as females tend to seek medical care earlier than males for suspicious, asymptomatic, and cosmetically disfiguring lesions. The greatest number of patients was in the age group of 61–80 years (47.2%) followed by 41–60 years (38.95%), 21–40 years (8.3%), and 81–100 years (5.6%), respectively (Figure 8). The youngest age of presentation in case of females was 29 years, while in males the corresponding age was 45 years. Correlation between gender and age group was not statistically significant (Fisher exact test P value being 0.177), implying that these two variables are independent (Table 1).

Out of all patients, 69.4% (25/36) hailed from rural areas. Majority of the patients were illiterate (80.6%) (Table 2). A

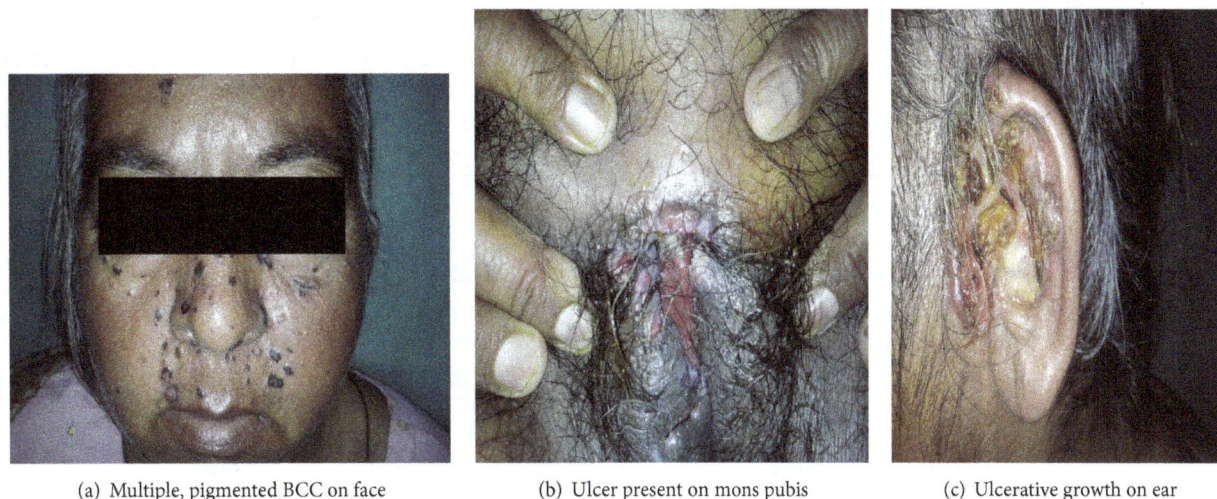

(a) Multiple, pigmented BCC on face   (b) Ulcer present on mons pubis   (c) Ulcerative growth on ear

FIGURE 1: Metastatic BCC.

TABLE 3: Sex-wise comparison of duration of sun exposure.

Gender	Number (n)	Mean duration (hours/day) of sun exposure	Standard deviation SD	χ^2 value (d.f.)	P value
Male	13	6	1.15	6.71 (1)	0.000[HS]
Female	23	2.91	1.41		

HS: highly significant.

statistically significant association was seen between duration of disease and illiteracy (χ^2 value = 6.95 and P value = 0.01). This meant that illiterate patients present at a later stage of disease attributable to lack of awareness about disease entity. Farming was the main occupation among male patients (92.3%), while housekeeping was the major job among female patients (95.7%).

3.2. Clinical Data.
The duration of disease before seeking medical care ranged from 5 months to as long as 15 years, with mean duration being 4.7 years. The average duration of sun exposure was 6 hours/day in case of males and 2.91 hours/day in female patients. This difference in duration of sun exposure was statistically significant (t-value being 6.71 and P value = 0.000) (Table 3). However, the females were intermittently exposed to high intensity sunlight due to work in open kitchens and fields during sowing and harvesting seasons.

None of the patients had been taking photoprotective measures such as use of sunscreens and protective clothing. There was no history of treatment with PUVA or NBUVB in any of the study cases. All the patients were nonalcoholics and nonsmokers. No patient had features suggestive of genodermatoses associated with predilection for cutaneous malignancies like xeroderma pigmentosa, albinism, and so forth. Out of 36 patients, one (2.8%) had been previously treated for breast and endometrial carcinoma. Family history of cutaneous and systemic malignancies was not present in any of them. All the cases belonged to Fitzpatrick skin types III and IV (calculated via Fitzpatrick scoring scale).

Majority of patients (88.9%) had a solitary lesion. Out of total 36 patients, two (5.6%) had 2 lesions at the time of presentation. One female (2.8%) patient had multiple lesions over face followed by development of ulcerative growths on ear and mons pubis. She was later diagnosed with BCC having noncontiguous and distant cutaneous metastasis (Figure 1). Another female patient had multifocal lesions on eyelid, temple, and nose. This patient was previously treated for breast and endometrial carcinoma.

The size of lesions ranged from as small as 0.5 cm to 5 cm in diameter. The size of lesions was found to have a statistically significant association with duration of disease (χ^2 = 11.10; P value = 0.004) (Table 4). Majority of cases (97.2%) had lesions confined to head and neck area. The distribution of lesions was as follows: nose (50%), cheeks (22.2%), ear and preauricular area (13.9%), lower eyelid (13.9%), temporal area (5.6%), upper lip (2.8%), forehead (2.8%), scalp (2.8%), and mons pubis (2.8%) (Table 5). Nose was the most significant site of involvement in our study (χ^2 = 14.43; P value = 0.01, while corresponding values without involving nose as site of BCC were 1.00 and 0.80). The most common morphological subtype of BCC was nodular/noduloulcerative growth (77.8%) (Figures 1 and 2). A significant percentage of BCC was clinically pigmented (22.2%) (Table 6). Other types observed were micronodular (19.4%) and morpheaform (2.8%) BCC.

3.3. Histopathological Data (Figure 3).
The most common histopathological variant was nodular subtype (77.8%) with a significant proportion of tumors being pigmented (16.7%)

TABLE 4: Association between duration of disease and size of lesion.

Duration (years)	Small size (<1 cm)	Medium size (1-2 cm)	Large size (>2 cm)	Total	χ^2 (d.f.)	P value
0–5	7	9	4	20		
More than 5	0	5	11	16	11.10 (2)	0.004^S
Total	**7**	**14**	**15**	**36**		

S: significant at 1% level of significance.

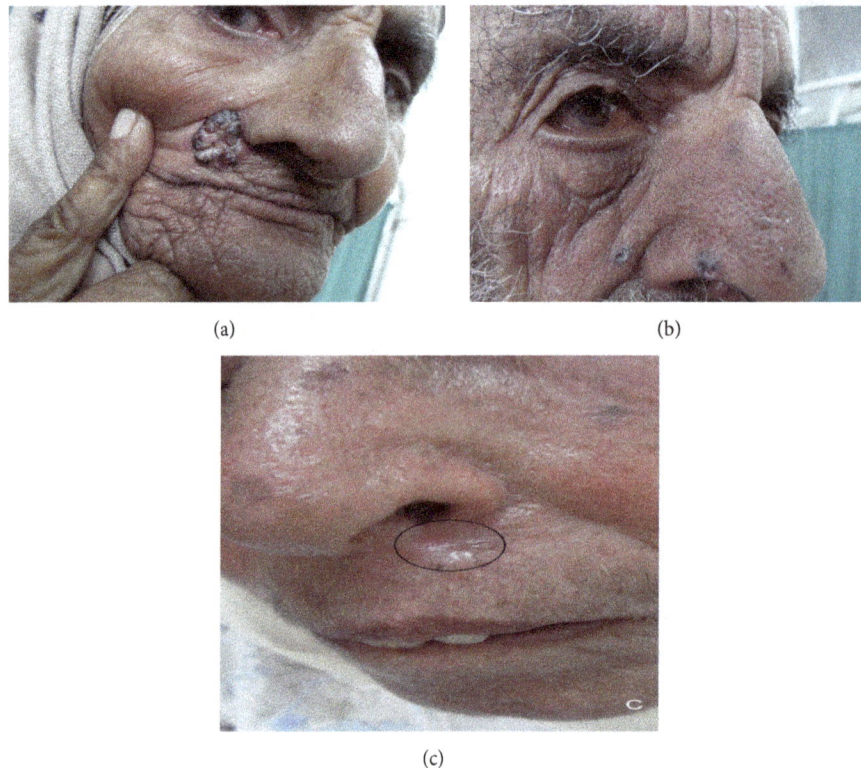

(a)

(b)

(c)

FIGURE 2: (a) Noduloulcerative, pigmented BCC in an elderly female. (b) Multiple, pigmented papular BCC on face. (c) Morpheaform BCC in an elderly woman.

TABLE 5: Distribution of BCC according to site.

Site	n	% age of patients	χ^2 (d.f.)	P value
Nose	18	50		
Cheeks	8	22.2		
Ear, preauricular area	5	13.9	14.43 (4)	0.01^s
Lower eyelid	5	13.9		
Others	6	16.8		
Total	**42**	**100**		

S: significant at 5% level of significance.

TABLE 6: Morphological types of BCC.

Morphology	n	% age of patients	χ^2 value (d.f.)	P value
Nodular/noduloulcerative	28	77.8		
Pigmented	8	22.2		
Micronodular	7	19.4	37.636 (3)	0.000^{HS}
Morpheaform	1	2.8		
Total	**44**	**100**		

HS: highly significant.

(Table 7). Other subtypes included basosquamous (8.3%), micronodular (2.8%), morpheaform (2.8%), keratotic (2.8%), and adenoid (2.8%) BCC and BCC with adnexal differentiation (2.8%).

4. Discussion

Basal cell carcinoma occurs worldwide (Table 8). So far, BCC has been considered as the disease of the White [14].

Consequently, most of the studies have focused on White populations in Europe, USA, and Australia with scarcity of data from developing countries (Table 9). Estimates of the incidence of BCC are imprecise since there is no cancer registry that collects data on BCC.

Although incidence rates of BCC vary significantly according to the ethnicity and geographic location, most studies show a rising trend in its incidence worldwide. This

(a)

(b)

(c)

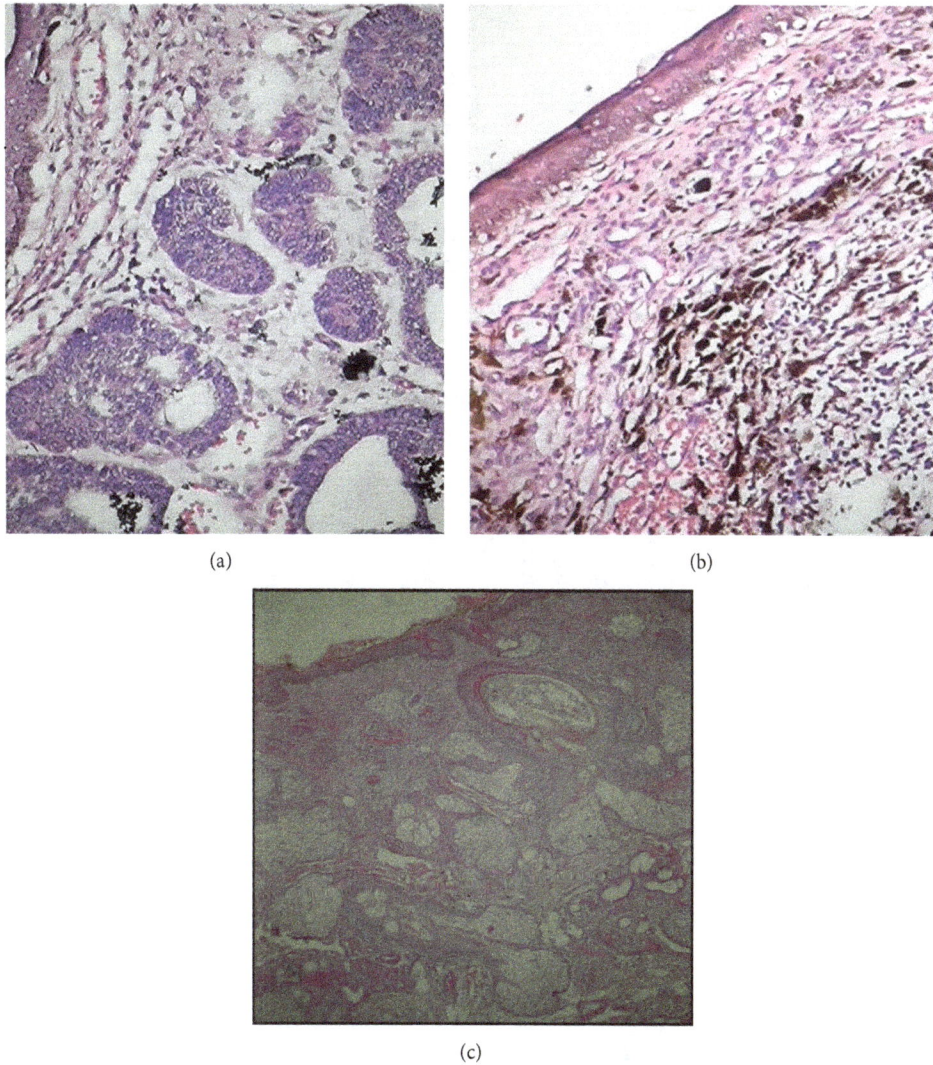

FIGURE 3: (a) Histopathology (hematoxylin and eosin, 40x): nodular BCC. (b) Histopathology (hematoxylin and eosin, 40x): pigmented BCC. (c) Histopathology (hematoxylin and eosin, 10x): adenoid BCC.

TABLE 7: Histopathological variants of BCC.

Histopathological variant	N	% age of cases	χ^2 value (d.f.)	P value
Nodular	28	77.8		
Pigmented	6	16.7	21.14 (2)	0.000[HS]
Others	8			
Total	**42**	22.3		

HS: highly significant.

TABLE 8: Worldwide incidence of BCC.

Country	Incidence of BCC (per 100,000 person-years)	Comment
Australia	>1600	Highest incidence
North America	~300	
Europe	40–80	
Africa	<1	Lowest rates

has been largely attributed to fair complexion and ozone layer depletion resulting in increased UV radiation reaching earth's surface. Similar increasing trend was noticed in our study as well. But factors other than the mentioned above need to be searched and verified as darker skin complexion in Indians should otherwise be protective against BCC. Moreover, ozone layer destruction is most evident over the temperate and polar regions, while India is a tropical country [15, 16].

Basal cell carcinoma is rare in young populations. An increased incidence has also been noticed in children and young adults [17]. This finding highlights the need for early institution of UV protection and skin cancer screening in the pediatric and young adult population. However, there was no case below the age of 20 years in our study. Radiotherapy is another risk factor for the development of BCC in younger age group. Relative risk of BCC is more for children who

TABLE 9: Studies regarding BCC in South Asia.

Study	n	Duration and type of study	M	F	M:F	Age	Highlights of the study — Sites	Subtype
Obaidullah and Aslam, 2008 [34]	100	4 years, prospective	45	55	0.8:1	Mean age = 56.3 years	—	24 pigmented nodular, 21 nonpigmented nodular, 30 ulcerative, and 6 lesions were of morphoeic type.
Asif et al., 2010 [35]	235	3 years, retrospective	53.2%	46.8%	1.2:1	32–90 years	Nose: 28.9% Eye: 24.7% Cheek: 20.4%	—
Laishram et al., 2010 [22]	30	5 years, retrospective	—	—	1:2	Median age = 70 years; most common age group is 61–70 years.	83.3% on head and neck, with predilection for face	Nodular subtype was the most frequent.
Malhotra et al., 2011 [23]	34	3 years	—	—	1.6:1	28 to 102 years. Majority in age group 40–60 years (44%)	91.2% on head and neck, with commonest site being medial/lateral canthus of eye	Most common histology subtype: nodular (64.7%); pigmented clinically (35.2%)
Chow et al., 2011 [36]	225	10 years, retrospective	94	132	0.7	Mean age = 73.1 (22–100) years	Nose: 31.6% Cheek: 16.5%	Ulcer: 64.8% Nodule: 19.3%
Deo et al. [3]	14	8 years, retrospective	—	—	—	—	—	—
Moore and Bennett, 2012 [37]	10	9 years, retrospective	5	5	—	68.9 years	100% on head region	Nodular: 50% Infiltrative: 10% Sclerosing: 10%
Janjua and Qureshi, 2012 [38]	171	3 years, retrospective	100	71	1.4:1	22–90 years (mean 61.3 ± 13.07 years)	Most common site: nose (31.5%) followed by cheek (26.9%)	Nodular variety: 46.2% and pigmented type: 18.7%
Chang and Gao, 2013 [39]	243	8 years, retrospective	118	125	0.94:1	65.16 ± 12.62 years	Head and neck region was the most common site (77.4%)	Nodular: 53.9% Superficial: 18.9% Infiltrative-morphoeic: 18.5%

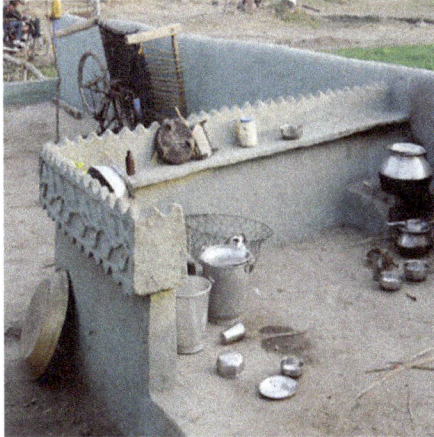

FIGURE 4: Open kitchen prevalent in rural India.

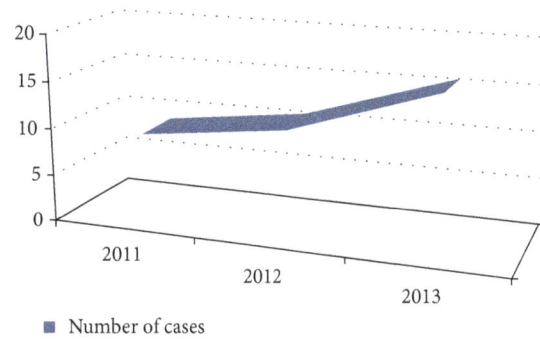

FIGURE 6: Year-wise diagnosed cases of BCC.

■ Number of cases

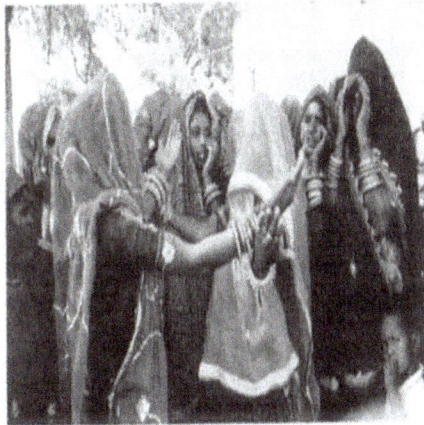

FIGURE 5: "Veil" custom (obsolete now): an old cultural practice in India in which face is kept hidden by a piece of cloth.

have undergone radiation therapy for enlarged thymus [18] or neoplasms such as medulloblastoma [19].

BCCs are more common in males as reported in most studies worldwide, presumably due to greater occupational and recreational exposure to ultraviolet radiation (UVR). However, an unusual female preponderance was noticed in our study which is consistent with findings of another Indian series [20]. Indian housewives especially rural women work in open kitchen (Figure 4) during their household chores and work in the fields during sowing and harvesting seasons exposing them to intermittent, high intensity UVR. It might explain higher frequency of BCC in females in our study as intermittent rather than constant, cumulative UVR exposure is implicated in the pathogenesis of BCC [21]. This female predilection may also be attributed to the changes in cultural practices like "veil" custom (Figure 5), structurally thinner skin with lower collagen density in the dermis when compared to men.

The most commonly affected age group in our study was 61–80 years (47.2%) followed by 41–60 years (38.95%), 21–40 years (8.3%), and 81–100 years (5.6%). This closely

resembles the findings of another study conducted in East India [22]. The cases belonged to age ranging from 29 to 92 years which is similar to study published from North India [23]. Higher rates of occurrence of BCC among elderly may be due to cumulative UVR induced DNA damage [24] as well as reduced efficiency of immune-surveillance and DNA repair mechanisms with aging [25].

In our study, higher frequency among rural inhabitants was seen when compared to urban residents. This can be explained on the basis of more outdoor activities (as agriculture is the main occupation), changes in clothing preferences, illiteracy, and infrequent use of sunscreens. The rural patients regard initial lesions of BCC as a minor cosmetic problem with insignificant impact on health and seek medical advice only when lesions become symptomatic or disfiguring. So, late presentation to health facilities is equally contributory. A study done in Punjab regarding cancer found that tap water contains high content of arsenic, chromium, iron, and mercury, whereas ground water has abundance of arsenic, chromium, nickel, and iron. Even pesticides have been detected in the locally grown vegetables as well. Tseng et al. found a dose-dependent relation between arsenic levels in drinking water and the prevalence of skin cancers [26]. Thus, exposure to harmful metals and pesticides may also add to the risk of skin cancers, but further clinical and research studies are needed to confirm their role in the pathogenesis of BCC and to delineate underlying mechanisms. Occupations at risk of BCC that are highlighted in our study include agricultural workers and housekeepers.

Use of tanning beds is associated with increased risk of BCC [27]. But their use is uncommon in our part of the world.

Immunocompromised patients like HIV positive patients or organ transplant recipients have a markedly increased risk of both typical and highly invasive NMSC. Interesting fact is that while the BCC/SCC incidence ratio is approximately 4 : 1 in the general population, SCCs become more prevalent in the transplant population with a BCC/SCC ratio of approximately 1 : 2. However, there was no HIV positive case seen amongst our study subjects.

The association between BCC and smoking remains unclear. Some studies refute any relationship between smoking and risk of BCC [28], while Boyd et al. found that BCC in young women is linked with past or current smoking [29]. Smith and Randle described an increased prevalence of

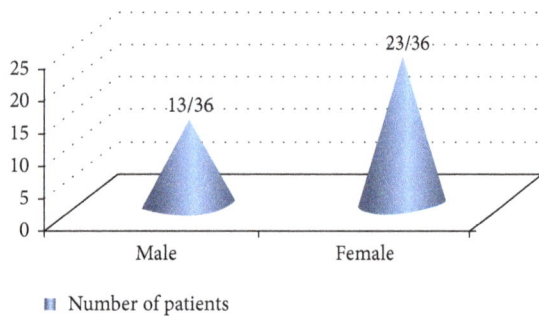

FIGURE 7: Gender distribution of BCC.

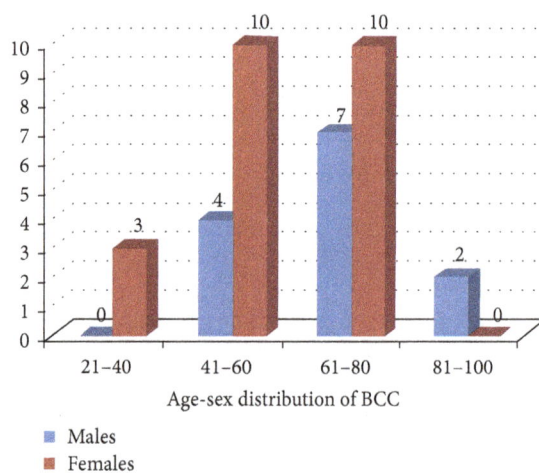

FIGURE 8: Age-sex distribution of BCC.

BCC larger than 1 cm in diameter among the smokers [30]. However, all the subjects in our study were nonsmokers.

Other iatrogenic risk factors associated with BCC include treatment with psoralens and UVA therapy and NBUVB for various ailments. None of the patients in our study had received such treatments. In a retrospective, nationwide cohort study of patients with psoriasis subjected to climatotherapy at the Dead Sea, it was found that the overall risk of cancer in patients treated at the Dead Sea was higher than that expected in the general population, owing to an excess risk of nonmelanoma skin cancer (NMSC), with multiple lesions being more common and predilection for younger individuals [31].

The most common location in our study was head and neck area (97.2%) which is close to what was observed by Malhotra et al. [23]. A significant proportion of cases were clinically pigmented (22.2%). This finding was in contrast to what has been seen in Western countries. This pigmentation might be misleading as, clinically, BCC may be misdiagnosed as melanoma.

Although most BCCs are slow-growing, relatively nonaggressive tumors, a minority have an aggressive behavior with local tissue destruction and, rarely, metastasis. Metastatic BCC has a reported incidence of only 0.0028–0.5% [32]. Risk factors for development of metastatic BCC include large primary tumor (>2 cm), location in head and neck region,

long standing lesion, multiple primary tumors and recurrences, prior radiation therapy, large tumor depth, invasion of perineural space and blood vessels, fair skin, male gender, and immunosuppression [33]. One of our patients was detected with metastatic BCC (Figure 1).

5. Conclusions

This study highlights a paradoxically increasing trend of BCC with female predilection and higher percentage of pigmented lesions in Indians. This skin malignancy tends to be commoner in rural and agriculture based population. Major contributory risk factors include intermittent rather than constant UV exposure, cultural and lifestyle changes, cosmetic indifference, possible role of arsenic and pesticides, improved clinical awareness, and diagnostic facilities. The increasing cancer burden calls for the need of introduction of national screening program including mandatory annual skin examination by trained health professionals at the national level. Since early detection and treatment of lesions are crucial to decrease functional and cosmetic morbidity and costs, this study highlights the importance of improving awareness among general practitioners, public health workers, and general population. The clinical and epidemiological data collected in this study would serve as a reference for future research and may be helpful in the development of preventive and educational strategies.

Acknowledgment

The authors are thankful to Dr. Ghansham, Department of Social and Preventive Medicine, GGS Medical College & Hospital, for help with the statistics.

References

[1] V. Malik, K. S. Goh, S. Leong, A. Tan, D. Downey, and D. O'Donovan, "Risk and outcome analysis of 1832 consecutively excised basal cell carcinoma's in a tertiary referral plastic surgery unit," *Journal of Plastic, Reconstructive and Aesthetic Surgery*, vol. 63, no. 12, pp. 2057–2063, 2010.

[2] P. T. Bradford, "Skin cancer in skin of color," *Dermatology Nursing*, vol. 21, no. 4, pp. 170–178, 2009.

[3] S. V. Deo, S. Hazarika, N. K. Shukla, S. Kumar, M. Kar, and A. Samaiya, "Surgical management of skin cancers: experience from a regional cancer centre in North India," *Indian Journal of Cancer*, vol. 42, no. 3, pp. 145–150, 2005.

[4] A. B. Hyman and A. J. Barsky, "Basal cell epithelioma of the palm," *Archives of Dermatology*, vol. 92, no. 5, pp. 571–573, 1965.

[5] G. Pearson, L. E. King Jr., and A. S. Boyd, "Basal cell carcinoma of the lower extremities," *International Journal of Dermatology*, vol. 38, no. 11, pp. 852–854, 1999.

[6] J. C. Newman and D. J. Leffell, "Correlation of embryonic fusion planes with the anatomical distribution of basal cell carcinoma," *Dermatologic Surgery*, vol. 33, no. 8, pp. 957–965, 2007.

[7] A. C. Markey, E. B. Lane, D. M. MacDonald, and I. M. Leigh, "Keratin expression in basal cell carcinomas," *British Journal of Dermatology*, vol. 126, no. 2, pp. 154–160, 1992.

[8] B. W. LeSueur, N. G. Silvis, and R. C. Hansen, "Basal cell carcinoma in children: report of 3 cases," *Archives of Dermatology*, vol. 136, no. 3, pp. 370–372, 2000.

[9] C. Roudier-Pujol, A. Auperin, T. Nguyen, P. Duvillard, E. Benhamou, and M.-F. Avril, "Basal cell carcinoma in young adults: not more aggressive than in older patients," *Dermatology*, vol. 199, no. 2, pp. 119–123, 1999.

[10] J. L. Lim and R. S. Stern, "High levels of ultraviolet B exposure increase the risk of non-melanoma skin cancer in psoralen and ultraviolet A-treated patients," *Journal of Investigative Dermatology*, vol. 124, no. 3, pp. 505–513, 2005.

[11] M. R. Wehner, M. L. Shive, M.-M. Chren, J. Han, A. A. Qureshi, and E. Linos, "Indoor tanning and non-melanoma skin cancer: systematic review and meta-analysis," *British Medical Journal*, vol. 345, no. 7877, Article ID e5909, 2012.

[12] M. R. Karagas, "Occurrence of cutaneous basal cell and squamous cell malignancies among those with a prior history of skin cancer," *Journal of Investigative Dermatology*, vol. 102, no. 6, pp. 10S–13S, 1994.

[13] C. Heal, P. Buettner, and S. Browning, "Risk factors for wound infection after minor surgery in general practice," *Medical Journal of Australia*, vol. 185, no. 5, pp. 255–258, 2006.

[14] A. Lomas, J. Leonardi-Bee, and F. Bath-Hextall, "A systematic review of worldwide incidence of nonmelanoma skin cancer," *The British Journal of Dermatology*, vol. 166, no. 5, pp. 1069–1080, 2012.

[15] "Myth: Ozone Depletion Occurs Only in Antarctica — Science — Ozone Layer Protection — US EPA," http://www.epa.gov/ozone/science/myths/glob_dep.html.

[16] World Meteorological Organization, *Assessment of Ozone Depletion*, World Meteorological Organization, 2010, http://search.usa.gov/search?affiliate=esrl.noaa.gov_csd&query=assessment+of+ozone+depletion.

[17] L. J. Christenson, T. A. Borrowman, C. M. Vachon et al., "Incidence of basal cell and squamous cell carcinomas in a population younger than 40 years," *The Journal of the American Medical Association*, vol. 294, no. 6, pp. 681–690, 2005.

[18] N. Meibodi, M. Maleki, Z. Javidi, and Y. Nahidi, "Clinicopathological evaluation of radiation induced basal cell carcinoma," *Indian Journal of Dermatology*, vol. 53, no. 3, pp. 137–139, 2008.

[19] M. Endo, K. Fujii, K. Sugita, K. Saito, Y. Kohno, and T. Miyashita, "Nationwide survey of nevoid basal cell carcinoma syndrome in Japan revealing the low frequency of basal cell carcinoma," *American Journal of Medical Genetics Part A*, vol. 158, no. 2, pp. 351–357, 2012.

[20] M. Mamata and R. Karuna, "Basal cell carcinoma: evaluation of clinical and histologic variables," *Indian Journal of Dermatology*, vol. 49, pp. 25–27, 2004.

[21] S. Rosso, F. Joris, and R. Zanetti, "Risk of basal and squamous cell carcinomas of the skin in Sion, Switzerland: a case-control study," *Tumori*, vol. 85, no. 6, pp. 435–442, 1999.

[22] R. S. Laishram, A. Banerjee, P. Punyabati, and L. D. C. Sharma, "Pattern of skin malignancies in Manipur, India: a 5-year histopathological review," *Journal of Pakistan Association of Dermatologists*, vol. 20, no. 3, pp. 128–132, 2010.

[23] P. Malhotra, A. Singh, and V. Ramesh, "Basal cell carcinoma in the North Indian population: clinicopathologic review and immunohistochemical analysis," *Indian Journal of Dermatology, Venereology and Leprology*, vol. 77, no. 3, pp. 328–330, 2011.

[24] R. P. Gallagher, G. B. Hill, C. D. Bajdik et al., "Sunlight exposure, pigmentary factors, and risk of nonmelanocytic skin cancer: I. Basal cell carcinoma," *Archives of Dermatology*, vol. 131, no. 2, pp. 157–163, 1995.

[25] R. L. Bariani, F. X. Nahas, M. V. Jardini Barbosa, A. B. Farah, and L. M. Ferreira, "Basal cell carcinoma: an updated epidemiological and therapeutically profile of an urban population," *Acta Cirurgica Brasileira*, vol. 21, no. 2, pp. 66–73, 2006.

[26] W. P. Tseng, H. M. Chu, S. W. How, J. M. Fong, C. S. Lin, and S. Yeh, "Prevalence of skin cancer in an endemic area of chronic arsenicism in Taiwan," *Journal of the National Cancer Institute*, vol. 40, no. 3, pp. 453–463, 1968.

[27] M. R. Karagas, V. A. Stannard, L. A. Mott, M. J. Slattery, S. K. Spencer, and M. A. Weinstock, "Use of tanning devices and risk of basal cell and squamous cell skin cancers," *Journal of the National Cancer Institute*, vol. 94, no. 3, pp. 224–226, 2002.

[28] R. Corona, E. Dogliotti, M. D'Errico et al., "Risk factors for basal cell carcinoma in a Mediterranean population: role of recreational sun exposure early in life," *Archives of Dermatology*, vol. 137, no. 9, pp. 1162–1168, 2001.

[29] A. S. Boyd, Y. Shyr, and L. E. King Jr., "Basal cell carcinoma in young women: an evaluation of the association of tanning bed use and smoking," *Journal of the American Academy of Dermatology*, vol. 46, no. 5, pp. 706–709, 2002.

[30] J. B. Smith and H. W. Randle, "Giant basal cell carcinoma and cigarette smoking," *Cutis*, vol. 67, no. 1, pp. 73–76, 2001.

[31] G. Frentz, J. H. Olsen, and W. W. Avrach, "Malignant tumours and psoriasis: climatotherapy at the Dead Sea," *British Journal of Dermatology*, vol. 141, no. 6, pp. 1088–1091, 1999.

[32] R. Shrivastava, K. Singh, and M. Shrivastava, "Soft tissue metastasis in basal cell carcinoma," *Indian Journal of Dermatology*, vol. 52, no. 4, pp. 206–208, 2007.

[33] S.-H. Seo, W.-H. Shim, D.-H. Shin, Y.-S. Kim, and H.-W. Sung, "Pulmonary metastasis of basal cell carcinoma," *Annals of Dermatology*, vol. 23, no. 2, pp. 213–216, 2011.

[34] Obaidullah and M. Aslam, "Preliminary report on recurrence of Basal Cell Carcinoma (bcc) after surgical excision in NWFP and Afghanistan," *Journal of Postgraduate Medical Institute*, vol. 22, no. 4, 2008.

[35] M. Asif, N. Mamoon, Z. Ali, and F. Akhtar, "Epidemiological and excision margin status of basal cell carcinoma—three years armed forces institute of pathology experience in pakistan," *Asian Pacific Journal of Cancer Prevention*, vol. 11, no. 5, pp. 1421–1423, 2010.

[36] V. L. Y. Chow, J. Y. W. Chan, R. C. L. Chan, J. H. P. Chung, and W. I. Wei, "Basal cell carcinoma of the head and neck region in ethnic Chinese," *International Journal of Surgical Oncology*, vol. 2011, Article ID 890908, 7 pages, 2011.

[37] M. G. Moore and R. G. Bennett, "Basal cell carcinoma in Asians: a retrospective analysis of ten patients," *Journal of Skin Cancer*, vol. 2012, Article ID 741397, 5 pages, 2012.

[38] O. S. Janjua and S. M. Qureshi, "Basal cell carcinoma of the head and neck region: an analysis of 171 cases," *Journal of Skin Cancer*, vol. 2012, Article ID 943472, 4 pages, 2012.

[39] J.-M. Chang and X.-M. Gao, "Clinical and histopathological characteristics of basal cell carcinoma in Chinese patients," *Chinese Medical Journal*, vol. 126, no. 2, pp. 211–214, 2013.

34

Sun Protection Beliefs among Hispanics in the US

Marimer Santiago-Rivas, Chang Wang, and Lina Jandorf

Department of Oncological Sciences, Cancer Prevention and Control Division, Icahn School of Medicine at Mount Sinai, One Gustave L. Levy Place, New York, NY 10029-6574, USA

Correspondence should be addressed to Marimer Santiago-Rivas; marimer.santiago-rivas@mssm.edu

Academic Editor: Marianne Berwick

Purpose. We reviewed the literature on sun protection beliefs in Hispanics living in the United States to explore what challenges are faced by area of research. *Method*. A review of PubMED, PsycINFO, and CINAHL databases was performed. Studies were published in peer-reviewed journals (in all years available) and written in English. The search terms used were ["skin cancer" OR "sun protection"] AND ["Latino" OR "Hispanic"] AND "beliefs." Eligible papers were included in the final analysis after meeting the following inclusion criteria: (1) the records had to quantitatively examine and report sun protection beliefs in Hispanics, (2) the number of Hispanic participants in the sample had to be clearly specified, and (3) studies reporting differences in sun protection beliefs between Hispanics and other racial and ethnic groups were included in the review. *Results*. Of the 92 articles identified, 11 met inclusion criteria and addressed sun protection beliefs regarding skin cancer seriousness and susceptibility, and benefits and barriers of sun protection and skin cancer risk behaviors. Characteristics of studies and results were examined. *Conclusion*. There is insufficient evidence to determine a pattern of sun protection beliefs among Hispanics in the United States. More quality studies are needed which focus on sun protection beliefs in Hispanics.

1. Introduction

Skin cancer is the most common cancer in the United States (US). It is estimated that close to 4 million skin cancer diagnoses (including basal cell and squamous cell carcinomas) are made every year [1]. Melanoma (an aggressive form of skin cancer) is diagnosed in more than 70,000 persons every year, creating a high health and economic burden with an estimated annual cost of $3.5 billion [2]. Risk factors for skin cancer include sun sensitivity (sunburning easily, difficulty tanning), a history of excessive sun exposure, sunburns, use of artificial tanning, and a past history of skin cancer [1]. Most of skin cancer cases could be prevented by protecting the skin from excessive sun exposure and avoiding indoor tanning. Results from an analysis of national data showed that the majority of the US population reported infrequent incidence of sun protection behaviors [3]. Characteristics of groups reporting lower incidence of sun protection include being young (under the age of 40), having a lower education level, being a smoker or a risky drinker, and being less sensitive to the sun [3]. Health research should focus on the identification of psychosocial and modifiable variables to promote sun protection among groups at higher risk for skin cancer and in the general population.

Even when it has been documented that the Hispanic/Latino (referred to as Hispanic) population suffers from a disparity regarding certain cancers compared to non-Hispanic whites (referred to as whites), the lifetime risk of developing skin cancer is higher among whites than other racial groups. For melanoma, it is higher among whites (2.9% in men, 1.9% in women) than in Hispanics (0.52% in men, 0.51% in women) [1, 4]. A study conducted in Miami showed that, among 3000 cases of nonmelanoma skin cancer reviewed, 60.1% were diagnosed in whites and 38.4% were diagnosed in Hispanics [5]. Findings using the Southeastern Arizona Skin Cancer Registry showed that the rates for nonmelanoma skin cancer in whites were approximately 11 times greater than rates for Latinos [6]. A case control study of nonmelanoma cancer diagnoses in Hispanics (with whites as control) showed that 15.3% of Latino patients reported recurrence of their malignancy as compared to 31.3% of controls [7]. Also, a lower proportion of Latinos (34.0% versus 61.3% controls) had a current diagnosis or prior history of actinic keratosis. On the other hand, skin cancer has been associated with considerable morbidity and mortality in the Hispanic population. Compared with whites, Hispanics have lower 5-year melanoma survival rates, 76.6% versus 87.0% for men and 88.3% versus 92.3 for women [4]. Hispanics are more likely to have advanced and thicker melanomas at diagnosis when compared with whites [8–16]. A greater percentage of melanomas occurred among Hispanics in younger age groups (24.4% less than 40 years old) compared with blacks and whites, 15.8% and 14.3%, respectively [16]. Also, Hispanics tend to report lower frequency of skin-related visits to dermatologists than their white counterparts [17]. Data obtained from cancer registries of Puerto Rico, New York, New Jersey, and Connecticut show that Puerto Ricans living in the US report higher melanoma rates than those residing in Puerto Rico [18]. At the same time, there are variations in the behaviors reported by Hispanics and non-Hispanics. A systematic review examined the incidence of sun protection behaviors among Hispanics in the US [19]. Overall, the prevalence of these behaviors is both low and mixed. While a slightly lower share of Hispanics (9.5–29.9%) report usage of sunscreen either most of the time or always compared to 16.5%–35.9% of whites, Hispanics reported slightly higher rates of wearing hats either most of the time or always (23.9–25.0% versus 20–20.7%). Recent studies of sun protection behaviors show that around 53% of Hispanics stay in shade, and around 20% use protective clothing when outside on a warm sunny day either most of the time or always [20, 21]. Hispanics who are less acculturated report lower rates of sunscreen use than those who are more acculturated [21]. Still, little is known about skin cancer risk factors in the Latino population. It is critical to identify psychosocial and modifiable factors influencing skin cancer morbidity and mortality in Hispanics in the US.

The Community Preventive Service Task Force reviewed skin cancer prevention evidence from a Community Guide systematic review published in 2004 combined with more recent evidence [22, 23]. The review found that education interventions in primary and middle schools (Kindergarten–8th grade), which include strategies to integrate parents, caregivers, and teachers, decrease sun exposure, sun protection, and formation of new moles. Multicomponent, communitywide interventions including a combination of individual-directed strategies (e.g., activities to change the knowledge, attitudes, beliefs, or behaviors), mass media campaigns, and policy changes are recommended based on evidence of effectiveness in increasing sunscreen use, but results for effects on other protective behaviors are mixed. Results also suggest benefits in reducing sunburns among children. In addition, findings illustrate that other approaches, such as mass media alone, provider education and media-based education sessions in health care settings, and educational activities in high school and colleges, did not provide sufficient evidence to determine their applicability for skin cancer prevention. Many of these studies were conducted outside of the US (i.e., Australia and the United Kingdom), but the Task Force suggests that findings are likely to be applicable to the US because results were similar across countries. Various interventions and education initiatives in the recent past have targeted minorities with the intention of improving skin

cancer, but these were not multicomponent initiatives [24–26]. A group of Hispanic women evaluated two educational videos to increase positive sun protection beliefs and behaviors [24]. There was an effect in skin cancer risk awareness postintervention, and participants reported they preferred the video emphasizing the benefits of sun protection for skin cancer prevention more than the video emphasizing its effect on photoaging. Little research has examined the association between sun protection behavioral outcomes and the health outcome of interest, that is, skin cancer incidence [23]. More research is needed to verify the efficacy of multicomponent, communitywide interventions addressing the effect of sun protection attitudes, perceptions, beliefs, and behaviors on increasing sun protection. In addition, research should evaluate its effect on decreasing sunburns (short-term effect) and skin cancer incidence (long-term effect) in the general public and in subgroups at particular risk for skin cancer.

This paper examines published studies that include health beliefs concerning skin cancer prevention and sun protection in Hispanics.

2. Materials and Methods

2.1. Search Strategy. We performed a search of the databases PubMed, PsycINFO, and CINAHL. All publication years and all search fields were included. The search was limited to articles in English and employed specific search keywords. One example of a search strategy used with the PubMED database is ((skin cancer) AND Hispanic) AND beliefs; ((skin cancer) AND Latino) AND beliefs; ((sun protection) AND Hispanic) AND beliefs; ((sun protection) AND Latino) AND beliefs. We decided to use broad search terms to make sure we would identify as many pertinent studies as possible. For our search, we decided to use the word "Hispanic" and "Latino" to indicate our population of interest, that is, US residents of Mexican, Cuban, Puerto Rican, Central American, South American, and other Spanish-speaking country origins. A search in PubMED demonstrated how research, with some exceptions (including US Census data and self-report), interchangeably uses these terms and lacks stratification of the members of this group [27]. A study by the Pew Hispanic Center found that more than half Hispanics (51%) have no preference for any of the two terms to describe their ethnicity [28]. At the same time, the term "Hispanic" was chosen to be used in this paper given that sun protection research applies this term more frequently compared with the term "Latino" (see Table 1 for list of the term(s) for ethnicity and raced used by each study included in this review). A manual secondary search of all bibliographies from relevant articles was performed to yield further relevant publications. We excluded studies conducted outside the US, as well as studies without data for Hispanic participants on the report of sun protection beliefs. Studies that compared the differences in sun protection beliefs between Hispanics and non-Hispanics were included as well.

2.2. Eligibility Criteria. Articles were reviewed for relevance with the criteria for inclusion being as follows. (1) The reports

TABLE 1: Findings related to sun protection and skin cancer risk beliefs in Hispanics.

Study	Sample	Design	Term used for ethnicity and race	Sun protection/skin cancer risk beliefs and findings (Hispanic)	Comments about quality of study
Andreeva et al. (2008) [36]	Total ($N = 1,782$) Hispanic ($N = 437$) *Adolescents*	Cross-sectional self-survey (no information about survey in Spanish)	Hispanic non-Hispanic	Results affect size in structural model (standardized solution): perceived peer norms for sun exposure and barriers to sun safety (0.459); barriers to sun safety and protanning attitudes (0.015), and barriers to sun safety and sun-safe behavior (0.142). Hispanics having lower scores on the tan-related measures and slightly higher scores on barriers.	Data were collected as part of sunny days, healthy ways program in Colorado, New Mexico, and Arizona. Information about validation of measurements in Hispanic sample was not reported. Original study reported low alpha reliability (less than 0.70) for measures of barriers to sun protection and peer norms for sun exposure.
Buster et al. (2012) [29]	Total ($N = 1,246$) Hispanic ($N = 161$) *Adults*	Population-based interviewer survey (no information about interview in Spanish)	Hispanic black, white	Results comparison with whites: likelihood of future skin cancer (OR 1.41); likelihood of skin cancer compared with average person of the same age (OR 0.83); worry about skin cancer (OR 0.83); there is not much you can do to lower chance of getting skin cancer (OR 3.87); there are so many recommendations about preventing skin cancer; it is hard to know which ones to follow (OR 3.35).	Data collected by Health Information National Trends Survey (HINTS). Statistical analyses were conducted with samples of different sizes (Hispanic $n = 161$ versus white $n = 966$). The HINTS is available in both Spanish and English (not mentioned in the paper), but there was no mention of possible influence of language preference.
Cheng et al. (2010) [37]	Total ($N = 1,214$) Hispanic ($N = 266$) *Adolescents*	Cross-sectional self-survey (no information about survey in Spanish)	Hispanic black, white	Percentages: tanning makes people look more attractive (true 61%); tanning makes people look older (True 27%).	The survey was part of an educational intervention which included a pretest, a 30-minute lesson on sun protection, and a posttest. There was no mention of this intervention being available in Spanish and English, or assessment of cultural competence. Limitations include a population surveyed from only New Jersey public schools and small Hispanic sample.
Coups et al. (2014) [30]	Total ($N = 787$) Hispanic) *Adults*	Cross-sectional self-survey/online (survey available in Spanish)	Hispanic	Weighted means (range 1–5) and standard deviations: suntan benefits = 2.58 (1.08); sunscreen benefits = 3.71 (0.94); shade seeking benefits = 3.62 (0.96); sun protective clothing benefits = 3.72 (0.94); sunscreen barriers = 2.51 (0.78); shade seeking barriers = 2.77 (0.71); sun protective clothing barriers = 2.70 (0.83); skin cancer worry = 2.51 (1.13); perceived skin cancer risk = 3.71 (1.06); photoaging concerns = 3.72 (1.02); perceived natural skin protection = 2.61 (1.26).	Participants completed an English- or Spanish-language online survey. Information about validity and reliability of measures by language preference was not provided. Authors mentioned survey items that were not already available in Spanish were translated, affecting the cultural appropriateness of the study for the Spanish-speaking Hispanic population. A large proportion of the sample was of Mexican origin (71%).

TABLE 1: Continued.

Study	Sample	Design	Term used for ethnicity and race	Sun protection/skin cancer risk beliefs and findings (Hispanic)	Comments about quality of study
Coups et al. (2013) [21, 31]	Total (N = 787 Hispanic) *Adults*	Cross-sectional self-survey/online (survey available in Spanish)	Hispanic	Correlates of sun protection beliefs and skin self-examination (and total body examination): perceived skin cancer risk AOR 1.34 (AOR 0.89); perceived skin cancer severity AOR 1.05 (1.91).	Participants completed an English- or Spanish-language online survey. Information about validity and reliability of measures by language preference was not provided. Participants' state of residence was as follows: California, *n* = 379; Texas, *n* = 231; Florida, *n* = 110; Arizona, *n* = 41; and New Mexico, *n* = 26.
Heckman and Cohen-Filipic (2012) [34]	Total (N = 74 Hispanic) *Adolescents and young adults*	Cross-sectional self-survey (survey available in Spanish)	Hispanic	Means (range 0–10 and 4–20) and standard deviations: how likely is it that you will develop skin cancer? = 3.70 (2.43); how likely is it that your skin will age too soon? = 3.69 (2.62); benefits of UV exposure (four items) = 11.10 (3.83); benefits of sun protection (four items) = 13.11 (3.87).	This pilot study was part of an educational collaboration between a high school science department and a cancer center in the suburbs of Philadelphia. A small Hispanic sample (*n* = 74) was studied. Items from original study were developed from a sample of parents and children (N = white = 55%, African American = 26%, and Hispanic = 15%). The sun protection benefits scales were originally developed as mixed sun protection knowledge and attitude scale, and it had low alpha reliability (less than 0.70). The reviewed study showed better reliability. Participants could choose to receive information and surveys in either English or Spanish, but no information about appropriateness of the measures for culture or language preference was provided.
Hernandez et al. (2014) [24]	Total study 1 (N = 52 Hispanic); total study 2 (N = 80 Hispanic; 67 women, 13 men) *Adults*	Qualitative (quantitative results reported); experimental phase (video) (study conducted in Spanish)	Hispanic	Study 1 frequencies: believes she can develop a skin cancer (Yes = 25/52); concerned about lentigines (Yes = 48/52) and wrinkles (Yes = 35/52). Study 2 frequencies: fair-skinned Hispanics are at risk for skin cancer (prevideo, agreement = 54/80; postvideo agreement = 72/80); dark-skinned Hispanics are at risk for skin cancer (preagreement = 44/80; postagreement = 69/80).	Effect of two short Spanish-language films on sun protection beliefs was tested (in Chicago, Illinois). One emphasized photoaging benefits of sun protection, while the second focused on its benefits for skin cancer prevention. Nine patients at a dermatology clinic, whose primary language was Spanish, were asked to view the videos and review the questionnaires before it being administered. The samples studied were small, and it is not clear how results would apply to English-speaking Hispanics. Authors developed the videos using primarily the opinions of women rather than men, and the male sample size in the intervention group was limited.

TABLE 1: Continued.

Study	Sample	Design	Term used for ethnicity and race	Sun protection/skin cancer risk beliefs and findings (Hispanic)	Comments about quality of study
Imahiyerobo-Ip et al. (2011) [35]	Total ($N = 165$) Hispanic ($N = 38$) *Patients*	Cross-sectional self-survey (no information about survey in Spanish)	Hispanic white, African American, Asian, and others	Frequency and percentage: believes that skin cancer can happen in darker skin types (29/37; 78%).	A survey was administered to 165 patients seeking care from a dermatology practice in New York City. Limitations include the small sample size and the inclusion of patients who may have had a history of actinic keratoses.
Ma et al. (2007) [32]	Total ($N = 369$) Hispanic ($N = 221$) *Adolescents*	Cross-sectional self-survey (no information about survey in Spanish)	White Hispanic white non-Hispanic	Frequencies, percentages, and results comparison with whites: chances of developing skin cancer in the future "higher than average" (4.1%), "average" (19%), "lower than average" (51.6%), and "don't know" (25.3%). Logistic regression "average or above" (OR 0.6) after controlling for age, sex, skin type, and family history of skin cancer.	A pilot survey study using 1 of the 33 public high schools located in the Miami-Dade County area of Florida. A self-administered, anonymous survey, which was derived from a tool used in a derivate of the national Nurses' Health Study (94% white). Information about validation of measurements in Hispanic sample, or clarification of the term "average risk of skin cancer" was not reported.
Mahler (2014) [38]	Total ($N = 1183$) Hispanic ($N = 65$) *Adults*	Baseline self-survey (no information about survey in Spanish)	Hispanic white, Asian/Pacific Islander	Significant differences in percentages of responses when compared with whites after controlling for skin sensitivity. Sunscreen benefits: avoid getting too dark (Hispanic 15.1%, white 5.8%). Sunscreen barriers: it is too much trouble (Hispanic 16.4%, white 30.6%); I am dark skinned (Hispanic 29.1%, white 3%).	The data were drawn from baseline questionnaires completed during 9 different sun protection experiments conducted in San Diego, California. Participants who indicated ever using sunscreen checked any of the listed sunscreen benefits/barriers. The authors mentioned that the list was developed through piloting, but no additional information is provided. No information about appropriateness of the measures for culture or language preference was provided. A small Hispanic sample was used for the statistical comparisons.
Pipitone et al. (2002) [33]	Total ($N = 153$) Hispanic ($N = 27$) *Adults*	Cross-sectional self-survey (no information about survey in Spanish)	White Hispanic white non-Hispanic	Frequencies perceived risk of melanoma or skin cancer "higher than average" (4%), "average" (59%), "lower than average" (22%), and "don't know" (15%).	Prospective survey of a group of suburban employees to evaluate perceptions of skin cancer risk. Low participation in the study and small Hispanic sample. Information about validation of measurements in Hispanic sample, or clarification of the term "average risk of skin cancer" for comparisons was not reported.

OR: odds ratio; AOR: adjusted odds ratio.

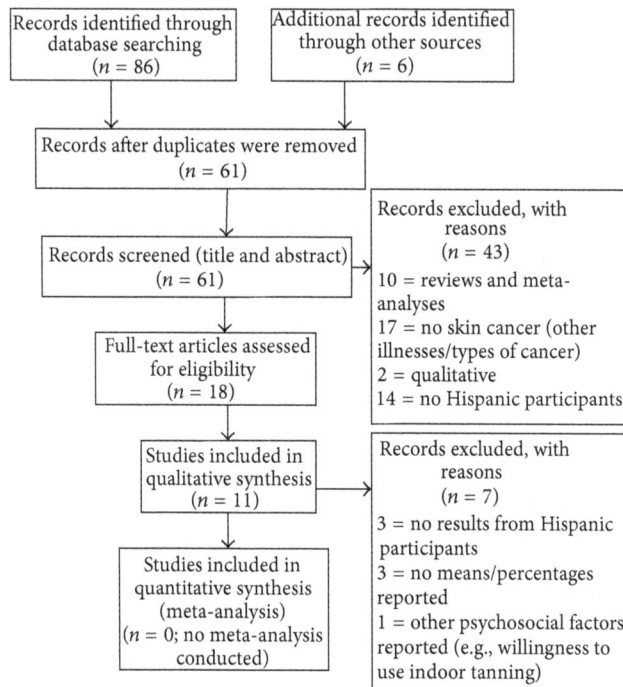

FIGURE 1: Flow diagram of literature search.

had to quantitatively examine and report (frequency, means, percentages, effect sizes, and/or odds ratio) sun protection beliefs in Hispanic samples, including constructs such as skin cancer risk/susceptibility and severity/seriousness, and sun protection beliefs (barriers and benefits of sun protection and skin cancer risk). (2) The number of Hispanic participants in the sample had to be stated. (3) Studies that reported the differences in sun protection beliefs between Hispanics and other racial and ethnic groups were used. Books, book chapters, meta-analyses, comments, and reviews were excluded.

3. Results

The first database searched was PubMED, followed by a search of PsycINFO and CINAHL. A total of 86 articles were identified from these databases, and 6 articles were identified from bibliographies, for a total of 92 records (see Figure 1). A search of duplicates was conducted, leaving 61 records that were title- and abstract-screened and 18 records that were screened in full. The title and abstract screening step evaluated the title and the abstract of each of the 61 articles to determine whether the abstracts met the following criteria: (1) informed about sun protection beliefs, (2) informed about the sample used (humans), (3) suggested that the study included Hispanics in the sample, (4) used English as publication language, and (5) indicated that the publication was peer-reviewed. As part of the full screening step, the manuscripts from the 18 abstracts were obtained and read in full to determine whether they met the eligibility criteria: (1) the records had to quantitatively examine and report sun protection beliefs in Hispanics, (2) the number of Hispanic participants in the sample had to

be clearly specified, and (3) studies reporting differences in sun protection beliefs between Hispanics and other racial and ethnic groups were included in the review. These manuscripts were read in full, and eleven were included in the final analysis (see Figure 1). Data on the author, year of publication, sample characteristics, methodology used, measures selected, and quantitative results from each of the articles were abstracted and evaluated.

Findings are illustrated in Table 1. Six studies included adult participants, and three studies included children and adolescents (students in middle school and high school). One study included both adolescents and adults, and one study did not report information regarding the inclusion of participants that were under 18 years old (participants were patients at a dermatology clinic). Three studies excluded participants with history of skin cancer, and five studies reported data on sun protection behaviors. One study was population-based. Two studies had survey materials available in Spanish, and one study was conducted entirely in Spanish. Two studies reported data on country origin/heritage. Five studies had relatively small Hispanic samples (less than 100 participants). Most studies ($n = 10$) were published during the last decade (2004–2014).

Skin cancer seriousness (severity, worry) was a belief considered in three studies [29–31]. Results from a population study showed that Hispanics and whites share similar levels of worry about skin cancer ($P > 0.05$) [29]. One study reported a midrange score in terms of skin cancer worry in Hispanics. Another study found that perceived skin cancer severity was associated with incidence of total body examination (i.e., a head-to-toe examination of the skin performed by a physician used to identify suspicious growths that may be cancer or growths that may develop into skin), but not with incidence of skin self-examination (i.e., a head-to-toe examination of the skin performed by the individual, not a physician) [30, 31].

Most studies included in the review ($n = 8$) considered skin cancer susceptibility (or risk) beliefs. One study found that Hispanics believe they have lower than average risk of developing skin cancer, and that their level of risk is lower when compared with whites [32]. A second study reported that most Hispanics described their skin cancer susceptibility as average [33]. A third study also found lower perception of skin cancer risk when Hispanics were compared with whites but the difference was not significant when participants were asked to compare their own likelihood of getting skin cancer compared with the risk of an average person of the same age [29]. Two studies reported similar scores on their skin cancer risk and photoaging (changes in skin appearance induced by sun exposure) concern measures but used different scales for the scores [30, 34]. Participants were inclined to not agree or disagree (midrange score) with the following statement: "The natural color of my skin protects me from the sun" [30]. After quantifying qualitative information from an all-female sample, it was found that less than half of the participants believe they can develop skin cancer [24]. On the other hand, almost all participants were concerned about the effect of sun exposure on their appearance. Using a different sample as part of an experiment within the same study, participants reported an increase in skin cancer susceptibility "of Hispanics with fair skin and Hispanics with dark skin" (not their own susceptibility) after watching an educational video about sun protection behaviors. Another study asked Hispanics about the skin cancer susceptibility of people "in darker skin types," and results showed that a slightly lower proportion of Hispanics (78%) endorsed this statement compared with white (91%) and black (86%) participants [35]. Another study reported that perceived skin cancer risk is associated with skin self-examination [31].

A strong effect size was reported for association between perceived peer norms for sun exposure and barriers to sun safety in Hispanic middle school students [36]. Hispanics are more likely to believe that there is not much they can do to lower their risk of getting skin cancer and that there are too many recommendations to prevent this illness [26]. It was also reported that more than half of Hispanics believe that tanning makes people look more attractive and do not endorse the belief that tanning makes people older [37]. One study showed that Hispanics tend to marginally agree more with statements regarding sun protection benefits than barriers [30]. Participants also indicated what were the most important benefits and barriers to engage in sun protection behaviors, with "avoid getting sunburn" and "not part of my daily routine" as frequently endorsed statements. Another study showed a similar pattern in terms of sun protection beliefs [34]. An additional reason Hispanics endorse for failing to use sunscreen is because they consider themselves "dark skinned" [38].

4. Discussion

This study examined published reports of sun protection beliefs in Hispanics, and we found eleven manuscripts that followed the established criteria. Results suggest that low skin cancer susceptibility is commonly found in this population and that Hispanics moderately perceive skin cancer as a serious health threat. Results also suggest that assessments of sun protection barriers and benefits vary significantly by study. Overall, findings illustrated that there are limited studies on psychosocial and modifiable factors that influence sun protection. Many of the studies included in this review have limited sample size or used samples that do not represent the heterogeneous Hispanic population (e.g., 70% of participants in one study were of Mexican origin) [30, 31]. Findings must be validated in larger, more comprehensive studies. Results also emphasize the need for comparable and consistent assessment regarding sun protection. This finding is consistent with previous skin cancer prevention results. An evaluation of interventions designed to educate primary care physicians about skin cancer showed a lack of uniformity across interventions and outcome assessments, preventing the direct comparison of intervention efficacy and the dissemination of effective components [39].

Skin cancer can be prevented by practicing sun protection, but skin cancer disparities might be associated with the perceptions, knowledge, attitudes, and beliefs Hispanics hold regarding skin cancer and sun protection. It has been found

that individuals who express the benefits of sun protection are likely to report sun protection behaviors consistently more than those who communicate the barriers of sun protection [40–42]. Hispanics are more likely to believe there is little they can do to lower their chances of getting skin cancer, that there are so many recommendations about skin cancer prevention that they do not know which one to believe and believe that they are below average risk for skin cancer compared with whites. It is critical to understand the sets of beliefs that underlie sun protection among Hispanics and improve health promotion initiatives to decrease sun protection disparities.

Most common types of skin cancer are squamous cell carcinoma and basal cell carcinoma (SCC and BCC, resp.; nonmelanoma), and melanoma. These cancers have different causes and presentations. Basal cell carcinoma diagnoses are more common in Hispanics than squamous cell carcinoma and melanoma diagnoses [43, 44]. While person characteristics (e.g., light skin, sun sensitivity, and blistering sunburns early in life) and intermittent sun exposure are strong risk factors for the diagnosis of melanoma, both cumulative and intermittent sun exposure are the most common cause of basal cell carcinoma. In terms of presentation, melanoma usually involves sites not exposed to the sun, including palmar, plantar, and mucosal surfaces, and the lower extremities [45]. Areas such as the head and the neck regions seem to be more prone for basal cell carcinoma. Literature in sun exposure at the workplace indicates an elevated risk for SCC but is less conclusive for BCC [46]. A population-based control-study among individuals diagnosed with invasive melanoma found that frequent sunscreen use when not planning to be in the sun during the last 20 years was strongly associated with lower likelihood of melanoma [47]. Also, those who reported use of sun protection (not sunscreen) were at lower risk of developing melanoma, even if its use was inconsistent. Consistent with the compensation hypothesis of sunscreen use and increased sun exposure, optimal use of sunscreen SPF+15 was associated with highest amount of sun exposure. Research directly associating sun protection behaviors to decreased skin cancer risk is limited and inconsistent. The present study shows that research still struggles to investigate and understand the specific factors that might be associated with melanoma and nonmelanoma skin cancer incidence, and disparities in skin cancer. Research should clarify the association between the disease, the target population, and the particular mechanisms to prevent the disease.

Previous research shows a moderate level of awareness about skin cancer risk factors and prevention behaviors among Hispanics. Using a qualitative approach, forty Hispanics were asked about their understanding of skin cancer risk terminology [26]. Results illustrated that participants did not recognize possible indicators of skin cancer risk (e.g., painful sunburns). One study showed that more Hispanics do not use sunscreen because they perceive themselves as dark skinned when compared with whites and Asian/Pacific Islanders (29% versus 3% versus 11.4%, $P < 0.05$) [38]. Results included in the present review emphasize the need for improved assessments of sun protection beliefs and to incorporate the evaluation of the meaning and significance Hispanics give to sun protection: do they know what protective clothing is?; what do they think about using sunscreen "all the time" when out in the sun, including cloudy days?; would they wear a hat at all?; do they know how their skin reacts to sun exposure? These are questions that future research should address if we want to report a more accurate analysis of sun protection. This review underscores the importance of developing culturally relevant, validated, and reliable measures of sun protection and skin cancer risk perception for Hispanic adults, adolescents, and children.

Our search was limited to peer-reviewed journals, which generally publish studies with significant results. It was also limited to results on sun protection beliefs in Hispanics living in the US. Findings cannot be generalized to studies conducted in other countries, and there is a possibility that important elements of sun protection were not captured in our review. A strength of this review is that it helped us realize that the full potentials of the assessment and applications of sun protection beliefs for the prevention of skin cancer in Hispanics remain largely unverified and untested. This finding should open the doors to many research initiatives to promote health in a growing minority population and to identify and understand factors that contribute to disparities in the incidence and mortality of cancer.

Hispanics are a diverse group that exhibit differences in terms of sun protection behaviors, sun sensitivity, level of acculturation, country of origin, access to health services, and socioeconomic status. Future research should develop comprehensive, culturally sensitive measures of sun protection beliefs, facilitators, and barriers. Measures should be grounded in theory, research evidence, and ethnographic study. Also, researchers must ensure that their recruitment strategy attains a more diverse sample than previous research. The National Cancer Institute states that overcoming cancer health disparities is one of the best opportunities we have for lessening the burden of cancer [48]. It is goal of the institute to improve the understanding of the causes of cancer health disparities as a way to eliminate them. It is critical to identify modifiable factors that can reduce skin cancer morbidity and mortality disparities in the US. There is a need for informed, culturally sensitive measures to assess sun protection in the Hispanic population in order to (1) directly inform the development of a study to investigate the ability of sun protection beliefs to predict the likelihood to engage in positive health outcomes (i.e., sun protection behaviors), (2) make informed assessments of the effect of sun protection on skin cancer morbidity and mortality, (3) contribute to the limited literature on sun protection in Hispanics, (4) inform the development of targeted public health recommendations and initiatives to increase sun protection, and (5) make a contribution to the identification and understanding of experiences Hispanics have regarding sun protection.

Acknowledgment

The authors acknowledge the support received by the Department of Oncological Sciences, Icahn School of Medicine at Mount Sinai (Grant R25-CA081137).

References

[1] American Cancer Society, *Cancer Facts & Figures 2013*, American Cancer Society, Atlanta, Ga, USA, 2013.

[2] D. U. Ekwueme, G. P. Guy Jr., C. Li, S. H. Rim, P. Parelkar, and S. C. Chen, "The health burden and economic costs of cutaneous melanoma mortality by race/ethnicity—United States, 2000 to 2006," *Journal of the American Academy of Dermatology*, vol. 65, no. 5, supplement 1, pp. S133.e1–S133.e12, 2011.

[3] E. J. Coups, S. L. Manne, and C. J. Heckman, "Multiple skin cancer risk behaviors in the U.S. population," *The American Journal of Preventive Medicine*, vol. 34, no. 2, pp. 87–93, 2008.

[4] American Cancer Society, *Datos y Estadísticas sobre el Cáncer entre los Hispanos/Latinos 2012-2014*, Sociedad Americana Contra El Cáncer, Atlanta, Ga, USA, 2012.

[5] M. P. McLeod, K. M. Ferris, S. Choudhary et al., "Contralateral distribution of nonmelanoma skin cancer between older Hispanic/Latino and non-Hispanic/non-Latino individuals," *British Journal of Dermatology*, vol. 168, no. 1, pp. 65–73, 2013.

[6] R. B. Harris, K. Griffith, and T. E. Moon, "Trends in the incidence of nonmelanoma skin cancers in southeastern Arizona, 1985–1996," *Journal of the American Academy of Dermatology*, vol. 45, no. 4, pp. 528–536, 2001.

[7] S. Javed, S. A. Javed, R. M. Mays, and S. K. Tyring, "Clinical characteristics and awareness of skin cancer in Hispanic patients," *Dermatology Online Journal*, vol. 19, no. 9, Article ID 19623, 2013.

[8] M. Clairwood, J. Ricketts, J. Grant-Kels, and L. Gonsalves, "Melanoma in skin of color in Connecticut: an analysis of melanoma incidence and stage at diagnosis in non-Hispanic blacks, non-Hispanic whites, and Hispanics," *International Journal of Dermatology*, vol. 53, no. 4, pp. 425–433, 2014.

[9] M. G. Cockburn, J. Zadnick, and D. Deapen, "Developing epidemic of melanoma in the hispanic population of California," *Cancer*, vol. 106, no. 5, pp. 1162–1168, 2006.

[10] S. Hu, Y. Parmet, G. Allen et al., "Disparity in melanoma: a trend analysis of melanoma incidence and stage at diagnosis among whites, Hispanics, and blacks in Florida," *Archives of Dermatology*, vol. 145, no. 12, pp. 1369–1374, 2009.

[11] S. Hu, R. M. Soza-Vento, D. F. Parker, and R. S. Kirsner, "Comparison of stage at diagnosis of melanoma among Hispanic, black, and white patients in Miami-Dade County, Florida," *Archives of Dermatology*, vol. 142, no. 6, pp. 704–708, 2006.

[12] S. Javed, S. A. Javed, R. M. Mays, and S. K. Tyring, "Clinical characteristics and awareness of skin cancer in Hispanic patients," *Dermatology Online Journal*, vol. 19, no. 9, article 19623, 2013.

[13] R. M. Merrill, J. D. Harris, and J. G. Merrill, "Differences in incidence rates and early detection of cancer among nonhispanic and hispanic whites in the united states," *Ethnicity and Disease*, vol. 23, no. 3, pp. 349–355, 2013.

[14] R. M. Merrill, N. D. Pace, and A. N. Elison, "Cutaneous malignant melanoma among white Hispanics and non-Hispanics in the United States," *Ethnicity and Disease*, vol. 20, no. 4, pp. 353–358, 2010.

[15] R. A. Pollitt, C. A. Clarke, S. M. Swetter, D. H. Peng, J. Zadnick, and M. Cockburn, "The expanding melanoma burden in California hispanics: importance of socioeconomic distribution, histologic subtype, and anatomic location," *Cancer*, vol. 117, no. 1, pp. 152–161, 2011.

[16] X.-C. Wu, M. J. Eide, J. King et al., "Racial and ethnic variations in incidence and survival of cutaneous melanoma in the United States, 1999–2006," *Journal of the American Academy of Dermatology*, vol. 65, no. 5, pp. S26–S37, 2011.

[17] S. A. Davis, S. Narahari, S. R. Feldman, W. Huang, R. O. Pichardo-Geisinger, and A. J. McMichael, "Top dermatologic conditions in patients of color: an analysis of nationally representative data," *Journal of Drugs in Dermatology*, vol. 11, no. 4, pp. 466–473, 2012.

[18] G. Y. F. Ho, N. R. Figueroa-Vallés, T. de La Torre-Feliciano et al., "Cancer disparities between Mainland and island Puerto Ricans," *Revista Panamericana de Salud Publica*, vol. 25, no. 5, pp. 394–400, 2009.

[19] J. Weiss, R. S. Kirsner, and S. Hu, "Trends in primary skin cancer prevention among US Hispanics: a systematic review," *Journal of Drugs in Dermatology*, vol. 11, no. 5, pp. 580–586, 2012.

[20] E. J. Coups, J. L. Stapleton, S. V. Hudson, A. Medina-Forrester, A. Natale-Pereira, and J. S. Goydos, "Sun protection and exposure behaviors among Hispanic adults in the United States: differences according to acculturation and among Hispanic subgroups," *BMC Public Health*, vol. 12, no. 1, article 985, 2012.

[21] E. J. Coups, J. L. Stapleton, S. V. Hudson et al., "Linguistic acculturation and skin cancer-related behaviors among hispanics in the southern and western united states," *JAMA Dermatology*, vol. 149, no. 6, pp. 679–686, 2013.

[22] Community Preventive Services Task Force—Cancer Prevention & Control, *The Guide to Community Preventive Services Website*, 2014, http://www.thecommunityguide.org/cancer/index.html.

[23] M. Saraiya, K. Glanz, P. A. Briss et al., "Interventions to prevent skin cancer by reducing exposure to ultraviolet radiation: a systematic review," *American Journal of Preventive Medicine*, vol. 27, no. 5, pp. 422–466, 2004.

[24] C. Hernandez, S. Wang, I. Abraham et al., "Evaluation of educational videos to increase skin cancer risk awareness and sun-safe behaviors among adult Hispanics," *Journal of Cancer Education*, vol. 29, no. 3, pp. 563–569, 2014.

[25] R. V. Kundu, M. Kamaria, S. Ortiz, D. P. West, A. W. Rademaker, and J. K. Robinson, "Effectiveness of a knowledge-based intervention for melanoma among those with ethnic skin," *Journal of the American Academy of Dermatology*, vol. 62, no. 5, pp. 777–784, 2010.

[26] J. K. Robinson, K. M. Joshi, S. Ortiz, and R. V. Kundu, "Melanoma knowledge, perception, and awareness in ethnic minorities in Chicago: recommendations regarding education," *Psycho-Oncology*, vol. 20, no. 3, pp. 313–320, 2011.

[27] N. Jaimes, V. Londono, and A. C. Halpern, "The term hispanic/latino: a note of caution," *JAMA Dermatology*, vol. 149, no. 3, pp. 274–275, 2013.

[28] P. Taylor, H. M. Lopez, J. H. Martinez, and G. Velasco, *When Labels Don't Fit: Hispanics and Their Views of Identity*, Pew Hispanic Center, Washington, DC, USA, 2012.

[29] K. J. Buster, Z. You, M. Fouad, and C. Elmets, "Skin cancer risk perceptions: a comparison across ethnicity, age, education, gender, and income," *Journal of the American Academy of Dermatology*, vol. 66, no. 5, pp. 771–779, 2012.

[30] E. J. Coups, J. L. Stapleton, S. L. Manne et al., "Psychosocial correlates of sun protection behaviors among U.S. Hispanic adults," *Journal of Behavioral Medicine*, pp. 1–9, 2014.

[31] E. J. Coups, J. L. Stapleton, S. V. Hudson et al., "Skin cancer surveillance behaviors among US Hispanic adults," *Journal of the American Academy of Dermatology*, vol. 68, no. 4, pp. 576–584, 2013.

[32] F. Ma, F. Collado-Mesa, S. Hu, and R. S. Kirsner, "Skin cancer awareness and sun protection behaviors in white Hispanic and white non-Hispanic high school students in Miami, Florida," *Archives of Dermatology*, vol. 143, no. 8, pp. 983–988, 2007.

[33] M. Pipitone, J. K. Robinson, C. Camara, B. Chittineni, and S. G. Fisher, "Skin cancer awareness in suburban employees: a hispanic perspective," *Journal of the American Academy of Dermatology*, vol. 47, no. 1, pp. 118–123, 2002.

[34] C. J. Heckman and J. Cohen-Filipic, "Brief report: ultraviolet radiation exposure, considering acculturation among hispanics (Project URECAH)," *Journal of Cancer Education*, vol. 27, no. 2, pp. 342–346, 2012.

[35] J. Imahiyerobo-Ip, I. Ip, S. Jamal, U. Nadiminti, and M. Sanchez, "Skin cancer awareness in communities of color," *Journal of the American Academy of Dermatology*, vol. 64, no. 1, pp. 198–200, 2011.

[36] V. A. Andreeva, K. D. Reynolds, D. B. Buller, C.-P. Chou, and A. L. Yaroch, "Concurrent psychosocial predictors of sun safety among middle school youth," *Journal of School Health*, vol. 78, no. 7, pp. 374–381, 2008.

[37] C. E. Cheng, B. Irwin, D. Mauriello, L. Hemminger, A. Pappert, and A. B. Kimball, "Health disparities among different ethnic and racial middle and high school students in sun exposure beliefs and knowledge," *Journal of Adolescent Health*, vol. 47, no. 1, pp. 106–109, 2010.

[38] H. I. Mahler, "Reasons for using and failing to use sunscreen: comparison among whites, Hispanics, and Asian/Pacific Islanders in Southern California," *JAMA Dermatology*, vol. 150, no. 1, pp. 90–91, 2014.

[39] J. M. Goulart, E. A. Quigley, S. Dusza et al., "Skin cancer education for primary care physicians: a systematic review of published evaluated interventions," *Journal of General Internal Medicine*, vol. 26, no. 9, pp. 1027–1035, 2011.

[40] V. K. Nahar, M. A. Ford, J. S. Hallam, M. A. Bass, A. Hutcheson, and M. A. Vice, "Skin cancer knowledge, beliefs, self-efficacy, and preventative behaviors among north mississippi landscapers," *Dermatology Research and Practice*, vol. 2013, Article ID 496913, 7 pages, 2013.

[41] N. A. Kasparian, J. K. McLoone, and B. Meiser, "Skin cancer-related prevention and screening behaviors: a review of the literature," *Journal of Behavioral Medicine*, vol. 32, no. 5, pp. 406–428, 2009.

[42] S. Manne and S. Lessin, "Prevalence and correlates of sun protection and skin self-examination practices among cutaneous malignant melanoma survivors," *Journal of Behavioral Medicine*, vol. 29, no. 5, pp. 419–434, 2006.

[43] W. E. Hoy, "Nonmelanoma skin carcinoma in Albuquerque, New Mexico: experience of a major health care provider," *Cancer*, vol. 77, no. 12, pp. 2489–2495, 1996.

[44] H. M. Gloster Jr. and K. Neal, "Skin cancer in skin of color," *Journal of the American Academy of Dermatology*, vol. 55, no. 5, pp. 741–760, 761–744, 2006.

[45] K. Byrd-Miles, E. L. Toombs, and G. L. Peck, "Skin cancer in individuals of African, Asian, Latin-American, and American-Indian descent: differences in incidence, clinical presentation,

and survival compared to Caucasians," *Journal of Drugs in Dermatology*, vol. 6, no. 1, pp. 10–16, 2007.

[46] S. Surdu, "Non-melanoma skin cancer: occupational risk from UV light and arsenic exposure," *Reviews on Environmental Health*, vol. 29, no. 3, pp. 255–265, 2014.

[47] D. Lazovich, R. I. Vogel, M. Berwick, M. A. Weinstock, E. M. Warshaw, and K. E. Anderson, "Melanoma risk in relation to use of sunscreen or other sun protection methods," *Cancer Epidemiology, Biomarkers & Prevention*, vol. 20, no. 12, pp. 2583–2593, 2011.

[48] National Cancer Institiute, *Cancer Health Disparities*, 2014, http://www.cancer.gov/cancertopics/disparities.

Permissions

All chapters in this book were first published in JSC, by Hindawi Publishing Corporation; hereby published with permission under the Creative Commons Attribution License or equivalent. Every chapter published in this book has been scrutinized by our experts. Their significance has been extensively debated. The topics covered herein carry significant findings which will fuel the growth of the discipline. They may even be implemented as practical applications or may be referred to as a beginning point for another development.

The contributors of this book come from diverse backgrounds, making this book a truly international effort. This book will bring forth new frontiers with its revolutionizing research information and detailed analysis of the nascent developments around the world.

We would like to thank all the contributing authors for lending their expertise to make the book truly unique. They have played a crucial role in the development of this book. Without their invaluable contributions this book wouldn't have been possible. They have made vital efforts to compile up to date information on the varied aspects of this subject to make this book a valuable addition to the collection of many professionals and students.

This book was conceptualized with the vision of imparting up-to-date information and advanced data in this field. To ensure the same, a matchless editorial board was set up. Every individual on the board went through rigorous rounds of assessment to prove their worth. After which they invested a large part of their time researching and compiling the most relevant data for our readers.

The editorial board has been involved in producing this book since its inception. They have spent rigorous hours researching and exploring the diverse topics which have resulted in the successful publishing of this book. They have passed on their knowledge of decades through this book. To expedite this challenging task, the publisher supported the team at every step. A small team of assistant editors was also appointed to further simplify the editing procedure and attain best results for the readers.

Apart from the editorial board, the designing team has also invested a significant amount of their time in understanding the subject and creating the most relevant covers. They scrutinized every image to scout for the most suitable representation of the subject and create an appropriate cover for the book.

The publishing team has been an ardent support to the editorial, designing and production team. Their endless efforts to recruit the best for this project, has resulted in the accomplishment of this book. They are a veteran in the field of academics and their pool of knowledge is as vast as their experience in printing. Their expertise and guidance has proved useful at every step. Their uncompromising quality standards have made this book an exceptional effort. Their encouragement from time to time has been an inspiration for everyone.

The publisher and the editorial board hope that this book will prove to be a valuable piece of knowledge for researchers, students, practitioners and scholars across the globe.

List of Contributors

A. I. Reeder
Cancer Society of New Zealand Social and Behavioural Research Unit, Department of Preventive and Social Medicine, Dunedin School of Medicine, University of Otago

G. F. H. McLeod
Department of Psychological Medicine, School of Medical and Health Sciences, University of Otago, Christchurch 8140, New Zealand

A. R. Gray and R. McGee
Department of Preventive and Social Medicine, Dunedin School of Medicine, University of Otago Dunedin 9054, New Zealand

Hui-Qing Yin, Joseph S. Rossi, Colleen A. Redding, Andrea L. Paiva, Steven F. Babbin and Wayne F. Velicer
Cancer Prevention Research Center, University of Rhode Island, 130 Flagg Road, Kingston, RI 02881, USA

Judith M. Fontana, Justin G. Mygatt, Katelyn L. Conant and Johnan A. R. Kaleeba
Department of Microbiology and Immunology, Uniformed Services University of the Health Sciences, 4301 Jones Bridge Road, Bethesda, MD 20814, USA

Chris H. Parsons
Department of Medicine and Microbiology, Stanley S. Scott Cancer Center, Louisiana State University Health Science Center, New Orleans, LA 70112, USA

Erin M. Burns, Kathleen L. Tober, Judith A. Riggenbach and Tatiana M. Oberyszyn
Department of Pathology, The Ohio State University, 1645 Neil Avenue, 129 Hamilton Hall, Columbus, OH 43210, USA

Donna F. Kusewitt
Department of Molecular Carcinogenesis, Science Park, UT MD Anderson Cancer Center, 1808 Park Road 1C, Smithville, TX 78957, USA

Gregory S. Young
Center for Biostatistics, The Ohio State University, 2012 Kenny Road, Columbus, OH 43221, USA

Marie-LaureMatthey-Giè, Nicolas Demartines andMaurice Matter
Department of Visceral Surgery, University Hospital CHUV, Lausanne, Switzerland

Ariane Boubaker
Department of Nuclear Medicine, University Hospital CHUV, Lausanne, Switzerland

Igor Letovanec
Department of Pathology, University Hospital CHUV, Lausanne, Switzerland

Donald B. Warren, Jason B. Hobbs and Richard F. Wagner Jr.
Department of Dermatology, The University of Texas Medical Branch, 301 University Boulevard, Galveston, TX 77555-0783, USA

Ryan R. Riahi
Department of Dermatology, Louisiana State University, New Orleans, LA 70112-2865, USA

Robert M. Samstein, Nancy Y. Lee and Christopher A. Barker
Department of Radiation Oncology, Memorial Sloan Kettering Cancer Center, 1275 York Avenue, New York, NY 10065, USA

Alan L. Ho
Department of Medicine, Memorial Sloan Kettering Cancer Center, New York, NY 10065, USA

Janine Mitchell, Peta Callaghan and Jackie Street
School of Population Health, Level 11 Terrace Towers, 178 North Terrace, The University of Adelaide

Susan Neuhaus and Taryn Bessen
Royal Adelaide Hospital, North Terrace, Adelaide, SA 5000, Australia

Ashok Singh, Anupama Singh, Bilal Bin Hafeez and Ajit K. Verma
Department of Human Oncology, Wisconsin Institutes for Medical Research, School of Medicine and Public Health, 1111 Highland Avenue, University of Wisconsin, Madison, WI 53705, USA

Jordan M. Sand
Department of Human Oncology, Wisconsin Institutes for Medical Research, School of Medicine and Public Health, 1111 Highland Avenue, University of Wisconsin, Madison, WI 53705, USA
Molecular and Environmental Toxicology Center, Wisconsin Institutes for Medical Research, Paul P. Carbone Comprehensive Cancer Center, School of Medicine and Public Health, University of Wisconsin, Madison, WI 53705, USA

Erika Heninger
UWCCC Flow Cytometry Core Facility, School of Medicine and Public Health, University of Wisconsin, Madison, WI 53705, USA

Vinayak K. Nahar, M. Allison Ford, Martha A. Bass and Michael A. Vice
Department of Health, Exercise Science and Recreation Management, The University of Mississippi, 215 Turner Center

Jeffrey S. Hallam
Department of Social and Behavioral Sciences, College of Public Health, Kent State University, 750 Hilltop Drive, Kent, OH 44242, USA

Sergio Umberto De Marchi, Serena Bonin, Nicola di Meo and Giusto Trevisan
Institute of Dermatology and Venereology, University of Trieste, Ospedale Maggiore, Piazza Ospedale 1, 34100 Trieste, Italy

Giuseppe Stinco and Enzo Errichetti
Institute of Dermatology, Department of Experimental and Clinical Medicine, University of Udine, Ospedale San Michele, Piazza Rodolone 1, 33013 Gemona del Friuli, Italy

Muhammed BeGir Öztürk
Department of Plastic Reconstructive and Aesthetic Surgery, Tekirdag Government Hospital, 59020 Tekirdag, Turkey

Arzu Akan
Department of General Surgery, Okmeydani Training and Research Hospital, 34445 Istanbul, Turkey

Özay Özkaya, Onur Egemen and Turgut Kayadibi
Department of Plastic Reconstructive and Aesthetic Surgery, Okmeydani Training and Research Hospital, 34445 Istanbul, Turkey

Ali RJza ÖreroLlu
Department of Plastic Reconstructive and Aesthetic Surgery, Prof. Dr. A. Ilhan Ozdemir State Hospital, 28000 Giresun, Turkey

Mithat Akan
Department of Plastic Reconstructive and Aesthetic Surgery, Medipol University Hospital, 34200 Istanbul, Turkey

Andrew L. Ji and Scott A. Davis
Galderma Center for Dermatology Research, Department of Dermatology, Wake Forest School of Medicine, Winston-Salem, NC 27157-1071, USA

Michael R. Baze
Nova Southeastern University/Broward Health Medical Center, Department of Dermatology, Fort Lauderdale, FL 33315, USA

Steven R. Feldman
Galderma Center for Dermatology Research, Department of Dermatology, Wake Forest School of Medicine, Winston-Salem, NC 27157-1071, USA
Galderma Center for Dermatology Research, Department of Pathology, Wake Forest School of Medicine, Winston-Salem, NC 27157-1071, USA
Galderma Center for Dermatology Research, Department of Public Health Sciences, Wake Forest School of Medicine, Winston-Salem, NC 27157-1071, USA

Alan B. Fleischer Jr.
Galderma Center for Dermatology Research, Department of Dermatology, Wake Forest School of Medicine, Winston-Salem, NC 27157-1071, USA
Wake Forest University School of Medicine, Department of Dermatology, Medical Center Boulevard, Winston-Salem, NC 27157-1071, USA

Kowichi Jimbow
Institute of Dermatology and Cutaneous Sciences, 1-27 Odori West 17, Chuo-ku, Sapporo 060-0042, Japan
Department of Dermatology, School of Medicine, Sapporo Medical University, South 1West 16, Chuo-ku, Sapporo 060-8556, Japan

Yasue Ishii-Osai, Akihiro Yoneta, Takafumi Kamiya and Toshiharu Yamashita
Department of Dermatology, School of Medicine, Sapporo Medical University, South 1West 16, Chuo-ku, Sapporo 060-8556, Japan

Shosuke Ito and Kazumasa Wakamatsu
Department of Chemistry, School of Health Sciences, Fujita Health University, 1-98 Dengakugakubo, Kutsukake-cho, Toyoake, Aichi 470-1192, Japan

Yasuaki Tamura
Department of Pathology 1, School of Medicine, Sapporo Medical University, South 1West 16, Chuo-ku, Sapporo 060-8556, Japan

Akira Ito
Department of Chemical Engineering, Faculty of Engineering, Kyushu University, 744 Motooka, Nishi-ku, Fukuoka 819-0395, Japan

Hiroyuki Honda
Department of Biotechnology, School of Engineering, Nagoya University, Furo-cho, Chikusa-ku, Nagoya 464-8603, Japan

Katsutoshi Murase and Satoshi Nohara
Meito Sangyo Co., Ltd., 25-5 Kaechi, Nishibiwajima-cho, Kiyosu, Aichi 452-0067, Japan

Eiichi Nakayama
Faculty of Health and Welfare, Kawasaki University of Medical Welfare, 288 Matsushimai, Kurashiki, Okayama 701-0193, Japan

Takeo Hasegawa
Department of Hyperthermia Medical Research Laboratory, Louis Pasteur Center for Medical Research, 103-5, Tanakamonzen-cho, Sakyo-ku, Kyoto 606-8225, Japan

Itsuo Yamamoto
Yamamoto Vinita Co., Ltd., 3-12 ueshio 6, Tennoji-ku, Osaka 543-0002, Japan

Takeshi Kobayashi
Department of Biological Chemistry, College of Bioscience and Biotechnology, Chubu University, 1200 Matsumoto-cho, Kasugai, Aichi 487-8501, Japan

Sarita Nibhoria, Kanwardeep Kaur Tiwana and Manmeet Kaur
Department of Pathology, G.G.S. Medical College and Hospital BFUHS, Faridkot, Punjab 151203, India

Sumir Kumar
Department of Skin and VD, G.G.S. Medical College and Hospital BFUHS, Faridkot, Punjab 151203, India

Rebecca G. Simmons, Kristi Smith, Meghan Balough and Michael Friedrichs
Utah Department of Health, Salt Lake City, UT 84116, USA

J. J. Cubitt
Stoke Mandeville Hospital, Mandeville Road, Aylesbury HP21 8AL, UK
TheWelsh Centre for Burns and Plastic Surgery, Morriston Hospital, Morriston, SA6 6NL, UK

A. A. Khan, E. Royston, M. Rughani and P. G Budny
Stoke Mandeville Hospital, Mandeville Road, Aylesbury HP21 8AL, UK

M. R. Middleton
Oxford NIHR Biomedical Research, Churchill Hospital, Old Road, Headington, OX3 7LE, UK

Stephanie H. Shirley, Kristine von Maltzan, Paige O. Robbins and Donna F. Kusewitt
Department of Molecular Carcinogenesis, Science Park, University of Texas MD Anderson Cancer Center, 1808 Park Road 1C, Smithville, TX 78957, USA

M. Fernández-Guarino, A. Harto, B. Pérez-García and P. Jaén
Dermatology Department, Ramon y Cajal Universitary Hospital, Carretera de Colmenar Km 9, 100, 28034Madrid, Spain

A. Royuela
Statistics Department, Ramon y Cajal Universitary Hospital, Carretera de Colmenar Km 9, 100, 28034 Madrid, Spain

Vera Teixeira, Inês Coutinho, Rita Cabral, David Serra, Maria Manuel Brites and Ricardo Vieira
Dermatology Department, Coimbra University Hospital, Praceta Mota Pinto, 3000-075 Coimbra, Portugal

Américo Figueiredo
Dermatology Department, Coimbra University Hospital, Praceta Mota Pinto, 3000-075 Coimbra, Portugal
Faculty of Medicine, University of Coimbra, 3000-075 Coimbra, Portugal

Maria José Julião
Pathology Department, Coimbra University Hospital, 3000-075 Coimbra, Portugal

Anabela Albuquerque
Nuclear Medicine Department, Coimbra University Hospital, 3000-075 Coimbra, Portugal

João Pedroso de Lima
Faculty of Medicine, University of Coimbra, 3000-075 Coimbra, Portugal
Nuclear Medicine Department, Coimbra University Hospital, 3000-075 Coimbra, Portugal

Rajani Katta
Department of Dermatology, Baylor College of Medicine, 1977 Butler Boulevard, Suite E6.200, Houston, TX 77030, USA

Danielle Nicole Brown
Department of Dermatology, Baylor College of Medicine, Houston, TX 77030, USA

Erica H. Lee, Nehal and Stephen W. Dusza
Department of Medicine, Dermatology Service, Memorial Sloan Kettering Cancer Center, New York, NY 10022, USA

Rajiv I. Nijhawan
Department of Medicine, Dermatology Service, Memorial Sloan Kettering Cancer Center, New York, NY 10022, USA
Department of Dermatology, University of Texas Southwestern Medical Center, Dallas, TX 75390, USA

Kishwer S. Amanda Levine, Amanda Hill and Christopher A. Barker
Department of Radiation Oncology, Memorial Sloan Kettering Cancer Center, New York, NY 10065, USA

Shalaka S. Hampras, Rhianna A. Reed and Dana E. Rollison
Department of Cancer Epidemiology, Moffitt Cancer Center, Tampa, Florida, USA

Spencer Bezalel and Michael Cameron
University of South Florida, Morsani College of Medicine, Tampa, Florida, USA

Basil Cherpelis and Neil Fenske
Department of Dermatology, University of South Florida, College of Medicine, Tampa, FL, USA
Department of Cutaneous Surgery, University of South Florida, College of Medicine, Tampa, FL, USA

Vernon K. Sondak
Cutaneous Oncology Program, Moffitt Cancer Center, Tampa, Florida, USA

Jane Messina
Department of Dermatology, University of South Florida, College of Medicine, Tampa, FL, USA
Cutaneous Oncology Program, Moffitt Cancer Center, Tampa, Florida, USA
Departments of Pathology and Cell Biology, University of South Florida, College of Medicine, Tampa, FL, USA

Massimo Tommasino and Tarik Gheit
Infections and Cancer Biology Group, International Agency for Research on Cancer-World Health Organization, Lyon 69372, France

Lori G. Strayer
Masonic Cancer Center, University of Minnesota, Minneapolis, MN, USA

Rachel I. Vogel
Masonic Cancer Center, University of Minnesota, Minneapolis, MN, USA
Division of Gynecologic Oncology, University of Minnesota, Minneapolis, MN, USA

Rehana L. Ahmed
Masonic Cancer Center, University of Minnesota, Minneapolis, MN, USA
Department of Dermatology, University of Minnesota, Minneapolis, MN, USA

Anne Blaes
Masonic Cancer Center, University of Minnesota, Minneapolis, MN, USA
Department of Medicine, Division of Hematology and Oncology, University of Minnesota, Minneapolis, MN, USA

DeAnn Lazovich
Masonic Cancer Center, University of Minnesota, Minneapolis, MN, USA
Division of Epidemiology and Community Health, University of Minnesota, Minneapolis, MN, USA

Sonia Kamath
Department of Dermatology, Keck School of Medicine of the University of Southern California (USC), 1200 N State Street, Room 3250, Los Angeles, CA 90033, USA

Kimberly A. Miller
Department of Preventive Medicine, Keck School of Medicine of USC, 2001 N. Soto Street, Suite 318-A, Los Angeles, CA 90032, USA

Myles G. Cockburn
Department of Dermatology, Keck School of Medicine of the University of Southern California (USC), 1200 N State Street, Room 3250, Los Angeles, CA 90033, USA
Department of Preventive Medicine, Keck School of Medicine of USC, 2001 N. Soto Street, Suite 318-A, Los Angeles, CA 90032, USA

Jessica N. Kimmel and Tiffany H. Taft
Department of Medicine, Division of Gastroenterology and Hepatology, Northwestern University School of Medicine, Arkes Family Pavilion Suite 1400, 676 North Saint Clair Street, Chicago, IL 60611, USA

Laurie Keefer
Department of Medicine, Division of Gastroenterology and Hepatology, Northwestern University School of Medicine, Arkes Family Pavilion Suite 1400, 676 North Saint Clair Street, Chicago, IL 60611, USA
Icahn School of Medicine, Mount Sinai Medical Center, Susan and Leonard Feinstein IBD Center, 17 East 102nd Street, 5th Floor, New York, NY 10029, USA

Robert A. Yockey
Department of Psychiatry and Behavioral Neuroscience and Department of Health Education and Promotion, University of Cincinnati, Cincinnati, OH 45221-0068, USA

Laura A. Nabors, Kristen Welker and Angelica M. Hardee
Health Promotion and Education Program, School of Human Services, University of Cincinnati, Cincinnati, OH 45221-0068, USA

Oladunni Oluwoye
Initiative for Research and Education to Advance Community Health (IREACH), Washington State University, Spokane, WA 99210-1495, USA

Olav A. Foss
Orthopaedic Research Centre, Clinic of Orthopaedy, Rheumatology and Dermatology, St. Olavs Hospital, Trondheim University Hospital, Trondheim 7030, Norway

Patricia Mjønes
Department of Cancer Research and Molecular Medicine, Faculty of Medicine, Norwegian University of Science and Technology (NTNU), Trondheim 7030, Norway
Department of Pathology and Medical Genetics, St. Olavs Hospital, Trondheim University Hospital, Trondheim 7030, Norway

Silje Fismen
Department of Pathology, University Hospital of North Norway, Tromsø 9019, Norway

Eidi Christensen
Department of Cancer Research and Molecular Medicine, Faculty of Medicine, Norwegian University of Science and Technology (NTNU), Trondheim 7030, Norway
Department of Dermatology, Clinic of Orthopaedy, Rheumatology and Dermatology, St. Olavs Hospital, Trondheim University Hospital, Trondheim 7030, Norway

I. Fernández-Canedo, M. Aguilar-Bernier, J. B. Repiso-Jiménez and J. C. Toribio-Montero, M. de Troya-Martín and N. Blázquez-Sánchez
Department of Dermatology, Agencia Sanitaria Costa del Sol, Marbella, Spain
Red de Investigación en Servicios de Salud en Enfermedades Crónicas (REDISSEC), Spain

F. Rivas-Ruiz
Red de Investigación en Servicios de Salud en Enfermedades Crónicas (REDISSEC), Spain
Unit of Investigation, Agencia Sanitaria Costa del Sol, Marbella, Spain

M. Jones-Caballero
Department of Dermatology, University of Sydney, Sydney, NSW, Australia

J. Rhee
Department of Otolaryngology and Communication, Sciences Medical College of Wisconsin, Milwaukee, WI, USA

Anna J. Lomax and Jennifer Lim
Chris O'Brien Lifehouse, Camperdown, NSW, Australia

Robert Cheng
Concord Repatriation General Hospital, Sydney, NSW, Australia

Centenary Institute, Sydney, NSW, Australia

Arianne Sweeting, Elizabeth L. Chua, Neil McGill and Patricia Lowe
Sydney Medical School, University of Sydney, Camperdown, NSW, Australia
Royal Prince Alfred Hospital, Camperdown, NSW, Australia

Nicholas Shackel
Centenary Institute, Sydney, NSW, Australia
Sydney Medical School, University of Sydney, Camperdown, NSW, Australia
Royal Prince Alfred Hospital, Camperdown, NSW, Australia

Catriona McNeil
Chris O'Brien Lifehouse, Camperdown, NSW, Australia
Sydney Medical School, University of Sydney, Camperdown, NSW, Australia
Royal Prince Alfred Hospital, Camperdown, NSW, Australia

Scott F. Lindsey, DianaM. Byrnes, Mark S. Eller, Ashley M. Rosa, Nitika Dabas and Julia Escandon
Department of Dermatology and Cutaneous Surgery, University of Miami Miller School of Medicine, Miami, FL 33136, USA

James M. Grichnik
Department of Dermatology and Cutaneous Surgery, University of Miami Miller School of Medicine, Miami, FL 33136, USA
Anna Fund Melanoma Program Sylvester Comprehensive Cancer Center, University of Miami Miller School of Medicine, Miami, FL 33136, USA
Frankel Family Division of Melanocytic Tumors, Department of Dermatology and Cutaneous Surgery, University of Miami Miller School of Medicine, Miami, FL 33136, USA
Interdisciplinary Stem Cell Institute, University of Miami Miller School of Medicine, University of Miami, FL 33136, USA

P. T. Lekalakala
Department of Maxillofacial and Oral Surgery, Sefako Makgatho Health Sciences University, Pretoria 0204, South Africa

R. A. G. Khammissa, J. Lemmer and L. Feller
Department of Periodontology and Oral Medicine, Sefako Makgatho Health Sciences University, Pretoria 0204, South Africa

B. Kramer
School of Anatomical Sciences, Faculty of Health Sciences, University of the Witwatersrand, Johannesburg 2000, South Africa

O. A. Ayo-Yusuf
School of Oral Health Sciences, Sefako Makgatho Health Sciences University, Pretoria 0204, South Africa

Sumir Kumar, Bharat BhushanMahajan, Sandeep Kaur and Amarbir Singh
Department of Dermatology, Venereology and Leprology, Guru Gobind Singh Medical College and Hospital, Sadiq Road, Faridkot, Punjab 151203, India Department of Skin&V.D., OPD Block, Guru Gobind Singh Medical College and Hospital, Sadiq Road, Faridkot, Punjab 151203, India

Ashish Yadav and Navtej Singh
Department of Skin&V.D., OPDBlock, Guru Gobind Singh Medical College and Hospital, Sadiq Road, Faridkot, Punjab 151203, India

Department of Pathology, Guru Gobind Singh Medical College and Hospital, Sadiq Road, Faridkot, Punjab 151203, India

Marimer Santiago-Rivas, Chang Wang and Lina Jandorf
Department of Oncological Sciences, Cancer Prevention and Control Division, Icahn School of Medicine at Mount Sinai, One Gustave L. Levy Place, New York, NY 10029-6574, USA

Index